ACP
ASIM

American College
of Physicians

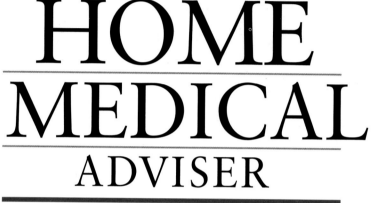

HOME
MEDICAL
ADVISER

American College of Physicians

HOME
MEDICAL
ADVISER

Medical Editors
DAVID R. GOLDMANN, MD FACP
DAVID A. HOROWITZ, MD

London, New York, Munich, Melbourne, Delhi

AMERICAN COLLEGE OF PHYSICIANS– AMERICAN SOCIETY OF INTERNAL MEDICINE

EDITORS-IN-CHIEF David R. Goldmann, MD FACP, David A. Horowitz, MD
PEDIATRIC CONSULTANT Mark D. Joffe, MD FAAP
Associate Professor of Pediatrics, University of Pennsylvania School of Medicine
Director, Community Pediatric Medicine, The Children's Hospital of Philadelphia
MANAGER, BOOKS PROGRAM David Myers
EDITORIAL ASSISTANT, BOOKS PROGRAM Alicia Dillihay

US EDITION
DK PUBLISHING, INC.
SENIOR EDITOR Jill Hamilton   SENIOR ART EDITOR Mandy Earey
EDITORIAL DIRECTOR Chuck Wills   CREATIVE DIRECTOR Tina Vaughan
PRODUCTION MANAGER Chris Avgherinos   DTP Russell Shaw, Milos Orlovic

UK EDITION
DORLING KINDERSLEY
Editorial Manager: Andrea Bagg; *Senior Art Editor*: Marianne Markham; *Senior Editors*: Mary Atkinson, Nicki Lampon,
Andrew Macintyre; *Editors*: Jolyon Goddard, Katie John, Janet Mohun, Teresa Pritlove, Hazel Richardson; *Art Editors*: Janice English,
Chris Walker; *Design Assistance*: Sara Freeman; *DTP Designers*: Julian Dams, John Goldsmid, Jason Little, Louise Paddick;
Picture Research Assistant: Marie Osborn; *Production Manager*: Michelle Thomas; *Out-of-house Technical Services Manager*:
Nicola Erdpresser; *Senior Managing Editor*: Martyn Page; *Managing Art Editor*: Louise Dick; *Art Director*: Bryn Walls

DK INDIA
Managing Editor: Prita Maitra; *Managing Art Editor*: Shuka Jain; *Project Editor*: Atanu Raychaudhuri; *Editors*: Chandana Chandra;
Sudhanshu Gupta; *Project Designer*: Sabyasachi Kundu; *Designer*: Sukanto Bhattacharjya; *DTP Coordinator and Software Trainer*:
Jacob Joshua; *DTP Designer*: Shailesh Sharma; *Head of Publishing*: Anita Roy

MEDICAL EDITORS AND CONSULTANTS
Medical Editors: Tony Smith MA BM BCH, Sue Davidson MB BS MRCP MRCGP DRCOG
Medical Consultants: Sir Peter Beale KBE FRCP FFCM FFOM DTM&H, Peter Cantillon MSc MRCGP,
Mark Furman MRCPCH, Stephen Hughes MRCPCH, Warren Hyer MB ChB MRCP MRCPCH, Penny Preston MB ChB MRCGP,
Andrew Shennan MB BS MRCOG MD, Frances Williams MA MB BChir MRCP DTM&H MRCPCH

First published in the United States in 2002 by DK Publishing, Inc.
375 Hudson Street, New York, New York 10014

2 4 6 8 10 9 7 5 3

Library of Congress Cataloging-in-Publication Data

American College of Physicians Home medical adviser / medical editors, David R. Goldmann and David A.
        Horowitz
        p. cm.
    Includes index.
    ISBN 978-0-7894-8933-3 (alk. paper)
    1. Medicine, Popular. I. Title: Home medical adviser. II. Goldmann, David. R. III Horowitz, David A.
RC81.A53872002
610--dc21

                                                                                        2002019482

Color reproduction by Colourscan, Singapore
Printed and bound in China by Toppan Printing.(ShenZhen)

see our complete catalog at **www.dk.com**

FOREWORD

We have entered a new era in medical science and health care delivery. With the recent explosion in medical information and technology has come tremendous change in the way that we communicate with each other. At the same time that researchers have been unlocking the secrets of the human genetic code, the Internet has entered our households. Not only have novel methods for diagnosis and therapy been advancing more rapidly than ever before, but so also has ease of access to medical information that affects our daily lives.

Now, as we enter the beginning of the twenty-first century, the explosion in medical information confronts us on all sides. In addition to the rapidly expanding universe of medical data, methods to disseminate it seem to multiply daily. This often makes it difficult to filter out what is reliable and what is not. Some of this new knowledge is literally being thrust upon us through "direct-to-consumer" marketing strategies. Today we are as likely to get information about disease states, symptoms, and treatments from television advertisements, newspapers and magazines, local health systems and pharmaceutical companies, and on-line "chat rooms" as from our personal physicians. This flood of unfiltered information has the potential to overwhelm us.

In bringing you the American College of Physicians HOME MEDICAL ADVISER, it is our desire to help you organize practical medical information for daily living. The easy-to-follow symptom charts are designed to lead you through rational approaches to common medical problems and to enable you to recognize what is serious and requires immediate action and what can be managed with self-help measures. The charts cover problems arising in both children and adults, with special sections on issues specific to men and women. Sections on normal growth and development and healthy living are included to emphasize the importance of prevention in staying well.

It is not our intention that this or any other book should replace the important relationship between people and their personal physicians or other health care providers. If providing reliable information, however, enables our readers to understand more about their symptoms in a way that allows them to communicate better with their doctors and to navigate the health care system more easily, we will have accomplished our goal. We hope that you find our work helpful and informative.

David R. Goldmann, MD   *David A. Horowitz, MD*

DAVID R. GOLDMANN, MD FACP & DAVID A. HOROWITZ, MD
MEDICAL EDITORS

CONTENTS

HOW TO USE THIS BOOK

The major part of this book consists of 150 question-and-answer symptom charts, which help you determine the possible cause of a symptom and what to do. Background information on how your body works and how to keep it healthy precedes the charts, and, after them, you can find information on dealing with major emergencies. The book concludes with useful information on drugs and how to contact support groups or find further health information.

Your body and health

You will find general information about the body and health in this highly illustrated section, which is divided into four parts. Your Body shows how major body systems function, and also covers pregnancy, birth, and child development. In Healthy Living, you can find out how to stay healthy and minimize the risks of common disorders. What to expect when you see your doctor and other healthcare professionals is covered in Professional Healthcare. Finally, Medical Tests covers procedures that doctors may use to diagnose and assess disorders.

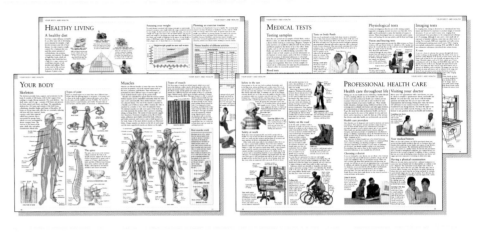

Symptom charts

The Symptom Charts are grouped according to age and/or sex: there are charts for children of different ages, charts for all adults, and charts specifically for men and women. The charts help you find a possible cause of many symptoms that may affect you or your child and tell you what steps you should take, whether it involves professional help or self-help. At the start of the charts section, there are detailed instructions on how to use the charts, along with two types of "chartfinder" to help you find the most appropriate chart for a particular symptom.

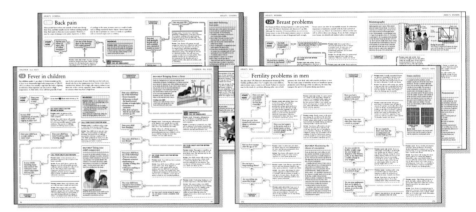

First aid

Here you will find step-by-step instructions for dealing with major emergencies, ranging from giving artificial respiration to someone who has stopped breathing to stopping severe bleeding. Techniques are described for treating infants, children, and adults. To help you find the first-aid information quickly, all the pages in this section have a red bar running down the edge.

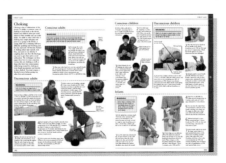

Drugs guide and useful addresses

The Drugs Guide tells you how drugs work and how to use them safely and includes concise profiles of over 35 major drug groups, including their main side effects. Useful Addresses provides addresses, telephone numbers, and online sites of support groups for different conditions and sources for additional health information.

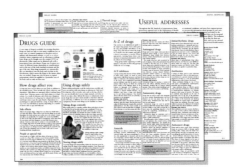

Finding information

You can find the information that you need from this book in several ways:

CONTENTS LISTS The comprehensive contents (pp.6–7) lists every symptom chart as well as the main headings in the other sections of the book. In addition, at the start of each group of charts, there is a contents list of the charts in that group.

CHARTFINDERS The system-by-system chartfinder (pp.46–47) groups the charts by body system or process, and the symptom-by-symptom chartfinder (p.48) alphabetically lists all the symptoms and can direct you to the appropriate chart.

CROSS-REFERENCES Throughout the book, there are cross-references to take you to pages with further information.

INDEX If you still cannot find what you need, the index (pp.314–319) covers every subject within the book.

YOUR BODY AND HEALTH

YOUR BODY
& HEALTH

Understanding how your body works and
how to look after yourself are essential if you
want to stay healthy. This section starts by
explaining the structure and function of the
major body systems. It then looks at how you
can modify your lifestyle to prevent health
problems from developing. The final parts of
the section describe how you can make the
best use of the help that health professionals
offer and how medical problems are
investigated should they occur.

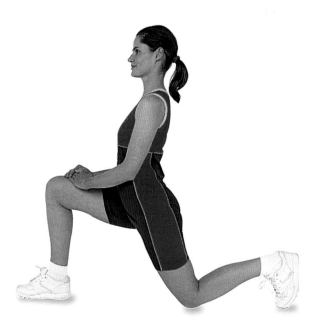

YOUR BODY

Skeleton

The skeleton provides form, support, and protection for the body. It consists of 206 bones, with further support from cartilage (a tough, fibrous material). The axial skeleton – the skull, spine, and rib cage – consists of 80 bones and protects the brain, spinal cord, heart, and lungs. The appendicular skeleton has 126 bones and consists of the limb bones, collarbones, shoulder blades, and bones of the pelvis. All bones are living tissue with cells that are constantly replacing old bone with new material. Bones contain a soft, fatty material called bone marrow; this is surrounded by spongy bone, which is in turn surrounded by denser compact bone. The marrow in the bones of the spine, skull, ribs, and pelvis manufactures blood cells.

Skull
Jawbone (mandible)
Collarbone (clavicle)
Shoulder blade (scapula)
Breastbone (sternum)
Humerus
Rib
Spine
Ulna
Radius
Wrist bones (carpals)
Hand bones (metacarpals)
Finger bones (phalanges)
Kneecap (patella)
Pelvis
Femur
Fibula
Tibia
Ankle bones (tarsals)
Foot bones (metatarsals)
Toe bones (phalanges)

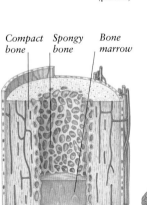

Compact bone   Spongy bone   Bone marrow

STRUCTURE OF BONE

Types of joint

Joints are formed where two or more bones meet. Different types of joint allow for differing degrees of movement. A few joints, such as those in the skull, are fixed. Semimovable joints, such as those in the spine, provide stability and some flexibility. The majority of joints, known as synovial joints, move freely. The main types of synovial joint, and their planes of movement, are illustrated below.

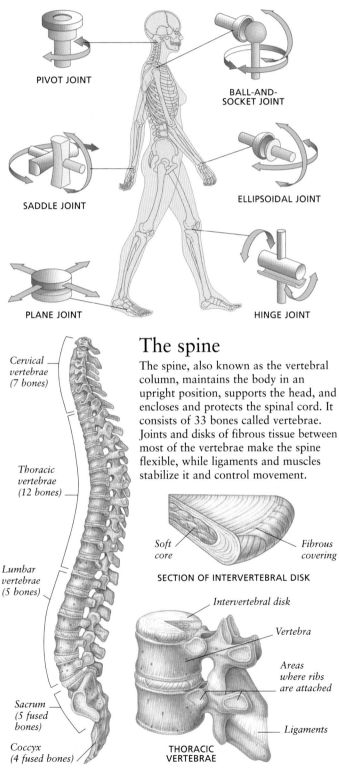

PIVOT JOINT

BALL-AND-SOCKET JOINT

SADDLE JOINT

ELLIPSOIDAL JOINT

PLANE JOINT

HINGE JOINT

The spine

The spine, also known as the vertebral column, maintains the body in an upright position, supports the head, and encloses and protects the spinal cord. It consists of 33 bones called vertebrae. Joints and disks of fibrous tissue between most of the vertebrae make the spine flexible, while ligaments and muscles stabilize it and control movement.

Cervical vertebrae (7 bones)
Thoracic vertebrae (12 bones)
Lumbar vertebrae (5 bones)
Sacrum (5 fused bones)
Coccyx (4 fused bones)

Soft core
Fibrous covering

SECTION OF INTERVERTEBRAL DISK

Intervertebral disk
Vertebra
Areas where ribs are attached
Ligaments

THORACIC VERTEBRAE

Muscles

Muscles are fibrous bundles of tissue that move the body, maintain its posture, and work internal organs such as the heart, intestines, and bladder. These functions are performed by three different types of muscle (right), of which skeletal muscle makes up the greatest bulk.

Muscles are controlled by signals from the nervous system. Skeletal muscle can be controlled consciously, while the other types work automatically. Most skeletal muscles connect two adjacent bones. One end of the muscle is attached by a flexible cord of fibrous tissue called a tendon; the other is attached by a tendon or by a sheet of connective tissue. The skeletal muscles not only move parts of the body but also help maintain the posture when a person is standing, sitting, or lying down. The names of some muscles suggest their functions. Extensors straighten joints, flexors bend joints, adductors move limbs toward the body, abductors pull limbs outward, and erectors raise or hold up parts of the body. Some of the main skeletal muscles are illustrated below. Deeper muscles are shown on the left of each image and the more superficial muscles are shown on the right.

Types of muscle

The three types of muscle are skeletal muscle, which covers and moves the skeleton; cardiac muscle, which forms the walls of the heart; and smooth muscle, found in the walls of the digestive tract, the blood vessels, and the genital and urinary tracts. Each type of muscle has a different function and consists of fibers of a particular shape. Skeletal muscle, which moves the limbs and body, is formed of long, strong, parallel fibers. This type of muscle is able to contract quickly and powerfully, but can work at maximum strength only for short periods of time. Heart muscle pumps blood around the body. It is composed of short, branching, interlinked fibers that form a network within the walls of the heart. This type of muscle can work continually without tiring. Smooth muscle carries out functions such as moving food through the digestive tract. It is composed of short, spindle-shaped fibers that are connected to form sheets and can work for prolonged periods.

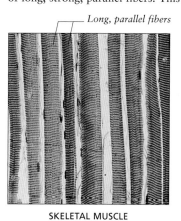

Long, parallel fibers

SKELETAL MUSCLE

How muscles work

Movement occurs when signals from the nervous system cause muscles to contract. Conscious movements of the body are produced by the interaction of skeletal muscles, bones, and joints. Most muscles connect one bone to another and cross a joint. When a muscle contracts, it pulls on the bones to move them. Many muscles are found in pairs, one on each side of a joint, and produce opposing movements. For example, in the upper arm, the triceps contracts to pull the arm straight and the biceps contracts to bend the arm.

Triceps contracts
Biceps relaxes
STRAIGHTENING THE ARM
Triceps relaxes
Biceps contracts
BENDING THE ARM

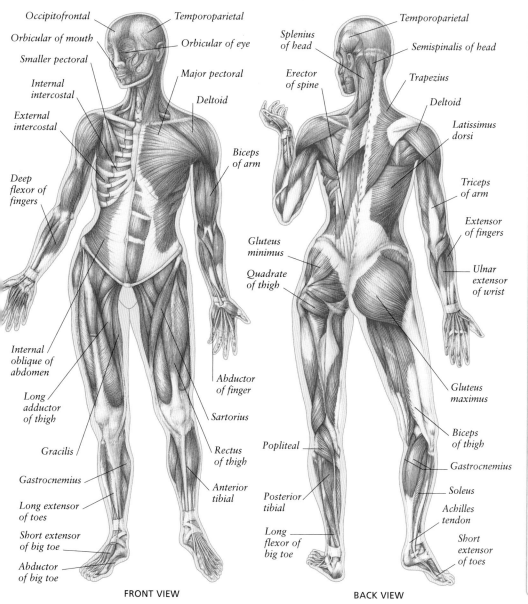

FRONT VIEW

BACK VIEW

11

Cardiovascular system

The cardiovascular system transports blood around the body, taking oxygen and nutrients to body tissues and removing waste products. The heart is a hollow, muscular organ that pumps all the body's blood – more than 10 pints (5 liters) – around the body about once a minute and faster during exercise. Blood flows through a network of vessels that reaches all parts of the body. Arteries carrying blood from the heart branch into smaller vessels and then into capillaries, which in turn join a network of veins that return blood to the heart.

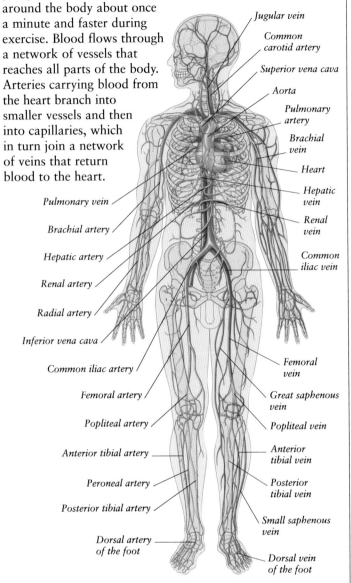

Jugular vein
Common carotid artery
Superior vena cava
Aorta
Pulmonary artery
Brachial vein
Heart
Hepatic vein
Renal vein
Common iliac vein
Pulmonary vein
Brachial artery
Hepatic artery
Renal artery
Radial artery
Inferior vena cava
Common iliac artery
Femoral artery
Femoral vein
Popliteal artery
Great saphenous vein
Anterior tibial artery
Popliteal vein
Peroneal artery
Anterior tibial vein
Posterior tibial artery
Posterior tibial vein
Dorsal artery of the foot
Small saphenous vein
Dorsal vein of the foot

Arteries and veins

Arteries have thick, muscular, elastic walls to withstand the high pressure of blood pumped out of the heart. Veins return blood to the heart. They have thinner walls that stretch easily, allowing them to expand and hold large volumes of blood when the body is at rest. The linings of many large veins have folds that act as one-way valves to stop blood from flowing in the wrong direction.

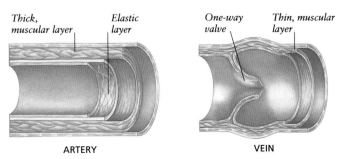

Thick, muscular layer
Elastic layer
One-way valve
Thin, muscular layer

ARTERY

VEIN

Structure of the heart

The heart is a double pump consisting mainly of muscle called myocardium. On each side, blood flows through veins into an upper chamber (atrium), then passes into a lower chamber (ventricle), which pumps the blood into the arteries. Blood flow through the chambers is controlled by one-way valves. The right side of the heart pumps blood into the pulmonary arteries and the lungs, and the left side pumps blood into the aorta and around the body.

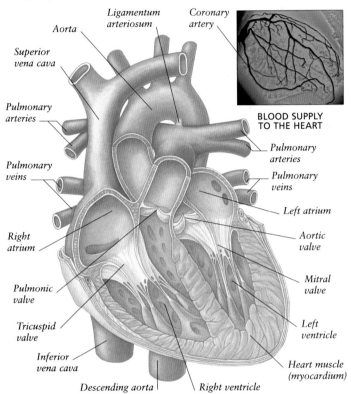

Ligamentum arteriosum
Coronary artery
Aorta
Superior vena cava
Pulmonary arteries
Pulmonary veins
Right atrium
Pulmonic valve
Tricuspid valve
Inferior vena cava
Descending aorta
Right ventricle

BLOOD SUPPLY TO THE HEART

Pulmonary arteries
Pulmonary veins
Left atrium
Aortic valve
Mitral valve
Left ventricle
Heart muscle (myocardium)

Blood circulation

The heart pumps blood into two linked circuits: the pulmonary and the systemic. The pulmonary circuit takes deoxygenated blood to the lungs, where it absorbs oxygen and releases carbon dioxide (a waste gas) through a network of capillaries; oxygenated blood is returned to the heart. The systemic circuit takes oxygenated blood to body tissues, where it releases oxygen and nutrients through capillary walls; carbon dioxide and other waste products pass from tissues into the blood, and the deoxygenated blood is returned to the heart.

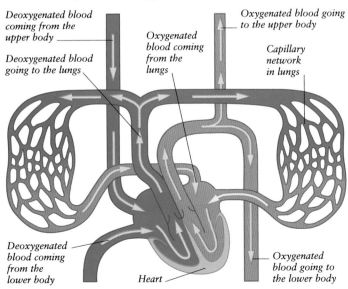

Deoxygenated blood coming from the upper body
Deoxygenated blood going to the lungs
Oxygenated blood coming from the lungs
Oxygenated blood going to the upper body
Capillary network in lungs
Deoxygenated blood coming from the lower body
Heart
Oxygenated blood going to the lower body

Respiratory system

Respiration is the process by which the body obtains oxygen, which it uses to produce energy, and expels carbon dioxide, the main waste product. Air inhaled through the nose or mouth passes down the trachea (windpipe) into the bronchi (lower airways), then into bronchioles (smaller airways) in the lungs. The bronchioles end in sacs called alveoli, which are surrounded by blood vessels. Here, oxygen passes into the blood and carbon dioxide enters the lungs to be exhaled. Breathing is powered by the diaphragm (a muscle) and the intercostal muscles. The respiratory system also includes the pharynx (throat), larynx (voicebox), and epiglottis. The tonsils and adenoids in the pharynx are thought to help fight infection. The larynx contains the vocal cords, which vibrate to produce sounds. The epiglottis seals the trachea during swallowing.

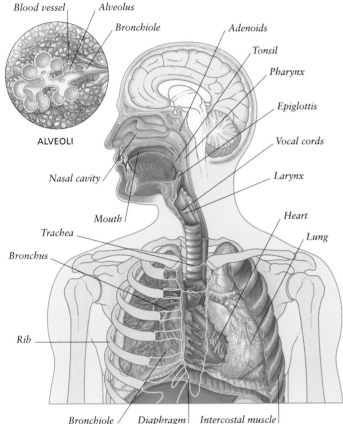

ALVEOLI

How breathing works

Breathing is the act by which the body takes in and expels air. The flow of air in and out of the body occurs because air moves from areas of high pressure to areas of low pressure. To breathe in (inhale), the diaphragm and the muscles between the ribs contract, causing the chest to enlarge. As a result the air pressure in the lungs decreases so that it is lower than the atmospheric pressure, and air is drawn into the lungs. To breathe out (exhale), the muscles relax, decreasing the volume of the lungs. The air pressure in the lungs becomes higher than that in the atmosphere, causing air to leave the body.

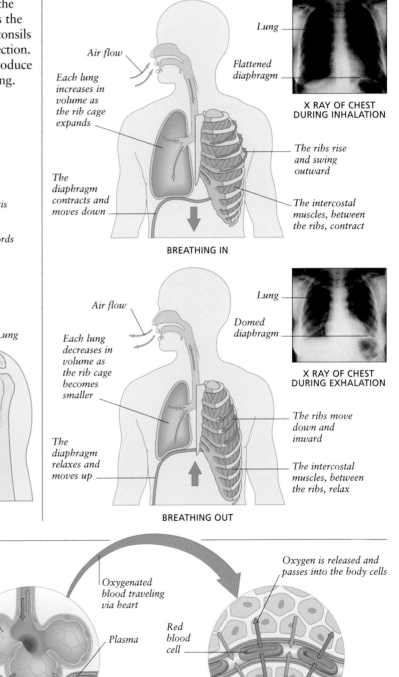

Gas exchange in the body

The body's tissues constantly take up oxygen from the blood and release carbon dioxide back into the blood. Oxygen is inhaled into the lungs, and passes from the alveoli (tiny sacs) into blood vessels called capillaries, where it binds to a substance called hemoglobin in the red blood cells. At the same time, carbon dioxide passes from the blood plasma (the fluid part of the blood) into the alveoli to be exhaled. In the capillaries in tissues, the red blood cells release oxygen, while carbon dioxide is absorbed into the plasma.

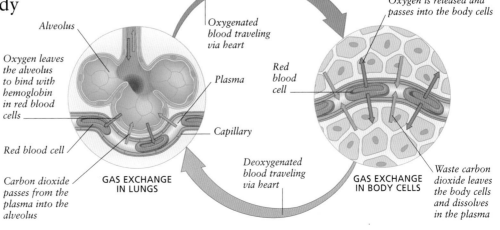

Nervous system

The nervous system gathers, analyzes, stores, and transmits information. It controls vital body functions and interacts with the outside world. There are two parts: the central nervous system, which is composed of the brain and spinal cord, and the peripheral nervous system, made up of nerves that branch from the brain and spinal cord to all areas of the body. Signals, in the form of tiny electrical impulses, are transmitted through the nervous system from the brain to the rest of the body and vice versa. The brain controls almost all activities – both conscious activities, such as movement, and unconscious functions, such as maintaining body temperature. It also receives information from the nerves about the environment and the condition of other parts of the body. For example, the nerves leading from the eyes register visual information and nerves beneath the surface of the skin transmit sensations such as pain. In addition, the brain is capable of complex processes such as learning, memory, thought, and emotion, and can instruct the body to act on the basis of these processes.

Structure and function of the brain

The brain is the most complex organ in the body. It has more than 100 billion nerve cells and billions of pathways. The largest part of the brain is the cerebrum. It is divided into two halves (hemispheres), which are connected by a bundle of nerve fibers called the corpus callosum. The outer layer (cerebral cortex) consists of tissue called gray matter, which generates and processes nerve signals. The inner layer consists of white matter, which transmits the signals. The cerebrum controls conscious thought and movement and interprets sensory information; different parts govern specific activities such as speech and vision. A structure at the base of the brain called the cerebellum controls balance, coordination, and posture. The brain is connected to the spinal cord by the brain stem, which controls vital functions such as respiration. Just above the brain stem is the hypothalamus, which links the nervous system and the endocrine system and helps regulate body temperature, sleep, and sexual behavior. The brain is protected by the skull and by membranes called meninges. Clear cerebrospinal fluid cushions the brain and spinal cord from injury.

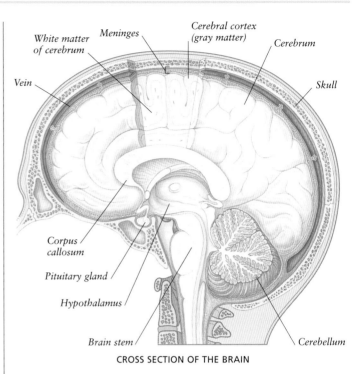

CROSS SECTION OF THE BRAIN

White matter of cerebrum · Meninges · Cerebral cortex (gray matter) · Cerebrum · Vein · Skull · Corpus callosum · Pituitary gland · Hypothalamus · Brain stem · Cerebellum

Organization of the nervous system

The central nervous system, comprising the brain and spinal cord, processes and coordinates nerve signals. The spinal cord forms the link between the brain and the rest of the body. Motor pathways, which carry messages from the brain, descend through the spinal cord, while sensory pathways from the skin and other sensory organs ascend through the spinal cord carrying messages to the brain. A network of peripheral nerves reaches all parts of the body. Each nerve is formed from hundreds of nerve fibers, which project from nerve cells, grouped in bundles. Thirty-one pairs of nerves branch off the spinal cord. These divide into smaller and smaller nerves throughout the torso and the limbs.

MAJOR SPINAL NERVES

Brain · Cervical nerves · Spinal cord · Thoracic nerves · Lumbar nerves · Sacral nerves

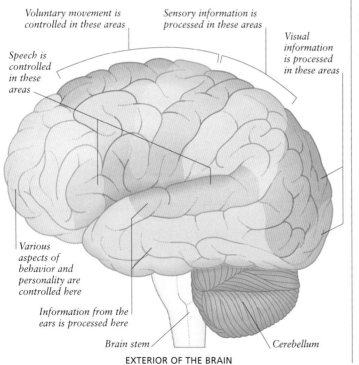

EXTERIOR OF THE BRAIN

Voluntary movement is controlled in these areas · Sensory information is processed in these areas · Visual information is processed in these areas · Speech is controlled in these areas · Various aspects of behavior and personality are controlled here · Information from the ears is processed here · Brain stem · Cerebellum

Gray matter · Spinal nerve · White matter · Meninges

Structure of the spinal cord
The spinal cord is made up of gray matter, which contains nerve cells and supporting cells, and white matter, which contains nerve fibers. The cord is enclosed by protective membranes called meninges.

The senses

Our senses enable us to monitor all aspects of our environment. The eyes provide visual information; the ears detect sound and also aid balance; the nose and tongue respond to different smells and tastes respectively; and the sensory nerves in the skin allow us to feel physical contact (touch), changes in temperature, and pain. In each case, information about the environment detected by the sense organs is transmitted by nerves to the brain, where it is then analyzed.

Vision

The organs of vision are the eyes. Light rays entering each eye are focused by the cornea and the lens so that they fall on the retina, producing an upside-down image on it. Cells in the retina convert this image into electrical impulses that pass along the optic nerve to the brain, where they are decoded to create vision. The iris alters the size of the pupil to control the amount of light reaching the retina. Blood vessels in the retina and a layer called the choroid supply the eye with nutrients.

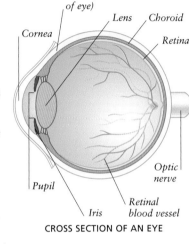

CROSS SECTION OF AN EYE

Sclera (white of eye) · Lens · Choroid · Retina · Cornea · Optic nerve · Pupil · Iris · Retinal blood vessel

View of the retina
The cells in the retina register color and light intensity. At the back of the retina is the optic disk, where nerve fibers converge to form the optic nerve and where blood vessels enter the eye. The disk contains no light-sensitive cells and is called the "blind spot." This photograph was taken through an ophthalmoscope, which magnifies and illuminates the inside of the eye.

Optic disk · Blood vessel

Hearing and balance

The ear is concerned not only with hearing but also with balance. It has outer, middle, and inner parts. The outer ear directs sound waves to the eardrum, causing it to vibrate. The bones of the middle ear transmit these vibrations to the inner ear, where they are converted into electrical signals. The signals pass along nerve cells to the brain, where they are analyzed. The inner ear also contains structures that aid balance by detecting the position and movements of the head, enabling us to stay upright and move without falling over.

Structure of the ear
The outer ear is composed of the pinna (the visible part) and the ear canal, which leads to the eardrum. The middle ear contains three tiny bones that connect the eardrum to a membrane separating the middle and inner ears. The inner ear houses the cochlea, which contains the sensory receptor for hearing, and structures that regulate balance.

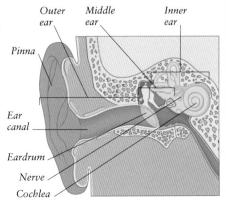

Outer ear · Middle ear · Inner ear · Pinna · Ear canal · Eardrum · Nerve · Cochlea

Smell

Smells are detected by specialized receptor cells in the roof of the nasal cavity. These receptor cells detect odor molecules in the air and convert the information into tiny electrical impulses. These impulses are transmitted along the olfactory nerve to the olfactory bulb (the end of the olfactory nerve) and then to the brain, where they are analyzed. The human sense of smell is highly sensitive, allowing us to detect more than 10,000 different odors.

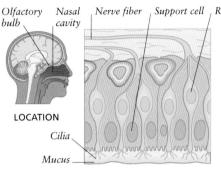

Olfactory bulb · Nasal cavity · Nerve fiber · Support cell · Receptor cell

LOCATION

Cilia · Mucus

Smell receptors
When odor molecules enter the nose, they stimulate cilia (tiny hairs) attached to receptor cells in the roof of the nasal cavity. The receptors transmit signals via nerve fibers to the olfactory bulb, which passes the signals to the brain.

Taste

Tastes are detected by the taste buds. These structures are located in the mouth and throat, with most – about 10,000 – on the upper surface of the tongue. They can distinguish only four basic tastes: sweet, sour, salty, and bitter. Each taste is detected by taste buds in a specific area of the tongue: bitterness is registered at the back, sourness at the sides, saltiness at the front, and sweetness at the tip. It is our sense of smell, in combination with these four basic tastes, that allows us to differentiate a great range of more subtle flavors.

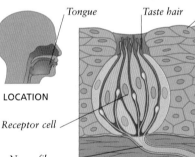

Tongue · Taste hair · Tongue surface

LOCATION

Receptor cell · Nerve fiber

Taste bud structure
Substances in the mouth come into contact with tiny hairs projecting from taste buds in the tongue. These hairs generate nerve impulses that travel along nerve fibers to a specialized area of the brain.

Touch

The sense of touch includes sensations such as pain, pressure, vibration, and temperature. These sensations are detected by two types of receptor under the surface of the skin: free (uncovered) nerve endings, and enclosed nerve endings called corpuscles. Different types of nerve ending or corpuscle monitor particular sensations. The number of receptors varies around the body: for example, the fingertips are highly sensitive and have many receptors, whereas the middle of the back has fewer receptors.

Touch receptors
Touch is detected by various receptors at different levels within the skin. Free (uncovered) nerve endings, near the skin surface, respond to touch, pain, pressure, and temperature. Merkel's and Meissner's corpuscles detect light touch, and Pacinian corpuscles detect deep pressure and vibration.

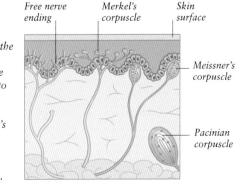

Free nerve ending · Merkel's corpuscle · Skin surface · Meissner's corpuscle · Pacinian corpuscle

Digestive system

The digestive system consists of the digestive tract and its associated organs. The digestive tract is a convoluted tube about 24 ft (7 m) long through which food passes while it is being broken down. The tract consists of the mouth, pharynx (throat), esophagus, stomach, small and large intestines, rectum, and anus. The associated digestive organs include three pairs of salivary glands, the liver, the pancreas, and the gallbladder. The digestive system breaks down food into simpler components that can be used by the cells of the body and eliminates the remaining substances as waste.

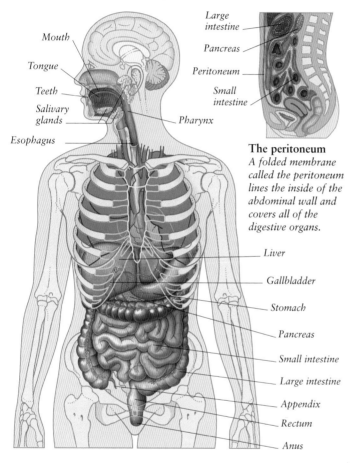

Mouth
Tongue
Teeth
Salivary glands
Esophagus

Large intestine
Pancreas
Peritoneum
Small intestine
Pharynx

The peritoneum
A folded membrane called the peritoneum lines the inside of the abdominal wall and covers all of the digestive organs.

Liver
Gallbladder
Stomach
Pancreas
Small intestine
Large intestine
Appendix
Rectum
Anus

Mouth and esophagus

The process of digestion begins in the mouth. The action of the teeth and tongue during chewing breaks food into small, soft pieces for swallowing, while substances in the saliva start to break down carbohydrates in the food. When you swallow, the tongue pushes the mixture of food and saliva, known as a bolus, down the throat into the esophagus. At the same time, the soft palate closes off the nasal cavity, and the epiglottis, a small flap of cartilage at the back of the tongue, helps close off the larynx.

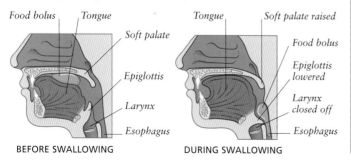

Food bolus
Tongue
Soft palate
Epiglottis
Larynx
Esophagus

Tongue
Soft palate raised
Food bolus
Epiglottis lowered
Larynx closed off
Esophagus

BEFORE SWALLOWING

DURING SWALLOWING

Stomach

Food moves down the esophagus into the stomach. There, it may spend up to 5 hours being churned and partially broken down by digestive juices until it becomes a semi-liquid substance called chyme. Swallowed fluids, such as water and alcohol, pass straight through the stomach and into the intestine in a few minutes.

Small intestine

Chyme enters the duodenum (the first part of the small intestine) and is further broken down by digestive juices from the liver and pancreas. The final stage of digestion takes place in the rest of the small intestine. Here, digestive juices released from the intestinal walls split nutrients into chemical units small enough to pass through the wall of the intestine into the surrounding network of blood vessels.

Large intestine

After nutrients have been absorbed in the small intestine, the remaining material passes into the large intestine. Most of the water content is absorbed back into the body, and the semi-solid waste that remains is called feces. It moves down into the rectum, where it is stored until it is released through the anus as a bowel movement.

Liver, gallbladder, and pancreas

The liver, gallbladder, and pancreas all help to break down food chemically. The liver uses the products of digestion to manufacture proteins such as antibodies (which help fight infection) and blood clotting factors. It also breaks down worn-out blood cells and excretes the wastes as bile, which is stored in the gallbladder and plays a part in the digestion of fats. The entry of food into the duodenum (the first part of the small intestine) stimulates the gallbladder to release the bile into the duodenum via the bile duct. The pancreas secretes powerful digestive juices, which are released into the duodenum when food enters it. Together with digestive juices produced by the intestinal lining, they help break down nutrients into substances that are absorbed into the blood and carried to the liver.

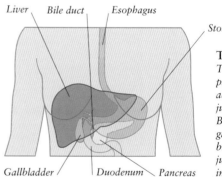

Liver
Bile duct
Esophagus
Stomach
Gallbladder
Duodenum
Pancreas

The digestive organs
The liver, gallbladder, and pancreas, in the upper abdomen, secrete digestive juices into the duodenum. Bile from the liver and gallbladder passes down the bile duct, and pancreatic juices are released directly into the duodenum.

Peristalsis

Food is propelled along the digestive tract by a continuous sequence of muscular contractions known as peristalsis. The walls of the digestive tract are lined with smooth muscle. To move a piece of food (bolus) forward, the muscle behind the food contracts while the muscle in front relaxes.

Peristaltic wave
To move pieces of food through the digestive tract, the muscles in the walls contract and relax in a sequence known as a peristaltic wave.

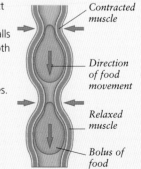

Contracted muscle
Direction of food movement
Relaxed muscle
Bolus of food

Endocrine system

The endocrine system produces hormones – chemicals that are carried in the bloodstream and control processes in other parts of the body. Such processes include metabolism (the chemical reactions constantly occurring in the body), responses to stress, growth, and sexual development.

The system comprises glands and other hormone-producing cells. Glands, such as the pituitary, adrenal, and thyroid glands, are organs whose only function is to produce specific hormones. Other organs and tissues, such as the ovaries, testes, heart, and kidneys, also contain hormone-producing cells.

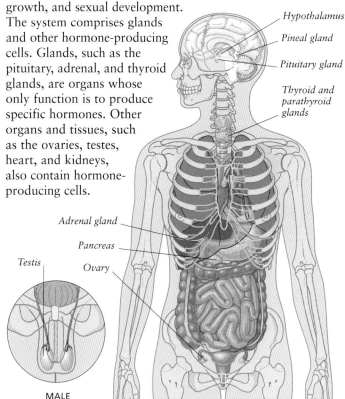

Hypothalamus
Pineal gland
Pituitary gland
Thyroid and parathyroid glands
Adrenal gland
Pancreas
Testis
Ovary
MALE

Pituitary gland and hypothalamus

The pituitary gland lies at the base of the brain. It is known as the "master gland" because it produces hormones that stimulate and control endocrine tissue in other glands and organs. It also secretes hormones that control growth, the volume of urine passed, and the contraction of the uterus during labor. The hypothalamus is a part of the brain that is linked to the pituitary gland. It secretes hormones called releasing factors that control the function of the pituitary, and also acts as a link between the nervous and endocrine systems.

Pineal gland

The pineal gland is situated deep inside the brain. Its precise function has yet to be clarified. However, the gland is known to produce a hormone called melatonin, which is thought to be associated with the daily cycle of sleep and waking.

Thyroid and parathyroid glands

The thyroid gland, in the neck, produces hormones that control metabolism. Some thyroid cells also secrete the hormone calcitonin, which lowers the blood level of calcium. The four parathyroid glands, behind the thyroid, produce a hormone that controls blood levels of calcium and phosphate. Calcium is vital for healthy bones and, with phosphate, plays an important part in nerve and muscle function.

Adrenal glands

The adrenal glands lie on top of the kidneys. Each gland has a cortex (outer layer) and a medulla (core). The cortex produces corticosteroid hormones, which help regulate blood levels of salt and glucose, and tiny amounts of male sex hormones, which promote the development of certain male sexual characteristics. The medulla secretes epinephrine (adrenaline) and norepinephrine (noradrenaline), which increase the heart rate and blood flow to the muscles in response to stress (a reaction called the "fight or flight response").

Pancreas

The pancreas lies behind the stomach. It produces digestive juices that help break down food. It also releases the hormones insulin and glucagon, which play an important part in regulating the level of glucose, a sugar that forms the body's main energy source.

Ovaries

The ovaries lie on either side of the uterus. They release eggs and produce the female sex hormones progesterone and estrogen, which regulate the menstrual cycle. Estrogen also encourages the development of some female sexual characteristics, such as enlargement of the breasts.

Testes

The testes hang in a bag of skin and muscles called the scrotum. They produce sperm and secrete the male sex hormone testosterone. This hormone is responsible for the onset of puberty and the development of male secondary sexual characteristics, such as facial hair.

Lymphatic system

The lymphatic system consists of a network of lymph vessels that runs throughout the body, clumps of bean-shaped lymph nodes (commonly called lymph glands), the spleen, the thymus gland, and other areas of lymphatic tissue, such as Peyer's patches in the wall of the intestine. The lymphatic system helps defend the body against infection and also to maintain the balance of body fluids.

Cervical lymph nodes
Lymph vessel
Axillary lymph nodes
Thoracic duct
Thymus gland
Spleen
Peyer's patch in intestine
Deep inguinal (groin) lymph nodes
Popliteal lymph nodes

Vessels and nodes

Lymph vessels carry a fluid called lymph around the body. Lymph helps maintain the body's fluid balance by collecting excess fluid from the tissues and returning it to the bloodstream. It also carries white blood cells, which fight infection. Lymph nodes, situated at junctions between lymph vessels, filter infectious organisms from the lymph. They are packed with lymphocytes, a type of white blood cell. Clusters of nodes are found in many parts of the body, including the neck, armpits, and groin.

Spleen and thymus

The spleen and the thymus gland produce certain types of lymphocytes (white blood cells). These cells produce antibodies, which help destroy infective organisms. The spleen also breaks down worn-out red blood cells.

Urinary system

The urinary system filters wastes from the blood, eliminating them together with excess water as urine. It also regulates body fluid levels and maintains the body's acid–base balance. The system consists of a pair of kidneys; the bladder; the ureters, which connect each kidney to the bladder; and the urethra, the tube through which urine leaves the body. The kidneys are red-brown, bean-shaped organs lying at the back of the abdomen, one on either side of the spine. They contain units called nephrons that filter the blood circulating through the kidneys and produce urine, which then passes down the ureters into the bladder. The bladder is kept closed by a ring of muscle (a sphincter) around its lower opening. This muscle can be relaxed voluntarily to allow urine to be expelled through the urethra. The male urethra is longer than the female urethra and also provides an outlet for semen (fluid that contains sperm and that is released during sexual activity). Because the female urethra is shorter and opens close to the vagina and anus, women are more prone to urinary infections than men.

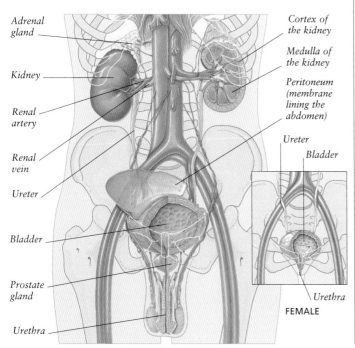

Adrenal gland
Kidney
Renal artery
Renal vein
Ureter
Bladder
Prostate gland
Urethra

Cortex of the kidney
Medulla of the kidney
Peritoneum (membrane lining the abdomen)
Ureter
Bladder
Urethra
FEMALE

Structure of the kidney

Inside the kidney, there are three regions: the cortex (outer layer), the medulla (middle layer), and the renal pelvis (inner region). The cortex contains functional units called nephrons. Each nephron consists of a glomerulus, a cluster of specialized capillaries in which the blood is filtered, and a renal tubule, through which the resulting waste fluids pass as they are turned into urine. The medulla consists of groups of urine-collecting ducts. Urine from these ducts passes into minor calyces and then into major calyces, which open into the renal pelvis. From here, the urine is funneled into the ureter.

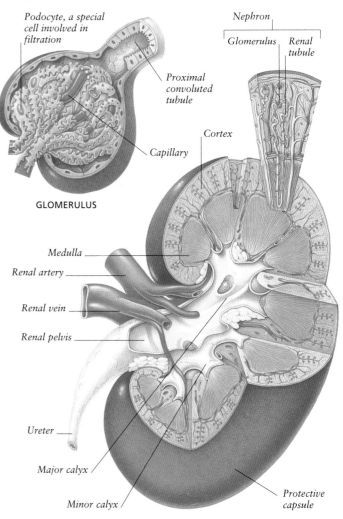

Podocyte, a special cell involved in filtration
Proximal convoluted tubule
Capillary
GLOMERULUS
Nephron
Glomerulus
Renal tubule
Cortex
Medulla
Renal artery
Renal vein
Renal pelvis
Ureter
Major calyx
Minor calyx
Protective capsule

How urine is made

Urine is composed of substances that have been filtered from the blood in the nephrons. A kidney has about a million nephrons. Each consists of a cluster of tiny capillaries called a glomerulus and a tube called the renal tubule. This has three parts: the proximal convoluted tubule, the loop of Henle, and the distal convoluted tubule. Blood first passes through the glomerulus. The capillary walls have pores that allow water and small particles (such as salts) to pass through, while retaining larger particles, such as proteins and red blood cells. The fluid that has been removed from the blood, called filtrate, enters the renal tubule, where water, and other useful substances such as glucose and salts are reabsorbed into the bloodstream as necessary.

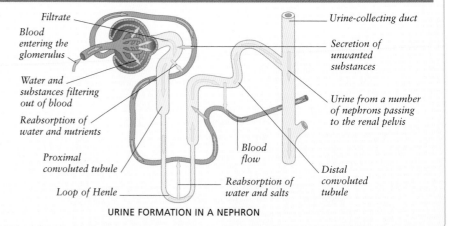

Filtrate
Blood entering the glomerulus
Water and substances filtering out of blood
Reabsorption of water and nutrients
Proximal convoluted tubule
Loop of Henle
Urine-collecting duct
Secretion of unwanted substances
Urine from a number of nephrons passing to the renal pelvis
Blood flow
Reabsorption of water and salts
Distal convoluted tubule
URINE FORMATION IN A NEPHRON

Male reproductive system

The male reproductive system produces sperm – cells that can fuse with eggs from a woman to form offspring. It also makes the male sex hormones needed for sperm production and for sexual development at puberty. The male genitals consist of the penis, the testes, and the scrotum, in which the testes are suspended. Each testis is packed with seminiferous tubules, which make sperm. The sperm are stored in the epididymis, a coiled tube that lies behind each testis. Another tube, the vas deferens, connects each epididymis to an ejaculatory duct, which in turn is connected to the urethra. Three glands – a pair of seminal vesicles and the prostate gland – secrete fluids to transport and nourish the sperm; the secretions and sperm form a fluid called semen. During sexual activity, the erectile tissue in the penis fills with blood, making the penis lengthen and stiffen in order to enter the woman's vagina. At orgasm, muscular contractions force semen along each vas deferens, down the urethra, and out of the penis.

Changes in boys during puberty

Puberty is the period during which sexual characteristics develop and sexual organs mature. In boys, puberty usually begins between the ages of about 12 and 15 and lasts for 3–4 years. The pituitary gland, at the base of the brain, starts to secrete hormones that stimulate the testes to produce the male sex hormone testosterone. This hormone stimulates changes such as enlargement of the genitals and the growth of body hair, and, later, sperm production and increased sex drive.

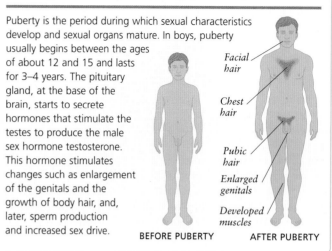

Facial hair

Chest hair

Pubic hair

Enlarged genitals

Developed muscles

BEFORE PUBERTY   **AFTER PUBERTY**

Bladder

Vas deferens

Scrotum

Prostate gland

Urethra

Penis

Testis

FRONT VIEW

Artery

Erectile tissue

Urethra

SECTION THROUGH THE PENIS

Vas deferens

Epididymis

Seminiferous tubule

CROSS SECTION OF A TESTIS

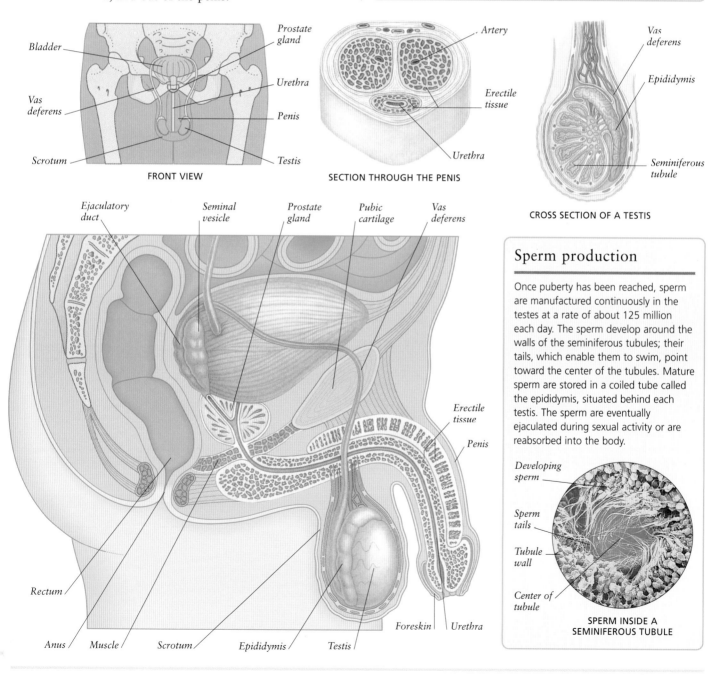

Ejaculatory duct

Seminal vesicle

Prostate gland

Pubic cartilage

Vas deferens

Erectile tissue

Penis

Rectum

Anus   *Muscle*   *Scrotum*   *Epididymis*   *Testis*

Foreskin   *Urethra*

Sperm production

Once puberty has been reached, sperm are manufactured continuously in the testes at a rate of about 125 million each day. The sperm develop around the walls of the seminiferous tubules; their tails, which enable them to swim, point toward the center of the tubules. Mature sperm are stored in a coiled tube called the epididymis, situated behind each testis. The sperm are eventually ejaculated during sexual activity or are reabsorbed into the body.

Developing sperm

Sperm tails

Tubule wall

Center of tubule

SPERM INSIDE A SEMINIFEROUS TUBULE

Female reproductive system

The internal structures of the female reproductive system – the ovaries, fallopian tubes, uterus, and vagina – lie in the lower third of the abdomen. The ovaries contain follicles that store eggs, the cells that fuse with the man's sperm to form offspring. Each month an egg matures and is released from an ovary; the fimbriae guide the egg into a fallopian tube, which propels it toward the uterus. The vagina, a passage with muscular walls, leads from the uterus to the outside of the body. The external structures, collectively known as the vulva, include the sensitive clitoris and folds of skin called the labia, which protect the entrances to the vagina and the urethra. Just inside the vaginal entrance lie the Bartholin's glands, which secrete a fluid for lubrication during sexual intercourse.

Changes in girls during puberty

Puberty is the period during which sexual characteristics develop and sexual organs mature. In girls, puberty begins between the ages of about 10 and 14 and lasts for 3–4 years. The pituitary gland starts to secrete hormones that stimulate the ovaries to produce the female sex hormones estrogen and progesterone. These hormones prompt physical changes such as enlargement of the breasts and hips and the growth of pubic and underarm hair. Later, they stimulate ovulation and menstruation.

Armpit hair
Enlarged breasts
Wider hips
Pubic hair
Thicker thighs

BEFORE PUBERTY   AFTER PUBERTY

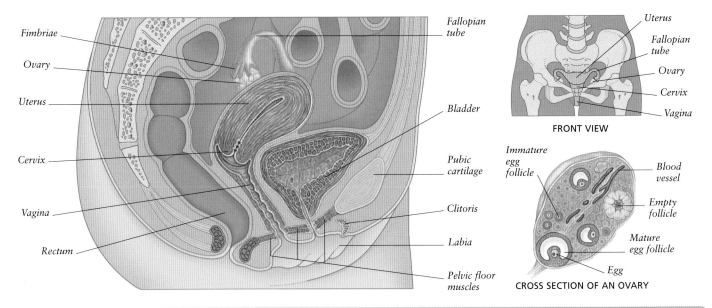

Fimbriae
Ovary
Uterus
Cervix
Vagina
Rectum

Fallopian tube
Bladder
Pubic cartilage
Clitoris
Labia
Pelvic floor muscles

Uterus
Fallopian tube
Ovary
Cervix
Vagina

FRONT VIEW

Immature egg follicle
Blood vessel
Empty follicle
Mature egg follicle
Egg

CROSS SECTION OF AN OVARY

The menstrual cycle

During the menstrual cycle, a woman's body is prepared for the possibility of pregnancy. The cycle is regulated by four sex hormones. Follicle-stimulating hormone and luteinizing hormone, which are secreted by the pituitary gland, cause an egg to mature in a follicle and be released. The egg and its follicle secrete estrogen and progesterone, which make the uterus lining thicken. If an egg is fertilized, it embeds itself in the lining. If it is not fertilized, it passes out of the body, together with blood and cells from the lining, during menstruation. The cycle lasts about 28 days, but this can vary from month to month and from woman to woman.

A complete menstrual cycle
The chart shows changes that occur in the endometrium (uterus lining) and the ovary during a menstrual cycle. The egg can be fertilized by a sperm at ovulation, the time when it is released from its follicle.

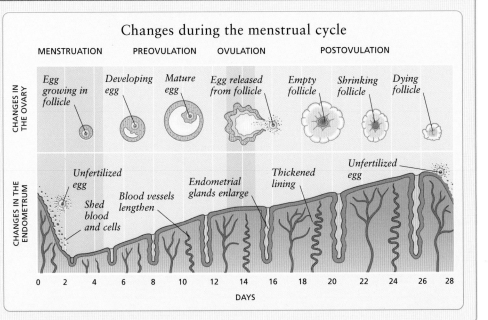

Changes during the menstrual cycle

MENSTRUATION | PREOVULATION | OVULATION | POSTOVULATION

CHANGES IN THE OVARY

Egg growing in follicle
Developing egg
Mature egg
Egg released from follicle
Empty follicle
Shrinking follicle
Dying follicle

CHANGES IN THE ENDOMETRIUM

Unfertilized egg
Shed blood and cells
Blood vessels lengthen
Endometrial glands enlarge
Thickened lining
Unfertilized egg

0 2 4 6 8 10 12 14 16 18 20 22 24 26 28

DAYS

Role of the breasts

Breasts play a part in sexual arousal, but their main role is to produce milk for babies. During puberty the hormone estrogen causes the breasts to grow and develop. During pregnancy, hormonal changes make the breasts enlarge further and, in late pregnancy, stimulate milk production in glands called lobules. These glands are connected to ducts that lead to channels called ampullae, which open onto the surface of the nipple. The rest of the breast tissue is mostly fat, with a small amount of connective tissue, which helps to support the breasts.

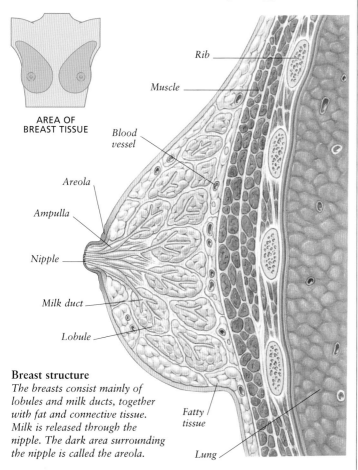

AREA OF BREAST TISSUE

Rib

Muscle

Blood vessel

Areola

Ampulla

Nipple

Milk duct

Lobule

Fatty tissue

Lung

Breast structure
The breasts consist mainly of lobules and milk ducts, together with fat and connective tissue. Milk is released through the nipple. The dark area surrounding the nipple is called the areola.

Menopause

Menopause is the time when menstrual cycles cease. It usually occurs between the ages of 45 and 55. The ovaries stop responding to follicle-stimulating hormone and produce less of the female sex hormones estrogen and progesterone. As a result, ovulation and menstruation end, and once a woman has reached menopause she is no longer fertile. In the years just before and after menopause, hormone changes produce symptoms such as mood swings, hot flashes, vaginal dryness, and night sweats. Menopause may also result in long-term physical changes, such as osteoporosis.

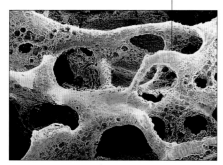

Thin, brittle bone

Osteoporotic bone
The sex hormone estrogen is needed to give bones strength. Low estrogen levels after menopause can worsen osteoporosis, a condition in which the bones lose density and may become thin and brittle, as shown in this microscopic image.

Conception and pregnancy

All organisms reproduce. In human beings, reproduction involves two types of cell: sperm, produced by the testes in men, and eggs, produced by the ovaries in women. These cells each contain half a set of DNA (genetic material). They are brought together by sexual intercourse; if a sperm penetrates and fertilizes an egg, the man's and woman's DNA combine to form new cells. Conception occurs when these cells embed themselves in the uterus. During pregnancy, which lasts for about 40 weeks (9 months), the cells develop into a baby.

Fertilization

During sexual intercourse, sperm are expelled into the woman's vagina, then swim up through the uterus and into the fallopian tubes. If the sperm meet an egg, they try to pierce its coating. If a sperm succeeds, it sheds its tail and fuses with the nucleus of the egg, while chemical changes in the egg stop any more sperm from entering. In this way a new cell is formed, combining DNA from the man and the woman.

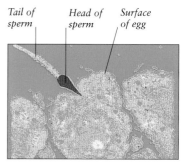

Tail of sperm

Head of sperm

Surface of egg

Sperm penetrating egg
The head of the sperm pushes through the egg's outer coating in order to reach the nucleus.

Beginning of pregnancy

The cell produced by the fusion of the egg and sperm is called a zygote. Within 2 days of fertilization, the zygote starts its journey along the fallopian tube toward the uterus, propelled by the muscular action of the tube's walls. At the same time, the zygote divides itself repeatedly to form a cluster of cells, which is called a morula. After 5–7 days, the cell cluster reaches the uterus. It embeds itself securely in the endometrium (the lining of the uterus) and continues to grow. From this moment onward, the pregnancy is properly established. One part of the cell cluster grows into the endometrium and becomes the placenta, which will nourish the developing baby. The rest of the cells, from which the baby will grow, become an embryo.

LOCATION

A single cell called a zygote is formed if an egg fuses with a sperm

The zygote begins to divide soon after it has been formed

The cluster of dividing cells, called a morula, grows as it travels along the fallopian tube

An embryo starts to form once the cluster of cells has embedded itself in the lining of the uterus wall

Fallopian tube

An unfertilized egg is released from an ovary

Ovary

Lining of the uterus

From egg to embryo
As the cells passing along the fallopian tube divide, their number doubles every 12 hours. When the cell cluster reaches the uterus, it contains hundreds of cells. Once embedded in the uterus lining, the cells start developing into an embryo.

How the baby is nourished

An unborn baby depends on its mother to supply it with oxygen, nutrients, and antibodies against infection, and to remove its waste products. These substances pass between the mother's blood and the baby's blood inside the placenta, an organ that is attached to the uterus lining and is connected to the baby by the umbilical cord. In the placenta, the mother's and baby's blood supplies are brought close together, although they do not actually mix.

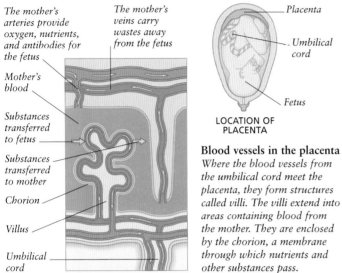

The mother's arteries provide oxygen, nutrients, and antibodies for the fetus

The mother's veins carry wastes away from the fetus

Mother's blood

Substances transferred to fetus

Substances transferred to mother

Chorion

Villus

Umbilical cord

Placenta

Umbilical cord

Fetus

LOCATION OF PLACENTA

Blood vessels in the placenta
Where the blood vessels from the umbilical cord meet the placenta, they form structures called villi. The villi extend into areas containing blood from the mother. They are enclosed by the chorion, a membrane through which nutrients and other substances pass.

The baby's development

The baby develops in a sac in the uterus. It is cushioned by amniotic fluid and nourished by blood from the umbilical cord. In the first 8 weeks, the baby is known as an embryo. During this time the limbs, head, and facial features appear, most of the organs form, and the heart begins to beat. From week 8, the baby is called a fetus. The body structures continue to develop throughout the pregnancy.

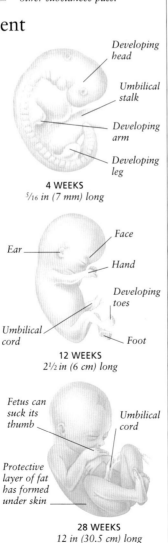

Developing head

Umbilical stalk

Developing arm

Developing leg

4 WEEKS
5/16 in (7 mm) long

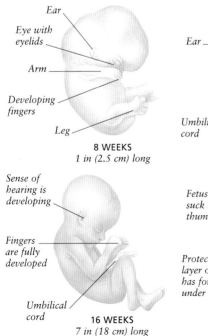

Ear

Eye with eyelids

Arm

Developing fingers

Leg

8 WEEKS
1 in (2.5 cm) long

Ear

Face

Hand

Developing toes

Umbilical cord

Foot

12 WEEKS
2½ in (6 cm) long

Sense of hearing is developing

Fingers are fully developed

Umbilical cord

16 WEEKS
7 in (18 cm) long

Fetus can suck its thumb

Umbilical cord

Protective layer of fat has formed under skin

28 WEEKS
12 in (30.5 cm) long

Changes in the mother's body

Pregnancy is divided into three stages (trimesters), each about 3 months long. During pregnancy, the mother's body undergoes major changes. The most noticeable are the swelling of the abdomen as the baby grows and the enlargement of the breasts as they prepare to produce milk. In addition, specific changes occur in each trimester.

In the first trimester, there are few visible changes. However, the mother's heart rate increases by about 8 beats per minute in order to increase the blood circulation. Changes in hormone levels may cause symptoms such as nausea. During the second trimester, the mother may begin to experience backache due to the weight of the fetus. Her appetite may increase. By 18–20 weeks the fetus starts to make noticeable movements, producing fluttering feelings in the mother's abdomen. In the third trimester, the mother rapidly gains weight as the fetus undergoes a growth spurt. The uterus eventually becomes so large that the top reaches almost to the mother's breastbone. In the last weeks the fetus changes position so that it is lying with its head pointing downward, ready for birth.

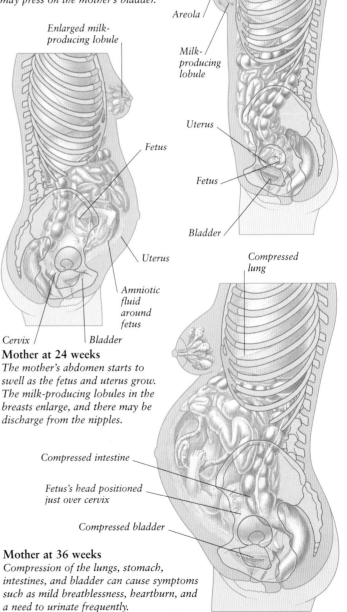

Mother at 12 weeks
The mother's breasts are tender and the areola (the area that surrounds the nipple) darkens. The enlarging uterus may press on the mother's bladder.

Enlarged milk-producing lobule

Areola

Milk-producing lobule

Uterus

Fetus

Fetus

Bladder

Uterus

Amniotic fluid around fetus

Cervix

Bladder

Compressed lung

Mother at 24 weeks
The mother's abdomen starts to swell as the fetus and uterus grow. The milk-producing lobules in the breasts enlarge, and there may be discharge from the nipples.

Compressed intestine

Fetus's head positioned just over cervix

Compressed bladder

Mother at 36 weeks
Compression of the lungs, stomach, intestines, and bladder can cause symptoms such as mild breathlessness, heartburn, and a need to urinate frequently.

The newborn baby

A newborn baby has to cope with dramatic physical changes as it leaves the total protection of the mother's uterus. In particular, the baby's body has to adapt in order to breathe air and function independently of the mother. The body systems can carry out the basic functions necessary for life, but they continue to develop and mature throughout childhood. A newborn baby also shows certain basic patterns of behavior that aid his or her survival, such as finding the mother's breast, sucking, responding to stimuli such as noise, and crying to gain attention and care.

The skin may be blotchy. It may also be covered with an oily substance called vernix, which protected the baby's skin in the uterus

The baby's hands may be clenched into fists

Many babies are born with hair. Premature babies may be covered with downy hair called lanugo hair, which disappears after about a month

The head may be temporarily misshapen due to pressure on the skull bones during birth. There are several soft areas called fontanelles, which are gaps between the bones

The nails may be long, and the ends may flake off by themselves

Babies born in the hospital are fitted with an identification bracelet

The genitals are large in proportion to the rest of the body, and may also appear red and swollen

Right after delivery, the umbilical cord is clipped and cut to leave a small stump. The stump falls off within 10 days

The edges of the lips may develop white blisters due to vigorous sucking as the baby feeds

The eyelids are puffy. The baby can see, but only to a distance of 8–10 in (20–25 cm)

Reflex actions and movements

Babies are born with certain automatic patterns of behavior. Some of these activities are involuntary actions, such as breathing, urinating, and passing feces, and others are reflex actions, instinctive movements designed to protect and to aid survival. The benefits of some reflex actions, such as sucking and "rooting" (searching for the mother's breast), are obvious. Others may be relics from a more primitive stage of human evolution; for example, the grasp reflex is thought to have originated with our ape ancestors, whose babies had to cling to their mothers as they were carried. The reflex actions, and involuntary actions such as urinating, are eventually replaced by voluntary, controlled actions as the baby's nervous system and muscles mature. Two typical reflex responses are shown below.

Walking reflex
If a newborn baby is held upright with the feet on a firm surface, he or she will make movements that resemble stepping or walking.

Arms and hands are stretched open

Legs make "stepping" motion

Startle (Moro) reflex
If a baby is startled, a protective movement occurs in which the baby flings the arms wide and stretches the legs out.

The heart before and after birth

In the fetus, the task of adding oxygen to the blood and filtering out waste gases is done by the placenta, but at birth the baby has to start breathing, obtaining oxygen from the lungs. Before birth, the fetus's heart pumps blood around the body and to the umbilical cord, but most of the blood bypasses the pulmonary arteries (the vessels leading to the lungs) by flowing through two special openings in the heart. With a baby's first breath the lungs expand and take in air; this triggers changes in the heart and circulation, causing the two openings in the heart to close so that all blood from the rest of the body then flows through the pulmonary arteries to the lungs to be oxygenated.

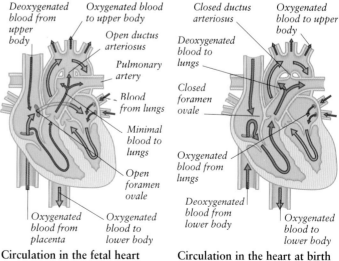

Deoxygenated blood from upper body

Oxygenated blood to upper body

Open ductus arteriosus

Pulmonary artery

Blood from lungs

Minimal blood to lungs

Open foramen ovale

Oxygenated blood from placenta

Oxygenated blood to lower body

Closed ductus arteriosus

Oxygenated blood to upper body

Deoxygenated blood to lungs

Closed foramen ovale

Oxygenated blood from lungs

Deoxygenated blood from lower body

Oxygenated blood to lower body

Circulation in the fetal heart
An opening called the foramen ovale and a channel called the ductus arteriosus divert most blood away from the pulmonary arteries.

Circulation in the heart at birth
The foramen ovale and ductus arteriosus close, so that all blood from the heart passes to the lungs to be oxygenated.

The growing child

Childhood is a time of dramatic physical, mental, and social development, during which a person grows from a dependent baby into a mature, self-sufficient individual. In addition, the child learns skills that allow him or her to interact with other people and with the environment. The rate of growth is fastest during the first year of life, and there is another period of rapid growth at puberty, the transition from childhood to adulthood. Children acquire many of the necessary physical, mental, and social skills during their first 5 years, but the learning process continues throughout life.

How bones grow and develop

At birth, much of the skeleton consists of tissue known as cartilage, with bone tissue only in the shafts of the largest bones. During childhood, the cartilage is gradually replaced by bone – a process called ossification. In the long bones of the limbs, areas called growth plates produce more cartilage to extend the bones, and this cartilage then turns to bone. By the beginning of adulthood, ossification is complete and the skeleton has reached its full size.

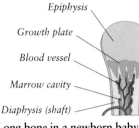

Epiphysis
Growth plate
Blood vessel
Marrow cavity
Diaphysis (shaft)

Long bone in a newborn baby
The diaphysis (shaft) is made of bone, while the epiphyses (ends) are made of cartilage.

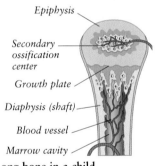

Epiphysis
Secondary ossification center
Growth plate
Diaphysis (shaft)
Blood vessel
Marrow cavity

Long bone in a child
Growth and ossification (bone formation) take place in the ends of the long bone.

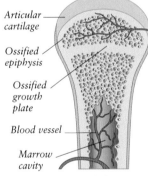

Articular cartilage
Ossified epiphysis
Ossified growth plate
Blood vessel
Marrow cavity

Long bone in an adult
All of the cartilage inside the bone has ossified. A layer of cartilage protects the ends of the bone.

How the skull and brain develop

A newborn baby has a full set of neurons (nerve cells), but the network of pathways between these cells is not yet mature. In the first 6 years, the brain grows and the neural (nerve) network rapidly becomes more complex, allowing a child to learn a wide range of skills and behavior. To allow for this expansion, the cranium (the part of the skull covering the brain) grows at soft gaps called fontanelles and at seams called sutures; these areas gradually turn to bone. During the rest of childhood the brain, neural network, and skull develop at a slower rate.

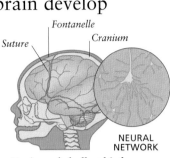

Fontanelle
Suture
Cranium

NEURAL NETWORK

Brain and skull at birth
The neural network is only partially developed. The skull bones are separated by sutures (seams) and fontanelles (soft gaps).

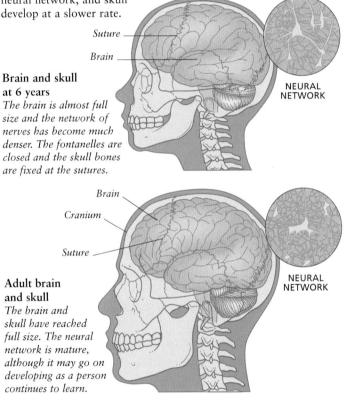

Suture
Brain

NEURAL NETWORK

Brain and skull at 6 years
The brain is almost full size and the network of nerves has become much denser. The fontanelles are closed and the skull bones are fixed at the sutures.

Brain
Cranium
Suture

NEURAL NETWORK

Adult brain and skull
The brain and skull have reached full size. The neural network is mature, although it may go on developing as a person continues to learn.

The growing body

Growth in childhood is controlled by hormones and is also influenced by factors such as diet and general health. A child's body grows continuously, but the rate of growth varies depending on the stage of life: the most rapid overall growth occurs during infancy and puberty. In addition, some parts of the body develop faster than others, causing the body proportions to alter as the child grows. At birth, the head makes up about one-quarter of the total body length, and until about age 6, it continues to grow quickly. The facial features change during childhood, as the face becomes larger in relation to the rest of the skull. The limbs, during infancy, are small in relation to the body and head, and lengthen as the child grows older, with especially rapid growth occurring during puberty. The body finally reaches its full size at around age 18. By this time, the head represents only about one-eighth of the body length, while the legs are about half.

Changing shape from birth to adulthood

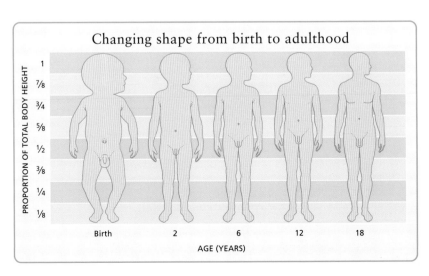

PROPORTION OF TOTAL BODY HEIGHT

1
7/8
3/4
5/8
1/2
3/8
1/4
1/8

Birth   2   6   12   18

AGE (YEARS)

Gaining skills during the first 5 years

Newborn babies can see, hear, perform reflex actions (such as sucking), and cry to gain their mother's attention. From birth to about age 5, young children learn a range of other essential skills. The four main areas of development are physical skills, manual dexterity, language, and social behavior. Achievement of these skills occurs in well-recognized steps known as "developmental milestones"; these occur in a certain order and at roughly predictable times, although the exact age at which they are reached varies from one child to another. The ability to learn particular skills, such as bladder and bowel control, depends upon the maturity of the child's nervous system. In addition, before acquiring certain complex skills, children need to develop a lesser ability first; for example, babies must learn to stand before they can walk.

Developmental milestones

Physical skills
The most important skills are control of posture, balance, and movement. Babies first learn how to lift and turn their heads, then to sit up. They later learn how to crawl, stand, walk, and run.

Can lift head to 45°
Can walk without help
Can catch a bounced ball
Can roll over
Can stand without help
Can crawl
Can throw a ball
Can balance on one foot for a second
Can stand by hoisting up own weight
Can kick a ball
Can sit unsupported
Can walk up stairs without help
Can bear weight on legs
Can walk holding on to furniture
Can pedal a tricycle
Can hop on one leg

Manual dexterity and vision
Children have to learn how to coordinate their hand movements and vision so that they can perform tasks such as picking up objects or drawing shapes.

Holds hands together
Likes to scribble
Can copy a circle
Plays with feet
Can build a tower of four bricks
Passes rattle from hand to hand
Can draw a straight line
Can copy a square
Reaches out for a rattle
Can pick up a small object
Can draw rudimentary likeness of a person
Can grasp object between finger and thumb

Hearing and language
Early on, babies turn toward voices and respond to sounds by cooing. At about 1 year, children can speak their first word and begin to understand the meaning of words. They later learn to form sentences.

Startled by loud sounds
Says "dada" and "mama" to parents
Can talk in full sentences
Turns toward voice
Can point to parts of the body
Squeals
Says "dada" and "mama" to anyone
Knows first and last names
Can define seven words
Can put two words together
Makes cooing noises
Starts to learn single words
Can name a color

Social behavior and play
The first social skill that babies master is smiling at people. They later learn to play with other children and tolerate separation from their parents. Children also acquire practical skills such as feeding and dressing themselves.

Smiles spontaneously
Can eat with a spoon and fork
Can eat with a knife and fork
Mimics housework
Separates easily from parent
Plays peekaboo
Can undress without help
Can dress without help
Eats with fingers
Stays dry in the day
Looks at own hands
Can drink from a cup
Stays dry at night

AGE (MONTHS)																
0	2	4	6	8	10	12	14	16	18	20	22	24	30	36	42	48	54	60

AGE (YEARS)				
0	1	2	3	4	5

Growth charts

Children have regular checkups during which their rate of growth is assessed. The weight and height (or, in a child under 2 years, length and head circumference), and the age, are plotted on charts with a shaded band to show the normal range of growth. There are different charts for boys and girls. Most children's measurements fall inside the band; if they fall outside, there may be a problem. You can also plot your child's growth yourself by measuring his or her height or, for babies, using measurements from the pediatrician.

Measuring your child's height
To measure your child, ask him or her to stand barefoot, against a wall. Rest a flat object, such as a book, on your child's head. Mark where the bottom of the book meets the wall. Measure the distance from the mark to the floor.

Using the charts

Find your child's age on the bottom of the chart and follow a vertical line up, then find the height, head circumference, or weight on the left of the chart and follow a horizontal line across. Mark the point at which these lines cross. If you plot these points at regular intervals, the points will form a curve showing your child's growth.

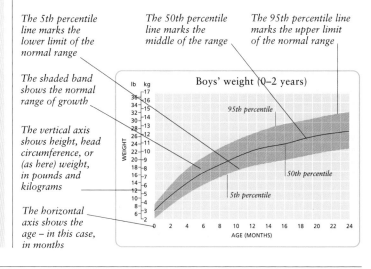

The 5th percentile line marks the lower limit of the normal range

The 50th percentile line marks the middle of the range

The 95th percentile line marks the upper limit of the normal range

The shaded band shows the normal range of growth

The vertical axis shows height, head circumference, or (as here) weight, in pounds and kilograms

The horizontal axis shows the age – in this case, in months

Children's head circumference 0–2 years

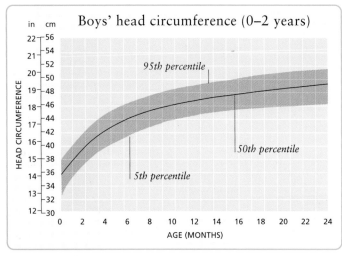

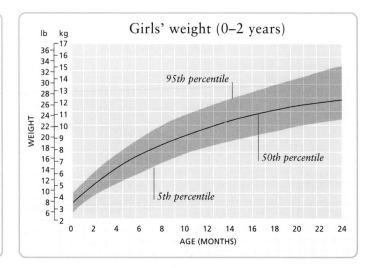

Children's weight 0–2 years

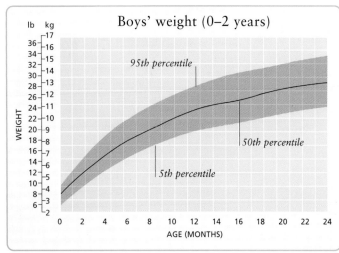

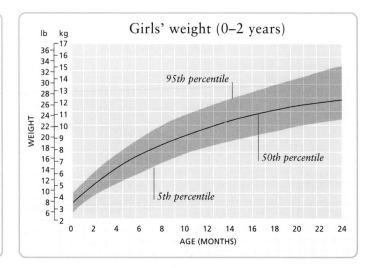

Children's length 0–2 years

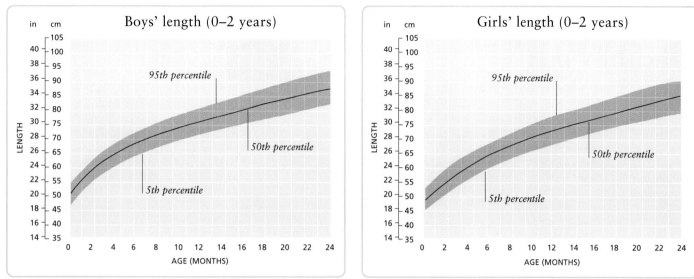

Children's weight 2–18 years

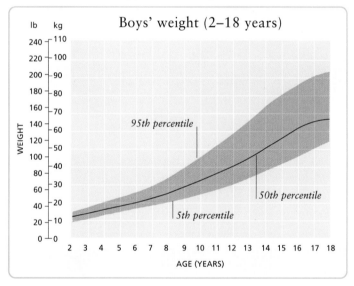
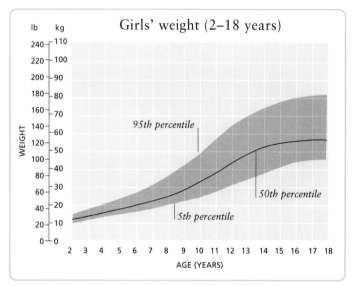

Children's height 2–18 years

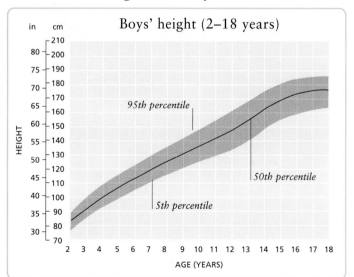
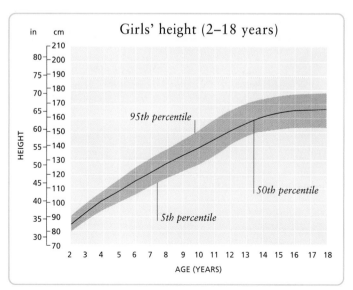

HEALTHY LIVING

A healthy diet

Diet has a major influence on health. It can affect your risk of developing many diseases; for example, a high-fat diet increases your risk of heart disease. It is also crucial in weight control. For a balanced diet you need the correct amounts of carbohydrates, fats, proteins, vitamins, and minerals. Eat plenty of high-fiber foods, which aid digestion; limit foods that have a high fat or sugar content; and avoid large amounts of salt, alcohol, and caffeine. Water is also vital for life, and you should try to drink at least 8 glasses (4 pints) a day.

Food groups

The food pyramid is widely used to represent the ideal proportion of the six food groups, shown here. in your diet. Eat more of the foods at the bottom of the pyramid and less of those at the top, following the suggested number of servings. The number of servings will vary in relation to your needs. For example, a very active person will need to eat more than someone who is sedentary.

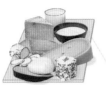
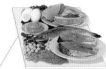
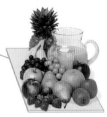
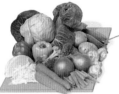
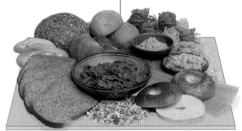

MILK, YOGURT, AND CHEESE (2–3 SERVINGS PER DAY)
Milk and dairy foods provide protein, calcium, and certain vitamins, such as B_2, B_{12}, and D. They can form a fairly large part of your diet, but choose low-fat varieties.

CANDIES, CAKES, AND OILS (MINIMAL SERVINGS)
Fatty foods, which are high in energy, and sugary foods, which can cause tooth decay, should be eaten in limited amounts.

MEAT, EGGS, FISH, NUTS, AND DRY BEANS (2–3 SERVINGS PER DAY)
Meat, fish, and nuts are rich in protein, essential for building and repairing cells, and provide B vitamins and minerals such as iron. They can also be high in fat, so eat them only in moderation.

VEGETABLES (3–5 SERVINGS PER DAY)
Vegetables are high in fiber (which aids digestion), natural sugar, and water, as well as a variety of vitamins and minerals.

FRUIT (2–4 SERVINGS PER DAY)
Fruit is high in fiber, natural sugars and complex carbohydrates, water, vitamins and minerals, and bioflavanoids.

BREAD, CEREAL, RICE, AND PASTA (6–11 SERVINGS PER DAY)
Bread, potatoes, and pasta are high in fiber, starches, and some vitamins and minerals, and can form a large proportion of your diet.

Vitamins and minerals

The body requires a range of vitamins and minerals because these substances play vital roles in growth and metabolism (the chemical processes that occur in the body). Vitamins D and K can be made in the body, but the other vitamins, and all minerals, must come from food. In affluent countries such as the US, most people's diets supply the Reference Daily Intake (RDIs) of vitamins and minerals, but certain people may need supplements. For example, pregnant women need extra folic acid for the health of the fetus, and vegans need extra vitamin B_{12} because they do not eat meat or other animal products (the usual source of this vitamin). Do not take more than the recommended amounts of vitamins A, D, E, and K, because the body stores these substances and they can become toxic if excessive amounts build up in body tissues. In addition, pregnant women should avoid foods that contain high levels of vitamin A because of potential harmful effects on the developing fetus.

Good sources of vitamins and minerals

Vitamin or mineral	RDI	Food sources	Necessary for
Vitamin A	0.8–1 mg	Eggs, carrots, liver	Eyes, hair, skin, bones
Vitamin B_1 (thiamine)	1.1–1.5 mg	Meat, peas, grains, cereals, breads	Energy production, nervous system
Vitamin B_2 (riboflavin)	1.3–1.7 mg	Eggs, meat, dairy products, leafy green vegetables	Nervous system, muscles
Vitamin B_3 (niacin)	15–19 mg	Fish, whole grains, peanuts, peas	Energy production, skin
Vitamin B_6 (pyridoxine)	1.6–2 mg	Meat, fish, whole grains, bananas	Blood formation, nervous system
Vitamin B_{12} (cobalamin)	2 mcg	Milk, fish, meat, eggs, yeast	Blood formation, nervous system
Vitamin C	60 mg	Many fruits and vegetables	Body's use of iron, immune system
Vitamin D	5–10 mcg	Dairy products, oily fish	Teeth and bones
Vitamin E	8–10 mcg	Vegetables, eggs, fish, margarine	Maintaining cell membranes
Vitamin K	60–80 mcg	Leafy green vegetables, formed by bacteria in intestines	Blood clotting, bone formation
Folic acid	180–200 mcg	Leafy green vegetables, organ meats, whole grains, breads, nuts	Fetal nervous system, keeping cells and blood healthy
Calcium	600–1,200 mg	Dairy products, eggs, peas, dry beans, edible fish bones	Bones, teeth, muscles, nervous system
Iron	10–15 mg	Eggs, meat, dairy products, leafy green vegetables	Red blood cell formation, muscles

Assessing your weight

To avoid diseases associated with being overweight or underweight, you need to maintain your weight within the range considered normal for your height. To find out if you are within this range, you can use a height and weight chart such as the one shown below. You can also assess your weight by calculating your body mass index (BMI). To do this, divide your weight in kilograms by the square of your height in meters. A BMI figure under 20 indicates that you are underweight, while a figure over 25 shows that you are overweight.

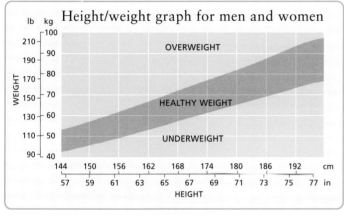

Height/weight graph for men and women

Exercise

Most people know that exercise is an important part of a healthy lifestyle. Regular exercise protects physical and mental health. It can also reduce your risk of developing long-term disease, increase your life expectancy, and improve your quality of life in later years. When you make exercise a part of your daily routine, you will probably find that you have a lot more energy for ordinary daily activities such as your professional work, shopping, housework, or child care.

How exercise benefits health

Regular exercise benefits most of the body's systems, especially the cardiovascular, musculoskeletal, and respiratory systems. It can also benefit mental health by providing pleasure, reducing stress, and producing physical changes that improve mood.

The supply of blood to the brain is increased, thus promoting mental alertness, and chemical changes occur that improve mood

Blood pressure is reduced, and this decrease helps to lower the risk of cardiovascular disease

The heart becomes stronger and can pump more blood with every heartbeat

The lungs can take in more oxygen from each breath and supply more oxygen to the body

Muscles become stronger and more efficient so that they can work for longer periods of time

Joints become stronger and more flexible and mobile as a result of exercise

Bones maintain their strength and density so that they are less prone to damage and disease

Planning an exercise routine

For exercise to be beneficial, it has to be regular. The recommended amount is at least 30 minutes of moderate exercise, such as a brisk walk, on at least 5 days of the week. To become more fit or lose weight, you will have to exercise harder. You need to do activities that work the heart and lungs (build stamina), improve joint mobility (increase flexibility), and increase muscle strength. If you have never exercised regularly before, or if you have any health concerns, consult your doctor before starting an exercise routine.

Fitness benefits of different activities

Activity	Fitness benefits		
	Stamina	Flexibility	Strength
Aerobics	★★★★	★★★	★★
Basketball	★★★★	★★★	★★
Cycling (fast)	★★★★	★★	★★★
Climbing stairs	★★★	★	★★★
Dancing (aerobic)	★★★	★★★★	★
Golf	★	★★	★
Hiking	★★★	★	★★
Jogging	★★★★	★★	★★
Swimming	★★★★	★★★★	★★★★
Tennis	★★	★★★	★★
Walking (briskly)	★★	★	★
Yoga	★	★★★★	★

KEY

★ Small effect	★★ Good effect	★★★ Very good effect	★★★★ Excellent effect

Exercising safely

To avoid overexertion or injury, start by setting realistic goals. If you are not in shape, begin exercising slowly and build up gradually. Take care to not overexert yourself and stop if you experience pain or feel ill. Make sure that you use the correct protective equipment, clothing, and footwear for your sport. Every time you exercise, start with a warming-up routine and finish with a cooling-down routine to prevent muscle cramps and stiffness and minimize the risk of injury. These types of routine involve gentle aerobic exercise, such as slow jogging, followed by a series of movements to stretch your muscles. Two typical stretches are shown here.

Keep your back straight while you move your hips

Rest your hands on your knee to steady yourself

Hip and thigh stretch
Kneel, then put one foot on the floor in front of you. Push your hips down and forward to stretch the back thigh. Repeat for the other thigh.

Lower back stretch
Kneel, sitting on your heels. Stretch your arms above your head, bend forward, and put your hands on the floor. Keep your arms, head, and body aligned.

Exercising at different ages

Most people, whatever their age, can derive physical and mental benefits from exercise. Apart from the overall improvements to your flexibility, strength, and stamina, exercise has different benefits for people at different stages of life. In children, it helps build strong bones and muscles, improves coordination, and can also be fun. In adults, exercise helps minimize the risk of heart disease. In older people, it helps slow processes associated with aging, such as loss of bone density, and enables people to stay mobile for longer. Regular exercise can also enable pregnant women to cope better with the demands of pregnancy and childbirth.

Activities for children
Games such as soccer can improve physical aspects such as strength, balance, and coordination. Such games can also be fun and enable children to make new friends with the other players.

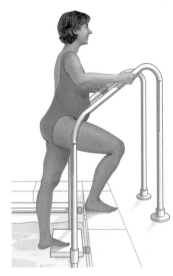

Pregnant women
During pregnancy, gentle swimming can allow you to stretch and exercise your muscles while the water supports your weight.

Older people
Activities such as walking can help lessen the effects of aging by maintaining your bone and muscle strength and joint flexibility.

Alcohol

Alcohol is a drug that alters your mental and physical state, reducing tension and facilitating social interaction. For this reason, it has been used socially for centuries. However, in excess, alcohol may cause loss of control over behavior and, in the long term, physical, psychological, and social problems.

Harmful effects of alcohol

Although moderate alcohol consumption makes you feel relaxed and can have a beneficial effect on health, excessive use of alcohol over a long period can result in serious health problems. When you have a drink, the alcohol is absorbed into the blood through the stomach and small intestine, reaching its maximum concentration in the blood 35–45 minutes afterward. This level depends on factors such as your weight and whether you have drunk the alcohol with food or on an empty stomach; if you take alcohol with food, your body will absorb the alcohol at a slower rate. Alcohol is broken down by

the liver at an average rate of about 1 unit per hour (*see* VOLUME OF DRINK EQUAL TO 1 UNIT OF ALCOHOL, below). Since your body cannot alter this rate, the more you drink, the longer it takes for your body to break down the alcohol. If you drink heavily at night, you may still be intoxicated the next morning. This situation can be dangerous if you plan to drive a vehicle or operate machinery.

In the short term, excessive drinking can cause intoxication and hangovers. In the longer term, alcohol damages most body systems. Regular, excessive drinking can also lead to alcohol dependence and social problems including domestic violence and vagrancy.

The brain's control of inhibitions and coordination is impaired by alcohol. Long-term drinking damages brain cells that control learning and memory

Drinking alcohol makes the blood vessels in the skin widen, causing the body to lose heat. Long-term drinking raises the risk of high blood pressure

The heart may be protected against disease by one or two drinks a day, but drinking more than this amount will increase the risk of cardiovascular disease

The liver may become inflamed (hepatitis) by excessive consumption of alcohol. Long-term drinking can seriously damage the liver and cause diseases such as cirrhosis and cancer

The stomach and the duodenum (the first part of the small intestine) may become ulcerated as a result of long-term drinking. In addition, stomach cancer is a risk

Sexual performance may be impaired by alcohol. In the long term, fertility may be reduced

Safe alcohol limits

To drink alcohol safely, you should limit your intake. Alcohol consumption is measured in units. Current guidelines in the US set by the medical profession state that, in general, men should drink no more than 3 units a day, and women no more than 2 units. Try to keep within these limits and have at least one or two alcohol-free days a week. The volume of a drink containing 1 unit depends on the percentage of alcohol by volume (ABV). The higher the ABV, the smaller the volume equivalent to 1 unit. The box below shows a selection of alcoholic drinks, each equal to 1 unit. Measures served at home or in bars may be larger than those shown here.

Volume of drink equal to 1 unit of alcohol

BEER	WINE	FORTIFIED WINE	HARD LIQUOR
(11 fl oz/330 ml; ABV 4%)	*(4½ fl oz/125 ml; ABV 13%)*	*(2½ fl oz/75 ml; ABV 20%)*	*(1½ fl oz/40 ml; ABV 40%)*

Tobacco

Tobacco is most commonly smoked in cigarettes but can also be smoked in cigars and pipes, inhaled as snuff, or chewed. Regardless of the form in which it is used, tobacco is harmful to health. In the US, smoking is one of the main causes of death in people under the age of 65. Smoking also damages the health of "passive smokers," who inhale other people's smoke. The only way to avoid these health risks is to avoid smoking or coming into contact with other people's smoke.

Health hazards of smoking

Tobacco smoke contains many substances damaging to health, such as tar, carbon monoxide, and nicotine. Tar irritates the airways; carbon monoxide attaches itself to red blood cells, reducing their ability to carry oxygen; and nicotine is addictive. Tobacco smoke also contains cancer-causing substances that can harm the lungs and other organs.

Inhaling smoke from smokers' cigarettes and exhalations is known as passive smoking. The smoke can irritate the eyes, nose, and throat. In the long term, it may cause lung cancer and cardiovascular disease. In children, exposure to smoke increases the risk of infections, such as ear infections, and can trigger asthma and allergies. Babies born to mothers who smoke are likely to be smaller than average and at greater risk of sudden infant death syndrome (crib death).

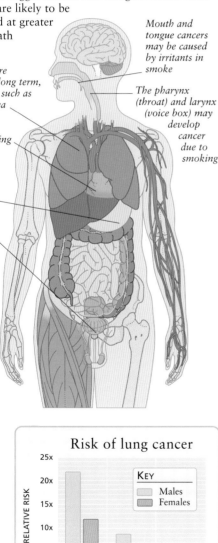

The airways to the lungs are irritated by smoke. In the long term, smoke can cause disorders such as lung cancer and emphysema

The risk of cardiovascular disease is increased by smoking

Smoke can irritate the stomach lining, leading to ulcers. Long-term smoking may cause stomach cancer

Bladder cancer may result from smoking

Cancer of the cervix may develop as a result of smoking

Mouth and tongue cancers may be caused by irritants in smoke

The pharynx (throat) and larynx (voice box) may develop cancer due to smoking

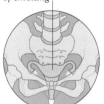

FEMALE

Smoking and lung cancer
This graph shows that male and female smokers are, respectively, over 20 and 10 times more likely to develop lung cancer than those who have never smoked. Ex-smokers have a much lower risk than current smokers; 15 years after giving up, they will have reduced their lung cancer risk by more than half.

Risk of lung cancer

KEY
- Males
- Females

RELATIVE RISK: 25x, 20x, 15x, 10x, 5x, 0

SMOKING STATUS: Current smokers, Ex-smokers, Non smokers

Giving up smoking

You can help prevent heart or lung disease by not smoking or by giving up before you begin to develop the diseases. No matter how long you have been smoking, you can prevent further damage by quitting. If you need help, consult your doctor for advice. If you want to try on your own, list the reasons why you want to stop smoking, then work out the reasons why you smoke. Plan ways to cope with temptation and ask your family and friends for support. Telephone hotlines staffed by ex-smokers can be helpful. Choose a fairly stress-free day and throw away cigarettes, lighters, and ashtrays. You may have withdrawal symptoms, such as irritability, and crave nicotine. Aids such as nicotine patches, gum, or the sustained release form of the antidepressant bupropion can help stop cravings. If you relapse, try to determine why, refer to your reasons for quitting, and try again.

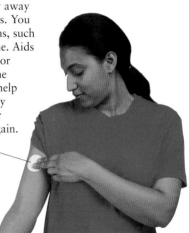

Nicotine patch in place

Using a nicotine patch
Nicotine patches deliver a constant supply of nicotine through the skin, helping stop cravings for cigarettes.

Drugs

A drug is any chemical that alters the function of an organ or a biochemical process in the body. Drugs that are used to improve body functions or to treat diseases and disorders are known as medicines. Certain drugs, such as the sleeping drug temazepam, may be both used as medicines and abused for recreation. Other drugs, such as ecstasy, have no medicinal value and are used only for recreational purposes. Drug abuse can cause serious physical and mental problems, particularly if the abuser becomes dependent on a drug or takes an overdose, and may even cause death. In addition, the use of recreational drugs is illegal.

Effects of drug use on the body

People use recreational drugs to alter their mood. The main types of drug are classified according to the usual mood change that they cause, but often they have a mixture of effects. Stimulants, such as cocaine, increase mental and physical activity; relaxants, such as marijuana and heroin, produce a feeling of calm; intoxicants, such as glue, make users feel giggly and dreamy; and hallucinogens, such as lysergic acid diethylamine (LSD), alter perception and cause hallucinations (seeing or hearing things that do not exist).

Extreme reactions and risks of drugs

Drugs pose serious health risks. Overdoses of drugs such as heroin and cocaine can be fatal; other drugs, such as ecstasy, can also cause death. Some drugs affect vital functions; for example, heroin can slow breathing and heart rate. In addition, extreme reactions or adverse interactions with substances such as alcohol may occur. Another common effect is dependence, a condition in which users experience physical and mental cravings when they do not take a drug. Some problems may arise soon after taking a drug (even for the first time); others are associated with long-term abuse. Injected drugs carry additional risks associated with the use of nonsterile needles, such as HIV infection, hepatitis B or C, or blood poisoning. If you or someone close to you abuses drugs, ask your doctor for information on health risks and advice on counseling and treatment.

Sex and health

Puberty, when the body makes the change from childhood to adulthood, prepares you physically for sexual activity and reproduction. The development of emotional maturity often takes much longer and involves both learning about yourself and gaining experience in dealing with other people.

Sex can be an intensely pleasurable experience that boosts the feeling of well-being. In addition, regular sex can improve cardiovascular fitness and help prolong life. However, you should be aware of the health risks of sex, such as unwanted pregnancy and diseases, called sexually transmitted diseases (STDs), that are spread only or mainly by sexual intercourse.

Sexual relationships

Sexual fulfillment depends on a blend of physical and psychological factors, and what is right for one person or couple may not suit another. You and your partner should be happy with the frequency of sexual activity and should be able to discuss which activities you enjoy or find unappealing. Anyone in a sexual relationship should be aware of transmitted diseases (STDs) and understand how to minimize the risk of exposure to such conditions by practicing safe sex (below). In addition, to avoid an unwanted pregnancy, you should be familiar with the options for contraception (*see* CONTRACEPTION CHOICES FOR MEN, p.254, and CONTRACEPTION CHOICES FOR WOMEN, p.276).

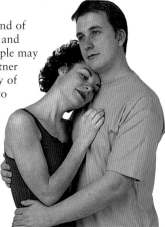

Physical and emotional benefits
Good sexual relationships fulfill both partners' needs for comfort and closeness as well as satisfying their physical desires.

It is common to experience a temporary lack of sexual desire or inability to perform sexually (*see* LOW SEX DRIVE IN MEN, p.250, and LOW SEX DRIVE IN WOMEN, p.272). Such problems are often due to stress or emotional difficulties, or to the use of alcohol, recreational drugs, or certain medications. Disorders such as diabetes mellitus can cause longer-term sexual problems. It is important to discuss concerns with your partner. Talk to your doctor if the problem is persistent.

Practicing safe sex

Sexually transmitted infections (STDs) are usually spread by contact with infected skin or body fluids such as semen, blood, and vaginal secretions. Many STDs are uncomfortable but curable, but some, such as HIV infection, are life-threatening. You can take simple steps to protect yourself. If you have sex with someone whom you do not know to be free of infection, use a condom, which gives protection against most STDs (apart from genital warts and pubic lice, which can affect body areas that are not covered by a condom). If you develop an STD, you should avoid sexual activity until you have been treated and are free of infection.

Stress

Stress is a physical or mental demand that provokes certain responses in us, allowing us to meet challenges or escape from danger. A moderate amount of stress can improve your performance in situations such as sports and work, but excessive stress can harm your health. You can minimize harmful stress by identifying situations that you find stressful and developing ways to cope with them.

Stress ratings of different life events

Very high	High
Death of a spouse	Retirement
Divorce or marital separation	Serious illness of family member
Personal injury or illness	Pregnancy
Loss of job	Change of job
Moving	Death of close friend

Moderate	Low
Big mortgage	Change in work conditions
Legal action over debt	Change in schools
Trouble with in-laws	Small mortgage or loan
Spouse begins or stops work	Change in eating habits
Trouble with boss	Christmas or other holidays

Sources of stress

Stress may result from external events or circumstances, your personal reactions to pressure, or a combination of these factors. Major external sources of stress include long-term problems, such as an unhappy relationship, debilitating illness, or unemployment; major changes, even desirable ones, such as marriage or moving; and a buildup of everyday stresses, such as being late for work or getting caught in a traffic jam. Behavior patterns that cause or aggravate stress include impatience and aggression, lack of confidence, and suppressing feelings of tension or anxiety.

Recognizing signs of stress

If signs of stress are recognized early, action can be taken to prevent health problems. These signs may include having less energy than usual, a reduced appetite, or eating more than you do normally. You may have headaches, mouth ulcers, or be unusually susceptible to minor infections, such as colds. If you feel very stressed, you may be anxious, tearful, irritable, or low in spirits. Sleep may be disrupted, and relationships may suffer. To distract yourself, you may rely on alcohol, tobacco, or drugs. If stress is causing any of these problems, seek help from your family, friends, or doctor.

Making lifestyle changes

If your lifestyle is stressful, try to minimize the harmful effects that stress may cause. Find time to keep up with your family and friends, and take up leisure activities. Exercising regularly can help relieve physical tension, as may learning to relax your body consciously (*see* RELAXATION EXERCISES, below). Break stressful tasks down into small, easy parts. Concentrate on important tasks and limit the number of less urgent ones to conserve your time and energy. If people make heavy demands on you, try to set limits on these demands.

Relaxation exercises

If you are under stress, your muscles tighten, the heart beats more rapidly, and breathing becomes fast and shallow. Relax both your mind and body by learning simple relaxation routines that slow down your body's stress responses. The breathing technique shown here may help reduce stress. For more information, ask your doctor if he or she can recommend any relaxation classes.

Breathing to relax
Breathe slowly and deeply, using your diaphragm and abdominal muscles. Rest one hand on your chest and one on your abdomen: the lower hand should move more than the upper one.

Safety and health

Your environment, like your personal habits, can affect your health but can be modified to some extent. Accidents are a major cause of death and serious injury, particularly in elderly people and small children. Other health hazards include factors such as certain weather conditions and features of your environment at home or work. However, you can easily avoid many risks to health and safety, whether at home, at work, or when traveling, by identifying potential hazards and taking steps to avoid them.

Home safety and health

Accidents are a major hazard to health. Almost half of all serious accidents happen in the home, with elderly people and young children having the highest rates of injury. Elderly people are particularly vulnerable to falling. Poor kitchen hygiene is also a significant risk to health since it can lead to food poisoning.

To prevent falls, install bright lighting, make rugs and mats secure, and keep floors clear. If you have a small child, install stair gates to prevent the child from falling down the stairs. Toddlers should be seated in a highchair with the harness securely fastened for meals.

Children are at significant risk from poisoning by medications, household plants, and toxic substances, including cleaning fluids and lead. Keep toxic

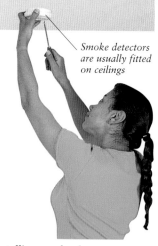

Smoke detectors are usually fitted on ceilings

Installing smoke detectors
Install smoke detectors on every floor of your home. Take care to keep them free of dust and test the batteries once a month.

substances out of their reach, and, to prevent lead poisoning, have lead-based paint removed professionally and lead pipes replaced. To prevent the buildup of carbon monoxide (a gas that is released by burning fuels), have chimneys, heating systems, and gas appliances inspected yearly, and never run machines with gasoline engines in a closed garage.

Use fire or hot items with care; for example, if you are a smoker, be sure to put out cigarettes and matches once you have finished with them. To prevent electrical fires, do not overload electrical sockets. Store flammable materials, such as paints, in a shed or garage. Keep a fire blanket or extinguisher in the kitchen, and install smoke detectors throughout your home, in case a fire breaks out.

To avoid food poisoning, keep your kitchen clean, cook food thoroughly, and store perishable foods in a refrigerator. Keep food in airtight containers, and use it by the recommended expiration date.

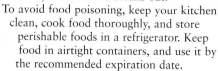

Keep surfaces clean to avoid food poisoning

Highchair straps should be fastened completely

Using a highchair
Children who have started feeding themselves should be placed in a highchair for their meals. Make sure that the harness is fastened securely to prevent falls, and do not leave your child alone.

Safety in the yard

The greatest risks associated with the outdoors are from ponds or pools, poisonous plants and chemicals, garden tools, barbecues, and play equipment. Ponds can pose a risk to small children, who can drown even in shallow water. Take care to supervise children when they are playing around these areas. Toxic plants may cause symptoms such as skin irritation and, if swallowed, internal irritation and vomiting. A few plants may be lethal. Teach children that touching or eating plants may be dangerous. If a child does eat anything poisonous, call your doctor immediately, or take the child to the hospital together with a sample of the plant. If you use poisonous garden chemicals, store them in a locked shed or cabinet. Consider safe alternatives, such as removing weeds by hand or applying chemical-free pesticides. Never leave dangerous machines or sharp tools where children can find them. When using such equipment yourself, wear the necessary protective clothing.

Insects such as bees, wasps, and mosquitoes can bite or sting. The venom may cause an allergic reaction. An extreme allergic reaction (anaphylaxis) can be life-threatening. To protect yourself, keep your arms and legs covered, and apply insect repellent to your skin.

Goggles *Ear protectors*

Thick gloves

Protective gear
Wear protective gear when using machinery such as a hedge cutter. For example, wear thick gloves, shield your eyes from flying debris with goggles, and use ear protectors to block out noise.

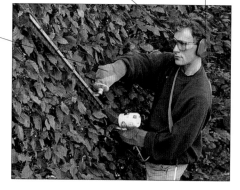

Pets and safety

Animals can cause allergies, and some infections and infestations may spread to people. Cat and dog feces may contain dangerous organisms such as the eggs of the toxocara worm. If ingested, these eggs may cause toxocariasis, a disease that may lead to blindness. Cat feces may also contain toxoplasma protozoa, which may cause serious harm to fetuses in pregnant women. Worm your pets regularly and dispose of their feces hygienically. Teach children to wash their hands after touching animals. Because pets such as dogs can bite, they should never be left alone with young children.

Handling dogs safely
Teach children how to approach and stroke dogs correctly. Even a normally friendly dog may bite if provoked.

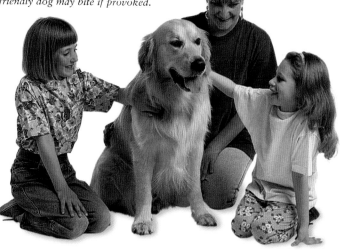

Safety in the sun

Overexposure to the sun may lead to sunburn, heatstroke, and, in the long term, serious problems such as skin cancer. You are at especially high risk if you have red or blond hair and green or blue eyes because your skin contains a low level of melanin, a pigment that absorbs ultraviolet light. To minimize the risk of sun damage, everyone should stay out of the sun in the middle of the day. If you are outdoors, make sure to protect your skin and eyes. Wear a wide-brimmed hat, a long-sleeved shirt, and long pants or skirt. Use a sunscreen with a suitable sun protection factor (SPF); the higher the factor, the greater the protection it gives you. Apply it 15–30 minutes before you go outside and reapply it every 2 hours. You should wear sunglasses that have an American National Standards Institute label and give maximum protection from ultraviolet light.

Apply sunscreen to uncovered areas

Protecting children's skin
Babies and children are at high risk of sunburn because of their delicate skin. Keep babies out of the sun and ensure that young children wear protective clothing and sunscreens.

Safety at work

Both office work and manual jobs can involve certain risks to health. It is wise to find out about any potential risks associated with your work and take action to prevent them. If necessary, ask your employer for help in minimizing these hazards.

Office work rarely poses risks to your physical safety, but it can give rise to various health problems. Two of the most common physical conditions are lower back pain, due to poor posture while sitting at a desk, and repetitive strain injury (RSI), a type of muscle strain caused by repetitive movements such as typing. Another common problem is psychological stress (p.32), which may be due to factors such as demanding situations or poor relationships with colleagues. To avoid physical problems, you should make sure that your work space is well ventilated and well lit. Sit with your back straight and feet on the floor. If you do a lot of typing, make sure that your wrists are supported while you work. If you are faced

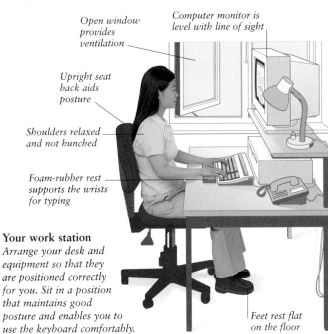

Open window provides ventilation

Computer monitor is level with line of sight

Upright seat back aids posture

Shoulders relaxed and not hunched

Foam-rubber rest supports the wrists for typing

Your work station
Arrange your desk and equipment so that they are positioned correctly for you. Sit in a position that maintains good posture and enables you to use the keyboard comfortably.

Feet rest flat on the floor

with stressful situations, try to resolve these problems, or seek help if necessary before they start to affect your health.

Many types of manual work are dangerous. Working with machinery or heavy objects may put you at risk of injury. Many chemicals are toxic or have other harmful effects such as burning the skin. Some forms of dust, such as silica (found in sand and some rocks) and asbestos, can damage the lungs if inhaled. Other hazards include loud noise and extreme temperatures. Your employer should inform you of any risks and supply protective equipment. If you are self-employed, find out about possible risks to protect yourself and ensure that you conform to safety regulations for your work.

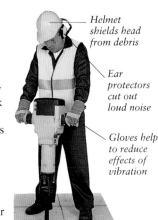

Helmet shields head from debris

Ear protectors cut out loud noise

Gloves help to reduce effects of vibration

Using equipment safely
When using tools such as a drill, you need clothing and equipment that protect you from noise, vibration, and flying debris.

Safety on the road

In the US, traffic accidents result in thousands of deaths and injuries each year. Nearly all accidents are due to human error rather than mechanical faults. A major cause of errors in drivers is alcohol abuse; other causes include lack of experience, use of medications, and fatigue. These factors can delay reactions and impair drivers' judgment. Drivers should ensure that they are not tired or under the influence of alcohol, and should make sure that any medications they are taking will not cause drowsiness. Every occupant of a car should wear a seat belt. Young children should have car seats that are appropriate for their size and weight.

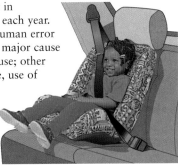

Child seats
A car seat for a child should cushion the child from possible injury and should allow the seat belt to fit correctly across his or her body.

Motorcyclists and cyclists need helmets and clothing that will protect them from adverse weather conditions and injury. They should ensure that their lights work properly, and wear reflectors or bright clothing to make them visible to other road users.

Pedestrians should use sidewalks or footpaths and should cross roads at pedestrian crossings. If there is no sidewalk, they should walk on the same side of the road as oncoming traffic. Anyone who has young children should ensure that they learn about road safety.

Bright clothing makes cyclists clearly visible to other road users

Cycle helmet protects head from impacts

Cycling safety
Cyclists should wear helmets to protect the skull and fluorescent or bright clothes to make them easily visible. Lights must be used at night. Always maintain your bicycle in good working order.

Tires should be inflated to the right pressure

Wheel reflectors for added visibility

Brakes must be checked regularly for wear and tear

PROFESSIONAL HEALTH CARE

Health care throughout life

Taking care of your health involves following a healthy lifestyle as well as making effective use of the health care system. Doctors and other professional health care workers provide treatment when you are sick and are also involved in some important elements of preventive health care. These include health education, checkups during childhood and later in life, screening tests to identify risk factors and early signs of disease, and immunizations to help prevent certain infectious diseases. To get the most from what professional health care has to offer, you need to be aware of the options for you and your family and to learn how to make the best use of the services that doctors and other health care professionals can provide.

Health care providers

Most disorders can be diagnosed and treated by internists and family practitioners. These doctors' practices provide a range of services, some of which include prenatal care, immunizations, and other preventive measures, as well as minor surgery such as wart removal. Other health care providers include nurses, dentists, physical therapists, and some practitioners of complementary and alternative therapy. In addition, organizations such as the National Institutes of Health provide advice on health by telephone or on the internet (*see* USEFUL ADDRESSES, p.311).

The usual way to obtain hospital care is by referral from your doctor. However, if you have a severe accident or a serious problem such as heavy bleeding, you should go straight to a hospital emergency department for treatment. If your injury or symptoms are not severe, you should consider waiting to see your doctor. Free-standing clinics such as those for the treatment of sexually transmitted infections are also available for self-referral.

Choosing a doctor

If you are looking for a new doctor, you can obtain a list of doctors in your area from your health insurance provider; you can also ask friends and neighbors if they can recommend anyone. When you find a practice, ask about their opening hours and how long, on average, you will have to wait for an appointment that is not urgent. In addition, ask whether the practice offers home visits, advice over the telephone, services provided by other healthcare professionals such as nurses, and access to special services, such as family planning clinics. You may also wish to ask if you can choose a female doctor rather than a male doctor (or vice versa) if you have a strong preference in this matter.

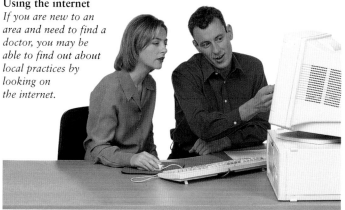

Using the internet
If you are new to an area and need to find a doctor, you may be able to find out about local practices by looking on the internet.

Visiting your doctor

Before your first appointment with a new doctor, you may be asked to complete a questionnaire about your health and lifestyle. On your first visit, your doctor will ask further questions and make sure that you are up to date with immunizations and screening. During later visits, the doctor will add notes to your medical records, which can be transferred if you change doctors. You have the right to see your own or your child's records. During a visit, do not hesitate to ask questions about your health and treatments.

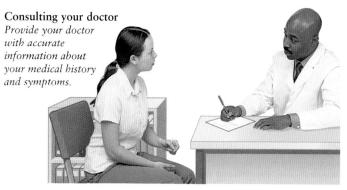

Consulting your doctor
Provide your doctor with accurate information about your medical history and symptoms.

Your medical history

When you first visit a doctor, you will be questioned about your present and past health; treatments that you are having or have had; disorders that could run in your family; and aspects of your lifestyle, such as diet and exercise. The information gathered from these questions is known as a medical history. If you then visit your doctor with a disorder or unexplained symptoms, your medical history can help him or her to reach a diagnosis. In addition, if there is evidence that you are at risk of developing certain disorders, your doctor will suggest preventive measures or screening to detect early signs.

Having a physical examination

When you see your doctor, you may have a physical examination to assess your state of health, look for abnormalities, or confirm or rule out a diagnosis. The examination usually begins with a check of external areas, such as the eyes, ears, skin, and nails, and a test of nervous reflexes. In some cases, the doctor can gather information about other areas apart from the one being examined; for example, a pale-colored tongue may be a sign of anemia. He or she may also check for abnormalities by listening to internal organs with a stethoscope (auscultation), by feeling (palpation), or by tapping areas and listening to the sounds produced (percussion).

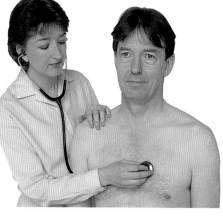

Listening to the chest
The doctor uses a stethoscope to listen to sounds within the chest, such as those made by the heart and lungs. A stethoscope is also used to listen to sounds made by the intestines or by blood flowing through vessels.

Checkups and screening

Checkups provide an opportunity to discuss with your doctor you or your child's general health. In the US, children have routine checkups that focus on healthy growth and development. In adults, checkups are usually given after beginning with a new doctor, for insurance purposes, or when starting a new job. In addition, pregnant women and those with a long-term illness, such as diabetes, should have regular checkups. Checkups for adults usually involve a physical examination (p.35) and basic screening, such as blood pressure measurement. Screening is important in preventing disease by looking for factors that increase the risk of disease and in detecting disease at an early stage when there is the greatest chance of treatment being successful. In some cases, screening may also be used to detect a rare inherited disease that may affect you or your children. Some tests may only be appropriate at certain ages. For example, newborn babies are screened for certain metabolic disorders, and the fecal occult blood test, which screens for colorectal cancer, is used for people over the age of 50.

Screening babies and children

In the uterus, babies may be tested for genetic disorders such as Down syndrome. Immediately after birth, a baby's appearance and responses are checked for abnormalities, and a few days later, a blood sample is taken from the heel to look for hypothyroidism (underactivity of the thyroid gland) and phenylketonuria (a metabolic defect that can cause brain damage). In early childhood, the acquisition of certain skills, known as developmental milestones, is monitored (see GAINING SKILLS DURING THE FIRST 5 YEARS, p.25), and, throughout childhood, growth is checked (see GROWTH CHARTS, pp.26–27). Children should also have regular eye and ear tests (see VISION TESTING IN CHILDREN, p.101, and HEARING TESTS IN CHILDREN, p.105).

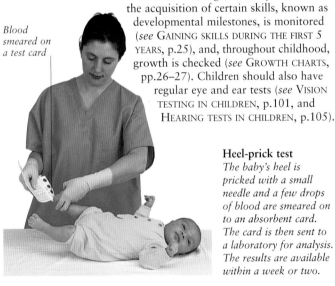

Blood smeared on a test card

Heel-prick test
The baby's heel is pricked with a small needle and a few drops of blood are smeared on to an absorbent card. The card is then sent to a laboratory for analysis. The results are available within a week or two.

Screening adults

Screening tests are advisable for adults at stages of life when the risk of certain diseases increases. For example, screening for early signs of breast cancer and cancer of the cervix is recommended for women in specific age groups (see COMMON SCREENING TESTS, right). Screening tests for other cancers, such as colorectal cancer and prostate cancer, are also available. One of the most common screening tests is blood pressure measurement. Usually, high blood pressure, or hypertension, does not produce symptoms but is a major risk factor for heart disease and stroke. Other screening tests that are recommended for adults include tests to check blood cholesterol levels, which also affect your risk of heart disease and stroke, and eye pressure measurement to check for glaucoma, a disorder that may cause blindness if left untreated. People with chronic disorders are usually advised to have regular screening to detect early signs of complications. For example, people with diabetes mellitus have regular screening for kidney disease, cardiovascular disorders, nerve damage, and problems in the blood vessels of the eye, which left untreated may lead to blindness.

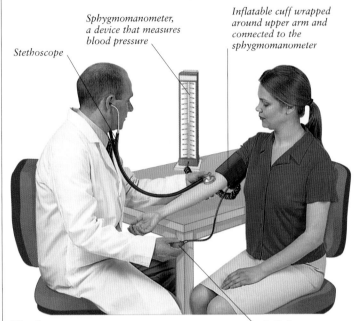

Stethoscope

Sphygmomanometer, a device that measures blood pressure

Inflatable cuff wrapped around upper arm and connected to the sphygmomanometer

Bulb for inflating and deflating cuff

Blood pressure measurement
To measure blood pressure, the doctor wraps an inflatable cuff around the upper arm and inflates it. The cuff is slowly deflated while the doctor uses a stethoscope to listen to blood flow through an artery.

Common screening tests

Test	When recommended	What it screens for
Heel-prick test (left); a blood sample is taken from the baby's heel	Shortly after birth	Hypothyroidism and phenylketonuria (a rare metabolic disorder)
Blood pressure measurement (above)	Every 2 years from about age 18	Hypertension (high blood pressure)
Blood cholesterol test; involves giving a blood sample for analysis	Every 5 years from age 20	High blood cholesterol
Pap smear test (p.264); a sample of cells is scraped from the cervix	Annually from first sexual activity to age 65	Precancerous changes in cells of the cervix or cancer of the cervix
Fecal occult blood test; involves providing a sample of feces for testing	Every year from age 50 on request from doctor	Colorectal cancer
Mammogram (p.257); an X ray of the breasts is taken	Annually from age 40, (recommendations vary, however)	Breast cancer
Screening for glaucoma (p.188); the pressure inside the eye is measured	Every 2 years from age 40; carried out by an opthalmologist	Glaucoma

Immunization

Immunization protects you from infectious disease for several months or years, or even for life. It can be conferred by using either vaccines or immunoglobulins. A vaccine contains a tiny amount of either a killed or modified infectious organism or a modified toxin (poison produced by bacteria). Once inside the body, the vaccine stimulates the immune system to make antibodies, proteins that help destroy the organism or toxin if encountered in the body. Immunoglobulins contain antibodies taken from the blood of a person or animal who has overcome a certain infection and give useful short-term protection. Most vaccines involve several injections over a period of months or years to build up adequate protection. Immunizations may have side effects, such as mild fever. However, serious side effects are extremely rare.

Routine immunizations

Most routine immunizations are given during infancy and childhood according to an immunization program (below). The immunization program begins shortly after birth because it is important to protect babies against infectious diseases that may be life-threatening in infancy. You should keep records of all your immunizations and those of your children in case a doctor other than your family doctor needs to know about your immune status.

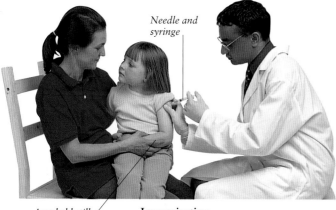

Needle and syringe

Arm held still during injection

Immunization
Most immunizations are given by injection.

Recommended immunization schedule

Disease	Number of doses	Timing of immunization
Hepatitis B (Hep B)	3	0–2 months; 1–4 months; 6–18 months
Diphtheria, Tetanus, and Pertussis (DTaP)	5	2 months; 4 months; 6 months; 15–18 months, 4–6 years
Haemophilus influenzae type b (Hib)	4	2 months; 4 months; 6 months; 12–15 months
Inactivated Polio (IPV)	4	2 months; 4 months; 6–18 months; 4–6 years
Pneumococcal Conjugate Vaccine (PCV)	4	2 months; 4 months; 6 months; 12–15 months
Measles, mumps, and rubella (MMR)	2	12–15 months; 4–6 years
Varicella	1	12–18 months
Tetanus and Diphtheria (Td)	1	11–12 years; booster every 10 years thereafter

Immunizations for adults

The immunity given by some immunizations wears off after several years, so it is important for adults to have repeat doses known as boosters. For example, you need a booster immunization for tetanus every 10 years because the bacterium responsible for this disease is very common in the environment, and you are at risk of infection if you sustain a dirty or deep cut. In addition, make sure that you have been immunized for poliomyelitis if you were not during childhood. Immunizations are often given to adults who are traveling to areas where certain diseases are common (*see* TRAVEL IMMUNIZATIONS, below) or if there is a high risk of an infectious disease for health or work reasons (*see* IMMUNIZATIONS FOR SPECIAL CASES, below).

Travel immunizations

The immunizations needed before you travel depend on destination, state of health, and current immune status, and the duration, type, and purpose of your travel. If you are planning to travel, make sure that you have been immunized against tetanus and poliomyelitis, and have booster doses if necessary. Most countries do not require visitors to have specific immunizations, but some may ask for a certification that you have been immunized against yellow fever, an infection that can cause severe jaundice. Consult your doctor, local travel clinic, or the CDC website (www.cdc.gov) about necessary immunizations at least 8 weeks before you travel because some need more than one dose to become effective. The table below shows the most common travel immunizations. Advice on immunizations for foreign travel changes frequently; always obtain current information.

Common travel immunizations

Disease	Dosage	Destination
Diphtheria	1 injection	Former USSR or developing countries
Hepatitis A	1 injection (immunoglobulin)	Developing countries (single visit)
	2 injections (vaccine)	Developing countries (frequent visits)
Hepatitis B	3 injections over 6 months	Areas where hepatitis B is endemic; necessary if you may need to receive medical or dental treatment in a developing country
Japanese B encephalitis	2–3 injections 1–2 weeks apart	Rural areas of the Indian subcontinent, China, Southeast Asia, and the Far East
Meningitis A and C	1 injection	Saudi Arabia, Sub-Saharan Africa, Nepal, Brazil; immunization certificate needed if traveling to Mecca
Rabies	3 injections over 4 weeks	Areas where rabies is endemic; necessary if you will be working with animals or traveling in remote areas
Typhoid	1 or 2 injections or 3 oral doses	Areas with poor sanitation
Yellow fever	1 injection	Parts of Africa and South America

Immunizations for special cases

In some circumstances, specific groups of people may need to be given immunizations that are not normally offered to most people. These immunizations are usually offered because these groups are at increased risk of developing a serious illness if they become infected. For example, immunizations against influenza and pneumococcal pneumonia are commonly given to people over the age of 65; to those who have reduced immunity, such as people with diabetes mellitus, HIV infection, or AIDS; and to those with long-term heart or lung disease. In addition, some people may need immunization if their type of work puts them at increased risk of an infectious disease. For example, people who work with animals may need to be vaccinated against the virus that causes rabies.

MEDICAL TESTS

Testing samples

Tests that are carried out on samples of body fluids, such as blood or urine, are often the first investigations requested by a doctor before making or confirming a diagnosis. Samples of urine and feces can usually be collected easily by the patient, and blood samples by the doctor in his or her office. Some samples, such as cell and tissue samples and certain body fluids, may need to be collected during a procedure. The results of tests on body samples can provide information on the function of certain organs, such as the liver or kidneys, or reveal the presence of abnormal substances or abnormal levels of normal substances, such as hormones, in the body. In addition, some tests can reveal the presence of disease-causing microorganisms. Most tests on body samples are carried out in a laboratory, but some may be performed in a doctor's office or even in the patient's home.

Blood tests

Blood tests can be used to find information about the blood itself and to assess the function of other parts of the body, such as the liver. The samples are usually taken from a vein, but may also be taken from capillaries (tiny blood vessels) by a finger prick, or occasionally from an artery. The most common blood tests performed are blood cell tests and blood chemistry tests. Blood cell tests include measuring the numbers of red and white blood cells and of platelets (cells that help blood clot). Blood carries many substances apart from cells, and blood chemistry tests can measure the levels of these substances. These tests are used to detect kidney, liver, and muscle damage, certain bone disorders, and inflammation. One type is carried out to measure the level of cholesterol in the blood. In addition, blood chemistry tests are performed to see if a gland, such as the thyroid gland in the neck, is producing abnormal amounts of a hormone.

Urine tests

Urine is most commonly tested for evidence of urinary tract infections or diabetes and can be used to help assess kidney function. Many urine tests are dipstick tests, which involve dipping a chemically treated stick into a sample of urine to show the presence or concentration of specific substances, such as glucose, or the presence of infectious organisms. Dipstick tests are usually performed in a doctor's office. If the test suggests an infection, the sample may be sent to a laboratory to grow and identify the microorganism. A specific test for a hormone produced in pregnancy is the basis of the urine pregnancy test, which can be performed at home (*see* HOME PREGNANCY TEST, p.260).

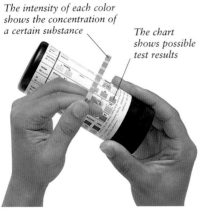

The intensity of each color shows the concentration of a certain substance

The chart shows possible test results

Testing with a dipstick
When a dipstick is put into a urine sample, chemicals in the squares along the stick react and cause a color change. Each square on the stick tests for a different chemical. After a specified amount of time, the colors of the squares, which indicate the concentration of substances in the urine, are compared to a chart.

Tests on body fluids

Tests may be performed on body fluids from wounds or abnormal areas of skin, from mucous membranes such as those of the nose and throat, or from internal areas such as the inside of a joint or around the brain and spinal cord. The tests may involve looking for infectious microorganisms, abnormal cells such as cancerous cells, or abnormal levels of certain chemicals. Other tests involve assessing cells or other substances that are normally found in the fluid, such as sperm in a sample of semen. Some samples, such as sputum, can be collected by the individual; others by a doctor. The samples are then usually sent to a laboratory for analysis.

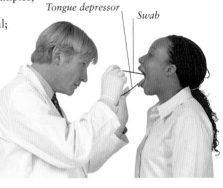

Tongue depressor   *Swab*

Having a swab taken
Fluids from wounds or from body cavities, such as the mouth, are usually collected with a swab – sterile cotton on a plastic stick.

Tests on feces

Samples of feces may be tested for infectious microorganisms or for evidence of digestive disorders. One common test is the fecal occult blood test, which can reveal tiny amounts of blood invisible to the naked eye. This test may be carried out if the doctor suspects that there may be bleeding in the digestive tract. The test may also be used to screen for colorectal cancer. Tests on samples of feces are usually carried out in a laboratory.

Cell and tissue tests

Microscopic studies of individual cells, or of a larger sample of tissue containing a variety of cells, can give a definitive diagnosis for many disorders. Tests on cells are often used to diagnose cancer or screen for genetic disorders. Cells may be obtained from body fluids such as sputum (fluid coughed up from the lungs) or scraped from tissue surfaces such as the cervix (*see* CERVICAL SMEAR TEST, p.264). Cells may also be withdrawn from the body using a needle and syringe. This process, called aspiration, is often used to take cells from the lungs, thyroid gland, or breasts (*see* ASPIRATION OF A BREAST LUMP, p.256). Tissue tests are used to detect areas of abnormal tissue such as cirrhosis of the liver or tumors. Samples are taken by biopsy, in which a small piece of tissue is removed from parts of the body such as the skin (*see* SKIN BIOPSY, p.183) or the liver (below).

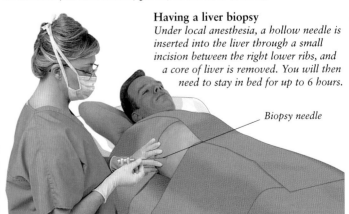

Having a liver biopsy
Under local anesthesia, a hollow needle is inserted into the liver through a small incision between the right lower ribs, and a core of liver is removed. You will then need to stay in bed for up to 6 hours.

Biopsy needle

Physiological tests

Certain investigations that do not involve testing samples (opposite) or imaging internal structures (see IMAGING TESTS, right) can be performed to assess the function of organs or systems. These physiological tests are commonly used to assess vision and hearing, the nervous system, and the heart and lungs.

Vision and hearing tests

The most common vision tests measure the ability to focus (see VISION TESTING, p.189, and VISION TESTING IN CHILDREN, p.101). Another test defines the visual field (the area that each eye can see independently). There is a range of tests for hearing. Some show how well sound is conducted through the ears; others measure how well sounds of varying pitch and volume can be heard or, in children, show the ability to hear speech (see HEARING TESTS, p.190, and HEARING TESTS IN CHILDHOOD, p.105).

Test area

Controls and touch-screen display

Response button

Visual field test
This test is used to map the visual field. You are asked to look at a screen and press a button when you see flashes in different areas of the screen.

Nervous system tests

Some tests are used to establish whether nerves can conduct impulses normally. Abnormalities may be the result of a compressed nerve or a disease such as diabetes mellitus. Another test, the electroencephalogram (EEG), records the electrical activity produced in the brain and is useful for the diagnosis of disorders such as epilepsy.

Heart and lung tests

Heart rhythm and rate can be monitored by tests in which the electrical activity in the heart muscle is recorded: electrocardiography (ECG; p.203), ambulatory ECG (p.205), and exercise ECG (below). Lung function can be tested in various ways. The simplest is measuring peak flow rate (p.197), which is the maximum rate at which you can breathe out. More complex tests show how quickly the lungs fill and empty (to detect narrowed airways), determine lung capacity (to check for disorders that cause the lungs to shrink), and measure blood levels of oxygen (see MEASURING BLOOD OXYGEN, p.201).

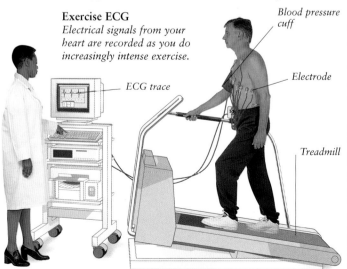

Exercise ECG
Electrical signals from your heart are recorded as you do increasingly intense exercise.

Blood pressure cuff

ECG trace

Electrode

Treadmill

Imaging tests

In imaging tests, energy is directed at or introduced into body tissues and detected by machines to produce images of internal structures. X rays are used in many tests, ranging from conventional X-ray procedures to the computerized technique of CT scanning. Although X rays carry a very small risk of exposure to harmful radiation, some tests use other forms of energy. For example, MRI uses magnetism and radio waves, and ultrasound scanning uses sound waves. Other imaging tests include radionuclide scanning, PET, and SPECT, which use radioactive substances introduced into certain tissues.

X rays

X rays are a form of radiation that can pass through body tissues to leave an image on photographic film. The ability of the rays to penetrate tissues depends on the density of those tissues. Solid, dense tissues such as bone let few rays through and appear white on the image. Muscular organs, such as the heart, appear gray. Tissues containing air, such as the lungs, and fluid-filled areas, such as the bladder, let most of the X rays through and appear black on the film. X-ray images are often used to assess bone injuries such as fractures or disorders such as arthritis. The images can also show disorders in some soft tissues, such as infection in the lungs, and breast X rays are used to screen women for breast cancer (see MAMMOGRAPHY, p.257). X rays may be used in other imaging techniques, such as bone densitometry (p.239).

Hollow or fluid-filled structures do not show clearly on plain X rays but can be imaged by introducing a contrast medium into the area before taking the X ray. The contrast medium blocks X rays and makes the area appear white on the image. Types of contrast X ray include barium contrast X rays (p.40), used to image the digestive tract; angiography (p.40), which shows blood vessels; and intravenous urography (p.227), which shows the urinary tract.

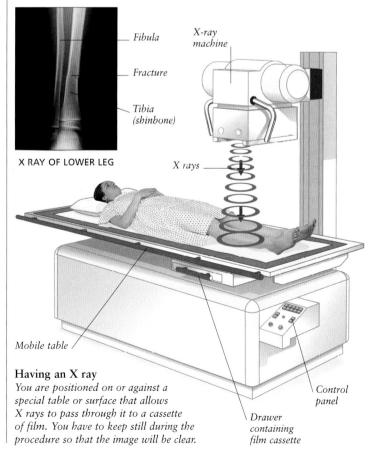

Fibula

Fracture

Tibia (shinbone)

X RAY OF LOWER LEG

X-ray machine

X rays

Mobile table

Control panel

Drawer containing film cassette

Having an X ray
You are positioned on or against a special table or surface that allows X rays to pass through it to a cassette of film. You have to keep still during the procedure so that the image will be clear.

Barium contrast X rays

Parts of the digestive tract that are not visible on plain X rays (p.39) can be imaged with barium contrast X rays. Barium sulfate, which is a contrast medium (a substance that blocks X rays), is introduced into the tract, then an X ray is taken. If the esophagus, stomach, or duodenum is to be investigated, the barium is swallowed in a drink, a procedure known as a barium swallow or meal. If the colon is to be viewed, the barium is given as an enema. These X rays can reveal abnormalities such as tumors and narrowed or blocked areas.

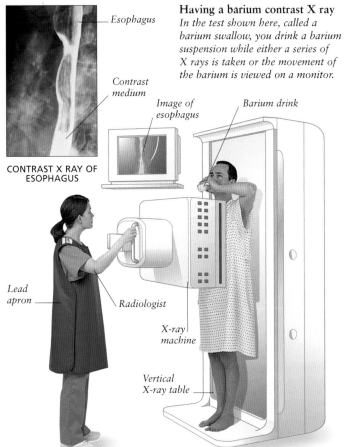

CONTRAST X RAY OF ESOPHAGUS

Esophagus

Contrast medium

Image of esophagus

Barium drink

Having a barium contrast X ray
In the test shown here, called a barium swallow, you drink a barium suspension while either a series of X rays is taken or the movement of the barium is viewed on a monitor.

Lead apron

Radiologist

X-ray machine

Vertical X-ray table

Angiography

In angiography, a dye is introduced into arteries to make them visible on X rays (p.39) and reveal problems such as narrowed areas. First, a catheter is inserted into an artery some distance away and passed through the body, under X-ray control, until it reaches the artery to be imaged. The dye is injected through the catheter directly into the vessel, so that it is not diluted by the blood, and a series of X rays is taken. Coronary angiography (below) shows the arteries supplying the heart muscle. Femoral angiography (p.233) shows arteries in the legs.

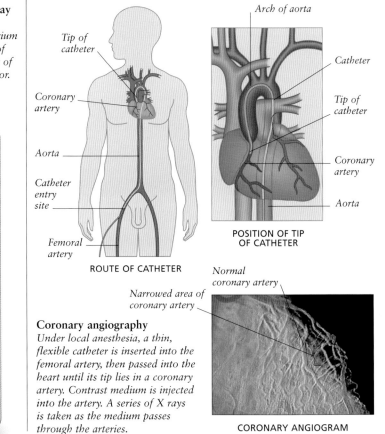

Tip of catheter

Coronary artery

Aorta

Catheter entry site

Femoral artery

ROUTE OF CATHETER

Arch of aorta

Catheter

Tip of catheter

Coronary artery

Aorta

POSITION OF TIP OF CATHETER

Normal coronary artery

Narrowed area of coronary artery

CORONARY ANGIOGRAM

Coronary angiography
Under local anesthesia, a thin, flexible catheter is inserted into the femoral artery, then passed into the heart until its tip lies in a coronary artery. Contrast medium is injected into the artery. A series of X rays is taken as the medium passes through the arteries.

CT scanning

Computed tomography (CT) scanning is an X-ray-based technique that produces detailed cross-sectional images of the body. The images show a wide range of tissues of varying densities that do not show clearly on plain X rays. CT scans reveal the anatomy of organs and other body structures, as well as abnormalities such as tumors or scar tissue inside organs. The scanner moves around the body; one section emits X rays, which pass through the body to a detector on the other side of the machine. This X-ray detector transmits data to a computer, which creates an image that is shown on a monitor or reproduced on X-ray film. Hollow or fluid-filled areas usually appear black on the images but can be shown with a contrast medium, which blocks the passage of X rays. In some cases, data from the scans can be used to create three-dimensional images. CT scans are most commonly used to investigate the brain or the solid abdominal organs but may also be carried out to view the lungs.

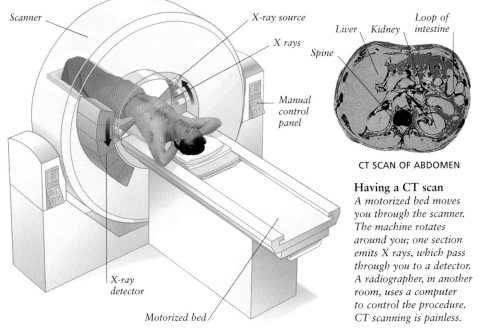

Scanner

X-ray source

X rays

Manual control panel

X-ray detector

Motorized bed

Liver   Kidney   Loop of intestine

Spine

CT SCAN OF ABDOMEN

Having a CT scan
A motorized bed moves you through the scanner. The machine rotates around you; one section emits X rays, which pass through you to a detector. A radiographer, in another room, uses a computer to control the procedure. CT scanning is painless.

MRI

Magnetic resonance imaging (MRI) uses magnetic force and radio waves to create images of internal structures and tissues. MRI can reveal fine details and abnormalities more clearly than other forms of imaging. The scanner contains two powerful magnets and a radiofrequency source. One magnet creates a powerful magnetic field, which causes hydrogen atoms throughout the body to line up. The radiofrequency source emits radio waves that briefly knock the atoms out of alignment. As the atoms realign, they emit signals (resonance) that are picked up by the other magnet placed around the area being scanned. Information about the signals is transmitted to a computer, which produces an image on a monitor. MRI is often used to examine the brain and spinal cord. It is also used to investigate sports injuries such as torn tendons.

Having an MRI scan
A motorized bed moves you into the scanner, and several scans are taken. You may be given earplugs because the machine is noisy. Some people find the machine claustrophobic, and if you feel nervous, you may be allowed to have someone with you.

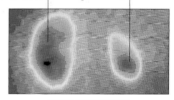

MRI SCAN OF KNEE JOINT

Skin
End of femur (thighbone)
Patella (kneecap)
Cartilage within joint
Fat
End of tibia (shinbone)

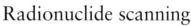

Radiofrequency source, which emits radio waves

Scanner

Manual control panel

Companion for patient

Motorized bed

Receiving magnet

Magnet that creates powerful magnetic field

Ultrasound scanning

In ultrasound scanning, images are created using ultrasound waves (high-frequency, inaudible sound waves). A device called a transducer is moved over the skin or, in some cases, inserted into a body opening such as the vagina or rectum, and sends ultrasound waves into the body. Where tissues of different densities meet, or where tissue meets fluid, the waves are reflected; the transducer picks up the echoes and passes them to a computer, which creates an image on a monitor. The images are updated continually so that movement can be seen. Doctors often use ultrasound to look at fetuses in the uterus (*see* ULTRASOUND SCANNING IN PREGNANCY, p.280) or the walls and valves of the heart, or to detect abnormalities such as cysts and kidney stones. A technique called Doppler ultrasound scanning (p.235), which shows the direction and speed of blood flow, is used to detect problems such as narrowed arteries or clots in veins.

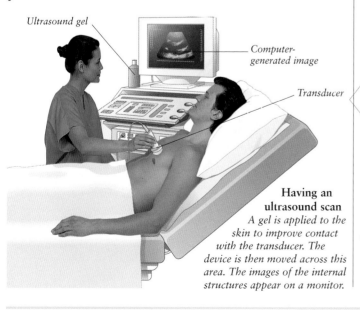

Ultrasound gel

Computer-generated image

Transducer

Having an ultrasound scan
A gel is applied to the skin to improve contact with the transducer. The device is then moved across this area. The images of the internal structures appear on a monitor.

Radionuclide scanning

Radionuclides are radioactive substances, and the radiation they emit can be used to create images. In radionuclide scanning, a tiny amount of the radionuclide is introduced into the body, usually by injection, then taken up by a specific type of tissue; for example, iodine is taken up by the thyroid gland. A device called a gamma camera detects the radiation and transmits data to a computer, which shows the tissue as areas of color. The higher the level of cell activity in the tissue, the more radiation is emitted and the more intensely colored the area appears. Radionuclide scans can show areas where cell activity is abnormally high, such as in tumors, or abnormally low, such as in damaged organs or cysts.

Having a radionuclide scan
Once your body has absorbed the radionuclide, you lie on a motorized bed that positions you over the gamma camera, which detects the radiation from the radionuclide. A computer interprets this as an image.

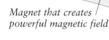

Normal kidney
Damaged kidney

SCAN OF KIDNEYS

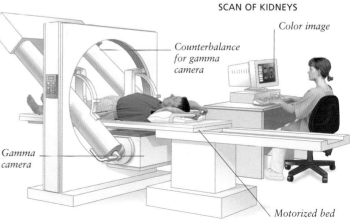

Counterbalance for gamma camera

Color image

Gamma camera

Motorized bed

PET and SPECT scanning

Positron emission tomography (PET) and single-photon-emission computerized tomography (SPECT) are forms of radionuclide scanning (p.41). In both, a radionuclide (radioactive substance) is introduced into the body and taken up by tissues, and the radiation emitted is detected by a scanner. PET uses a radionuclide attached to glucose or other molecules essential to cell metabolism and can show the functioning of individual cells within tissues. It is mainly used to assess the heart and the brain. SPECT uses radionuclides that emit photons (a form of energy), whose movements can be traced by the scanner. The technique can show blood flow within organs and is used to assess if they are functioning normally. SPECT is chiefly used to assess the brain, heart, liver, and lungs.

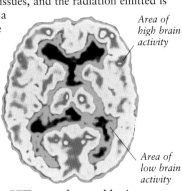

Area of high brain activity

Area of low brain activity

PET scan of normal brain
In this cross section of the brain, the yellow and red patches are highly active areas, and the blue and black patches are less active areas.

Endoscopy

Endoscopy is a procedure in which a doctor views internal structures using a tubelike instrument called an endoscope, which includes a fiberoptic light source and magnifying lenses. The tip of the endoscope is passed through a natural body opening, such as the mouth, or a small incision in the skin. A rigid or flexible endoscope may be used, depending on the area to be examined. The view may be seen directly through an eyepiece or shown on a monitor. Endoscopy may be used for diagnosis or for treatments.

Rigid endoscopes

A rigid endoscope is a short, straight metal viewing tube. It may be introduced through an incision in the skin and used for areas such as the abdominal cavity or the inside of joints, where the structures are near the skin surface. Endoscopy of joints is termed arthroscopy, and the endoscopes used are arthroscopes. Rigid endoscopes may also be inserted into natural orifices, such as the rectum. Procedures involving rigid endoscopes introduced through skin incisions are usually performed under general anesthesia, but local anesthesia may be used. Instruments may be passed down the endoscope or introduced through separate incisions made in the skin.

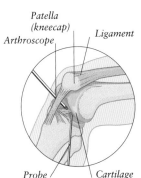

Patella (kneecap)
Arthroscope
Ligament
Probe
Cartilage
POSITION OF INSTRUMENTS

Arthroscopy
Small incisions are made on either side of the knee. The arthroscope is inserted through one incision, and a probe is inserted through the other. The probe is used to move tissues so that certain structures can be viewed more clearly.

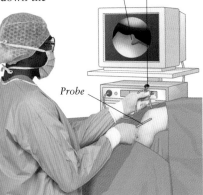

Image of knee joint
Endoscope
Probe

Flexible endoscopes

A flexible endoscope has a long, thin tube that can be steered around angles in internal passages, such as the esophagus and the colon, and enter deep into the body. These endoscopes are often used for viewing inside the digestive and respiratory tracts. The instrument is inserted through a natural opening such as the mouth or anus. The person undergoing the procedure is first given a sedative or a local anesthetic, sprayed, for example, onto the back of the throat. The endoscope incorporates a system of lights, lenses, and optical fibers, and usually a video camera at the tip, allowing the doctor to view structures either directly through an eyepiece or on a video screen. If procedures, such as taking tissue samples, need to be carried out, very fine instruments can be passed down the tube, and the doctor can use the view from the tip as a guide during the procedure. The view may be recorded on videotape.

Upper digestive tract endoscopy
Before the procedure, you may be given a sedative. The endoscope is then passed into the body through the mouth. The view from the tip of the endoscope allows the doctor to detect abnormalities in the lining of the digestive tract.

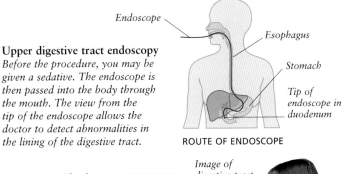

Endoscope
Esophagus
Stomach
Tip of endoscope in duodenum

ROUTE OF ENDOSCOPE

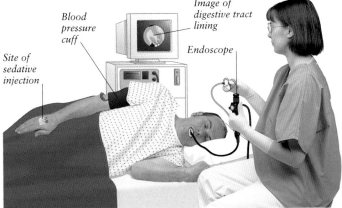

Blood pressure cuff
Image of digestive tract lining
Site of sedative injection
Endoscope

Endoscopic treatments

Endoscopy can be used for surgical treatments, often referred to as minimally invasive surgery. These treatments may even occur at the same time as the endoscopy is being used to make a diagnosis. Surgery is performed by using instruments passed down the endoscope. Endoscopic treatments include removal of intestinal polyps or diseased tissue (such as an inflamed gallbladder) and laser surgery to treat endometriosis. The doctor uses the endoscopic view as a guide during the procedure. Such operations are usually better for the patient than conventional surgery because the patient recovers faster and spends less time in the hospital. In some procedures, such as laparoscopy (investigation of the abdomen), gas may be pumped into the abdomen to create more space and provide a better view.

Area of endometriosis
Probe
Uterus
Ovary

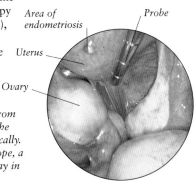

View of endometriosis
Endometriosis, in which tissue from the uterus lining grows outside the uterus, can be treated endoscopically. In this view through the endoscope, a probe holds tissues out of the way in preparation for laser surgery.

SYMPTOM CHARTS

The charts help you identify the possible causes of a symptom, tell you when to seek medical help, and, if appropriate, suggest how you can treat the symptom or its cause yourself. The section consists of charts for children of different ages, charts for all adults, and charts specifically for men or women. The information at the beginning of the section explains how to use the charts most effectively and how to identify the most appropriate chart for your symptom.

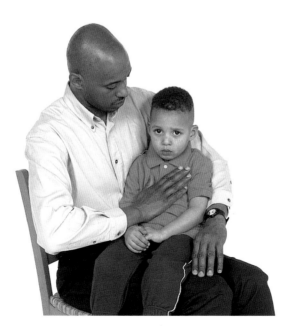

HOW TO USE THE CHARTS

Each of the 150 charts in this section covers a symptom or group of related symptoms and is similar to the example below. The chartfinders on pages 46–48 will help you find the chart you need for your symptom. If you have more than one symptom, choose the chart that deals with the symptom that bothers you the most. To use a chart, follow the pathway of questions with yes/no answers until it leads to a possible cause or causes (there may be several possible diagnoses for a given set of symptoms) and action. The action tells you what your doctor may do or what might happen in the hospital and, if self-help measures are appropriate, what you can do yourself. Many charts have boxes that give further self-help advice or provide information about dieases, tests, or treatments.

Warning box
This box highlights danger signs that need urgent medical attention or provides key information. Read the box first before working through the chart

Starting point
The starting point for each chart is always located in the top left corner of the page

Question boxes
These boxes ask for further information about your symptoms and can be answered YES or NO. Make sure that you read the questions carefully

Yes and No options
You can leave each question box by answering either YES or NO. YES is always to the right of a box, and NO is always at the bottom of a box

Pathway
The arrowed pathways lead you from one question to the next and eventually to a possible diagnosis

How the charts are organized

The charts are divided into four groups, each group indicated by a different color bar down the edge of the page. The groups are:
- Charts for children: problems affecting children of all ages, as well as charts specifically for babies under one or adolescents.
- General charts for adults: problems that can affect both men and women
- Charts for men: specific problems affecting men
- Charts for women: specific problems affecting women, including symptoms during pregnancy.

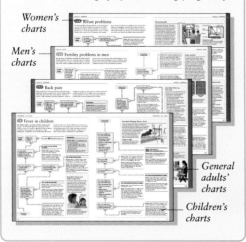

Women's charts

Men's charts

General adults' charts

Children's charts

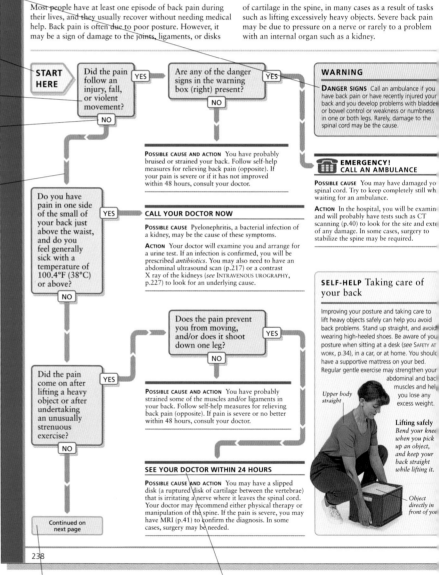

ADULTS: GENERAL

117 Back pain

Most people have at least one episode of back pain during their lives, and they usually recover without needing medical help. Back pain is often due to poor posture. However, it may be a sign of damage to the joints, ligaments, or disks of cartilage in the spine, in many cases as a result of tasks such as lifting excessively heavy objects. Severe back pain may be due to pressure on a nerve or rarely to a problem with an internal organ such as a kidney.

START HERE → Did the pain follow an injury, fall, or violent movement? — YES → Are any of the danger signs in the warning box (right) present? — YES →

NO

NO

WARNING
DANGER SIGNS Call an ambulance if you have back pain or have recently injured your back and you develop problems with bladder or bowel control or weakness or numbness in one or both legs. Rarely, damage to the spinal cord may be the cause.

EMERGENCY! CALL AN AMBULANCE
POSSIBLE CAUSE You may have damaged yo spinal cord. Try to keep completely still wh waiting for an ambulance.
ACTION In the hospital, you will be examin and will probably have tests such as CT scanning (p.40) to look for the site and exte of any damage. In some cases, surgery to stabilize the spine may be required.

POSSIBLE CAUSE AND ACTION You have probably bruised or strained your back. Follow self-help measures for relieving back pain (opposite). If your pain is severe or if it has not improved within 48 hours, consult your doctor.

Do you have pain in one side of the small of your back just above the waist, and do you feel generally sick with a temperature of 100.4°F (38°C) or above? — YES →

NO

CALL YOUR DOCTOR NOW
POSSIBLE CAUSE Pyelonephritis, a bacterial infection of a kidney, may be the cause of these symptoms.
ACTION Your doctor will examine you and arrange for a urine test. If an infection is confirmed, you will be prescribed *antibiotics*. You may also need to have an abdominal ultrasound scan (p.217) or a contrast X ray of the kidneys (*see* INTRAVENOUS UROGRAPHY, p.227) to look for an underlying cause.

Does the pain prevent you from moving, and/or does it shoot down one leg? — YES →

NO

Did the pain come on after lifting a heavy object or after undertaking an unusually strenuous exercise? — YES →

NO

POSSIBLE CAUSE AND ACTION You have probably strained some of the muscles and/or ligaments in your back. Follow self-help measures for relieving back pain (opposite). If pain is severe or no better within 48 hours, consult your doctor.

SEE YOUR DOCTOR WITHIN 24 HOURS
POSSIBLE CAUSE AND ACTION You may have a slipped disk (a ruptured disk of cartilage between the vertebrae) that is irritating a nerve where it leaves the spinal cord. Your doctor may recommend either physical therapy or manipulation of the spine. If the pain is severe, you may have MRI (p.41) to confirm the diagnosis. In some cases, surgery may be needed.

Continued on next page

238

SELF-HELP Taking care of your back

Improving your posture and taking care to lift heavy objects safely can help you avoid back problems. Stand up straight, and avoid wearing high-heeled shoes. Be aware of you posture when sitting at a desk (see SAFETY AT WORK, p.34), in a car, or at home. You shoulc have a supportive mattress on your bed. Regular gentle exercise may strengthen your abdominal and bacl muscles and helf you lose any excess weight.

Upper body straight

Lifting safely
Bend your knee when you pick up an object, and keep your back straight while lifting it.

Object directly in front of you

Continuation box
On two-page charts, these boxes show that the pathway continues onto the second page. Another box appears on the second page in a matching color to tell you where to pick up the pathway

Instructions for obtaining urgent medical help
These instructions tell you what to do when you need prompt medical help rather than a routine appointment with your doctor. They say whether to call an ambulance or how quickly to get in touch with your doctor

Possible cause or causes
This text tells you which condition or conditions are most likely to be responsible for your symptoms and whether you should consult your doctor

Action
This text tells you what can be done for your condition. If medical help is needed, it will tell you about tests you may have and likely treatments. If medical help is not necessary, information may be given on what you can do yourself

Color bar
Each group of charts is identified by a color bar, helping you find the chart you want more easily

Self-help box
This type of box may outline practical measures that you can take to relieve symptoms or cope with your problem. Alternatively, there may be advice on how to assess the severity of a symptom; for example, by taking body temperature during a fever

Instructions for obtaining urgent medical help

If your symptoms suggest that you need urgent medical attention rather than just a routine appointment with your doctor, the instructions at the end of a pathway will tell you what to do. There are three different levels of urgency. In the most urgent cases that are potentially life-threatening, you will be told to call an ambulance. For other urgent cases, you will be told to get help from your doctor either at once or within 24 hours. The instructions are fully explained below.

EMERGENCY! CALL AN AMBULANCE

Your condition may be life-threatening unless you receive immediate medical attention in the hospital. Usually, the best way to achieve this is by calling an ambulance so that you can be given medical care in transit. In some cases, going by car to the emergency department of the nearest hospital may be a better option, especially if an ambulance cannot reach you quickly.

CALL YOUR DOCTOR NOW

Your symptoms may indicate a serious problem that needs urgent medical assessment. Even if it is the middle of the night or the weekend, you should call your doctor immediately. He or she may visit you at home or want to see you at the office immediately. If you cannot get in touch with your doctor within 1 hour, go to the emergency department of your nearest hospital. If possible, go by car or taxi; if not, call for an ambulance.

SEE YOUR DOCTOR WITHIN 24 HOURS

You need prompt medical attention, but a short delay is unlikely to be damaging. Telephone your doctor and ask for an urgent appointment within the next 24 hours.

ADULTS: GENERAL

Continued from previous page

Are you over 50? YES / NO

POSSIBLE CAUSE You may have ankylosing spondylitis (inflammation of the joints between the vertebrae, resulting in the spinal column gradually becoming hard and inflexible). This is especially likely if you are between 20 and 40. Consult your doctor.

ACTION Your doctor will examine you and arrange for you to have a blood test and X rays (p.39) of your back and pelvic areas. If you are found to have ankylosing spondylitis, you will probably be given *nonsteroidal anti-inflammatory drugs*. You will also be referred to a physical therapist, who will teach you exercises to help keep your back mobile. These mobility exercises are an essential part of the treatment for this disorder and can be supplemented by other physical activities, such as swimming.

Has your back gradually become stiff as well as painful over a period of months or years? YES / NO

SEE YOUR DOCTOR WITHIN 24 HOURS

POSSIBLE CAUSE You may have a compression fracture of a vertebra as a result of osteoporosis, in which bones throughout the body become thin and weak. Osteoporosis is symptomless unless a fracture occurs. The disorder is most common in women who have passed menopause. A prolonged period of immobility may also lead to the development of osteoporosis.

ACTION Initial treatment for the pain is with *analgesics*. Your doctor may also request bone densitometry (below). Specific treatment for osteoporosis depends on the underlying cause. However, in all cases, it is important that you try to remain active and do weight-bearing exercise, such as walking.

Did the pain come on suddenly after an extended stay in bed or confinement to a wheelchair, or are you over 60? YES / NO

Are you female and pregnant? YES / NO

CONSULT YOUR DOCTOR IF YOU ARE UNABLE TO MAKE A DIAGNOSIS FROM THIS CHART AND YOUR BACK PAIN IS SEVERE OR IF THE NATURE OF LONG-STANDING BACK PAIN SUDDENLY CHANGES.

to chart **147** BACK PAIN IN PREGNANCY (p.284)

SELF-HELP Relieving back pain

Most back pain is the result of minor sprains or strains and can usually be helped by simple measures. Try the following:
- If possible, keep moving and carry out your normal daily activities.
- Rest in bed if the pain is severe, but do not stay in bed for more than 2 days.
- Take over-the-counter *nonsteroidal anti-inflammatory drugs*.
- Place a heating pad or wrapped hot-water bottle against the painful area.
- If heat does not provide relief, try using an ice pack (or a wrapped pack of frozen peas); place it over the painful area for 15 minutes every 2–3 hours.

If your backache is severe or is no better within 2 days, consult your doctor.

Once your back pain has cleared up, you should take steps to prevent a recurrence by following the self-help advice for taking care of your back (opposite).

POSSIBLE CAUSE Osteoarthritis of the spine is probably the cause of your symptoms. In this condition, joints between the vertebrae in the spine are progressively damaged. This is particularly likely if you are over 50 and you are overweight. Consult your doctor.

ACTION Your doctor may arrange for blood tests and an X ray (p.39) to confirm the diagnosis. Over-the-counter *analgesics* should help relieve your symptoms. If you are overweight, it will help to lose weight (see HOW TO LOSE WEIGHT SAFELY, p.151). Your doctor may refer you for physical therapy to help you strengthen the muscles that support the spine.

Bone densitometry

This technique uses low-intensity X rays (p.39) to measure the density of bone. The X rays are passed through the body, and their absorption is interpreted by a computer and displayed as an image. The computer calculates the average bone density and compares it with the normal range for the person's age and sex. The procedure takes about 20 minutes and is painless.

During the procedure
The X-ray generator and detector move along the length of the spine, and information is displayed on a monitor.

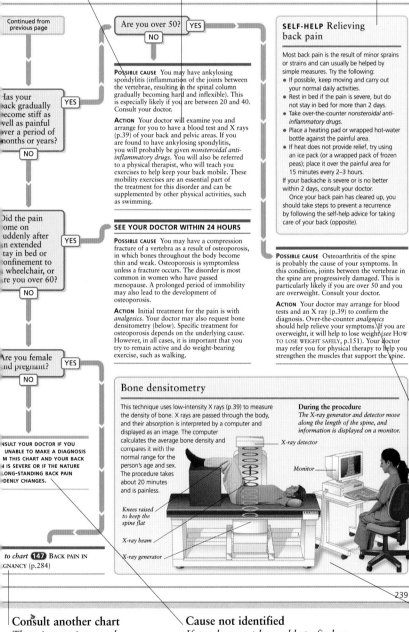

X-ray detector
Monitor
Knees raised to keep the spine flat
X-ray beam
X-ray generator

239

Consult another chart
These instructions send you to another chart in this book that may be more appropriate for your symptoms or may give you additional information

Cause not identified
If you have not been able to find an explanation for your symptoms, you will usually be told to consult your doctor. In some cases, you will be given a suggested time, such as 48 hours, within which to consult your doctor if symptoms are not improved

Drug treatments
If a type of drug, such an pain medication or sedative, is in italic typeface, additional information can be found in the A–Z of drugs (pp.305–310)

Information box
This type of box gives further information on what is involved in having a particular test or treatment that is mentioned elsewhere in the chart. In addition, some information boxes have key facts on a disease or extra detail of anatomy that is relevant to the chart

CHARTFINDERS

To help you find the chart you need, the charts have been listed here in two ways. The system-by-system chartfinder (below) groups the symptom charts under the affected body part or process, such as ear and hearing symptoms or pregnancy and childbirth symptoms. You should use this chartfinder if you know the affected body system but cannot clearly define your symptom. However, if you can identify your symptom, you should use the symptom-by-symptom chartfinder (p.48). This alphabetical list covers all the symptoms in the book and can direct you to the page of the right chart. In addition, the contents (pp.6–7) has a complete list of the symptom charts, and, at the start of each group of charts, such as charts for children, there is a list of the charts in that group.

System-by-system chartfinder

Symptom-by-symptom chartfinder

CHARTS FOR CHILDREN

1 Sleeping problems in babies

For children over 1 year, see chart 11, SLEEPING PROBLEMS IN CHILDREN (p.70).

Most babies wake at regular intervals through the day and night for feedings during the first few months of life. This is perfectly normal, and there is no point in trying to force a baby of this age into a routine that is more convenient for you. Consult this chart only if you think your baby is waking more frequently than is normal for him or her, if you have difficulty settling your baby at night, or if a baby who has previously slept well starts to wake during the night.

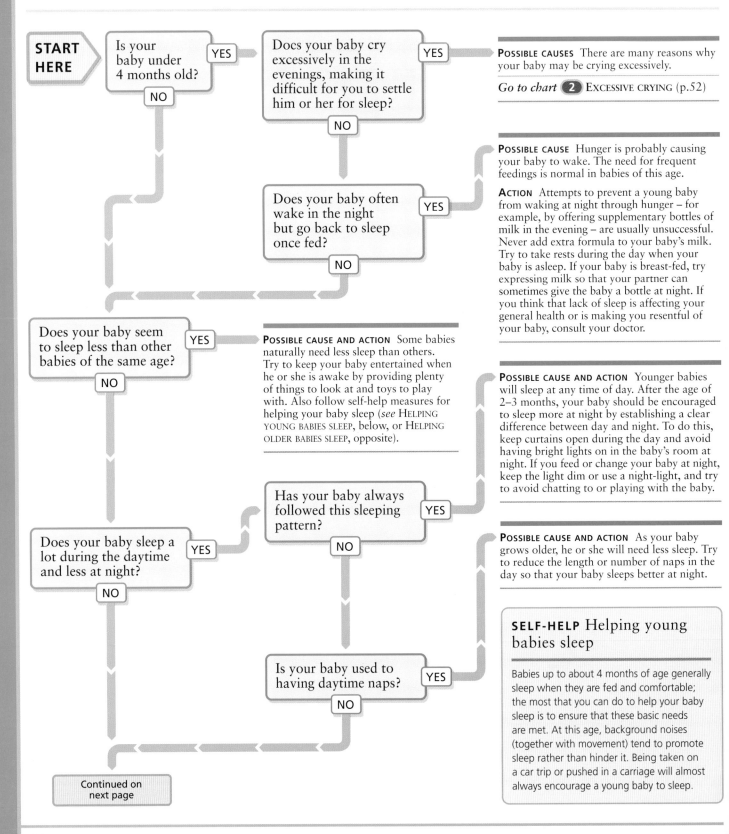

START HERE

Is your baby under 4 months old? — YES → **Does your baby cry excessively in the evenings, making it difficult for you to settle him or her for sleep?** — YES → **POSSIBLE CAUSES** There are many reasons why your baby may be crying excessively.

Go to chart 2 EXCESSIVE CRYING (p.52)

NO

Does your baby often wake in the night but go back to sleep once fed? — YES → **POSSIBLE CAUSE** Hunger is probably causing your baby to wake. The need for frequent feedings is normal in babies of this age.

ACTION Attempts to prevent a young baby from waking at night through hunger – for example, by offering supplementary bottles of milk in the evening – are usually unsuccessful. Never add extra formula to your baby's milk. Try to take rests during the day when your baby is asleep. If your baby is breast-fed, try expressing milk so that your partner can sometimes give the baby a bottle at night. If you think that lack of sleep is affecting your general health or is making you resentful of your baby, consult your doctor.

NO

Does your baby seem to sleep less than other babies of the same age? — YES → **POSSIBLE CAUSE AND ACTION** Some babies naturally need less sleep than others. Try to keep your baby entertained when he or she is awake by providing plenty of things to look at and toys to play with. Also follow self-help measures for helping your baby sleep (*see* HELPING YOUNG BABIES SLEEP, below, or HELPING OLDER BABIES SLEEP, opposite).

NO

Has your baby always followed this sleeping pattern? — YES → **POSSIBLE CAUSE AND ACTION** Younger babies will sleep at any time of day. After the age of 2–3 months, your baby should be encouraged to sleep more at night by establishing a clear difference between day and night. To do this, keep curtains open during the day and avoid having bright lights on in the baby's room at night. If you feed or change your baby at night, keep the light dim or use a night-light, and try to avoid chatting to or playing with the baby.

NO

Does your baby sleep a lot during the daytime and less at night? — YES ↑

NO

Is your baby used to having daytime naps? — YES → **POSSIBLE CAUSE AND ACTION** As your baby grows older, he or she will need less sleep. Try to reduce the length or number of naps in the day so that your baby sleeps better at night.

NO

Continued on next page

SELF-HELP Helping young babies sleep

Babies up to about 4 months of age generally sleep when they are fed and comfortable; the most that you can do to help your baby sleep is to ensure that these basic needs are met. At this age, background noises (together with movement) tend to promote sleep rather than hinder it. Being taken on a car trip or pushed in a carriage will almost always encourage a young baby to sleep.

Continued from previous page

Does your baby sleep in the same room as you? — YES

NO

POSSIBLE CAUSES You may find that sharing a room with your baby results in disturbed nights for both you and your baby. The problem may be that you make sounds that disturb your baby. However, it is more likely that you will be overaware of your baby's movements during sleep and may think that the little noises that babies often make in their sleep are signs of wakefulness. Many babies are restless sleepers and, if left undisturbed, will continue to sleep.

ACTION If possible, move your baby into a different room. It is unlikely that you would fail to hear a true cry, but you are not as likely to be disturbed by less urgent sounds.

Is your baby waking repeatedly at night after previously sleeping well? — YES

NO

CONSULT YOUR BABY'S DOCTOR IF YOU ARE UNABLE TO MAKE A DIAGNOSIS FROM THIS CHART.

Does your baby seem unwell in any way? — YES

NO

POSSIBLE CAUSES AND ACTION If your baby has specific symptoms, such as fever, diarrhea, or vomiting, consult the relevant chart in this book. If there are no specific symptoms but your baby continues to seem unwell, you should contact your baby's doctor.

Could your baby be waking because he or she is hungry? — YES

NO

POSSIBLE CAUSE AND ACTION As your baby grows, he or she will need more food. Increasing feedings in the evening may keep your baby from waking during the night. Alternatively, you may need to start weaning your baby (p.63) if you have not already done so. Consult your baby's doctor for advice.

Could your baby be too cold or hot during the night? — YES

NO

POSSIBLE CAUSE Being too hot or cold may be causing your baby to wake in the night.

ACTION Try to keep the temperature in your baby's room at about 65°F (18°C). Your baby should need no more covers than you would in similar circumstances. Letting your baby get too hot may increase the risk of sudden infant death syndrome (SIDS, left). If your baby kicks off the bedcovers and gets cold, try dressing him or her in a sleep suit at night.

Has there been any recent domestic stress or other possible cause of anxiety? — YES

NO

POSSIBLE CAUSE Babies sense anxiety or stress in their parents and can be disturbed by it.

ACTION It may take some time to reassure your baby. If you can, try to keep your baby's routine as stable as possible, even if your own life is unsettled. When your baby wakes at night, offer a drink and a cuddle, but make sure that your baby understands that he or she will be put back in the crib; otherwise, there is a danger that the baby will get into the habit of waking during the night and expecting to play (*see* HELPING OLDER BABIES SLEEP, above).

POSSIBLE CAUSE AND ACTION A need for the reassurance of your presence is the most common explanation for waking at night when a baby is past the stage of needing night feedings. Try to stick to a bedtime routine (*see* HELPING OLDER BABIES SLEEP, above).

SELF-HELP Helping older babies sleep

Babies older than about 4 months are past the stage of needing frequent night feedings and benefit from a bedtime routine. It is best to be consistent and firm, but this should not prevent bedtimes from being fun. Your baby needs reassurance that separation from you at bedtime is not a punishment. Here are some tips for problem-free nights:

- Avoid too much excitement in the hour or so before bed.
- Provide a night-light if your baby seems frightened of the dark.
- Do not be too ready to go to your baby if you hear whimpering in the night. He or she may be making noises while asleep.
- If your baby cries at night, settle him or her as quickly and quietly as possible.

SELF-HELP Reducing the risk of SIDS

There are things you can do to reduce the risk of sudden infant death syndrome (SIDS), also known as crib death. They are:

- Always put your baby to sleep on his or her back near the foot of the crib. This position is the safest, since he or she cannot wriggle under the bedcovers.
- Use a firm mattress with no pillow.
- Do not overwrap your baby in bedcovers.
- Do not place your baby's crib close to a radiator or other type of heater.
- Do not smoke in the presence of your baby.

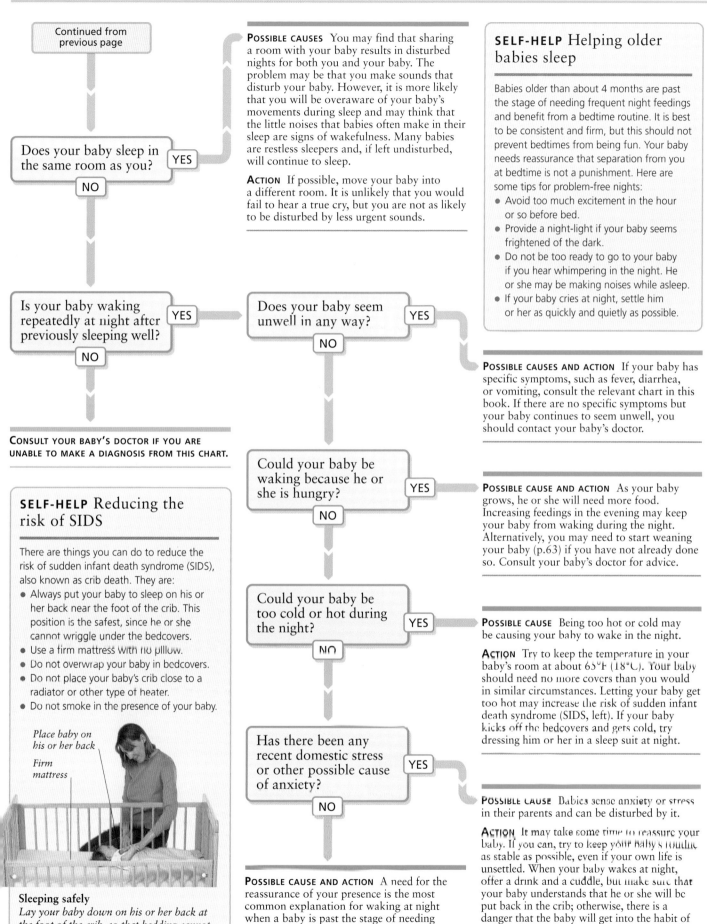

Place baby on his or her back

Firm mattress

Sleeping safely
Lay your baby down on his or her back at the foot of the crib, so that bedding cannot cover the face. Do not overwrap the baby.

2 Excessive crying

Crying is a young baby's only means of communicating physical discomfort or emotional distress. All babies sometimes cry when they are hungry, wet, upset, or in pain, and some babies occasionally cry for no obvious reason. Most parents soon learn to recognize the most common causes of their baby's crying and are usually able to deal with them according to need. You should consult this chart if your baby cries more often than you think is normal or if your baby suddenly starts to cry in an unusual way. In some cases, you may be advised to seek medical help.

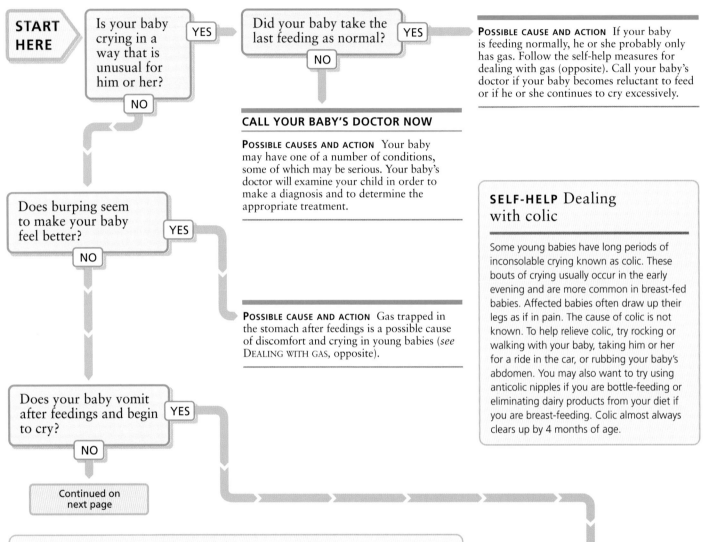

START HERE

Is your baby crying in a way that is unusual for him or her? — YES → **Did your baby take the last feeding as normal?** — YES →

POSSIBLE CAUSE AND ACTION If your baby is feeding normally, he or she probably only has gas. Follow the self-help measures for dealing with gas (opposite). Call your baby's doctor if your baby becomes reluctant to feed or if he or she continues to cry excessively.

Is your baby crying... NO ↓

Did your baby take the last feeding as normal? NO ↓

CALL YOUR BABY'S DOCTOR NOW

POSSIBLE CAUSES AND ACTION Your baby may have one of a number of conditions, some of which may be serious. Your baby's doctor will examine your child in order to make a diagnosis and to determine the appropriate treatment.

Does burping seem to make your baby feel better? — YES →

NO ↓

POSSIBLE CAUSE AND ACTION Gas trapped in the stomach after feedings is a possible cause of discomfort and crying in young babies (*see* DEALING WITH GAS, opposite).

Does your baby vomit after feedings and begin to cry? — YES →

NO ↓

Continued on next page

SELF-HELP Dealing with colic

Some young babies have long periods of inconsolable crying known as colic. These bouts of crying usually occur in the early evening and are more common in breast-fed babies. Affected babies often draw up their legs as if in pain. The cause of colic is not known. To help relieve colic, try rocking or walking with your baby, taking him or her for a ride in the car, or rubbing your baby's abdomen. You may also want to try using anticolic nipples if you are bottle-feeding or eliminating dairy products from your diet if you are breast-feeding. Colic almost always clears up by 4 months of age.

SELF-HELP Coping with crying

Many parents find it very stressful and feel unable to cope if their baby cries for hours on end. Such feelings are normal and do not mean that you are a bad parent. Ask neighbors or friends to look after your baby for an hour so that you can relax. If there is no one to ask, put your baby safely in his or her crib, close the door, and leave him or her for half an hour or so, until you feel better. Being left for a short while will not harm your baby. If the crying becomes unbearable and you are afraid that you might hit or shake your baby, put the baby in his or her crib and call your doctor or a self-help group (*see* USEFUL ADDRESSES, p.311).

Help with caring for your baby
Ask a neighbor or friend to look after your baby for a while if you have problems coping with his or her crying.

SEE YOUR BABY'S DOCTOR WITHIN 24 HOURS

POSSIBLE CAUSE Gastroesophageal reflux, in which the stomach contents leak back into the esophagus, may be the cause.

ACTION Your baby's doctor will examine your baby to exclude other causes. You may be advised to put your baby to sleep on his or her side with the head higher than the feet. If your baby is old enough, spending more time sitting in a baby chair may help. If your baby is bottle-fed, try thickening his or her feedings with rice cereal. The doctor may also suggest a drug that increases the muscular activity of the esophagus. Most babies grow out of this condition by age 1.

Continued from previous page

Is your baby under 4 months old? — **NO** / **YES**

Does your baby seem content for most of the day but cry a great deal during the late afternoon and evening? — **NO** / **YES**

POSSIBLE CAUSE Colic is the term often used to describe this common type of crying. It usually starts when a baby is about 2 weeks old and ceases by the age of 4 months. The precise cause of colic is not known.

ACTION There is no effective cure for colic. However, some self-help measures may give you and your baby temporary relief (*see* DEALING WITH COLIC, opposite). The main priority for parents is to find a way of coping with a constantly crying baby (*see* COPING WITH CRYING, opposite).

Does your baby usually stop crying when picked up and given your full attention? — **NO** / **YES**

POSSIBLE CAUSE The need for attention and physical comfort is a common cause of crying. Some babies are quite happy when left alone in their crib or playpen, but others need the constant reassurance of their parents' presence.

ACTION Cuddle your baby as much as he or she seems to want. At this age, there is no danger of "spoiling," and your baby will be happier as a result of an increased feeling of security. To enable you to get on with your everyday chores, you can try putting a young baby in a carrying sling while you go about the house. An older baby may be content if placed in a bouncing cradle or propped up on some cushions where he or she can see you. Once your baby seems content, you should avoid fussing over him or her.

Could your baby be teething? — **NO** / **YES**

POSSIBLE CAUSE AND ACTION Teething can cause babies some discomfort. A hard, cooled object to chew on, such as a teething ring cooled in the refrigerator, may help. You can also give the recommended dose of *analgesics* to relieve the discomfort (*see* TEETHING, p.115).

Has your baby been immunized recently? — **NO** / **YES**

POSSIBLE CAUSE Some babies may feel uncomfortable or have a mild fever in the week after a routine immunization (p.37).

ACTION Take your baby's temperature (p.54). If he or she has a fever, follow the advice for dealing with fever after immunization (p.55). If your baby does not have a fever and his or her crying is still worrying you, consult your baby's doctor.

POSSIBLE CAUSE Even young babies can be upset by increased tension in the home, particularly if the mother is affected.

ACTION Your baby will need more attention and reassurance than usual but should settle down within a week or so. Try to keep your baby's routine as stable as possible, even if other aspects of life are changing. If you think that your baby's crying could be a reaction to your own tension, try to find ways of reducing any strain you are under. Your baby's doctor may be able to suggest ways of helping.

Has there been recent major domestic stress? — **NO** / **YES**

SELF-HELP Dealing with gas

All babies swallow air when feeding. This air may then get trapped in the intestine, causing discomfort. Gas may be worse if your baby cries just before a feeding or feeds greedily. Here are some tips that may prevent gas from occurring or may help release the gas:

- If your baby is bottle-fed, make sure that the hole in the nipple is the right size.
- Support your baby in a semi-upright position when feeding so that swallowed air rises to the top of the stomach.
- Burp your baby at intervals during each feeding. Hold your baby upright against your shoulder or on your lap. Gently rub or pat his or her back to encourage gas to come up.

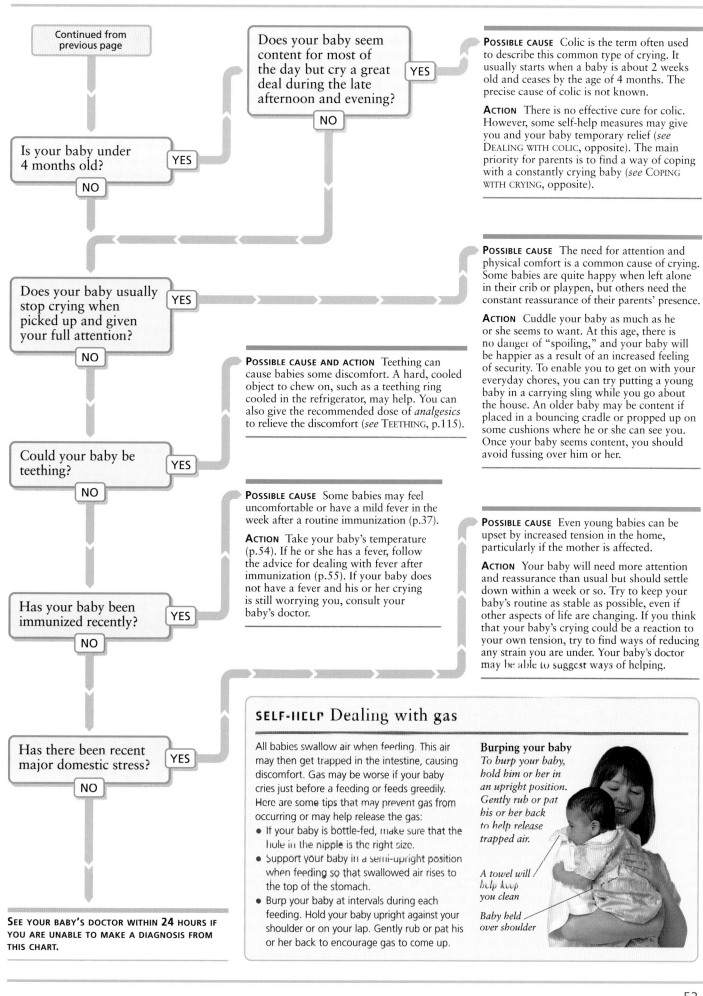

Burping your baby
To burp your baby, hold him or her in an upright position. Gently rub or pat his or her back to help release trapped air.

A towel will help keep you clean

Baby held over shoulder

SEE YOUR BABY'S DOCTOR WITHIN 24 HOURS IF YOU ARE UNABLE TO MAKE A DIAGNOSIS FROM THIS CHART.

③ Fever in babies

For children over 1, see chart 14, FEVER IN CHILDREN (p.76). A fever is an abnormally high body temperature of 100.4°F (38°C) or above. A baby that has a fever will have a hot forehead and is likely to seem unhappy and fretful. If you think your baby may be unwell, take his or her temperature (*see* TAKING YOUR BABY'S TEMPERATURE, below). Some babies are at risk for a seizure when they develop a high fever (*see* FEBRILE CONVULSIONS IN BABIES AND CHILDREN, opposite). If your baby has a fever, take steps to reduce it (*see* BRINGING DOWN A FEVER, p.77), and consult this chart.

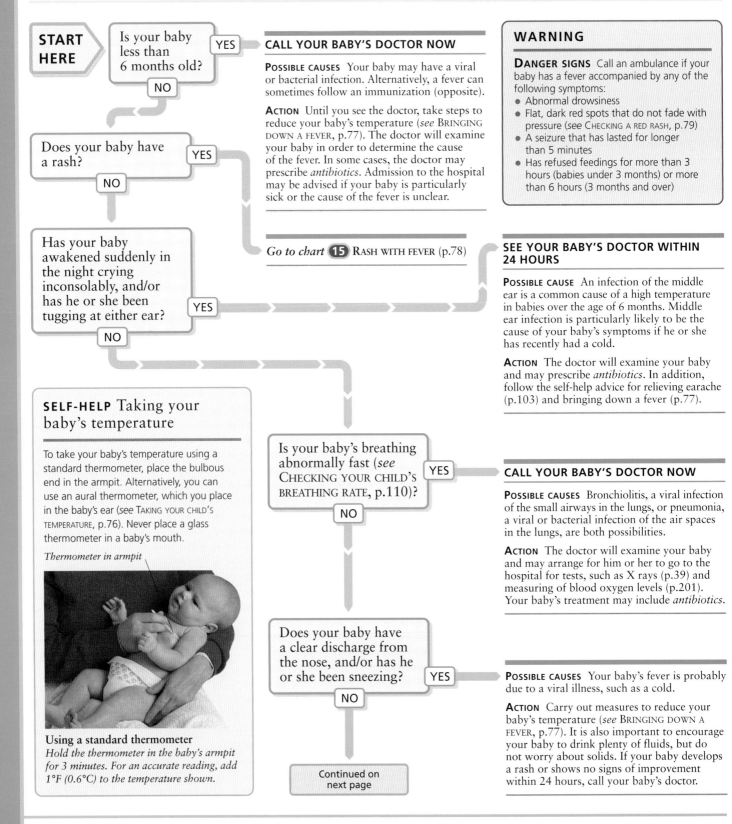

START HERE ▶ **Is your baby less than 6 months old?** — **YES**

NO

Does your baby have a rash? — **YES**

NO

Has your baby awakened suddenly in the night crying inconsolably, and/or has he or she been tugging at either ear? — **YES**

NO

CALL YOUR BABY'S DOCTOR NOW

POSSIBLE CAUSES Your baby may have a viral or bacterial infection. Alternatively, a fever can sometimes follow an immunization (opposite).

ACTION Until you see the doctor, take steps to reduce your baby's temperature (*see* BRINGING DOWN A FEVER, p.77). The doctor will examine your baby in order to determine the cause of the fever. In some cases, the doctor may prescribe *antibiotics*. Admission to the hospital may be advised if your baby is particularly sick or the cause of the fever is unclear.

Go to chart **⑮** RASH WITH FEVER (p.78)

WARNING

DANGER SIGNS Call an ambulance if your baby has a fever accompanied by any of the following symptoms:
- Abnormal drowsiness
- Flat, dark red spots that do not fade with pressure (*see* CHECKING A RED RASH, p.79)
- A seizure that has lasted for longer than 5 minutes
- Has refused feedings for more than 3 hours (babies under 3 months) or more than 6 hours (3 months and over)

SEE YOUR BABY'S DOCTOR WITHIN 24 HOURS

POSSIBLE CAUSE An infection of the middle ear is a common cause of a high temperature in babies over the age of 6 months. Middle ear infection is particularly likely to be the cause of your baby's symptoms if he or she has recently had a cold.

ACTION The doctor will examine your baby and may prescribe *antibiotics*. In addition, follow the self-help advice for relieving earache (p.103) and bringing down a fever (p.77).

SELF-HELP Taking your baby's temperature

To take your baby's temperature using a standard thermometer, place the bulbous end in the armpit. Alternatively, you can use an aural thermometer, which you place in the baby's ear (*see* TAKING YOUR CHILD'S TEMPERATURE, p.76). Never place a glass thermometer in a baby's mouth.

Thermometer in armpit

Is your baby's breathing abnormally fast (*see* CHECKING YOUR CHILD'S BREATHING RATE, p.110)? — **YES**

NO

CALL YOUR BABY'S DOCTOR NOW

POSSIBLE CAUSES Bronchiolitis, a viral infection of the small airways in the lungs, or pneumonia, a viral or bacterial infection of the air spaces in the lungs, are both possibilities.

ACTION The doctor will examine your baby and may arrange for him or her to go to the hospital for tests, such as X rays (p.39) and measuring of blood oxygen levels (p.201). Your baby's treatment may include *antibiotics*.

Does your baby have a clear discharge from the nose, and/or has he or she been sneezing? — **YES**

NO

POSSIBLE CAUSES Your baby's fever is probably due to a viral illness, such as a cold.

ACTION Carry out measures to reduce your baby's temperature (*see* BRINGING DOWN A FEVER, p.77). It is also important to encourage your baby to drink plenty of fluids, but do not worry about solids. If your baby develops a rash or shows no signs of improvement within 24 hours, call your baby's doctor.

Using a standard thermometer
Hold the thermometer in the baby's armpit for 3 minutes. For an accurate reading, add 1°F (0.6°C) to the temperature shown.

Continued on next page

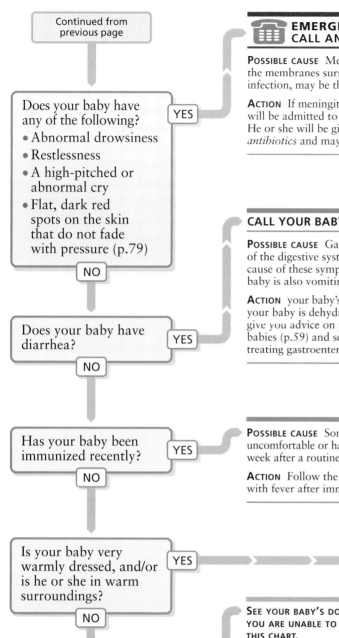

Continued from previous page

Does your baby have any of the following?
• Abnormal drowsiness
• Restlessness
• A high-pitched or abnormal cry
• Flat, dark red spots on the skin that do not fade with pressure (p.79)

YES → **EMERGENCY! CALL AN AMBULANCE**

POSSIBLE CAUSE Meningitis, inflammation of the membranes surrounding the brain due to infection, may be the cause of these symptoms.

ACTION If meningitis is suspected, your baby will be admitted to the hospital immediately. He or she will be given urgent treatment with *antibiotics* and may need intensive care.

NO

Does your baby have diarrhea?

YES → **CALL YOUR BABY'S DOCTOR NOW**

POSSIBLE CAUSE Gastroenteritis, an infection of the digestive system, is the most likely cause of these symptoms, especially if your baby is also vomiting.

ACTION your baby's doctor will check whether your baby is dehydrated. He or she may also give you advice on preventing dehydration in babies (p.59) and self-help measures for treating gastroenteritis in babies (p.57).

NO

Has your baby been immunized recently?

YES → **POSSIBLE CAUSE** Some babies may feel uncomfortable or have a mild fever in the week after a routine immunization (p.37).

ACTION Follow the advice for dealing with fever after immunization (right).

NO

Is your baby very warmly dressed, and/or is he or she in warm surroundings?

YES → **POSSIBLE CAUSE** Overheating, caused by too much clothing or by being in excessively warm surroundings, can result in a fever.

ACTION A baby does not need to wear much more clothing than an adult would in similar conditions and will be comfortable in a room temperature of 60–68°F (15–20°C). A baby's crib should never be placed next to a radiator. Remove any excess clothing and move your baby to a slightly cooler (although not cold) place. If your baby's temperature is not down to normal within an hour, follow the advice for reducing a fever (p.77) and call your baby's doctor.

NO

SEE YOUR BABY'S DOCTOR WITHIN 24 HOURS IF YOU ARE UNABLE TO MAKE A DIAGNOSIS FROM THIS CHART.

Fever after immunizations

Some babies and young children develop a mild fever after an immunization. Routine immunizations (p.37) are usually given at the ages of 2, 3, 4, and 12–15 months. If your child develops a fever after an immunization, you should follow the self-help advice for reducing his or her fever (see BRINGING DOWN A FEVER, p.77). Call your baby's doctor immediately if your child's temperature rises above 102°F (39°C) or if he or she has other symptoms, such as an unusual or high-pitched cry. You should also call the doctor if self-help measures are not successful in reducing your child's temperature.

If your child has been sick after having an immunization, mention it to the doctor before the next immunization is due. He or she can advise you on how to deal with any symptoms that may develop.

If your child has a fever at the time of a scheduled immunization, it should be postponed until he or she is better.

Febrile convulsions in babies and children

A febrile convulsion is a type of seizure that affects some children aged 6 months to 5 years. It is triggered by an abrupt rise in body temperature, often at the onset of a feverish illness. During a convulsion, the child may:
• Lose consciousness
• Shake or jerk violently
• Stop breathing temporarily or breathe shallowly, which may result in a bluish tinge to the skin
• Urinate and/or pass feces
• Roll back his or her eyes
Febrile convulsions usually last for less than 5 minutes and, although frightening, are not often serious. About one-third of the children who have had a febrile convulsion have

another one within 6 months. Most affected children stop having convulsions at about 5 years of age. Febrile convulsions are rarely an indication of epilepsy in later life.

Convulsions may be avoided by keeping your child's temperature down (see BRINGING DOWN A FEVER, p.77). If he or she does have a febrile convulsion, remove excess clothes, try to reduce his or her temperature by sponging with tepid water, and surround him or her with soft objects, such as pillows, to prevent injury.

After the seizure has ended, place your child in the recovery position (p.292). He or she may fall asleep shortly afterward. Call your baby's doctor if your child has a convulsion. If it lasts more than 5 minutes, call an ambulance.

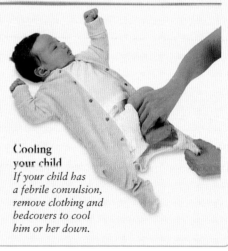

Cooling your child
If your child has a febrile convulsion, remove clothing and bedcovers to cool him or her down.

4 Vomiting in babies

For children over 1 year, see chart 38, VOMITING IN CHILDREN (**p.118**).
In young babies, it is easy for parents to confuse vomiting, which may indicate an illness, with regurgitation (spitting up), the effortless bringing up of small amounts of milk. Almost any minor upset can cause a baby to vomit once, and this is unlikely to be cause for concern. However, persistent vomiting in babies can be a sign of an underlying problem.

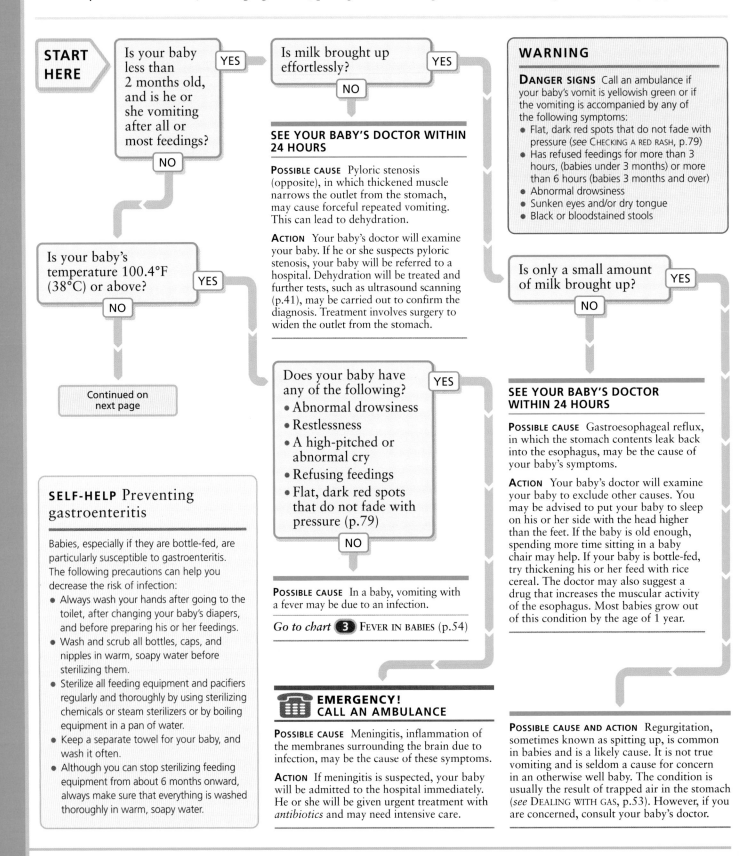

START HERE

Is your baby less than 2 months old, and is he or she vomiting after all or most feedings?
YES / NO

Is your baby's temperature 100.4°F (38°C) or above?
YES / NO

Continued on next page

Is milk brought up effortlessly?
YES / NO

SEE YOUR BABY'S DOCTOR WITHIN 24 HOURS

POSSIBLE CAUSE Pyloric stenosis (opposite), in which thickened muscle narrows the outlet from the stomach, may cause forceful repeated vomiting. This can lead to dehydration.

ACTION Your baby's doctor will examine your baby. If he or she suspects pyloric stenosis, your baby will be referred to a hospital. Dehydration will be treated and further tests, such as ultrasound scanning (p.41), may be carried out to confirm the diagnosis. Treatment involves surgery to widen the outlet from the stomach.

Does your baby have any of the following?
- **Abnormal drowsiness**
- **Restlessness**
- **A high-pitched or abnormal cry**
- **Refusing feedings**
- **Flat, dark red spots that do not fade with pressure (p.79)**
YES / NO

POSSIBLE CAUSE In a baby, vomiting with a fever may be due to an infection.

Go to chart **3** FEVER IN BABIES (p.54)

WARNING

DANGER SIGNS Call an ambulance if your baby's vomit is yellowish green or if the vomiting is accompanied by any of the following symptoms:
- Flat, dark red spots that do not fade with pressure (*see* CHECKING A RED RASH, p.79)
- Has refused feedings for more than 3 hours, (babies under 3 months) or more than 6 hours (babies 3 months and over)
- Abnormal drowsiness
- Sunken eyes and/or dry tongue
- Black or bloodstained stools

Is only a small amount of milk brought up?
YES / NO

SEE YOUR BABY'S DOCTOR WITHIN 24 HOURS

POSSIBLE CAUSE Gastroesophageal reflux, in which the stomach contents leak back into the esophagus, may be the cause of your baby's symptoms.

ACTION Your baby's doctor will examine your baby to exclude other causes. You may be advised to put your baby to sleep on his or her side with the head higher than the feet. If the baby is old enough, spending more time sitting in a baby chair may help. If your baby is bottle-fed, try thickening his or her feed with rice cereal. The doctor may also suggest a drug that increases the muscular activity of the esophagus. Most babies grow out of this condition by the age of 1 year.

SELF-HELP Preventing gastroenteritis

Babies, especially if they are bottle-fed, are particularly susceptible to gastroenteritis. The following precautions can help you decrease the risk of infection:
- Always wash your hands after going to the toilet, after changing your baby's diapers, and before preparing his or her feedings.
- Wash and scrub all bottles, caps, and nipples in warm, soapy water before sterilizing them.
- Sterilize all feeding equipment and pacifiers regularly and thoroughly by using sterilizing chemicals or steam sterilizers or by boiling equipment in a pan of water.
- Keep a separate towel for your baby, and wash it often.
- Although you can stop sterilizing feeding equipment from about 6 months onward, always make sure that everything is washed thoroughly in warm, soapy water.

EMERGENCY! CALL AN AMBULANCE

POSSIBLE CAUSE Meningitis, inflammation of the membranes surrounding the brain due to infection, may be the cause of these symptoms.

ACTION If meningitis is suspected, your baby will be admitted to the hospital immediately. He or she will be given urgent treatment with *antibiotics* and may need intensive care.

POSSIBLE CAUSE AND ACTION Regurgitation, sometimes known as spitting up, is common in babies and is a likely cause. It is not true vomiting and is seldom a cause for concern in an otherwise well baby. The condition is usually the result of trapped air in the stomach (*see* DEALING WITH GAS, p.53). However, if you are concerned, consult your baby's doctor.

Continued from
previous page

**Does your baby
have a cough?** YES

NO

**Does your baby
have diarrhea?** YES

NO

**Is your baby's
vomit yellow
green?** YES

NO

SELF-HELP Treating gastroenteritis in babies

Gastroenteritis does not require treatment with
drugs such as *antibiotics*; giving rehydrating
solutions will prevent dehydration (p.59) and
aid recovery. If your baby is breast-fed, you
should gradually reduce the amount of
rehydrating solution as he or she gets better. If
your baby is bottle-fed, give only rehydrating
solutions at first; on the second day give
feedings that are half rehydrating solution and
half milk. Gradually return to normal feeding
over the next 24 hours. If diarrhea recurs at any
stage, temporary lactose intolerance (p.122)
may be the cause. Go back to rehydrating
solutions and call your baby's doctor.

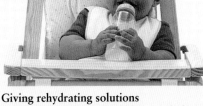

Giving rehydrating solutions
*Rehydrating solution should be given before
or with a breast- or bottle-feeding to ensure
that your baby receives the necessary amount.*

CALL YOUR BABY'S DOCTOR NOW

POSSIBLE CAUSE Gastroenteritis, an infection
of the digestive system, is the most likely
cause of these symptoms. In some cases, a
baby may also develop a fever.

ACTION Your baby's doctor will check
whether your baby is dehydrated and will
give you advice on preventing dehydration in
babies (p.59) and treating gastroenteritis in
babies (above). To prevent future attacks,
follow the advice for preventing gastroenteritis
(opposite).

CALL YOUR BABY'S DOCTOR NOW

POSSIBLE CAUSES Bronchiolitis, a viral infection
affecting the small airways in the lungs, or
pertussis (whooping cough), an infectious
disease that causes bouts of severe coughing,
may be the cause.

ACTION Your baby may be admitted to the
hospital, where his or her blood oxygen
levels can be measured (p.201). If bronchiolitis
is diagnosed, treatment may include
bronchodilator drugs and oxygen. If pertussis
is diagnosed, he or she may need *antibiotics*
to prevent the spread of the infection,
although these do not always affect the
severity of the symptoms.

CALL YOUR BABY'S DOCTOR NOW

POSSIBLE CAUSE Intussusception, in which the
intestine telescopes in on itself, causing an
obstruction, is a possibility.

ACTION Your baby may be admitted to the
hospital, where he or she can be fully
examined and an exact diagnosis made.
Treatment for intussusception usually involves
an enema to force the displaced intestinal
tissue back into the right position. If the enema
is not successful, surgery will be necessary.

**Does the vomiting only
occur during or after
travel in a vehicle?** YES

NO

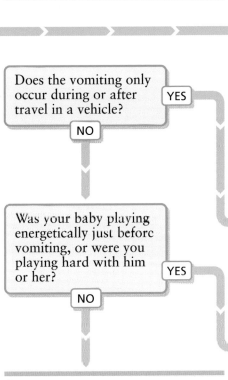

**Was your baby playing
energetically just before
vomiting, or were you
playing hard with him
or her?** YES

NO

Pyloric stenosis

Pyloric stenosis is a disorder that occurs in
babies under 2 months and is more common
in boys. In this condition, the ring of muscle
forming the outlet from the stomach into
the small intestine becomes narrowed and
thickened due to overgrowth of the muscle
tissue. The cause is unknown. Because the
stomach cannot empty into the intestine, the
stomach contents build up until repeated,
forceful vomiting occurs. Without treatment,
the baby will lose weight and develop
potentially life-threatening dehydration.
Treatment involves surgery, in which the
thickened muscle is cut to widen the
stomach outlet. The baby should be able to
resume normal feeding within 2–3 days and
have no permanent ill effects.

POSSIBLE CAUSE AND ACTION Motion sickness
is probably the cause. Although uncommon
in children under the age of 1 year, some
babies are particularly susceptible. The
condition may run in families. For self-help
measures, follow the advice on coping with
motion sickness (p.119).

POSSIBLE CAUSE AND ACTION In babies, the
muscles around the top of the stomach are
relatively lax compared with those of older
children, and enthusiastic playing may cause
vomiting. This is no cause for concern and
will be less of a problem as your baby grows
older. In the meantime, try to avoid rough
games, particularly after feedings.

**AN ISOLATED ATTACK OF VOMITING IS UNLIKELY
TO BE A SIGN OF A SERIOUS PROBLEM IN AN
OTHERWISE WELL BABY. HOWEVER, IF YOUR BABY
VOMITS MORE THAN ONCE IN A DAY OR SEEMS
OTHERWISE SICK, CALL YOUR BABY'S DOCTOR.**

5 Diarrhea in babies

For children over 1 year, see chart 40, DIARRHEA IN
CHILDREN **(p.122).**
Diarrhea is the frequent passing of abnormally loose or
watery stools. It is normal for a breast-fed baby to pass soft

stools up to 6 times a day, and this situation should not be
mistaken for diarrhea. If your baby does have diarrhea,
give him or her plenty of fluids to prevent dehydration (*see*
PREVENTING DEHYDRATION IN BABIES, opposite).

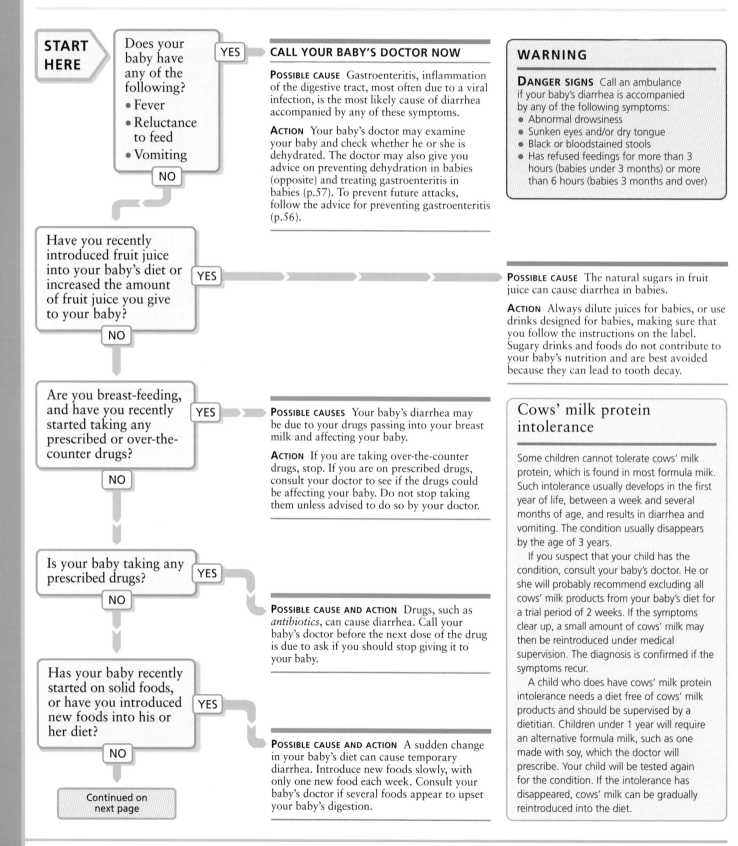

START HERE

Does your baby have any of the following?
- Fever
- Reluctance to feed
- Vomiting

YES →

NO

CALL YOUR BABY'S DOCTOR NOW

POSSIBLE CAUSE Gastroenteritis, inflammation
of the digestive tract, most often due to a viral
infection, is the most likely cause of diarrhea
accompanied by any of these symptoms.

ACTION Your baby's doctor may examine
your baby and check whether he or she is
dehydrated. The doctor may also give you
advice on preventing dehydration in babies
(opposite) and treating gastroenteritis in
babies (p.57). To prevent future attacks,
follow the advice for preventing gastroenteritis
(p.56).

WARNING

DANGER SIGNS Call an ambulance
if your baby's diarrhea is accompanied
by any of the following symptoms:
- Abnormal drowsiness
- Sunken eyes and/or dry tongue
- Black or bloodstained stools
- Has refused feedings for more than 3
  hours (babies under 3 months) or more
  than 6 hours (babies 3 months and over)

Have you recently introduced fruit juice into your baby's diet or increased the amount of fruit juice you give to your baby?

YES →

NO

POSSIBLE CAUSE The natural sugars in fruit
juice can cause diarrhea in babies.

ACTION Always dilute juices for babies, or use
drinks designed for babies, making sure that
you follow the instructions on the label.
Sugary drinks and foods do not contribute to
your baby's nutrition and are best avoided
because they can lead to tooth decay.

Are you breast-feeding, and have you recently started taking any prescribed or over-the-counter drugs?

YES →

NO

POSSIBLE CAUSES Your baby's diarrhea may
be due to your drugs passing into your breast
milk and affecting your baby.

ACTION If you are taking over-the-counter
drugs, stop. If you are on prescribed drugs,
consult your doctor to see if the drugs could
be affecting your baby. Do not stop taking
them unless advised to do so by your doctor.

Cows' milk protein intolerance

Some children cannot tolerate cows' milk
protein, which is found in most formula milk.
Such intolerance usually develops in the first
year of life, between a week and several
months of age, and results in diarrhea and
vomiting. The condition usually disappears
by the age of 3 years.

If you suspect that your child has the
condition, consult your baby's doctor. He or
she will probably recommend excluding all
cows' milk products from your baby's diet for
a trial period of 2 weeks. If the symptoms
clear up, a small amount of cows' milk may
then be reintroduced under medical
supervision. The diagnosis is confirmed if the
symptoms recur.

A child who does have cows' milk protein
intolerance needs a diet free of cows' milk
products and should be supervised by a
dietitian. Children under 1 year will require
an alternative formula milk, such as one
made with soy, which the doctor will
prescribe. Your child will be tested again
for the condition. If the intolerance has
disappeared, cows' milk can be gradually
reintroduced into the diet.

Is your baby taking any prescribed drugs?

YES →

NO

POSSIBLE CAUSE AND ACTION Drugs, such as
antibiotics, can cause diarrhea. Call your
baby's doctor before the next dose of the drug
is due to ask if you should stop giving it to
your baby.

Has your baby recently started on solid foods, or have you introduced new foods into his or her diet?

YES →

NO

POSSIBLE CAUSE AND ACTION A sudden change
in your baby's diet can cause temporary
diarrhea. Introduce new foods slowly, with
only one new food each week. Consult your
baby's doctor if several foods appear to upset
your baby's digestion.

Continued on next page

Continued from previous page

Did the diarrhea begin abroad, and has it persisted since returning home?

NO

YES

Have you just started to reintroduce milk into your baby's diet after a bout of gastroenteritis?

NO

YES

Has your baby's diarrhea lasted for more than 2 weeks?

NO

YES

Are your baby's height and weight within the normal range for his or her age (*see* GROWTH CHARTS, p.26)?

YES

NO

GIVE YOUR BABY PLENTY OF FLUIDS, AND SEE YOUR BABY'S DOCTOR WITHIN 24 HOURS.

Babies' stools

The first stools that a baby passes after birth are known as meconium, which is a sticky greenish black substance consisting mainly of mucus and bile. Within a day or two, the stools change to a brown color, then settle to a regular color. Most babies pass stools several times a day, although some can go for a few days without passing any. As long as your baby does not seem sick, there is probably nothing wrong.

Breast-fed babies can pass stools frequently. The stools are very soft and usually orange-yellow, like mustard, and there may be visible mucus. They may smell of sour milk.

Bottle-fed babies pass bulkier and more substantial stools than breast-fed babies. The stools are usually light brown and smell strongly, more like the stools of an adult.

Green stools are a sign that food has passed through the intestines very rapidly.

POSSIBLE CAUSE AND ACTION Your baby may have acquired an infection abroad. Consult your baby's doctor, and make sure that you mention any foreign travel.

POSSIBLE CAUSE Temporary intolerance to lactose (p.122), which is a natural sugar found in milk, is a possible cause of recurrent or persistent diarrhea. If milk is reintroduced into your baby's diet too soon after an episode of gastroenteritis, the diarrhea can recur.

ACTION Go back to giving your baby rehydrating solutions while he or she has diarrhea. Then gradually reintroduce milk (*see* TREATING GASTROENTERITIS IN BABIES, p.57). If diarrhea recurs, see your baby's doctor within 24 hours. The doctor will advise a lactose-free diet until your baby recovers.

POSSIBLE CAUSES Your baby may not be absorbing food normally. The cause may be a food intolerance, such as cows' milk protein intolerance (opposite), or a disorder such as cystic fibrosis or celiac disease. Consult your baby's doctor.

ACTION The doctor will examine your baby and may arrange for his or her stools to be tested for evidence of an infection. Your baby may be referred to a specialist to establish the underlying cause.

POSSIBLE CAUSE AND ACTION Some babies normally produce very soft stools but do not have diarrhea (*see* BABIES' STOOLS, above). If you are not sure whether or not your baby's stools are normal, you should consult your baby's doctor for advice.

SELF-HELP Preventing dehydration in babies

Diarrhea, vomiting, or fever can cause dehydration, a potentially life-threatening condition in babies. It is therefore important to give your baby extra fluids before breast-feeding or instead of bottle-feeding if he or she has any of these conditions. Rehydrating solutions can be bought over the counter as premixed liquid preparations that contain sodium, potassium, and glucose. While your baby still has symptoms, give him or her frequent feedings of rehydrating solution; see the table below for the total amount to give per day. If your baby is vomiting, give small sips of fluid every few minutes with a spoon or small cup.

Baby's weight		Daily intake of rehydrating solution	
lb	kg	fl.oz	ml
Under 9	Under 4	17	500
9	4	20	600
11	5	25	750
13	6	30	900
15	7	36	1050
18	8	41	1200
20	9	46	1350
Over 22	Over 10	51	1500

Daily intake of rehydrating solution
Use this table to determine the appropriate total daily intake of rehydrating solution for your baby's weight.

6 Feeding problems

For children over 1, see chart 37, EATING PROBLEMS (p.116). Feeding problems are a common source of irritability and crying in young babies as well as concern in their parents. Such problems may include a reluctance to feed, constant hungry crying, and swallowing too much air, leading to regurgitation. There may also be special problems for mothers who are breast-feeding. This chart deals with most of the common problems that may arise.

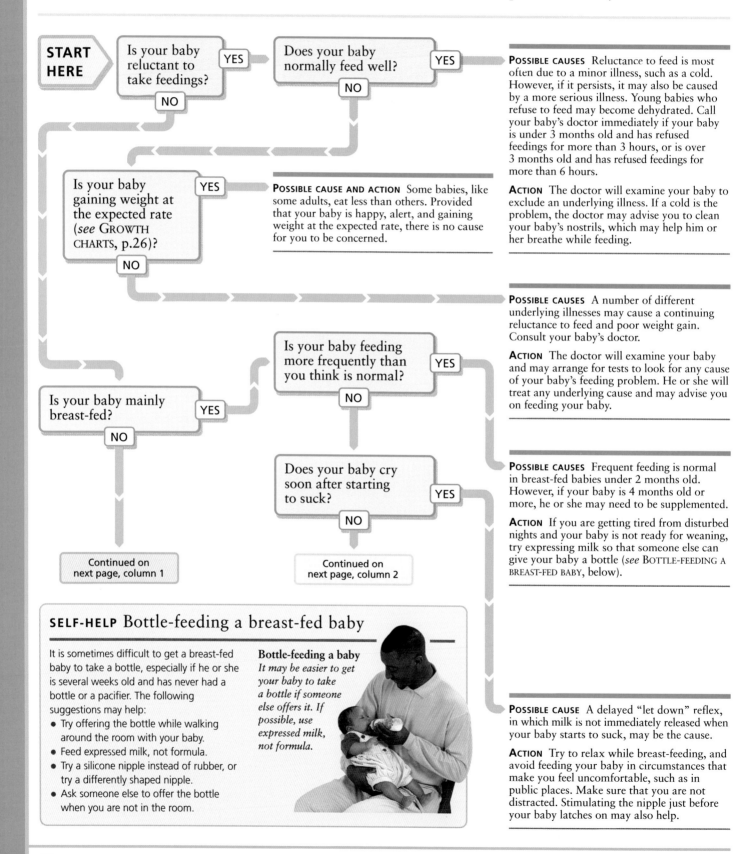

START HERE → Is your baby reluctant to take feedings? → **YES** → Does your baby normally feed well? → **YES**

POSSIBLE CAUSES Reluctance to feed is most often due to a minor illness, such as a cold. However, if it persists, it may also be caused by a more serious illness. Young babies who refuse to feed may become dehydrated. Call your baby's doctor immediately if your baby is under 3 months old and has refused feedings for more than 3 hours, or is over 3 months old and has refused feedings for more than 6 hours.

ACTION The doctor will examine your baby to exclude an underlying illness. If a cold is the problem, the doctor may advise you to clean your baby's nostrils, which may help him or her breathe while feeding.

Is your baby reluctant to take feedings? → **NO**

Does your baby normally feed well? → **NO**

Is your baby gaining weight at the expected rate (*see* GROWTH CHARTS, p.26)? → **YES**

POSSIBLE CAUSE AND ACTION Some babies, like some adults, eat less than others. Provided that your baby is happy, alert, and gaining weight at the expected rate, there is no cause for you to be concerned.

Is your baby gaining weight at the expected rate? → **NO**

POSSIBLE CAUSES A number of different underlying illnesses may cause a continuing reluctance to feed and poor weight gain. Consult your baby's doctor.

ACTION The doctor will examine your baby and may arrange for tests to look for any cause of your baby's feeding problem. He or she will treat any underlying cause and may advise you on feeding your baby.

Is your baby feeding more frequently than you think is normal? → **YES**

Is your baby mainly breast-fed? → **YES**

Is your baby feeding more frequently than you think is normal? → **NO**

Is your baby mainly breast-fed? → **NO**

POSSIBLE CAUSES Frequent feeding is normal in breast-fed babies under 2 months old. However, if your baby is 4 months old or more, he or she may need to be supplemented.

ACTION If you are getting tired from disturbed nights and your baby is not ready for weaning, try expressing milk so that someone else can give your baby a bottle (*see* BOTTLE-FEEDING A BREAST-FED BABY, below).

Does your baby cry soon after starting to suck? → **YES**

Does your baby cry soon after starting to suck? → **NO**

Continued on next page, column 1

Continued on next page, column 2

SELF-HELP Bottle-feeding a breast-fed baby

It is sometimes difficult to get a breast-fed baby to take a bottle, especially if he or she is several weeks old and has never had a bottle or a pacifier. The following suggestions may help:
- Try offering the bottle while walking around the room with your baby.
- Feed expressed milk, not formula.
- Try a silicone nipple instead of rubber, or try a differently shaped nipple.
- Ask someone else to offer the bottle when you are not in the room.

Bottle-feeding a baby
It may be easier to get your baby to take a bottle if someone else offers it. If possible, use expressed milk, not formula.

POSSIBLE CAUSE A delayed "let down" reflex, in which milk is not immediately released when your baby starts to suck, may be the cause.

ACTION Try to relax while breast-feeding, and avoid feeding your baby in circumstances that make you feel uncomfortable, such as in public places. Make sure that you are not distracted. Stimulating the nipple just before your baby latches on may also help.

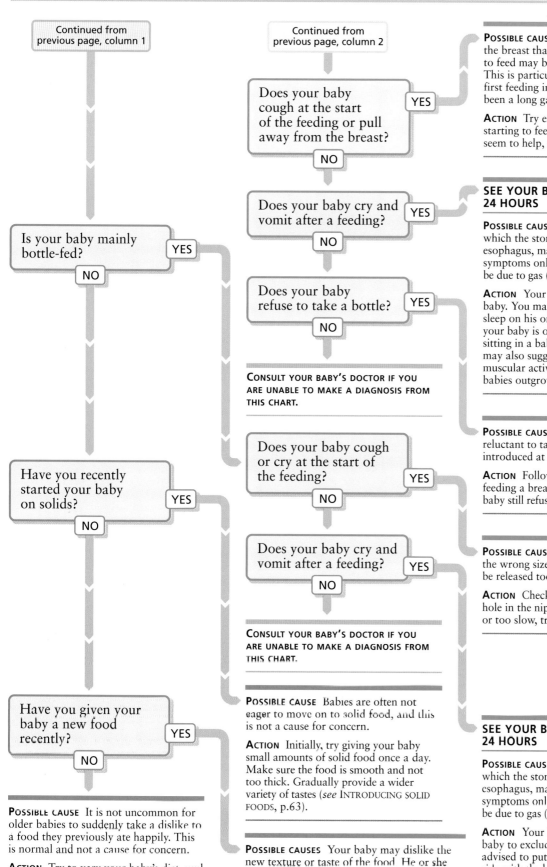

Continued from previous page, column 1

Continued from previous page, column 2

Does your baby cough at the start of the feeding or pull away from the breast? **YES**

NO

POSSIBLE CAUSE The initial rush of milk from the breast that occurs when your baby starts to feed may be causing him or her to choke. This is particularly likely to occur during the first feeding in the morning after there has been a long gap between feedings.

ACTION Try expressing a little milk before starting to feed your baby. If this does not seem to help, consult your baby's doctor.

Does your baby cry and vomit after a feeding? **YES**

NO

SEE YOUR BABY'S DOCTOR WITHIN 24 HOURS

POSSIBLE CAUSE Gastroesophageal reflux, in which the stomach contents leak back into the esophagus, may be the cause. However, if the symptoms only occur occasionally, they may be due to gas (*see* DEALING WITH GAS, p.53).

ACTION Your baby's doctor will examine your baby. You may be advised to put your baby to sleep on his or her side with the head raised. If your baby is old enough, spending more time sitting in a baby chair may help. Your doctor may also suggest a drug that increases the muscular activity of the esophagus. Most babies outgrow this condition by the age of 1.

Is your baby mainly bottle-fed? **YES**

NO

Does your baby refuse to take a bottle? **YES**

NO

CONSULT YOUR BABY'S DOCTOR IF YOU ARE UNABLE TO MAKE A DIAGNOSIS FROM THIS CHART.

POSSIBLE CAUSE Breast-fed babies may be reluctant to take a bottle unless it is introduced at an early stage.

ACTION Follow the self-help advice for bottle-feeding a breast-fed baby (opposite). If your baby still refuses a bottle, try using a feeder cup.

Have you recently started your baby on solids? **YES**

NO

Does your baby cough or cry at the start of the feeding? **YES**

NO

POSSIBLE CAUSE The hole in the nipple may be the wrong size for your baby, causing milk to be released too quickly or too slowly.

ACTION Check the flow of milk through the hole in the nipple. If the flows seems too quick or too slow, try using a different nipple.

Does your baby cry and vomit after a feeding? **YES**

NO

CONSULT YOUR BABY'S DOCTOR IF YOU ARE UNABLE TO MAKE A DIAGNOSIS FROM THIS CHART.

POSSIBLE CAUSE Babies are often not eager to move on to solid food, and this is not a cause for concern.

ACTION Initially, try giving your baby small amounts of solid food once a day. Make sure the food is smooth and not too thick. Gradually provide a wider variety of tastes (*see* INTRODUCING SOLID FOODS, p.63).

SEE YOUR BABY'S DOCTOR WITHIN 24 HOURS

POSSIBLE CAUSE Gastroesophageal reflux, in which the stomach contents leak back into the esophagus, may be the cause. However, if the symptoms only occur occasionally, they may be due to gas (*see* DEALING WITH GAS, p.53).

ACTION Your baby's doctor will examine your baby to exclude other causes. You may be advised to put your baby to sleep on his or her side with the head higher than the feet. If your baby is old enough, spending more time sitting in a baby chair may help, as will thickening his or her feedings with rice cereal. The doctor may also suggest a drug that increases the muscular activity of the esophagus. Most babies outgrow this condition by the age of 1.

Have you given your baby a new food recently? **YES**

NO

POSSIBLE CAUSE It is not uncommon for older babies to suddenly take a dislike to a food they previously ate happily. This is normal and not a cause for concern.

ACTION Try to vary your baby's diet, and gradually introduce a wider variety of tastes and textures. If your baby refuses to eat one particular food, stop offering it to him or her and reintroduce it at a later date. However, if you are concerned, consult your baby's doctor.

POSSIBLE CAUSES Your baby may dislike the new texture or taste of the food. He or she may also be less willing to eat something new if he or she is tired.

ACTION Stop giving your baby the new food for a while. Try it again at a later date, preferably at breakfast time when your baby is less likely to be tired.

7 Slow weight gain

For children over 1, see chart 12, GROWTH PROBLEMS (p.72).
Consult this chart if you are worried that your baby is gaining
weight too slowly. Most babies lose some weight in their
first week of life (*see* WEIGHT LOSS IN THE NEWBORN,
opposite), and this is not usually a cause for concern. After
this, babies should put on weight at a steady rate. Your baby
will be weighed and measured regularly at the doctor's
office, and his or her growth will be plotted on growth
charts (*see* GROWTH CHARTS, p.26) so that any problems
can be detected early. In the first year of life, growth is
faster than at any other time, and key body systems such
as the nervous system are developing rapidly. For this
reason, nutrition is particularly important at this time (*see*
NUTRITIONAL REQUIREMENTS OF BABIES, below).

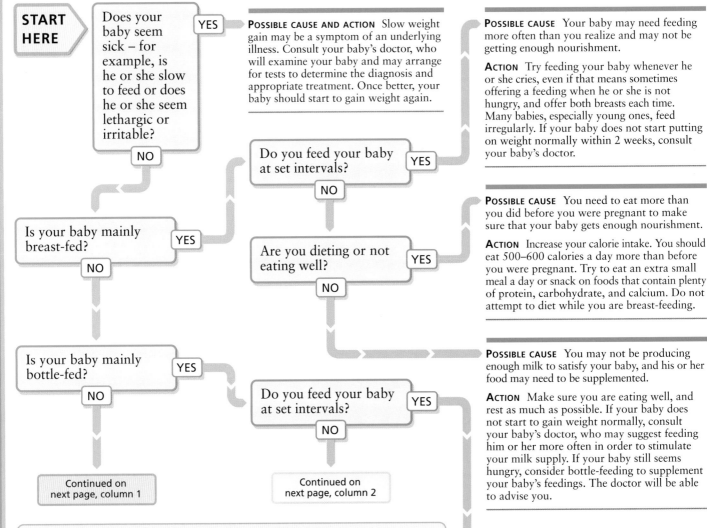

START HERE

Does your baby seem sick – for example, is he or she slow to feed or does he or she seem lethargic or irritable?

YES → **POSSIBLE CAUSE AND ACTION** Slow weight gain may be a symptom of an underlying illness. Consult your baby's doctor, who will examine your baby and may arrange for tests to determine the diagnosis and appropriate treatment. Once better, your baby should start to gain weight again.

NO

Is your baby mainly breast-fed?

YES

NO

Do you feed your baby at set intervals?

YES → **POSSIBLE CAUSE** Your baby may need feeding more often than you realize and may not be getting enough nourishment.

ACTION Try feeding your baby whenever he or she cries, even if that means sometimes offering a feeding when he or she is not hungry, and offer both breasts each time. Many babies, especially young ones, feed irregularly. If your baby does not start putting on weight normally within 2 weeks, consult your baby's doctor.

NO

Are you dieting or not eating well?

YES → **POSSIBLE CAUSE** You need to eat more than you did before you were pregnant to make sure that your baby gets enough nourishment.

ACTION Increase your calorie intake. You should eat 500–600 calories a day more than before you were pregnant. Try to eat an extra small meal a day or snack on foods that contain plenty of protein, carbohydrate, and calcium. Do not attempt to diet while you are breast-feeding.

NO

Is your baby mainly bottle-fed?

YES

NO

Do you feed your baby at set intervals?

YES → **POSSIBLE CAUSE** You may not be producing enough milk to satisfy your baby, and his or her food may need to be supplemented.

ACTION Make sure you are eating well, and rest as much as possible. If your baby does not start to gain weight normally, consult your baby's doctor, who may suggest feeding him or her more often in order to stimulate your milk supply. If your baby still seems hungry, consider bottle-feeding to supplement your baby's feedings. The doctor will be able to advise you.

NO

Continued on next page, column 1

Continued on next page, column 2

POSSIBLE CAUSE Your baby may need feeding more often than you realize and may not be getting enough nourishment.

ACTION Try feeding your baby whenever he or she cries, even if that means sometimes offering a feeding when he or she is not hungry. Many babies, especially young ones, feed irregularly. If your baby is not putting on weight normally within 2 weeks, consult your baby's doctor.

Nutritional requirements of babies

Babies need a diet relatively high in calories, high in fat, low in fiber, and low in salt. It should contain enough protein for growth and carbohydrate for energy. If you are vegetarian, you can bring your baby up on the same type of diet as yourself but need to be careful to include sufficient iron. A vegan diet without supplements is not nutritionally complete for a baby. From 4 weeks of age, babies benefit from supplements of vitamins A, C, and D. This is most conveniently achieved by using vitamin drops available from your baby's doctor.

Age in months	Approximate daily requirements			
	Calories	Protein	Fat	Iron
Up to 3	530 cal.	13 g	4 g	2 mg
3–6	700 cal.	13 g	4 g	4 mg
6–9	800 cal.	14 g	4 g	8 mg
9–12	1200 cal.	20 g	4 g	9 mg

SELF-HELP Introducing solid foods

By the time your baby is 4–6 months, he or she should be ready for solid foods in addition to breast milk or formula. Start by introducing your baby to puréed fruit or vegetables and baby rice. Try giving him or her a taste after a milk feeding. Gradually introduce other foods and textures. Your own food can be strained or puréed, but do not add salt or sugar when preparing it. Do not give eggs, wheat-based foods such as wheat cereals, citrus fruits, or fatty foods until your baby is at least 6 months old. Do not give cows' milk, honey, or foods with nuts until he or she is at least 12 months.

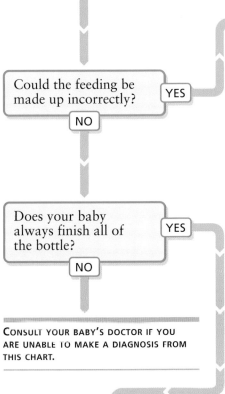

Eating from a spoon
As part of the process, introduce your baby to the idea of taking food from a spoon.

Age	Suggested feeding program
4–6 months	Offer your baby yogurt and puréed foods, including fruit, such as bananas, vegetables, legumes, and rice.
6–9 months	You can now give mashed or minced food, including eggs (as long as they are hard-boiled), fish, and chicken. You can also offer finger foods, such as toast, cubes of apple, or bits of hard cheese.
9–12 months	Introduce more variety into the diet, and provide food that contains small pieces, such as peas and chopped carrots.
Over 12 months	Your baby can now have the same diet as the rest of the family; but avoid salt and sugar, and give him or her whole, rather than low-fat, milk.

Continued from previous page, column 1

Continued from previous page, column 2

POSSIBLE CAUSE If there is too little powder or too much water in the feeding, your baby will not be receiving enough nourishment.

ACTION Always follow the manufacturer's instructions exactly when mixing feeds. Never add extra powder to your baby's feedings. If your baby does not start putting on weight normally within 2 weeks, consult your baby's doctor.

Have you continued bottle- or breast-feeding since introducing solid foods for your baby? YES / NO

Could the feeding be made up incorrectly? YES / NO

POSSIBLE CAUSE It is very difficult for babies to get sufficient nourishment from solid food alone; breast milk or formula feedings are still essential.

ACTION Offer your baby breast milk or formula in addition to solid foods (see INTRODUCING SOLID FOODS, above). If your baby does not start putting on weight normally within 2 weeks or if you have trouble getting him or her to take solid food, consult your baby's doctor.

Does your baby always finish all of the bottle? YES / NO

Weight loss in the newborn

Your baby may lose weight in the first week of life; however, this is unlikely to be a cause for concern. Most babies, particularly if they are breast fed, may lose up to 7 oz (200 g) in the first few days after delivery. This weight loss is normal and is partly due to the relatively small amount of food they take in initially. In addition, newborn babies need to adjust to life outside the uterus and now have to take in, digest, and absorb their food, rather than have it supplied through the placenta. Most babies start to gain weight by the 5th day and are usually back to their birth weight by about 10 days after delivery.

Your baby will probably be weighed by the midwife or doctor in the first 2 weeks. Once your baby has regained his or her birth weight, he or she should continue to put on weight at a steady rate. For the first 3 months, your baby should gain about 6 oz (170 g) a week. By 4–6 months, a baby should have roughly doubled his or her birth weight.

CONSULT YOUR BABY'S DOCTOR IF YOU ARE UNABLE TO MAKE A DIAGNOSIS FROM THIS CHART.

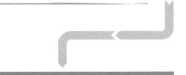

POSSIBLE CAUSE Check that you are giving your baby the right foods for his or her age. He or she may need more nourishment.

ACTION Follow the advice for introducing solid foods for your baby (above), and offer food or milk whenever your baby seems hungry. If your baby does not start putting on weight normally within 2 weeks or if you are not sure what foods he or she should have, consult your baby's doctor.

POSSIBLE CAUSE As your baby grows, his or her appetite will increase, and he or she may need more food than you are now offering, even if you are giving the recommended amount for your baby's age.

ACTION Offer more breast milk or formula than usual, and let your baby feed until he or she is satisfied. If your baby is over 4 months, he or she may be ready to start on solids (see INTRODUCING SOLID FOODS, above). If your baby does not start to gain weight normally or if you need further advice on weaning, consult your baby's doctor.

8 Skin problems in babies

If your baby has a rash with a temperature, see chart 15, RASH WITH FEVER *(p.78).*
The skin of newborn babies is very sensitive and can easily become irritated from rubbing on clothes or bedding. Such minor skin problems are usually no cause for concern. One of the most common skin problems in babies is diaper rash, which can be treated easily. Other rashes and skin abnormalities that occur for no apparent reason or persist longer than a few days should be brought to your baby's doctor's attention, especially if your baby seems sick.

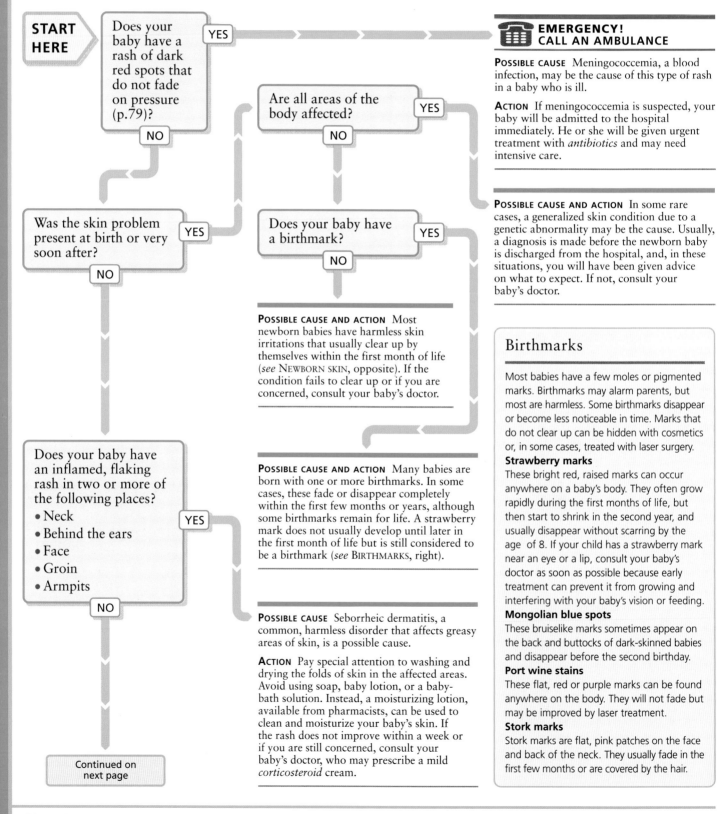

START HERE

Does your baby have a rash of dark red spots that do not fade on pressure (p.79)? — **YES** →

NO ↓

Was the skin problem present at birth or very soon after? — **YES** →

NO ↓

Does your baby have an inflamed, flaking rash in two or more of the following places?
• Neck
• Behind the ears
• Face
• Groin
• Armpits
— **YES** →

NO ↓

Continued on next page

Are all areas of the body affected? — **YES** →

NO ↓

Does your baby have a birthmark? — **YES** →

NO ↓

POSSIBLE CAUSE AND ACTION Most newborn babies have harmless skin irritations that usually clear up by themselves within the first month of life (*see* NEWBORN SKIN, opposite). If the condition fails to clear up or if you are concerned, consult your baby's doctor.

POSSIBLE CAUSE AND ACTION Many babies are born with one or more birthmarks. In some cases, these fade or disappear completely within the first few months or years, although some birthmarks remain for life. A strawberry mark does not usually develop until later in the first month of life but is still considered to be a birthmark (*see* BIRTHMARKS, right).

POSSIBLE CAUSE Seborrheic dermatitis, a common, harmless disorder that affects greasy areas of skin, is a possible cause.

ACTION Pay special attention to washing and drying the folds of skin in the affected areas. Avoid using soap, baby lotion, or a baby-bath solution. Instead, a moisturizing lotion, available from pharmacists, can be used to clean and moisturize your baby's skin. If the rash does not improve within a week or if you are still concerned, consult your baby's doctor, who may prescribe a mild *corticosteroid* cream.

EMERGENCY! CALL AN AMBULANCE

POSSIBLE CAUSE Meningococcemia, a blood infection, may be the cause of this type of rash in a baby who is ill.

ACTION If meningococcemia is suspected, your baby will be admitted to the hospital immediately. He or she will be given urgent treatment with *antibiotics* and may need intensive care.

POSSIBLE CAUSE AND ACTION In some rare cases, a generalized skin condition due to a genetic abnormality may be the cause. Usually, a diagnosis is made before the newborn baby is discharged from the hospital, and, in these situations, you will have been given advice on what to expect. If not, consult your baby's doctor.

Birthmarks

Most babies have a few moles or pigmented marks. Birthmarks may alarm parents, but most are harmless. Some birthmarks disappear or become less noticeable in time. Marks that do not clear up can be hidden with cosmetics or, in some cases, treated with laser surgery.

Strawberry marks
These bright red, raised marks can occur anywhere on a baby's body. They often grow rapidly during the first months of life, but then start to shrink in the second year, and usually disappear without scarring by the age of 8. If your child has a strawberry mark near an eye or a lip, consult your baby's doctor as soon as possible because early treatment can prevent it from growing and interfering with your baby's vision or feeding.

Mongolian blue spots
These bruiselike marks sometimes appear on the back and buttocks of dark-skinned babies and disappear before the second birthday.

Port wine stains
These flat, red or purple marks can be found anywhere on the body. They will not fade but may be improved by laser treatment.

Stork marks
Stork marks are flat, pink patches on the face and back of the neck. They usually fade in the first few months or are covered by the hair.

Continued from previous page

Does your baby have yellowish brown crusts on the scalp?
YES

POSSIBLE CAUSE Your baby may have cradle cap, a form of seborrheic dermatitis. It is a common, harmless condition.

ACTION You can soften the crusts by rubbing your baby's scalp with baby or olive oil at night and then washing off the crusts the next morning. Alternatively, special shampoos to treat the condition are available over the counter. However, the condition usually clears up by itself within a few weeks. If it does not or if you are concerned, consult your baby's doctor.

NO

Does your baby have a red, itchy rash on the face, arms, or legs?
YES

POSSIBLE CAUSE Your child may have atopic eczema, an allergic condition. This diagnosis is most likely if any other family members also suffer from eczema or other allergic conditions. Consult your baby's doctor.

ACTION If the diagnosis is confirmed, the doctor will advise you on dealing with atopic eczema (p.80). He or she may also prescribe a *corticosteroid* cream. If the rash is widespread or weepy, your child should see the doctor within 24 hours. Many children with atopic eczema grow out of it by the age of 8.

NO

Has your baby got an inflamed area of skin on his or her bottom with or without spots spreading from it?
YES

Is the skin broken or ulcerated?
YES

POSSIBLE CAUSE AND ACTION Your baby may have diaper rash that has become infected. Consult your baby's doctor, who may prescribe an anti-infective cream or a *corticosteroid* cream. In the meantime, follow the advice on treating diaper rash (below).

NO

NO

Are there several red spots outside the main area of the rash?
YES

NO

CONSULT YOUR BABY'S DOCTOR IF YOU ARE UNABLE TO MAKE A DIAGNOSIS FROM THIS CHART

Newborn skin

A newborn baby's skin is very delicate and easily irritated. Do not use soap or wipes to clean your baby until he or she is at least 6 weeks old because these can dry the skin. Water is usually sufficient for cleansing the diaper area, and a few drops of baby oil in the bathwater will help avoid dry skin.

There are several harmless skin problems that commonly affect babies. These include:
- Blotchy skin, partly due to blood vessels being visible because there is little fat below the skin, and partly because circulation is not mature, resulting in uneven blood flow.
- Milia – white spots on the nose and cheeks caused by blocked sebaceous glands in the skin. The spots clear up without treatment within the first couple of weeks.
- Peeling or flaking skin on the hands and feet. Gently rub moisturizing lotion into the affected areas.
- Heat rash – small red spots, often on the upper chest. Make sure that your baby is not too warm. No treatment is needed.

SEE YOUR BABY'S DOCTOR WITHIN 24 HOURS

POSSIBLE CAUSE A skin infection with the yeast that causes thrush is a possibility. It may accompany diaper rash and oral thrush.

ACTION Your baby's doctor will probably prescribe an *antifungal* cream and will possibly also prescribe a *corticosteroid* cream.

POSSIBLE CAUSE Your baby probably has diaper rash, which affects most babies at some time, particularly when they have diarrhea. Some babies seem more susceptible than others.

ACTION Follow the advice on treating diaper rash (left). If the rash does not clear up within a few days or if it becomes worse, consult your baby's doctor, who may prescribe a *corticosteroid* cream to reduce the inflammation.

SELF-HELP Diaper rash

Diaper rash affects most babies at some time. It is particularly common after diarrhea but can also develop if the skin becomes irritated from wearing a wet or soiled diaper for a long time. You can help clear up your baby's diaper rash by following these steps:
- Let your baby play without wearing a diaper as often as possible, preferably at least once a day.
- Wash the baby's diaper area with water, dry it carefully, and avoid scented wipes.
- Change your baby's diaper often.
- Make sure that you dry the creases in your baby's skin thoroughly.
- Apply a water-repellent cream such as zinc and castor oil or petroleum jelly.
- If you use cloth diapers, make sure they are thoroughly rinsed, and avoid using biological detergents.

Consult your baby's doctor if the rash becomes blistery, weepy, or ulcerated or if it does not clear up within a few days.

9 Not feeling well

For unusual or excessive fatigue in a child, see chart 10, FATIGUE (p.68).

A child may sometimes complain of feeling sick without giving you a clear idea of what exactly the matter is. At other times, you may suspect that your child is not well if he or she seems quieter or more irritable than usual. Use this chart to look for specific signs of illness. Such signs may lead you to a more specific chart within this book or to consult a doctor.

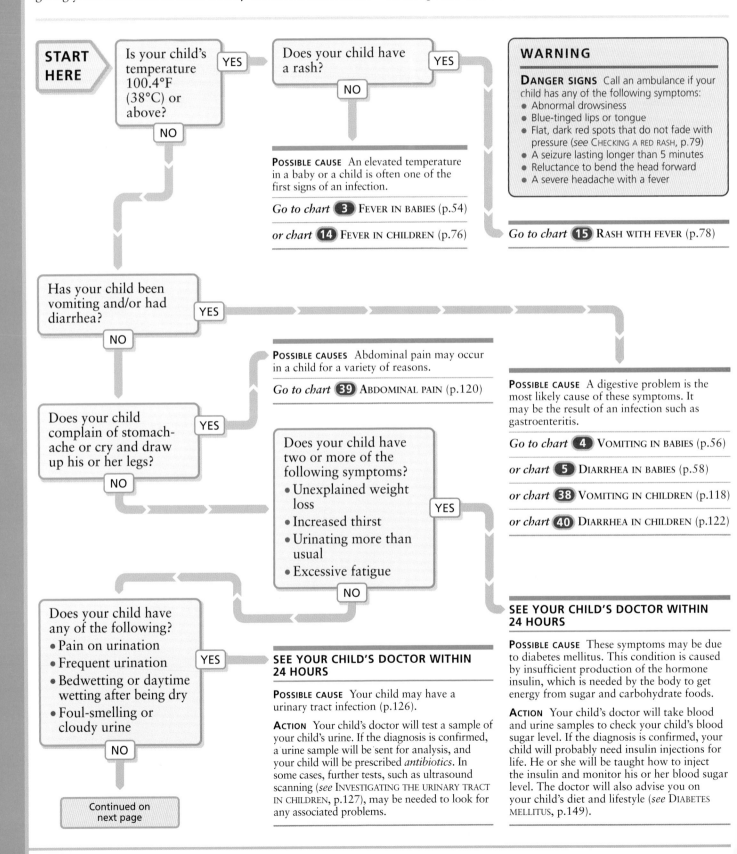

START HERE

Is your child's temperature 100.4°F (38°C) or above? — YES → **Does your child have a rash?** — YES → **WARNING**

NO (temperature)

POSSIBLE CAUSE An elevated temperature in a baby or a child is often one of the first signs of an infection.

Go to chart **3** FEVER IN BABIES (p.54)

or chart **14** FEVER IN CHILDREN (p.76)

NO (rash)

WARNING

DANGER SIGNS Call an ambulance if your child has any of the following symptoms:
- Abnormal drowsiness
- Blue-tinged lips or tongue
- Flat, dark red spots that do not fade with pressure (see CHECKING A RED RASH, p.79)
- A seizure lasting longer than 5 minutes
- Reluctance to bend the head forward
- A severe headache with a fever

Go to chart **15** RASH WITH FEVER (p.78)

Has your child been vomiting and/or had diarrhea? — YES →

NO

POSSIBLE CAUSES Abdominal pain may occur in a child for a variety of reasons.

Go to chart **39** ABDOMINAL PAIN (p.120)

POSSIBLE CAUSE A digestive problem is the most likely cause of these symptoms. It may be the result of an infection such as gastroenteritis.

Go to chart **4** VOMITING IN BABIES (p.56)

or chart **5** DIARRHEA IN BABIES (p.58)

or chart **38** VOMITING IN CHILDREN (p.118)

or chart **40** DIARRHEA IN CHILDREN (p.122)

Does your child complain of stomach-ache or cry and draw up his or her legs? — YES →

NO

Does your child have two or more of the following symptoms?
- Unexplained weight loss
- Increased thirst
- Urinating more than usual
- Excessive fatigue

— YES →

NO

SEE YOUR CHILD'S DOCTOR WITHIN 24 HOURS

POSSIBLE CAUSE These symptoms may be due to diabetes mellitus. This condition is caused by insufficient production of the hormone insulin, which is needed by the body to get energy from sugar and carbohydrate foods.

ACTION Your child's doctor will take blood and urine samples to check your child's blood sugar level. If the diagnosis is confirmed, your child will probably need insulin injections for life. He or she will be taught how to inject the insulin and monitor his or her blood sugar level. The doctor will also advise you on your child's diet and lifestyle (see DIABETES MELLITUS, p.149).

Does your child have any of the following?
- Pain on urination
- Frequent urination
- Bedwetting or daytime wetting after being dry
- Foul-smelling or cloudy urine

— YES →

NO

SEE YOUR CHILD'S DOCTOR WITHIN 24 HOURS

POSSIBLE CAUSE Your child may have a urinary tract infection (p.126).

ACTION Your child's doctor will test a sample of your child's urine. If the diagnosis is confirmed, a urine sample will be sent for analysis, and your child will be prescribed *antibiotics*. In some cases, further tests, such as ultrasound scanning (see INVESTIGATING THE URINARY TRACT IN CHILDREN, p.127), may be needed to look for any associated problems.

Continued on next page

Continued from
previous page

SELF-HELP Encouraging your child to drink

If your child is sick, it is better to concentrate
on encouraging him or her to drink rather than
worrying about a poor appetite. The following
measures may encourage your child to drink:
- Offer him or her interesting drinks, such as
  fruit-flavored drinks, rather than plain water.
- Offer him or her ice pops or ice cubes to suck.
- Offer small drinks frequently. Encourage your
  child to drink before an activity, such as a story.
- Use straws, bright or unusual cups, or "grown-
  up" cups to add interest.
- Let your child help prepare drinks or ice pops.

Eating ice popsicles
*If your child is
reluctant to drink,
offer him or her
an alternative
such as a
flavored ice
pop instead.*

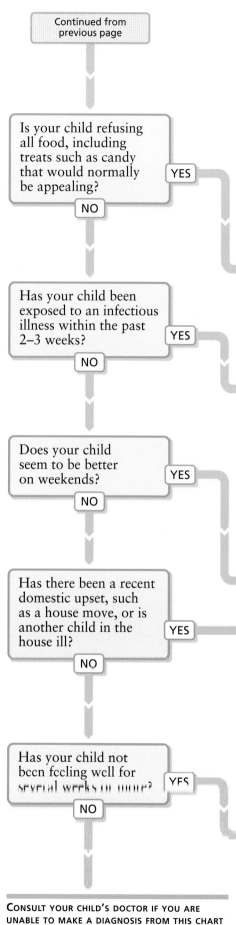

**Is your child refusing
all food, including
treats such as candy
that would normally
be appealing?**
NO / YES

**Is your child also
refusing to drink?**
YES / NO

**SEE YOUR CHILD'S DOCTOR WITHIN
24 HOURS**

POSSIBLE CAUSE AND ACTION A sore mouth or
throat is likely. However, refusing to drink can
lead to dehydration. Your child's doctor will
examine your child to establish the cause.
Encourage your child to drink (above). If he or
she is under 3 months and has refused feedings
for 3 hours or is under 12 months and has
refused to drink for 6 hours, contact the
doctor immediately.

**Has your child been
exposed to an infectious
illness within the past
2–3 weeks?**
NO / YES

POSSIBLE CAUSE Your child may be in the
very early stages of a childhood infectious
disease. It is common for children who
are coming down with an infectious
disease to feel sick and listless for
2 or 3 days before any specific symptoms
develop.

ACTION If your child develops any other
symptoms, consult the relevant chart
in this book. If your child is still not
feeling well after 48 hours and there
is no obvious cause, consult your
child's doctor.

POSSIBLE CAUSE A refusal to eat is common in
a child who is not well for any reason.

ACTION Do not worry about your child's
refusal to eat as long as he or she is drinking
plenty (*see* ENCOURAGING YOUR CHILD TO
DRINK, above). However, if your child is still
not eating after 48 hours, and there is no
obvious cause, consult your child's doctor.

**Does your child
seem to be better
on weekends?**
NO / YES

**Has there been a recent
domestic upset, such
as a house move, or is
another child in the
house ill?**
NO / YES

POSSIBLE CAUSE Some children are easily
unsettled by changes around them. They
may express this by changes in behavior
or not feeling well. An illness in another
child in the family may cause conflicting
feelings; your child may be anxious
about the other child but also jealous of
the extra attention given to him or her.

ACTION Talk to your child to find out
what the problem is. Extra reassurance
may help. If your child still does not feel
well, consult your child's doctor.

POSSIBLE CAUSE Your child may be anxious
about something at school, such as exams.
Many children express anxiety by behaving
in different ways than they normally do.

ACTION Talk to your child to find out what
the problem is. You should also talk to his or
her teachers to see if there is a problem you
are not aware of, such as bullying. If your
child continues to complain of feeling sick,
consult your child's doctor.

**Has your child not
been feeling well for
several weeks or more?**
NO / YES

POSSIBLE CAUSE AND ACTION Your child may be
unhappy or worried rather than physically ill.
Some children find it hard to express feelings
and may seem sick instead. Take time to talk
to your child, and, if necessary, consult
your child's doctor, who may refer him or her
to a specialist.

**Are your child's height
and weight within the
normal range for his or
her age (*see* GROWTH
CHARTS, p.26)?**
YES / NO

POSSIBLE CAUSE AND ACTION Your child may
have an underlying disorder, such as a urinary
tract infection. Consult your child's doctor,
who may arrange for tests to look for an
underlying cause and determine the
appropriate treatment. Your child may be
referred to a specialist.

**CONSULT YOUR CHILD'S DOCTOR IF YOU ARE
UNABLE TO MAKE A DIAGNOSIS FROM THIS CHART
AND YOUR CHILD IS NO BETTER IN 48 HOURS.**

10 Fatigue

*For **unusual drowsiness**, see chart 22,* CONFUSION AND/OR DROWSINESS **(p.90)**.

It is normal for a child to be tired if he or she has slept badly the night before or had a particularly long or energetic day. It is also common for children to need more sleep than normal during growth spurts and at puberty. If your child seems tired most of the time or fatigue is preventing him or her from taking part in social activities or keeping up at school, there may be an underlying medical problem. In many cases, such fatigue is short-lived and may be the result of a recent infection. However, you should consult your child's doctor to rule out a more serious problem.

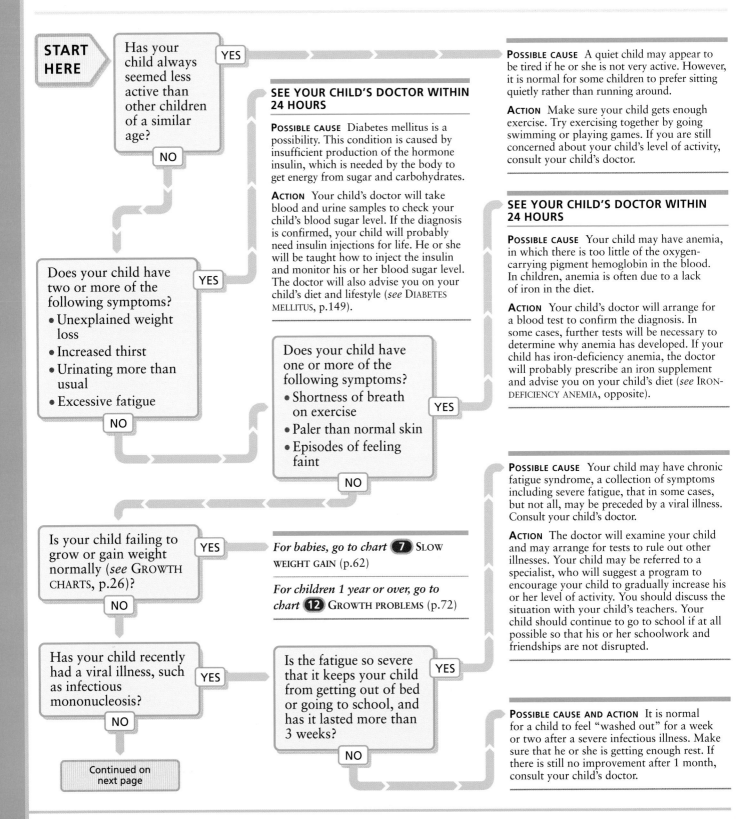

START HERE

Has your child always seemed less active than other children of a similar age? — **YES** →

POSSIBLE CAUSE A quiet child may appear to be tired if he or she is not very active. However, it is normal for some children to prefer sitting quietly rather than running around.

ACTION Make sure your child gets enough exercise. Try exercising together by going swimming or playing games. If you are still concerned about your child's level of activity, consult your child's doctor.

NO ↓

Does your child have two or more of the following symptoms?
- Unexplained weight loss
- Increased thirst
- Urinating more than usual
- Excessive fatigue

— **YES** →

SEE YOUR CHILD'S DOCTOR WITHIN 24 HOURS

POSSIBLE CAUSE Diabetes mellitus is a possibility. This condition is caused by insufficient production of the hormone insulin, which is needed by the body to get energy from sugar and carbohydrates.

ACTION Your child's doctor will take blood and urine samples to check your child's blood sugar level. If the diagnosis is confirmed, your child will probably need insulin injections for life. He or she will be taught how to inject the insulin and monitor his or her blood sugar level. The doctor will also advise you on your child's diet and lifestyle (*see* DIABETES MELLITUS, p.149).

NO ↓

Does your child have one or more of the following symptoms?
- Shortness of breath on exercise
- Paler than normal skin
- Episodes of feeling faint

— **YES** →

SEE YOUR CHILD'S DOCTOR WITHIN 24 HOURS

POSSIBLE CAUSE Your child may have anemia, in which there is too little of the oxygen-carrying pigment hemoglobin in the blood. In children, anemia is often due to a lack of iron in the diet.

ACTION Your child's doctor will arrange for a blood test to confirm the diagnosis. In some cases, further tests will be necessary to determine why anemia has developed. If your child has iron-deficiency anemia, the doctor will probably prescribe an iron supplement and advise you on your child's diet (*see* IRON-DEFICIENCY ANEMIA, opposite).

NO ↓

Is your child failing to grow or gain weight normally (*see* GROWTH CHARTS, p.26)? — **YES** →

*For **babies**, go to chart **7** SLOW WEIGHT GAIN (p.62)*

*For **children 1 year or over**, go to chart **12** GROWTH PROBLEMS (p.72)*

NO ↓

POSSIBLE CAUSE Your child may have chronic fatigue syndrome, a collection of symptoms including severe fatigue, that in some cases, but not all, may be preceded by a viral illness. Consult your child's doctor.

ACTION The doctor will examine your child and may arrange for tests to rule out other illnesses. Your child may be referred to a specialist, who will suggest a program to encourage your child to gradually increase his or her level of activity. You should discuss the situation with your child's teachers. Your child should continue to go to school if at all possible so that his or her schoolwork and friendships are not disrupted.

Has your child recently had a viral illness, such as infectious mononucleosis? — **YES** →

Is the fatigue so severe that it keeps your child from getting out of bed or going to school, and has it lasted more than 3 weeks? — **YES** →

NO ↓

POSSIBLE CAUSE AND ACTION It is normal for a child to feel "washed out" for a week or two after a severe infectious illness. Make sure that he or she is getting enough rest. If there is still no improvement after 1 month, consult your child's doctor.

NO →

Continued on next page

Continued from previous page

Is your child taking any prescribed drugs? **YES**

NO

POSSIBLE CAUSE AND ACTION Certain drugs, such as *antihistamines* and *anticonvulsants*, can cause fatigue as a side effect. Consult your child's doctor. Meanwhile, make sure your child does not stop taking his or her prescribed drugs.

POSSIBLE CAUSES Children often snore if they have a cold, and this is nothing to worry about. However, if your child snores all the time, he or she may have enlarged tonsils or adenoids (p.107), which may block the airway during sleep. Consult your child's doctor.

ACTION The doctor will examine your child's throat. In some cases, your doctor may refer your child to a specialist. Surgical removal of the tonsils and adenoids may improve the situation.

Does your child snore? **YES**

NO

Does your child sleep badly? **YES**

NO

Is your child's sleep disturbed by symptoms such as a cough or itchy skin? **YES**

NO

POSSIBLE CAUSE Symptoms of conditions such as asthma or eczema that do not bother a child during the day can disturb his or her sleep. Consult your child's doctor.

ACTION The doctor will examine your child and prescribe appropriate treatment. If your child is already receiving treatment for a condition such as asthma or eczema, it may need to be adjusted. Once the symptoms have been treated, your child should sleep better.

Could your child be getting too little sleep because of going to bed late or rising early? **YES**

NO

Go to chart **1** SLEEPING PROBLEMS IN BABIES (p.50)

or go to chart **11** SLEEPING PROBLEMS IN CHILDREN (p.70)

POSSIBLE CAUSE A lack of sleep is one of the most common causes of fatigue. Difficulty getting your child to sleep is usually temporary and caused by lack of a fixed bedtime routine or anxiety. However, persistent problems may be the result of a behavioral problem.

ACTION Impose a regular bedtime routine, and be firm with your child (*see* GETTING YOUR CHILD TO SLEEP, p.70). If he or she is old enough, talk about any concerns he or she may have. If your child is still not sleeping properly within a few weeks, consult your child's doctor.

Has there been a recent upset at home or at school? **YES**

NO

POSSIBLE CAUSE Fatigue may be one sign of anxiety or depression as the result of a temporary upset.

ACTION Try to discover and deal with any underlying worries that your child has. Mild anxiety or depression can often be cleared up with extra reassurance and support. However, if your child's fatigue persists or becomes severe, consult your child's doctor.

POSSIBLE CAUSE It is likely that your child is overdoing things due to long days or pressure to take part in various activities.

ACTION Talk to your child about dropping or rotating any optional activities. Encourage him or her to spend more time at home, playing quietly. Most children adjust to increased levels of activity at school within a term.

Do any of the following apply? **YES**
- Your child is one of the youngest in his or her school year
- Your child has recently started going to a play group or school
- Your child has increased his or her afterschool activities

NO

CONSULT YOUR CHILD'S DOCTOR IF YOU ARE UNABLE TO MAKE A DIAGNOSIS FROM THIS CHART AND YOUR CHILD'S FATIGUE IS PERSISTENT OR SEVERE.

Iron-deficiency anemia

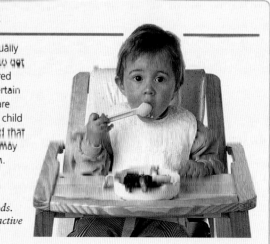

In children, iron-deficiency anemia is usually caused by a lack of iron in the diet. Try to get your child to eat green vegetables and red meat, although this may be difficult. Certain foods, such as some breakfast cereals, are fortified with iron and are useful if your child will not eat other iron-rich foods. A child that is not eating solids by 6 months of age may need a formula milk with additional iron. Ask your child's doctor for advice.

Providing an iron-rich diet
Offer your child plenty of iron-rich foods. Try to make green vegetables look attractive to encourage your child to eat them.

11 Sleeping problems in children

For children under 1 year, see chart 1, SLEEPING PROBLEMS IN BABIES (p.50).

The amount of sleep a child needs at night varies from about 9 to 12 hours according to age and individual requirements (*see* SLEEP REQUIREMENTS IN CHILDHOOD, right). Lack of sleep rarely affects health but may affect behavior during the day or performance at school. However, refusal to go to sleep at what you think is a reasonable time and/or waking in the middle of the night can be disruptive and distressing for the family if it occurs regularly. A number of factors, including physical illness, emotional upset, nightmares, and lack of a regular bedtime routine, may cause such sleeping problems.

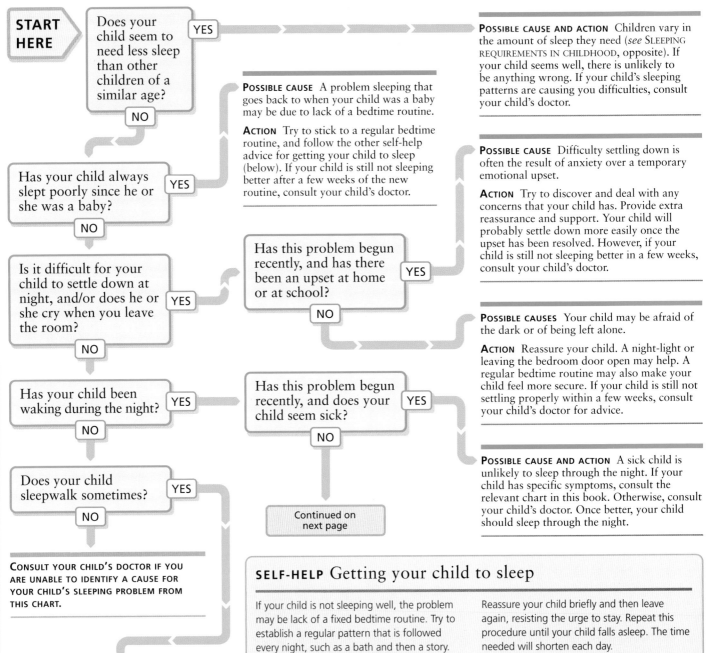

START HERE

Does your child seem to need less sleep than other children of a similar age?
YES →

POSSIBLE CAUSE AND ACTION Children vary in the amount of sleep they need (*see* SLEEPING REQUIREMENTS IN CHILDHOOD, opposite). If your child seems well, there is unlikely to be anything wrong. If your child's sleeping patterns are causing you difficulties, consult your child's doctor.

NO ↓

Has your child always slept poorly since he or she was a baby?
YES →

POSSIBLE CAUSE A problem sleeping that goes back to when your child was a baby may be due to lack of a bedtime routine.

ACTION Try to stick to a regular bedtime routine, and follow the other self-help advice for getting your child to sleep (below). If your child is still not sleeping better after a few weeks of the new routine, consult your child's doctor.

NO ↓

Is it difficult for your child to settle down at night, and/or does he or she cry when you leave the room?
YES →

Has this problem begun recently, and has there been an upset at home or at school?
YES →

POSSIBLE CAUSE Difficulty settling down is often the result of anxiety over a temporary emotional upset.

ACTION Try to discover and deal with any concerns that your child has. Provide extra reassurance and support. Your child will probably settle down more easily once the upset has been resolved. However, if your child is still not sleeping better in a few weeks, consult your child's doctor.

NO ↓

POSSIBLE CAUSES Your child may be afraid of the dark or of being left alone.

ACTION Reassure your child. A night-light or leaving the bedroom door open may help. A regular bedtime routine may also make your child feel more secure. If your child is still not settling properly within a few weeks, consult your child's doctor for advice.

NO ↓

Has your child been waking during the night?
YES →

Has this problem begun recently, and does your child seem sick?
YES →

NO ↓

POSSIBLE CAUSE AND ACTION A sick child is unlikely to sleep through the night. If your child has specific symptoms, consult the relevant chart in this book. Otherwise, consult your child's doctor. Once better, your child should sleep through the night.

Does your child sleepwalk sometimes?
YES →

NO ↓

Continued on next page

CONSULT YOUR CHILD'S DOCTOR IF YOU ARE UNABLE TO IDENTIFY A CAUSE FOR YOUR CHILD'S SLEEPING PROBLEM FROM THIS CHART.

POSSIBLE CAUSE AND ACTION Sleepwalking is most common between the ages of 6 and 12. There is no need to worry as long as you ensure that your child is safe, for example by locking all outer doors. Do not try to wake your child, but guide him or her back to bed if necessary. Children usually grow out of it by age 12.

SELF-HELP Getting your child to sleep

If your child is not sleeping well, the problem may be lack of a fixed bedtime routine. Try to establish a regular pattern that is followed every night, such as a bath and then a story. Often, children do not sleep well because they are afraid of the dark. This problem can be solved by a night-light or leaving the bedroom door open. If you have difficulty in getting your child to sleep, settle him or her, say goodnight, and leave the room. If your child cries, leave him or her for a few minutes before returning.

Reassure your child briefly and then leave again, resisting the urge to stay. Repeat this procedure until your child falls asleep. The time needed will shorten each day.

If your child wakes during the night, only get up if he or she is truly crying. (A child who is only whimpering may drift back to sleep.) Go into the room to make sure nothing is wrong, reassure your child, and leave again. If your child still cries, try the method above. He or she will eventually settle back to sleep.

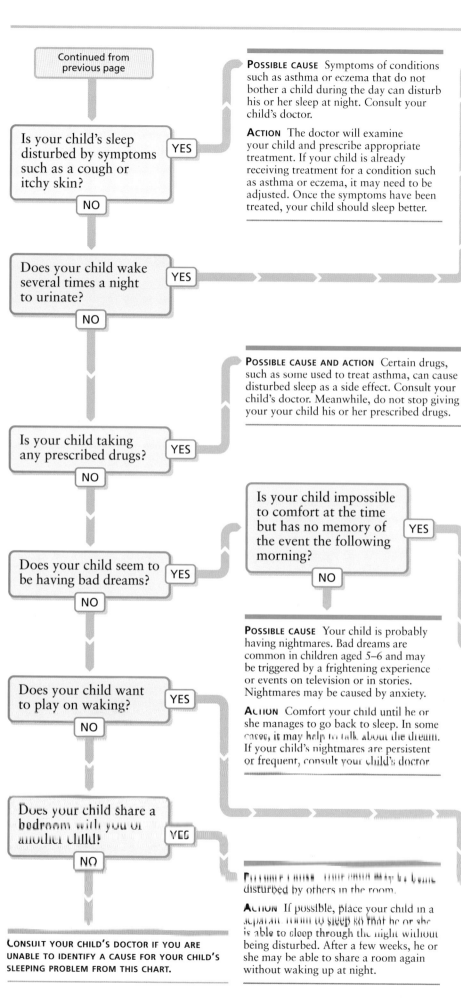

Continued from previous page

Is your child's sleep disturbed by symptoms such as a cough or itchy skin?
— YES →

POSSIBLE CAUSE Symptoms of conditions such as asthma or eczema that do not bother a child during the day can disturb his or her sleep at night. Consult your child's doctor.

ACTION The doctor will examine your child and prescribe appropriate treatment. If your child is already receiving treatment for a condition such as asthma or eczema, it may need to be adjusted. Once the symptoms have been treated, your child should sleep better.

NO ↓

Does your child wake several times a night to urinate?
— YES →

POSSIBLE CAUSES Waking more than once or twice during the night to pass urine may be a sign of an underlying disorder, such as a urinary tract infection. However, the most common cause is drinking too many fluids.

Go to chart **43** URINARY PROBLEMS (p.126)

NO ↓

Is your child taking any prescribed drugs?
— YES →

POSSIBLE CAUSE AND ACTION Certain drugs, such as some used to treat asthma, can cause disturbed sleep as a side effect. Consult your child's doctor. Meanwhile, do not stop giving your your child his or her prescribed drugs.

NO ↓

Does your child seem to be having bad dreams?
— YES →

Is your child impossible to comfort at the time but has no memory of the event the following morning?
— YES →
— NO ↓

POSSIBLE CAUSE Your child is probably having nightmares. Bad dreams are common in children aged 5–6 and may be triggered by a frightening experience or events on television or in stories. Nightmares may be caused by anxiety.

ACTION Comfort your child until he or she manages to go back to sleep. In some cases, it may help to talk about the dream. If your child's nightmares are persistent or frequent, consult your child's doctor.

NO ↓

Does your child want to play on waking?
— YES →

NO ↓

Does your child share a bedroom with you or another child?
— YES →

POSSIBLE CAUSE Your child may be being disturbed by others in the room.

ACTION If possible, place your child in a separate room to sleep so that he or she is able to sleep through the night without being disturbed. After a few weeks, he or she may be able to share a room again without waking up at night.

NO ↓

CONSULT YOUR CHILD'S DOCTOR IF YOU ARE UNABLE TO IDENTIFY A CAUSE FOR YOUR CHILD'S SLEEPING PROBLEM FROM THIS CHART.

Sleep requirements in childhood

Children vary in the amount of sleep that they need, and it is normal for some children to sleep more than others of a similar age. In general, children sleep less as they grow up. The proportion of sleep spent dreaming also goes down, from about half in a newborn to about one-fifth in a teenager. You should only worry about your child's sleeping if he or she seems sick or if excessive sleepiness interferes with his or her activities.

Age	Average total sleep per 24 hours
Up to 3 months	16 hours
3–5 months	14 hours
5–24 months	13 hours
2–3 years	12 hours
3–5 years	11 hours
5–9 years	10½ hours
9–13 years	10 hours

Amount of sleep according to age
This table shows the average number of hours of sleep needed by babies and children of different ages.

POSSIBLE CAUSE Your child is probably having night terrors, a condition in which a child seems to be awake and terrified, although he or she is actually asleep and will not remember the incident in the morning. Night terrors are most common in 4–7 year olds.

ACTION You may be able to prevent a night terror by waking your child in the restless period that often precedes it. Night terrors usually occur about 2 hours after falling asleep. However, once one has started, there is little you can do except stay with your child. If he or she has frequent night terrors, consult your child's doctor. Night terrors will become less frequent as your child grows older.

POSSIBLE CAUSE AND ACTION Children are often ready to start their day earlier than their parents and may go through a phase of early waking. If you want your child to go back to sleep, follow the self-help advice for getting your child to sleep (opposite). If your child is old enough, you may wish to leave him or her to play quietly instead.

12 Growth problems

For children under 1, see chart 7, SLOW WEIGHT GAIN *(p.62). For weight problems in adolescents, see chart 51,* ADOLESCENT WEIGHT PROBLEMS *(p.139).*
Many parents worry that their child is too short or too thin; others worry that their child or is too tall or has put on too much weight. However, some children are naturally smaller or bigger than average, and serious disorders affecting growth are rare. The best way to avoid unnecessary anxiety is to keep a regular record of your child's height and weight so that you can check that his or her growth rate is within the normal range (*see* GROWTH CHARTS, p.26). Consult this chart if your child is losing weight or is gaining weight at a much slower rate than you would expect, or if your child fails to grow in height as much as expected.

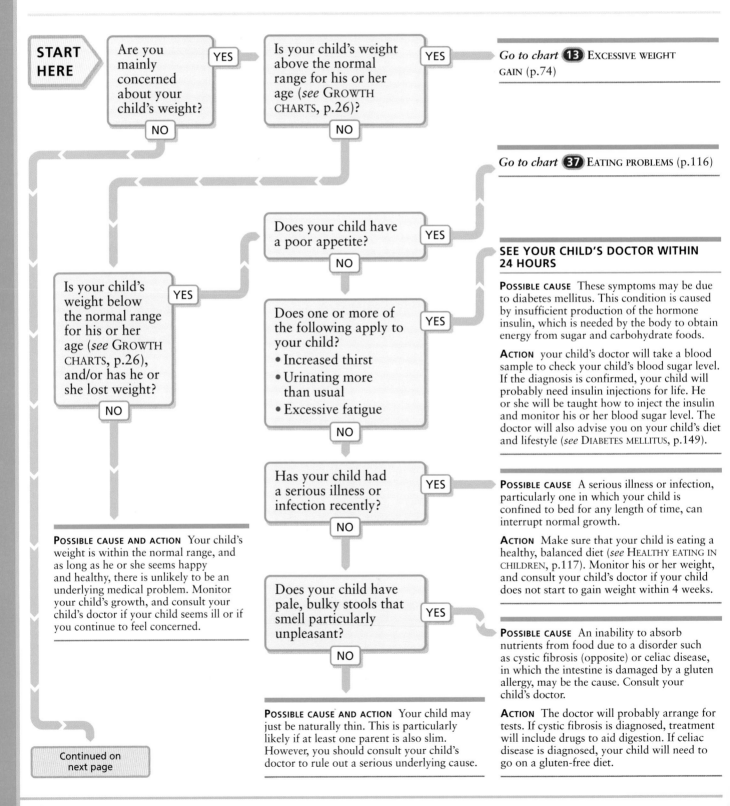

START HERE

Are you mainly concerned about your child's weight? YES → **Is your child's weight above the normal range for his or her age (*see* GROWTH CHARTS, p.26)?** YES → *Go to chart* **13** EXCESSIVE WEIGHT GAIN (p.74)

NO / NO

Go to chart **37** EATING PROBLEMS (p.116)

Is your child's weight below the normal range for his or her age (*see* GROWTH CHARTS, p.26), and/or has he or she lost weight? YES →

Does your child have a poor appetite? YES →

NO

Does one or more of the following apply to your child?
• Increased thirst
• Urinating more than usual
• Excessive fatigue
YES →

NO

SEE YOUR CHILD'S DOCTOR WITHIN 24 HOURS

POSSIBLE CAUSE These symptoms may be due to diabetes mellitus. This condition is caused by insufficient production of the hormone insulin, which is needed by the body to obtain energy from sugar and carbohydrate foods.

ACTION your child's doctor will take a blood sample to check your child's blood sugar level. If the diagnosis is confirmed, your child will probably need insulin injections for life. He or she will be taught how to inject the insulin and monitor his or her blood sugar level. The doctor will also advise you on your child's diet and lifestyle (*see* DIABETES MELLITUS, p.149).

Has your child had a serious illness or infection recently? YES →

NO

POSSIBLE CAUSE A serious illness or infection, particularly one in which your child is confined to bed for any length of time, can interrupt normal growth.

ACTION Make sure that your child is eating a healthy, balanced diet (*see* HEALTHY EATING IN CHILDREN, p.117). Monitor his or her weight, and consult your child's doctor if your child does not start to gain weight within 4 weeks.

POSSIBLE CAUSE AND ACTION Your child's weight is within the normal range, and as long as he or she seems happy and healthy, there is unlikely to be an underlying medical problem. Monitor your child's growth, and consult your child's doctor if your child seems ill or if you continue to feel concerned.

Does your child have pale, bulky stools that smell particularly unpleasant? YES →

NO

POSSIBLE CAUSE An inability to absorb nutrients from food due to a disorder such as cystic fibrosis (opposite) or celiac disease, in which the intestine is damaged by a gluten allergy, may be the cause. Consult your child's doctor.

ACTION The doctor will probably arrange for tests. If cystic fibrosis is diagnosed, treatment will include drugs to aid digestion. If celiac disease is diagnosed, your child will need to go on a gluten-free diet.

POSSIBLE CAUSE AND ACTION Your child may just be naturally thin. This is particularly likely if at least one parent is also slim. However, you should consult your child's doctor to rule out a serious underlying cause.

Continued on next page

Continued from previous page

Are you mainly concerned about your child's height? **YES**

NO

CONSULT YOUR CHILD'S DOCTOR IF YOU ARE UNABLE TO MAKE A DIAGNOSIS FROM THIS CHART.

Cystic fibrosis

Cystic fibrosis is a genetic disorder in which secretions from the glands are abnormally thick. This results in a range of problems; in particular, thick mucus in the lungs causes a persistent cough and recurrent chest infections. Abnormal secretions from the pancreas interfere with the child's ability to digest food and cause him or her to pass pale, bulky, strong-smelling feces. Children with cystic fibrosis frequently fail to grow normally and are often underweight. The condition is present from birth but is sometimes undetected for months or years, during which time the lungs may have become damaged. Regular chest physical therapy performed by a parent, *antibiotics*, and drugs to aid digestion now enable most affected children to survive well into adulthood.

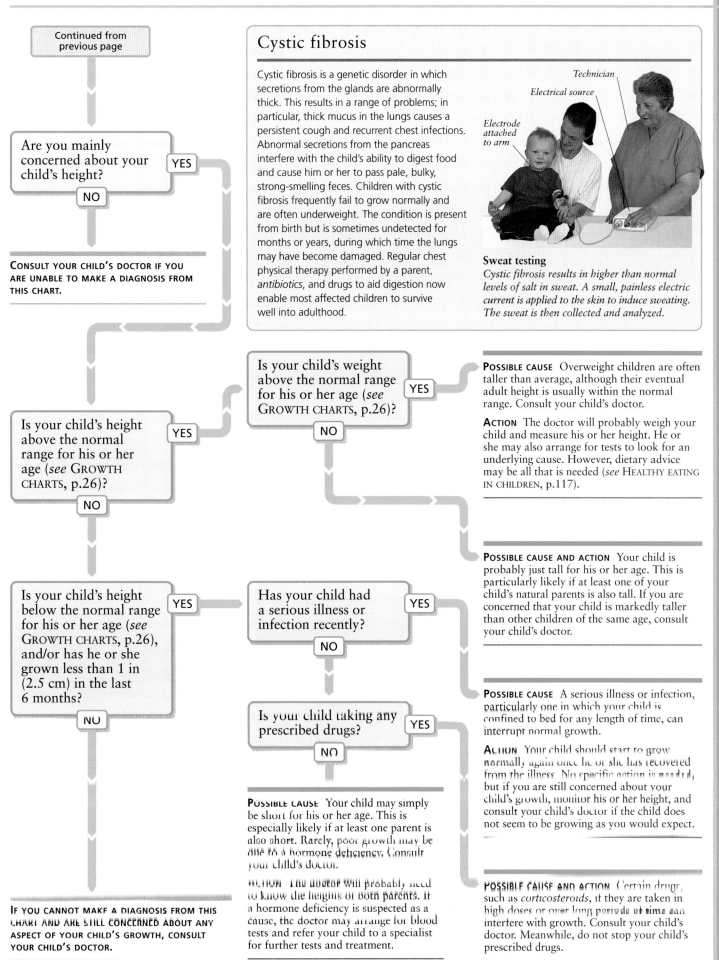

Technician
Electrical source
Electrode attached to arm

Sweat testing
Cystic fibrosis results in higher than normal levels of salt in sweat. A small, painless electric current is applied to the skin to induce sweating. The sweat is then collected and analyzed.

Is your child's height above the normal range for his or her age (*see* GROWTH CHARTS, p.26)? **YES**

NO

Is your child's weight above the normal range for his or her age (*see* GROWTH CHARTS, p.26)? **YES**

NO

POSSIBLE CAUSE Overweight children are often taller than average, although their eventual adult height is usually within the normal range. Consult your child's doctor.

ACTION The doctor will probably weigh your child and measure his or her height. He or she may also arrange for tests to look for an underlying cause. However, dietary advice may be all that is needed (*see* HEALTHY EATING IN CHILDREN, p.117).

Is your child's height below the normal range for his or her age (*see* GROWTH CHARTS, p.26), and/or has he or she grown less than 1 in (2.5 cm) in the last 6 months? **YES**

NO

Has your child had a serious illness or infection recently? **YES**

NO

Is your child taking any prescribed drugs? **YES**

NO

POSSIBLE CAUSE AND ACTION Your child is probably just tall for his or her age. This is particularly likely if at least one of your child's natural parents is also tall. If you are concerned that your child is markedly taller than other children of the same age, consult your child's doctor.

POSSIBLE CAUSE A serious illness or infection, particularly one in which your child is confined to bed for any length of time, can interrupt normal growth.

ACTION Your child should start to grow normally again once he or she has recovered from the illness. No specific action is needed, but if you are still concerned about your child's growth, monitor his or her height, and consult your child's doctor if the child does not seem to be growing as you would expect.

IF YOU CANNOT MAKE A DIAGNOSIS FROM THIS CHART AND ARE STILL CONCERNED ABOUT ANY ASPECT OF YOUR CHILD'S GROWTH, CONSULT YOUR CHILD'S DOCTOR.

POSSIBLE CAUSE Your child may simply be short for his or her age. This is especially likely if at least one parent is also short. Rarely, poor growth may be due to a hormone deficiency. Consult your child's doctor.

ACTION The doctor will probably need to know the heights of both parents. If a hormone deficiency is suspected as a cause, the doctor may arrange for blood tests and refer your child to a specialist for further tests and treatment.

POSSIBLE CAUSE AND ACTION Certain drugs, such as *corticosteroids*, if they are taken in high doses or over long periods of time can interfere with growth. Consult your child's doctor. Meanwhile, do not stop your child's prescribed drugs.

13 Excessive weight gain

Consult this chart if you think your child is overweight. Being overweight carries health risks and may contribute to emotional and social problems (*see* THE DANGERS OF CHILDHOOD OBESITY, opposite). It is therefore important to be alert to the possibility of excessive weight gain in your child. Appearance is not always a reliable sign of obesity because babies and toddlers are naturally chubby. The best way of ensuring that you notice any weight problem in your child is to keep a regular record of your child's growth (*see* GROWTH CHARTS, p.26). Increasing appreciation of the dangers of obesity in adults has led to a growing awareness that the problem often starts in childhood, when bad eating habits are established. It is extremely rare for excess weight to be due to a hormone problem.

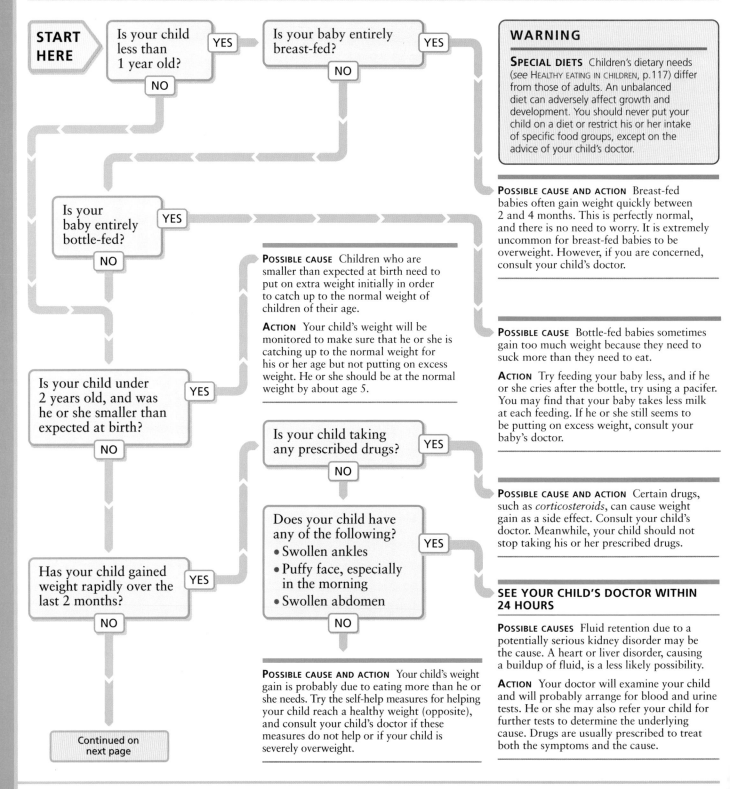

START HERE

Is your child less than 1 year old? — YES — **Is your baby entirely breast-fed?** — YES

NO / NO

Is your baby entirely bottle-fed? — YES

NO

POSSIBLE CAUSE Children who are smaller than expected at birth need to put on extra weight initially in order to catch up to the normal weight of children of their age.

ACTION Your child's weight will be monitored to make sure that he or she is catching up to the normal weight for his or her age but not putting on excess weight. He or she should be at the normal weight by about age 5.

Is your child under 2 years old, and was he or she smaller than expected at birth? — YES

NO

Is your child taking any prescribed drugs? — YES

NO

Does your child have any of the following?
- Swollen ankles
- Puffy face, especially in the morning
- Swollen abdomen

— YES

NO

Has your child gained weight rapidly over the last 2 months? — YES

NO

Continued on next page

POSSIBLE CAUSE AND ACTION Your child's weight gain is probably due to eating more than he or she needs. Try the self-help measures for helping your child reach a healthy weight (opposite), and consult your child's doctor if these measures do not help or if your child is severely overweight.

WARNING

SPECIAL DIETS Children's dietary needs (*see* HEALTHY EATING IN CHILDREN, p.117) differ from those of adults. An unbalanced diet can adversely affect growth and development. You should never put your child on a diet or restrict his or her intake of specific food groups, except on the advice of your child's doctor.

POSSIBLE CAUSE AND ACTION Breast-fed babies often gain weight quickly between 2 and 4 months. This is perfectly normal, and there is no need to worry. It is extremely uncommon for breast-fed babies to be overweight. However, if you are concerned, consult your child's doctor.

POSSIBLE CAUSE Bottle-fed babies sometimes gain too much weight because they need to suck more than they need to eat.

ACTION Try feeding your baby less, and if he or she cries after the bottle, try using a pacifer. You may find that your baby takes less milk at each feeding. If he or she still seems to be putting on excess weight, consult your baby's doctor.

POSSIBLE CAUSE AND ACTION Certain drugs, such as *corticosteroids*, can cause weight gain as a side effect. Consult your child's doctor. Meanwhile, your child should not stop taking his or her prescribed drugs.

SEE YOUR CHILD'S DOCTOR WITHIN 24 HOURS

POSSIBLE CAUSES Fluid retention due to a potentially serious kidney disorder may be the cause. A heart or liver disorder, causing a buildup of fluid, is a less likely possibility.

ACTION Your doctor will examine your child and will probably arrange for blood and urine tests. He or she may also refer your child for further tests to determine the underlying cause. Drugs are usually prescribed to treat both the symptoms and the cause.

Continued from previous page

Has your child been overweight since early childhood? **NO** / **YES**

Are other members of the family overweight? **NO** / **YES**

POSSIBLE CAUSE Overcating within the entire family is the most likely cause, although genetic factors also play a part.

ACTION Look at the way the whole family eats. By changing your own eating patterns, you can encourage your child to lose weight. Follow the advice for helping your child achieve a healthy weight (below), and consult your child's doctor if these measures do not help or if your child is severely overweight.

Is your child always expected to finish all the food on his or her plate? **NO** / **YES**

POSSIBLE CAUSE Your child is probably eating more than he or she needs.

ACTION Never force your child to eat. Allow him or her to stop eating, even if there is some food left, and serve smaller portions to avoid waste. Follow the advice for helping your child reach a healthy weight (below), and consult your child's doctor if these measures do not help or if your child is severely overweight.

Has your child been overweight for less than 6 months? **NO** / **YES**

POSSIBLE CAUSE AND ACTION Your child's weight gain is probably due to eating more than he or she needs. Try the self-help measures for helping your child reach a healthy weight (below), and consult your child's doctor if these measures do not help or if your child is severely overweight.

POSSIBLE CAUSE AND ACTION Your child's weight gain is probably due to eating more than he or she needs. Try the self-help measures for helping your child reach a healthy weight (right), and consult your child's doctor if these measures do not help or if your child is severely overweight.

Could your child be comfort-eating, for example, because of stressful events at home or school? **NO** / **YES**

POSSIBLE CAUSE Erratic weight gain is common just before a growth spurt, especially in girls.

ACTION Monitor your child's weight. If he or she does not grow in height to balance the weight gain, follow the advice for helping your child reach a healthy weight (right). Consult your child's doctor if these measures do not help or if your child is severely overweight.

POSSIBLE CAUSE Overeating when under stress is common and can cause weight gain.

ACTION Try to discover and deal with any underlying worries that your child has. If necessary, talk to your child's teachers. Follow the advice for helping your child reach a healthy weight (right), and consult your child's doctor if these measures do not help or if your child is severely overweight.

The dangers of childhood obesity

Being overweight can have a wide range of negative effects. Excess weight tends to reduce physical activity, which may compound the weight problem as well as contribute to poor fitness. Many overweight children also suffer from teasing or bullying from other children, making them insecure and unhappy. Low self-esteem, as a result of childhood teasing, often persists into adulthood.

Children who are overweight are likely to remain overweight as adults, putting them at increased risk for various disorders in later life, including life-threatening heart and circulatory disorders, such as a stroke or heart attack. Overweight adults are also more likely to suffer from joint problems, such as back or knee pain. Diabetes is more common in people who are overweight, as are some forms of cancer.

SELF-HELP Helping your child reach a healthy weight

Most overweight children eat more food than they need. To help your child lose weight, follow the advice for losing weight in adults (*see* HOW TO LOSE WEIGHT SAFELY, p.151) as well as the following measures:

- Make sure your child does not lose weight too quickly. He or she should lose a maximum of 1 lb (0.5 kg) per week.
- Involve your child, and let him or her take responsibility for losing weight.
- Stop buying high-fat and high-calorie foods, such as chocolate and soft drinks, so that the temptation is removed.
- Encourage your child to take up active leisure pursuits that he or she enjoys, such as soccer or dancing, instead of mostly watching TV or playing computer games.
- Encourage and reward your child for losing weight.

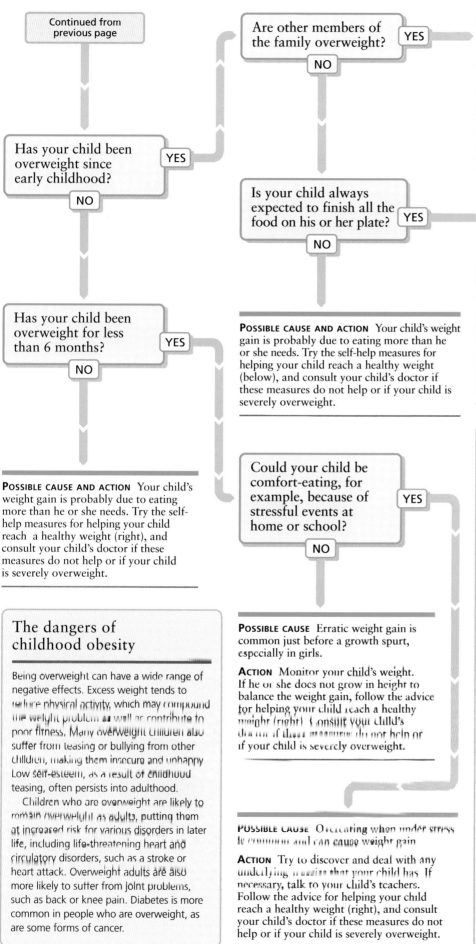

Eating healthily
High-fiber foods, such as whole-wheat bread and granola bars, are a healthy way to relieve hunger.

14 Fever in children

For children under 1, see chart 3, FEVER IN BABIES (p.54).
A fever is an abnormally high body temperature of 100.4°F (38°C) or above. It is usually a sign that the body is fighting an infection. Heat exposure can also lead to a high temperature. A child with a fever will feel generally ill and may be hot and sweaty. If your child does not feel well, you should take his or her temperature (*see* TAKING YOUR CHILD'S TEMPERATURE, below). If it is high, take steps to reduce it (*see* BRINGING DOWN A FEVER, opposite). Some children are at risk for seizures when they have a high fever.

START HERE → **Does your child have a rash?**
- YES → *Go to chart* **15** RASH WITH FEVER (p.78)
- NO ↓

Is your child complaining of earache, and/or is he or she tugging at either ear?
- YES →
- NO ↓

SEE YOUR CHILD'S DOCTOR WITHIN 24 HOURS

POSSIBLE CAUSE An infection of the middle ear is a possible cause of your child's symptoms.

ACTION Your child's doctor will examine your child. If the diagnosis is confirmed, he or she may prescribe *analgesics* and/or *antibiotics*. You can also try self-help measures for relieving earache (p.103).

Does your child have a cough and/or a runny nose?
- YES →
- NO ↓

Does your child have noisy breathing and/or a barking cough?
- YES →
- NO ↓

CALL YOUR CHILD'S DOCTOR NOW

POSSIBLE CAUSE A condition such as croup, in which the throat becomes swollen and narrowed due to a viral infection, is possible.

ACTION Your child's doctor may give your child a *corticosteroid* drug to ease his or her breathing. You should also try self-help measures for relieving a cough (p.108). If your child's symptoms are severe, he or she may need to be admitted to the hospital for monitoring and further treatment.

Is your child's breathing faster than normal? *See* CHECKING YOUR CHILD'S BREATHING RATE (p.110).
- YES →
- NO ↓

CALL YOUR CHILD'S DOCTOR NOW

POSSIBLE CAUSE A chest infection such as pneumonia (infection of the air spaces in the lungs) is possible.

ACTION If your child's doctor confirms the diagnosis, he or she will probably prescribe *antibiotics* and may arrange for a chest X ray (p.39). Take steps to reduce your child's temperature (*see* BRINGING DOWN A FEVER, opposite), and make sure he or she drinks plenty of fluids. Occasionally, hospital admission is necessary.

POSSIBLE CAUSES Many viral infections, such as a cold, can cause a cough and runny nose.

ACTION Take steps to reduce your child's temperature (*see* BRINGING DOWN A FEVER, opposite), and give him or her plenty to drink. Call your child's doctor if a rash develops, if your child develops difficulty breathing, or if there is no improvement within 48 hours.

Continued on next page

WARNING

DANGER SIGNS Call an ambulance if your child has a fever that is associated with any of the following symptoms:
- A seizure lasting more than 5 minutes
- Flat, dark red spots that do not fade with pressure (*see* CHECKING A RED RASH, p.79)
- Abnormal drowsiness
- A severe headache

While waiting for medical help, follow the advice for bringing down a fever (p.77).

SELF-HELP Taking your child's temperature

An aural thermometer, placed in the ear, is a convenient, although not precise, method of taking your child's temperature. You can also use a standard thermometer placed in the armpit or in the mouth. Do not put a glass thermometer in the mouth of a child aged under 7. For the correct result, add 1°F (0.6°C) to a reading from the armpit.

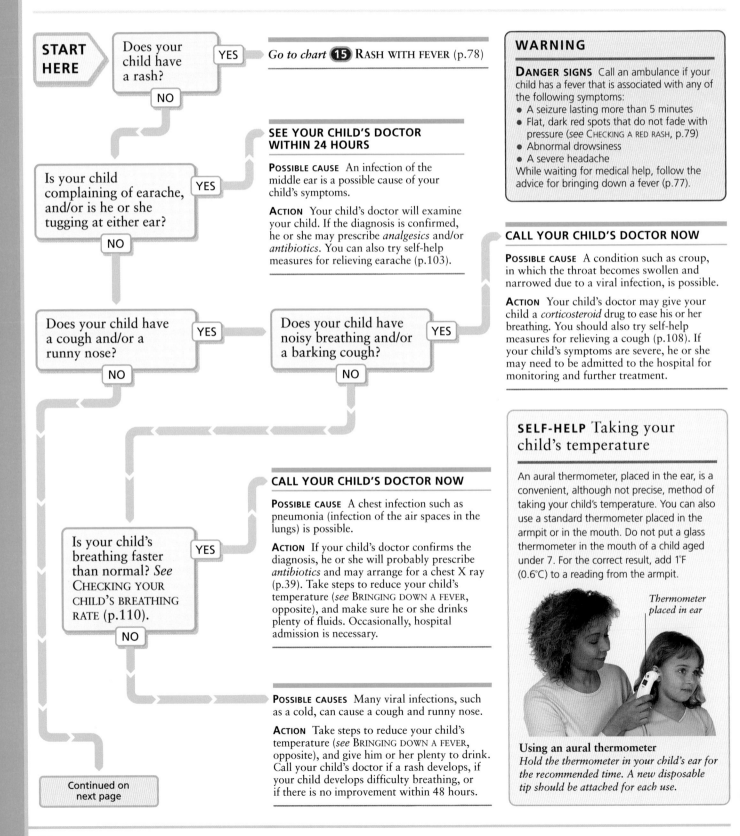

Thermometer placed in ear

Using an aural thermometer
Hold the thermometer in your child's ear for the recommended time. A new disposable tip should be attached for each use.

Continued from previous page

SELF-HELP Bringing down a fever

Lowering a temperature will help your child feel more comfortable and lessens the likelihood of a febrile convulsion occurring (p.55). Remove your child's clothes and give him or her plenty of cold drinks. If your child is over 2 months old, give him or her the recommended dose of acetaminophen. If the fever doesn't fall and your child is over 6 months old, give him or her the recommended dose of ibuprofen as well. The doses of both drugs can be repeated every 4 hours.

Wet face cloth *Drink* *Fan*

Cooling your child
Undress your child, lie him or her in a cool room, and sponge his or her head and body with tepid water.

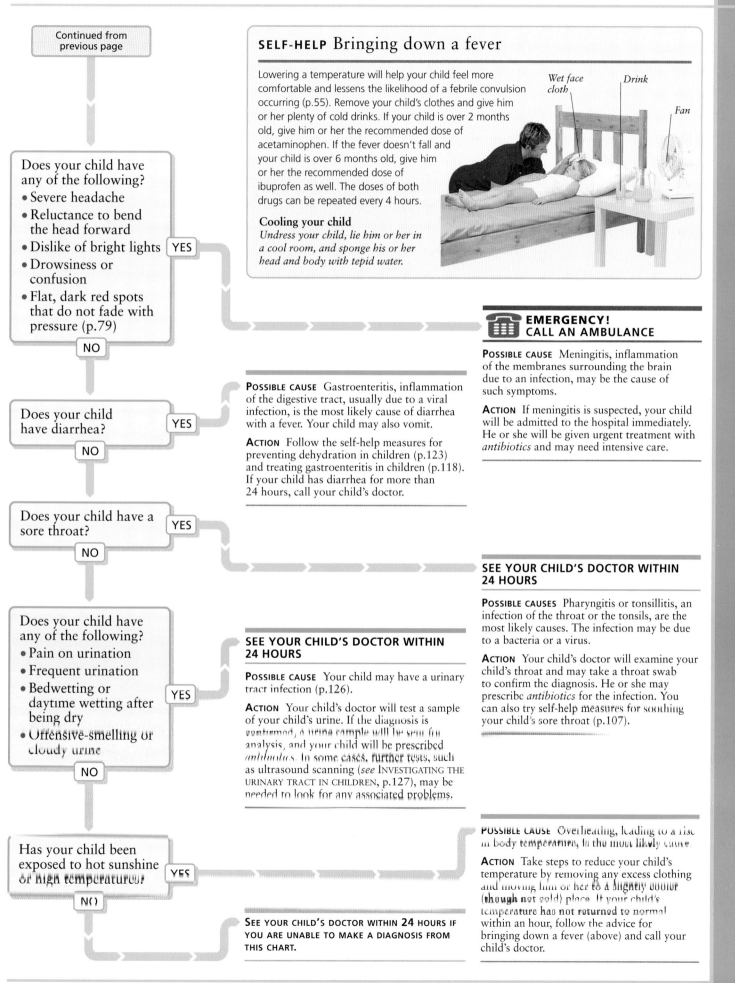

Does your child have any of the following?
- Severe headache
- Reluctance to bend the head forward
- Dislike of bright lights
- Drowsiness or confusion
- Flat, dark red spots that do not fade with pressure (p.79)

YES

NO

EMERGENCY! CALL AN AMBULANCE

POSSIBLE CAUSE Meningitis, inflammation of the membranes surrounding the brain due to an infection, may be the cause of such symptoms.

ACTION If meningitis is suspected, your child will be admitted to the hospital immediately. He or she will be given urgent treatment with *antibiotics* and may need intensive care.

Does your child have diarrhea?

YES

NO

POSSIBLE CAUSE Gastroenteritis, inflammation of the digestive tract, usually due to a viral infection, is the most likely cause of diarrhea with a fever. Your child may also vomit.

ACTION Follow the self-help measures for preventing dehydration in children (p.123) and treating gastroenteritis in children (p.118). If your child has diarrhea for more than 24 hours, call your child's doctor.

Does your child have a sore throat?

YES

NO

SEE YOUR CHILD'S DOCTOR WITHIN 24 HOURS

POSSIBLE CAUSES Pharyngitis or tonsillitis, an infection of the throat or the tonsils, are the most likely causes. The infection may be due to a bacteria or a virus.

ACTION Your child's doctor will examine your child's throat and may take a throat swab to confirm the diagnosis. He or she may prescribe *antibiotics* for the infection. You can also try self-help measures for soothing your child's sore throat (p.107).

Does your child have any of the following?
- Pain on urination
- Frequent urination
- Bedwetting or daytime wetting after being dry
- Offensive-smelling or cloudy urine

YES

NO

SEE YOUR CHILD'S DOCTOR WITHIN 24 HOURS

POSSIBLE CAUSE Your child may have a urinary tract infection (p.126).

ACTION Your child's doctor will test a sample of your child's urine. If the diagnosis is confirmed, a urine sample will be sent for analysis, and your child will be prescribed *antibiotics*. In some cases, further tests, such as ultrasound scanning (*see* INVESTIGATING THE URINARY TRACT IN CHILDREN, p.127), may be needed to look for any associated problems.

Has your child been exposed to hot sunshine or high temperatures?

YES

NO

POSSIBLE CAUSE Overheating, leading to a rise in body temperature, is the most likely cause.

ACTION Take steps to reduce your child's temperature by removing any excess clothing and moving him or her to a slightly cooler (though not cold) place. If your child's temperature has not returned to normal within an hour, follow the advice for bringing down a fever (above) and call your child's doctor.

SEE YOUR CHILD'S DOCTOR WITHIN 24 HOURS IF YOU ARE UNABLE TO MAKE A DIAGNOSIS FROM THIS CHART.

15 Rash with fever

Consult this chart if your child develops a rash anywhere on the body associated with a temperature of 100.4°F (38°C) or higher. In children, this combination of symptoms is often caused by a viral infection, but, in some cases, it can be caused by a serious bacterial infection, such as meningitis, that needs urgent medical attention. Routine immunizations will protect your child against most serious infections. However, your child will still be at risk of developing a number of less serious infections and may even develop a mild form of diseases against which he or she has been immunized.

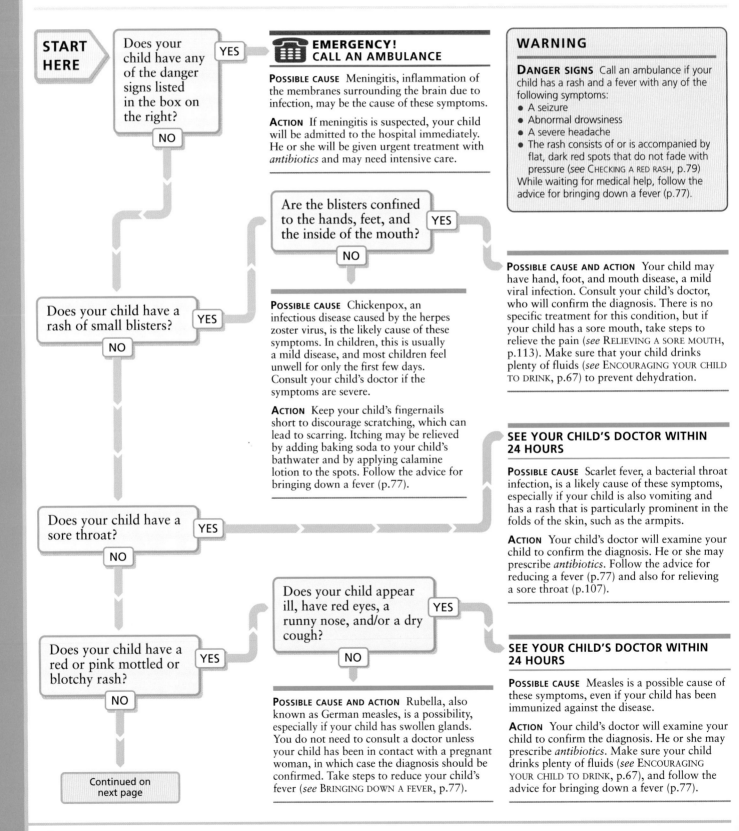

START HERE

Does your child have any of the danger signs listed in the box on the right? YES / NO

YES → **EMERGENCY! CALL AN AMBULANCE**

POSSIBLE CAUSE Meningitis, inflammation of the membranes surrounding the brain due to infection, may be the cause of these symptoms.

ACTION If meningitis is suspected, your child will be admitted to the hospital immediately. He or she will be given urgent treatment with *antibiotics* and may need intensive care.

WARNING

DANGER SIGNS Call an ambulance if your child has a rash and a fever with any of the following symptoms:
- A seizure
- Abnormal drowsiness
- A severe headache
- The rash consists of or is accompanied by flat, dark red spots that do not fade with pressure (*see* CHECKING A RED RASH, p.79)

While waiting for medical help, follow the advice for bringing down a fever (p.77).

Does your child have a rash of small blisters? YES / NO

YES → **Are the blisters confined to the hands, feet, and the inside of the mouth?** YES / NO

NO → **POSSIBLE CAUSE** Chickenpox, an infectious disease caused by the herpes zoster virus, is the likely cause of these symptoms. In children, this is usually a mild disease, and most children feel unwell for only the first few days. Consult your child's doctor if the symptoms are severe.

ACTION Keep your child's fingernails short to discourage scratching, which can lead to scarring. Itching may be relieved by adding baking soda to your child's bathwater and by applying calamine lotion to the spots. Follow the advice for bringing down a fever (p.77).

YES → **POSSIBLE CAUSE AND ACTION** Your child may have hand, foot, and mouth disease, a mild viral infection. Consult your child's doctor, who will confirm the diagnosis. There is no specific treatment for this condition, but if your child has a sore mouth, take steps to relieve the pain (*see* RELIEVING A SORE MOUTH, p.113). Make sure that your child drinks plenty of fluids (*see* ENCOURAGING YOUR CHILD TO DRINK, p.67) to prevent dehydration.

Does your child have a sore throat? YES / NO

YES → **SEE YOUR CHILD'S DOCTOR WITHIN 24 HOURS**

POSSIBLE CAUSE Scarlet fever, a bacterial throat infection, is a likely cause of these symptoms, especially if your child is also vomiting and has a rash that is particularly prominent in the folds of the skin, such as the armpits.

ACTION Your child's doctor will examine your child to confirm the diagnosis. He or she may prescribe *antibiotics*. Follow the advice for reducing a fever (p.77) and also for relieving a sore throat (p.107).

Does your child have a red or pink mottled or blotchy rash? YES / NO

YES → **Does your child appear ill, have red eyes, a runny nose, and/or a dry cough?** YES / NO

NO → **POSSIBLE CAUSE AND ACTION** Rubella, also known as German measles, is a possibility, especially if your child has swollen glands. You do not need to consult a doctor unless your child has been in contact with a pregnant woman, in which case the diagnosis should be confirmed. Take steps to reduce your child's fever (*see* BRINGING DOWN A FEVER, p.77).

YES → **SEE YOUR CHILD'S DOCTOR WITHIN 24 HOURS**

POSSIBLE CAUSE Measles is a possible cause of these symptoms, even if your child has been immunized against the disease.

ACTION Your child's doctor will examine your child to confirm the diagnosis. He or she may prescribe *antibiotics*. Make sure your child drinks plenty of fluids (*see* ENCOURAGING YOUR CHILD TO DRINK, p.67), and follow the advice for bringing down a fever (p.77).

Continued on next page

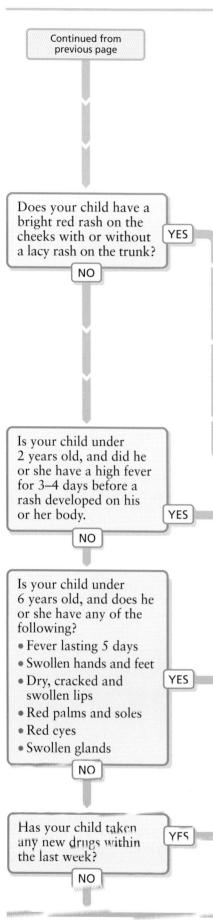

Continued from previous page

Does your child have a bright red rash on the cheeks with or without a lacy rash on the trunk? — YES

NO

Is your child under 2 years old, and did he or she have a high fever for 3–4 days before a rash developed on his or her body. — YES

NO

Is your child under 6 years old, and does he or she have any of the following?
- Fever lasting 5 days
- Swollen hands and feet
- Dry, cracked and swollen lips
- Red palms and soles
- Red eyes
- Swollen glands

YES

NO

Has your child taken any new drugs within the last week? — YES

NO

SEE YOUR CHILD'S DOCTOR WITHIN **24 HOURS** IF YOU ARE UNABLE TO MAKE A DIAGNOSIS FROM THIS CHART.

Infections that cause a rash

Many viral infections cause a fever and a rash. The more serious ones, such as measles, have become much less common as a result of routine immunizations. Many of these infections can also affect adults, whose symptoms can be more severe than children's. The incubation period is the time between acquiring an infection and first developing symptoms.

Disease (incubation period)	Symptoms	Period when infectious
Chickenpox (7–21 days)	Crops of raised, red, itchy spots that turn into blisters and then scabs, mainly on face and trunk	From 2 days before the rash develops until all the blisters have scabs
Erythema infectiosum (4–20 days)	Bright red cheeks; lacy rash, mainly on trunk	Until the rash develops
Hand, foot, and mouth disease (4 days)	Mild fever; rash of small blisters on hands, feet, and inside of mouth	For duration of blisters
Measles (7–14 days)	Cough; runny nose; red eyes; mottled or blotchy red rash, first on the face, then trunk and arms	Until 5 days after the rash develops
Roseola infantum (variable)	High fever followed by flat, light-red rash on the trunk; swollen glands in the neck	Until 5 days after the onset of the symptoms
Rubella (14–19 days)	Mild fever; swollen glands in the neck; flat pink mottled or blotchy rash, mainly on face and trunk	From 1 week before the rash develops until 5 days after the rash develops or until the rash disappears
Scarlet fever (2–5 days)	High fever; severe sore throat; vomiting; red rash on body, most obvious in skin folds	Until 24 hours after antibiotics are started

POSSIBLE CAUSE AND ACTION Your child may have roseola infantum, a common early childhood infection. This condition is difficult to diagnose before the rash appears as the fever is the only symptom. By the time the rash appears, the child is usually better. If you suspect that your child has this condition and he or she still has a fever, consult your child's doctor. He or she will examine your child and may do tests to exclude more serious problems.

CALL YOUR CHILD'S DOCTOR NOW

POSSIBLE CAUSE Kawasaki disease, a rare condition of unknown cause, which can damage the heart and joints, is a possibility.

ACTION If your child's doctor suspects that your child has Kawasaki disease, your child will be admitted to the hospital, where his or her condition can be monitored and treatment given to reduce the risk of heart complications.

CALL YOUR CHILD'S DOCTOR NOW

POSSIBLE CAUSES Your child may have an allergy to the prescribed medicine, or he or she may have a viral illness unrelated to the drug.

ACTION Your child's doctor will examine your child to determine the cause of the symptoms. If your child does have a drug allergy, the doctor will be able to tell you whether your child should avoid this drug in the future.

POSSIBLE CAUSE AND ACTION Your child may have erethema infectiosum, although 70–85 percent of the time, this viral infection is not accompanied by fever. Also known as slapped-cheek disease or fifth disease, this condition is usually mild. Follow the advice on reducing a fever (p.77). The diagnosis should be confirmed if your child has been in contact with a pregnant woman. If you are worried or your child is no better in 48 hours, call the doctor.

Checking a red rash

If you or your child develops dark red or purple blotches, check whether they fade with pressure by pressing a clear glass against them. If the rash is visible through the glass, it may be a form of purpura, which is caused by bleeding under the skin and may occur in meningitis. If you or your child has a nonfading rash, call an ambulance.

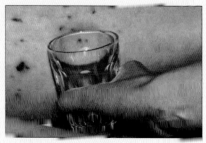

Checking a rash
Here, the rash is still visible when the glass is pressed against the skin, a sign that it may be caused by an illness such as meningitis.

16 Skin problems in children

For skin problems in children under 1, see chart 8, SKIN
PROBLEMS IN BABIES (p.64).
Childhood spots and rashes are usually due to irritation or
inflammation of the skin as a result of a local problem such as
an allergic reaction. However, a rash associated with a fever

may be due to a generalized infection (*see* VIRAL INFECTIONS
THAT CAUSE A RASH, p.79). A rash without a fever or feeling
sick is probably no cause for concern; but if it is itchy or
sore, consult your child's doctor. Call an ambulance if a rash
is accompanied by difficulty breathing and/or facial swelling.

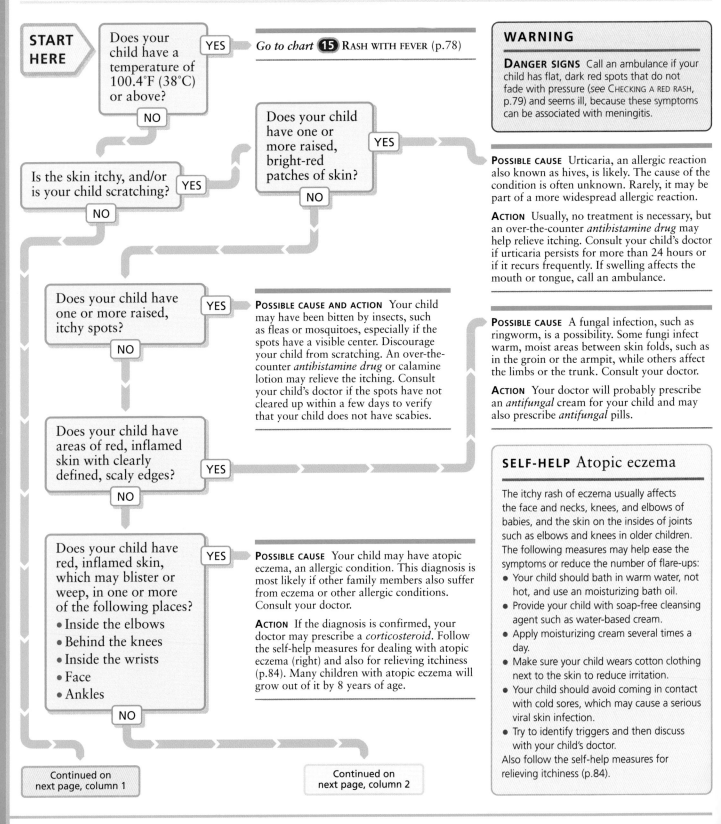

START HERE

Does your child have a temperature of 100.4°F (38°C) or above?
— **YES** → *Go to chart* **15** RASH WITH FEVER (p.78)
— **NO**

Is the skin itchy, and/or is your child scratching?
— **YES** → Does your child have one or more raised, bright-red patches of skin?
  — **YES**
  — **NO**
— **NO**

Does your child have one or more raised, itchy spots?
— **YES** → **POSSIBLE CAUSE AND ACTION** Your child may have been bitten by insects, such as fleas or mosquitoes, especially if the spots have a visible center. Discourage your child from scratching. An over-the-counter *antihistamine drug* or calamine lotion may relieve the itching. Consult your child's doctor if the spots have not cleared up within a few days to verify that your child does not have scabies.
— **NO**

Does your child have areas of red, inflamed skin with clearly defined, scaly edges?
— **YES**
— **NO**

Does your child have red, inflamed skin, which may blister or weep, in one or more of the following places?
- Inside the elbows
- Behind the knees
- Inside the wrists
- Face
- Ankles
— **YES** → **POSSIBLE CAUSE** Your child may have atopic eczema, an allergic condition. This diagnosis is most likely if other family members also suffer from eczema or other allergic conditions. Consult your doctor.

ACTION If the diagnosis is confirmed, your doctor may prescribe a *corticosteroid*. Follow the self-help measures for dealing with atopic eczema (right) and also for relieving itchiness (p.84). Many children with atopic eczema will grow out of it by 8 years of age.
— **NO**

WARNING

DANGER SIGNS Call an ambulance if your child has flat, dark red spots that do not fade with pressure (*see* CHECKING A RED RASH, p.79) and seems ill, because these symptoms can be associated with meningitis.

POSSIBLE CAUSE Urticaria, an allergic reaction also known as hives, is likely. The cause of the condition is often unknown. Rarely, it may be part of a more widespread allergic reaction.

ACTION Usually, no treatment is necessary, but an over-the-counter *antihistamine drug* may help relieve itching. Consult your child's doctor if urticaria persists for more than 24 hours or if it recurs frequently. If swelling affects the mouth or tongue, call an ambulance.

POSSIBLE CAUSE A fungal infection, such as ringworm, is a possibility. Some fungi infect warm, moist areas between skin folds, such as in the groin or the armpit, while others affect the limbs or the trunk. Consult your doctor.

ACTION Your doctor will probably prescribe an *antifungal* cream for your child and may also prescribe *antifungal* pills.

SELF-HELP Atopic eczema

The itchy rash of eczema usually affects the face and necks, knees, and elbows of babies, and the skin on the insides of joints such as elbows and knees in older children. The following measures may help ease the symptoms or reduce the number of flare-ups.
- Your child should bath in warm water, not hot, and use an moisturizing bath oil.
- Provide your child with soap-free cleansing agent such as water-based cream.
- Apply moisturizing cream several times a day.
- Make sure your child wears cotton clothing next to the skin to reduce irritation.
- Your child should avoid coming in contact with cold sores, which may cause a serious viral skin infection.
- Try to identify triggers and then discuss with your child's doctor.
Also follow the self-help measures for relieving itchiness (p.84).

Continued on next page, column 1

Continued on next page, column 2

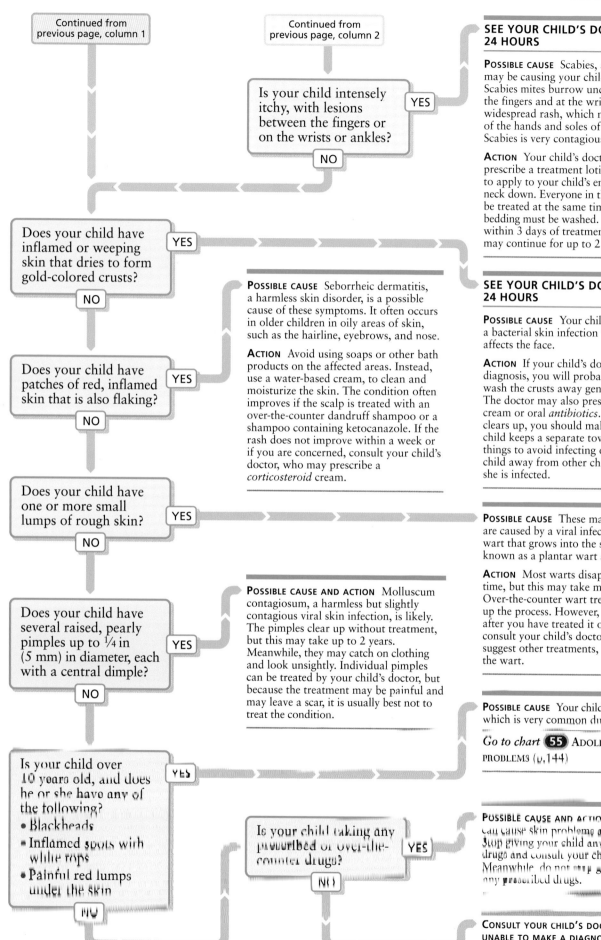

Continued from previous page, column 1

Continued from previous page, column 2

Is your child intensely itchy, with lesions between the fingers or on the wrists or ankles? **YES** / **NO**

Does your child have inflamed or weeping skin that dries to form gold-colored crusts? **YES** / **NO**

Does your child have patches of red, inflamed skin that is also flaking? **YES** / **NO**

Does your child have one or more small lumps of rough skin? **YES** / **NO**

Does your child have several raised, pearly pimples up to ¼ in (5 mm) in diameter, each with a central dimple? **YES** / **NO**

Is your child over 10 years old, and does he or she have any of the following?
• Blackheads
• Inflamed spots with white tops
• Painful red lumps under the skin
YES / **NO**

Is your child taking any prescribed or over-the-counter drugs? **YES** / **NO**

POSSIBLE CAUSE Seborrheic dermatitis, a harmless skin disorder, is a possible cause of these symptoms. It often occurs in older children in oily areas of skin, such as the hairline, eyebrows, and nose.

ACTION Avoid using soaps or other bath products on the affected areas. Instead, use a water-based cream, to clean and moisturize the skin. The condition often improves if the scalp is treated with an over-the-counter dandruff shampoo or a shampoo containing ketocanazole. If the rash does not improve within a week or if you are concerned, consult your child's doctor, who may prescribe a *corticosteroid* cream.

POSSIBLE CAUSE AND ACTION Molluscum contagiosum, a harmless but slightly contagious viral skin infection, is likely. The pimples clear up without treatment, but this may take up to 2 years. Meanwhile, they may catch on clothing and look unsightly. Individual pimples can be treated by your child's doctor, but because the treatment may be painful and may leave a scar, it is usually best not to treat the condition.

SEE YOUR CHILD'S DOCTOR WITHIN 24 HOURS

POSSIBLE CAUSE Scabies, a parasitic infection, may be causing your child's symptoms. Scabies mites burrow under the skin between the fingers and at the wrists and can cause a widespread rash, which may affect the palms of the hands and soles of the feet in babies. Scabies is very contagious.

ACTION Your child's doctor will probably prescribe a treatment lotion, which you need to apply to your child's entire body from the neck down. Everyone in the household must be treated at the same time, and clothing and bedding must be washed. The mites should die within 3 days of treatment, but the itching may continue for up to 2 weeks.

SEE YOUR CHILD'S DOCTOR WITHIN 24 HOURS

POSSIBLE CAUSE Your child may have impetigo, a bacterial skin infection that commonly affects the face.

ACTION If your child's doctor confirms the diagnosis, you will probably be advised to wash the crusts away gently with warm water. The doctor may also prescribe an *antibiotic* cream or oral *antibiotics*. Until the infection clears up, you should make sure that your child keeps a separate towel and other wash things to avoid infecting others. Keep your child away from other children while he or she is infected.

POSSIBLE CAUSE These may be warts, which are caused by a viral infection of the skin. A wart that grows into the sole of the foot is known as a plantar wart and may be painful.

ACTION Most warts disappear naturally in time, but this may take months or years. Over-the-counter wart treatments may speed up the process. However, if a wart persists after you have treated it or if it is painful, consult your child's doctor. He or she may suggest other treatments, such as freezing the wart.

POSSIBLE CAUSE Your child may have acne, which is very common during adolescence.

Go to chart **55** ADOLESCENT SKIN PROBLEMS (p.144)

POSSIBLE CAUSE AND ACTION Certain drugs can cause skin problems as a side effect. Stop giving your child any over-the-counter drugs and consult your child's doctor. Meanwhile, do not stop giving your child any prescribed drugs.

CONSULT YOUR CHILD'S DOCTOR IF YOU ARE UNABLE TO MAKE A DIAGNOSIS FROM THIS CHART.

17 Hair, scalp, and nail problems

Consult this chart if your child has any problems affecting the hair, scalp, fingernails, or toenails. In general, eating a well-balanced diet will help keep your child's hair and nails strong and healthy. Use a soft hairbrush on a young child's hair because it can be easily damaged. If your child's hair is long, avoid braiding it tightly or using uncovered rubber bands to tie it back. In children, the most common hair problems needing treatment are fungal infections and head lice.

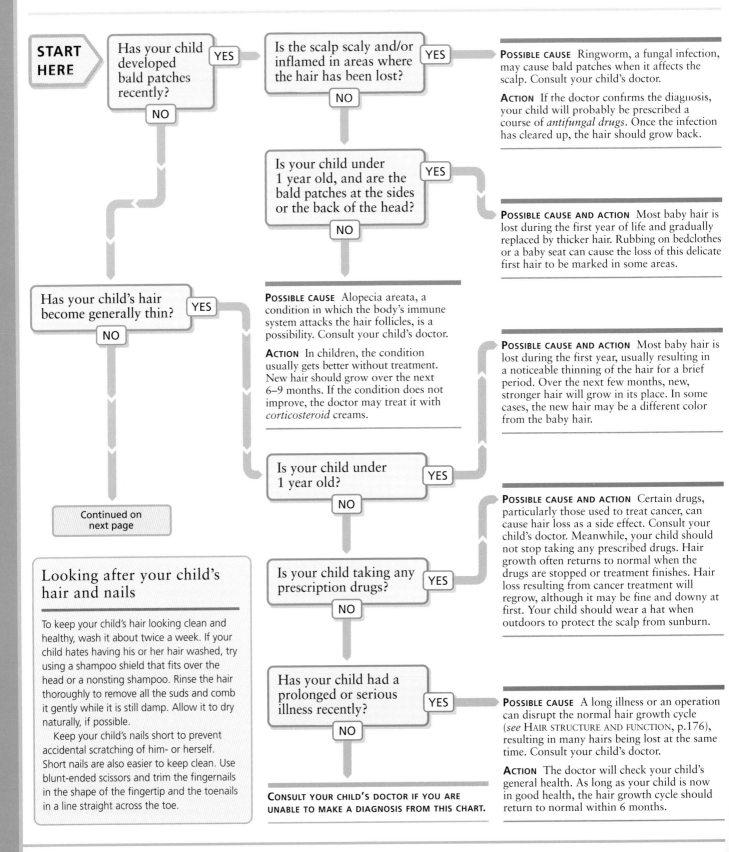

START HERE

Has your child developed bald patches recently? — **YES** → **Is the scalp scaly and/or inflamed in areas where the hair has been lost?** — **YES** → **POSSIBLE CAUSE** Ringworm, a fungal infection, may cause bald patches when it affects the scalp. Consult your child's doctor.

ACTION If the doctor confirms the diagnosis, your child will probably be prescribed a course of *antifungal drugs*. Once the infection has cleared up, the hair should grow back.

NO → **Is your child under 1 year old, and are the bald patches at the sides or the back of the head?** — **YES** → **POSSIBLE CAUSE AND ACTION** Most baby hair is lost during the first year of life and gradually replaced by thicker hair. Rubbing on bedclothes or a baby seat can cause the loss of this delicate first hair to be marked in some areas.

POSSIBLE CAUSE Alopecia areata, a condition in which the body's immune system attacks the hair follicles, is a possibility. Consult your child's doctor.

ACTION In children, the condition usually gets better without treatment. New hair should grow over the next 6–9 months. If the condition does not improve, the doctor may treat it with *corticosteroid* creams.

Has your child's hair become generally thin? — **YES** →

NO → Continued on next page

Is your child under 1 year old? — **YES** → **POSSIBLE CAUSE AND ACTION** Most baby hair is lost during the first year, usually resulting in a noticeable thinning of the hair for a brief period. Over the next few months, new, stronger hair will grow in its place. In some cases, the new hair may be a different color from the baby hair.

NO → **Is your child taking any prescription drugs?** — **YES** → **POSSIBLE CAUSE AND ACTION** Certain drugs, particularly those used to treat cancer, can cause hair loss as a side effect. Consult your child's doctor. Meanwhile, your child should not stop taking any prescribed drugs. Hair growth often returns to normal when the drugs are stopped or treatment finishes. Hair loss resulting from cancer treatment will regrow, although it may be fine and downy at first. Your child should wear a hat when outdoors to protect the scalp from sunburn.

NO → **Has your child had a prolonged or serious illness recently?** — **YES** → **POSSIBLE CAUSE** A long illness or an operation can disrupt the normal hair growth cycle (*see* HAIR STRUCTURE AND FUNCTION, p.176), resulting in many hairs being lost at the same time. Consult your child's doctor.

ACTION The doctor will check your child's general health. As long as your child is now in good health, the hair growth cycle should return to normal within 6 months.

NO → **CONSULT YOUR CHILD'S DOCTOR IF YOU ARE UNABLE TO MAKE A DIAGNOSIS FROM THIS CHART.**

Looking after your child's hair and nails

To keep your child's hair looking clean and healthy, wash it about twice a week. If your child hates having his or her hair washed, try using a shampoo shield that fits over the head or a nonsting shampoo. Rinse the hair thoroughly to remove all the suds and comb it gently while it is still damp. Allow it to dry naturally, if possible.

Keep your child's nails short to prevent accidental scratching of him- or herself. Short nails are also easier to keep clean. Use blunt-ended scissors and trim the fingernails in the shape of the fingertip and the toenails in a line straight across the toe.

Continued from
previous page

SELF-HELP Treating head lice

Contrary to popular belief, head lice prefer clean, not dirty, hair. Head lice can be treated with an over-the-counter lotion or shampoo. Follow the directions on the package, and then remove the dead lice and their eggs, known as nits, by combing through the hair with a fine-toothed nit comb. Alternatively, try coating the hair in conditioner and combing it through with a nit comb daily, or using a battery-operated comb that electrocutes the lice. Whichever method you use, treat everyone in the household and wash all combs and towels in hot water to prevent reinfestations.

Removing lice and eggs
Carefully combing through your child's hair with a fine-toothed nit comb will remove eggs and dead lice.

Fine-toothed nit comb

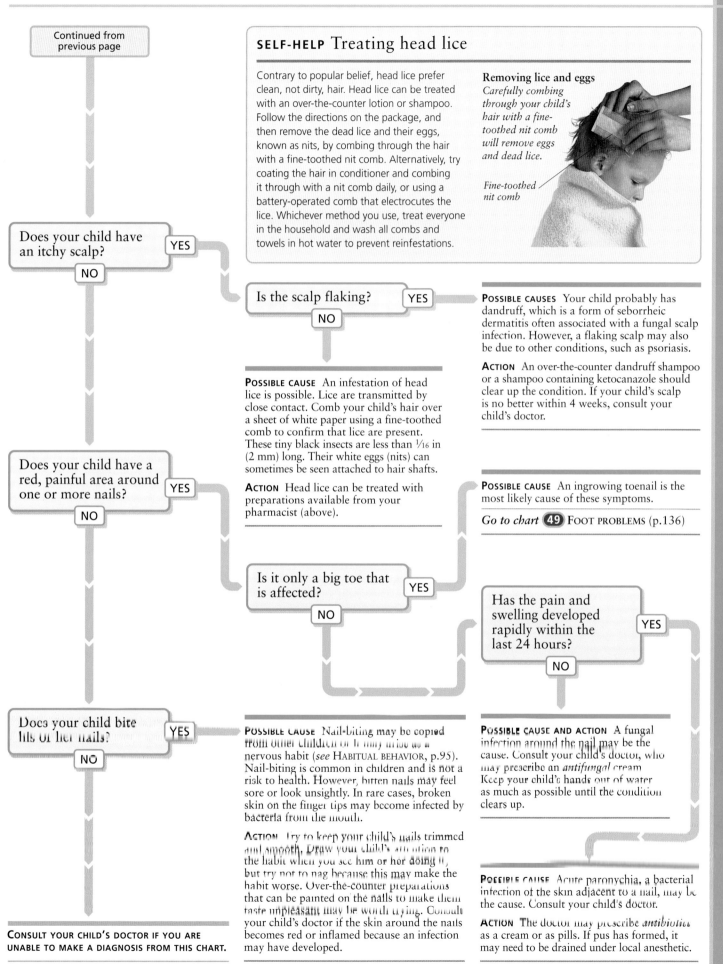

Does your child have an itchy scalp? — YES

NO

Is the scalp flaking? — YES

NO

POSSIBLE CAUSES Your child probably has dandruff, which is a form of seborrheic dermatitis often associated with a fungal scalp infection. However, a flaking scalp may also be due to other conditions, such as psoriasis.

ACTION An over-the-counter dandruff shampoo or a shampoo containing ketocanazole should clear up the condition. If your child's scalp is no better within 4 weeks, consult your child's doctor.

POSSIBLE CAUSE An infestation of head lice is possible. Lice are transmitted by close contact. Comb your child's hair over a sheet of white paper using a fine-toothed comb to confirm that lice are present. These tiny black insects are less than 1/16 in (2 mm) long. Their white eggs (nits) can sometimes be seen attached to hair shafts.

ACTION Head lice can be treated with preparations available from your pharmacist (above).

Does your child have a red, painful area around one or more nails? — YES

NO

POSSIBLE CAUSE An ingrowing toenail is the most likely cause of these symptoms.

Go to chart **49** FOOT PROBLEMS (p.136)

Is it only a big toe that is affected? — YES

NO

Has the pain and swelling developed rapidly within the last 24 hours? — YES

NO

Does your child bite his or her nails? — YES

NO

POSSIBLE CAUSE Nail-biting may be copied from other children or it may arise as a nervous habit (*see* HABITUAL BEHAVIOR, p.95). Nail-biting is common in children and is not a risk to health. However, bitten nails may feel sore or look unsightly. In rare cases, broken skin on the finger tips may become infected by bacteria from the mouth.

ACTION Try to keep your child's nails trimmed and smooth. Draw your child's attention to the habit when you see him or her doing it, but try not to nag because this may make the habit worse. Over-the-counter preparations that can be painted on the nails to make them taste unpleasant may be worth trying. Consult your child's doctor if the skin around the nails becomes red or inflamed because an infection may have developed.

POSSIBLE CAUSE AND ACTION A fungal infection around the nail may be the cause. Consult your child's doctor, who may prescribe an *antifungal* cream. Keep your child's hands out of water as much as possible until the condition clears up.

POSSIBLE CAUSE Acute paronychia, a bacterial infection of the skin adjacent to a nail, may be the cause. Consult your child's doctor.

ACTION The doctor may prescribe *antibiotics* as a cream or as pills. If pus has formed, it may need to be drained under local anesthetic.

CONSULT YOUR CHILD'S DOCTOR IF YOU ARE UNABLE TO MAKE A DIAGNOSIS FROM THIS CHART.

18 Itching

Itching is a common and distressing symptom for a child and can have a variety of causes, including external irritants or infestation by parasites. It is important to deal promptly with any disorder that produces itching because, if it persists, scratching can lead to an infection or changes in the skin, which can, in turn, lead to further itching.

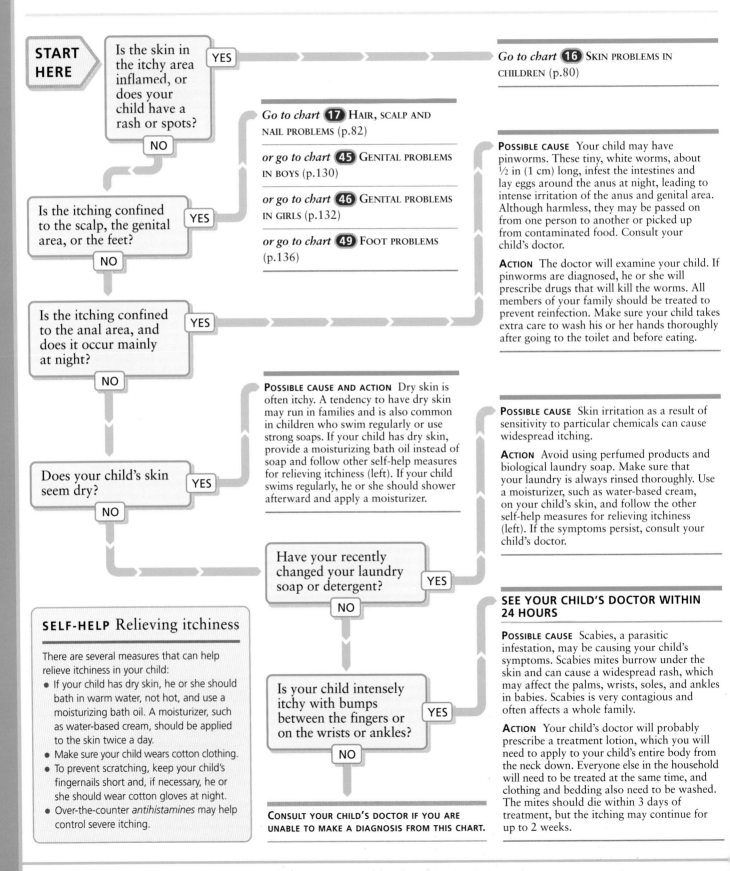

START HERE

Is the skin in the itchy area inflamed, or does your child have a rash or spots?

YES → *Go to chart* **16** SKIN PROBLEMS IN CHILDREN (p.80)

NO

Is the itching confined to the scalp, the genital area, or the feet?

YES → *Go to chart* **17** HAIR, SCALP AND NAIL PROBLEMS (p.82)

or go to chart **45** GENITAL PROBLEMS IN BOYS (p.130)

or go to chart **46** GENITAL PROBLEMS IN GIRLS (p.132)

or go to chart **49** FOOT PROBLEMS (p.136)

NO

Is the itching confined to the anal area, and does it occur mainly at night?

YES → **POSSIBLE CAUSE** Your child may have pinworms. These tiny, white worms, about ½ in (1 cm) long, infest the intestines and lay eggs around the anus at night, leading to intense irritation of the anus and genital area. Although harmless, they may be passed on from one person to another or picked up from contaminated food. Consult your child's doctor.

ACTION The doctor will examine your child. If pinworms are diagnosed, he or she will prescribe drugs that will kill the worms. All members of your family should be treated to prevent reinfection. Make sure your child takes extra care to wash his or her hands thoroughly after going to the toilet and before eating.

NO

Does your child's skin seem dry?

YES → **POSSIBLE CAUSE AND ACTION** Dry skin is often itchy. A tendency to have dry skin may run in families and is also common in children who swim regularly or use strong soaps. If your child has dry skin, provide a moisturizing bath oil instead of soap and follow other self-help measures for relieving itchiness (left). If your child swims regularly, he or she should shower afterward and apply a moisturizer.

NO

Have your recently changed your laundry soap or detergent?

YES → **POSSIBLE CAUSE** Skin irritation as a result of sensitivity to particular chemicals can cause widespread itching.

ACTION Avoid using perfumed products and biological laundry soap. Make sure that your laundry is always rinsed thoroughly. Use a moisturizer, such as water-based cream, on your child's skin, and follow the other self-help measures for relieving itchiness (left). If the symptoms persist, consult your child's doctor.

NO

Is your child intensely itchy with bumps between the fingers or on the wrists or ankles?

YES → **SEE YOUR CHILD'S DOCTOR WITHIN 24 HOURS**

POSSIBLE CAUSE Scabies, a parasitic infestation, may be causing your child's symptoms. Scabies mites burrow under the skin and can cause a widespread rash, which may affect the palms, wrists, soles, and ankles in babies. Scabies is very contagious and often affects a whole family.

ACTION Your child's doctor will probably prescribe a treatment lotion, which you will need to apply to your child's entire body from the neck down. Everyone else in the household will need to be treated at the same time, and clothing and bedding also need to be washed. The mites should die within 3 days of treatment, but the itching may continue for up to 2 weeks.

NO

CONSULT YOUR CHILD'S DOCTOR IF YOU ARE UNABLE TO MAKE A DIAGNOSIS FROM THIS CHART.

SELF-HELP Relieving itchiness

There are several measures that can help relieve itchiness in your child:
- If your child has dry skin, he or she should bath in warm water, not hot, and use a moisturizing bath oil. A moisturizer, such as water-based cream, should be applied to the skin twice a day.
- Make sure your child wears cotton clothing.
- To prevent scratching, keep your child's fingernails short and, if necessary, he or she should wear cotton gloves at night.
- Over-the-counter *antihistamines* may help control severe itching.

19 Lumps and swellings

For lumps and swellings in the scrotum, see chart 45, GENITAL PROBLEMS IN BOYS (p.130).
Consult this chart if your child has lumps or swellings on any area of the body. Lumps and swellings under the surface of the skin are often lymph nodes, commonly known as glands, that have enlarged in response to an infection. Other lumps and swellings may be due to injuries, bites, or stings. A persistent lump or swelling should always be examined by a doctor so that the cause can be established. However, there is rarely cause for serious concern in a child.

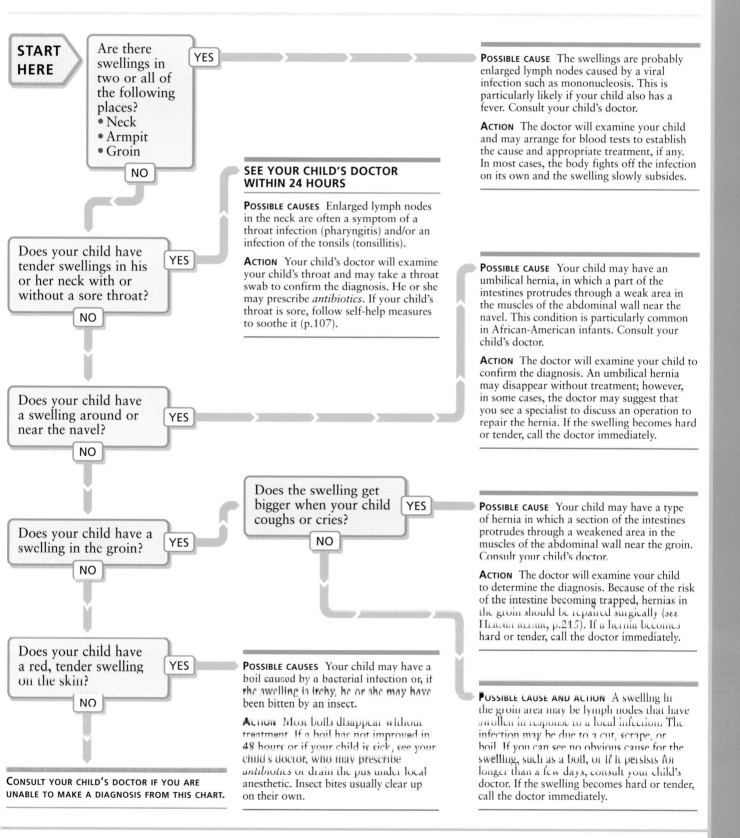

START HERE

Are there swellings in two or all of the following places?
• Neck
• Armpit
• Groin

YES →

POSSIBLE CAUSE The swellings are probably enlarged lymph nodes caused by a viral infection such as mononucleosis. This is particularly likely if your child also has a fever. Consult your child's doctor.

ACTION The doctor will examine your child and may arrange for blood tests to establish the cause and appropriate treatment, if any. In most cases, the body fights off the infection on its own and the swelling slowly subsides.

NO ↓

Does your child have tender swellings in his or her neck with or without a sore throat?

YES →

SEE YOUR CHILD'S DOCTOR WITHIN 24 HOURS

POSSIBLE CAUSES Enlarged lymph nodes in the neck are often a symptom of a throat infection (pharyngitis) and/or an infection of the tonsils (tonsillitis).

ACTION Your child's doctor will examine your child's throat and may take a throat swab to confirm the diagnosis. He or she may prescribe *antibiotics*. If your child's throat is sore, follow self-help measures to soothe it (p.107).

NO ↓

Does your child have a swelling around or near the navel?

YES →

POSSIBLE CAUSE Your child may have an umbilical hernia, in which a part of the intestines protrudes through a weak area in the muscles of the abdominal wall near the navel. This condition is particularly common in African-American infants. Consult your child's doctor.

ACTION The doctor will examine your child to confirm the diagnosis. An umbilical hernia may disappear without treatment; however, in some cases, the doctor may suggest that you see a specialist to discuss an operation to repair the hernia. If the swelling becomes hard or tender, call the doctor immediately.

NO ↓

Does your child have a swelling in the groin?

YES →

Does the swelling get bigger when your child coughs or cries?

YES →

POSSIBLE CAUSE Your child may have a type of hernia in which a section of the intestines protrudes through a weakened area in the muscles of the abdominal wall near the groin. Consult your child's doctor.

ACTION The doctor will examine your child to determine the diagnosis. Because of the risk of the intestine becoming trapped, hernias in the groin should be repaired surgically (see INGUINAL HERNIA, p.215). If a hernia becomes hard or tender, call the doctor immediately.

NO ↓ (from groin question)

NO (from coughs/cries question)

Does your child have a red, tender swelling on the skin?

YES →

POSSIBLE CAUSES Your child may have a boil caused by a bacterial infection or, if the swelling is itchy, he or she may have been bitten by an insect.

ACTION Most boils disappear without treatment. If a boil has not improved in 48 hours or if your child is sick, see your child's doctor, who may prescribe *antibiotics* or drain the pus under local anesthetic. Insect bites usually clear up on their own.

NO ↓

CONSULT YOUR CHILD'S DOCTOR IF YOU ARE UNABLE TO MAKE A DIAGNOSIS FROM THIS CHART.

POSSIBLE CAUSE AND ACTION A swelling in the groin area may be lymph nodes that have swollen in response to a local infection. The infection may be due to a cut, scrape, or boil. If you can see no obvious cause for the swelling, such as a boil, or if it persists for longer than a few days, consult your child's doctor. If the swelling becomes hard or tender, call the doctor immediately.

20 Dizziness, fainting, and seizures

A brief loss of consciousness in a child is usually due to fainting and is seldom serious. However, if the loss of consciousness is accompanied by abnormal movements, such as jerking limbs, the child may be having a seizure. There are several possible causes for a seizure, some of which need urgent treatment. Children often become dizzy as a result of games that involve spinning or amusement park rides, but dizziness for no obvious reason could be due to problems with the balance mechanism in the ear. If your child has regular episodes of dizziness or a seizure, consult your child's doctor. Keep an accurate account of the episode and any related symptoms to help the doctor establish the cause.

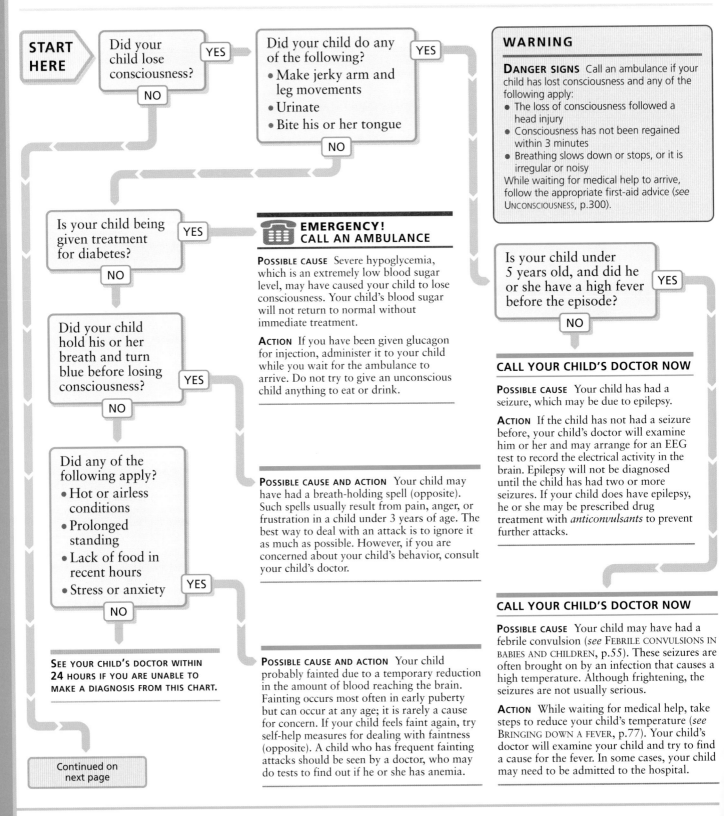

START HERE → **Did your child lose consciousness?** — YES → **Did your child do any of the following?**
• Make jerky arm and leg movements
• Urinate
• Bite his or her tongue
— YES →

NO ↓ (from "Did your child lose consciousness?")

NO ↓ (from "Did your child do any of the following?")

WARNING

DANGER SIGNS Call an ambulance if your child has lost consciousness and any of the following apply:
• The loss of consciousness followed a head injury
• Consciousness has not been regained within 3 minutes
• Breathing slows down or stops, or it is irregular or noisy
While waiting for medical help to arrive, follow the appropriate first-aid advice (see UNCONSCIOUSNESS, p.300).

Is your child being given treatment for diabetes? — YES →

NO ↓

☎ **EMERGENCY! CALL AN AMBULANCE**

POSSIBLE CAUSE Severe hypoglycemia, which is an extremely low blood sugar level, may have caused your child to lose consciousness. Your child's blood sugar will not return to normal without immediate treatment.

ACTION If you have been given glucagon for injection, administer it to your child while you wait for the ambulance to arrive. Do not try to give an unconscious child anything to eat or drink.

Is your child under 5 years old, and did he or she have a high fever before the episode? — YES →

NO ↓

Did your child hold his or her breath and turn blue before losing consciousness? — YES →

NO ↓

POSSIBLE CAUSE AND ACTION Your child may have had a breath-holding spell (opposite). Such spells usually result from pain, anger, or frustration in a child under 3 years of age. The best way to deal with an attack is to ignore it as much as possible. However, if you are concerned about your child's behavior, consult your child's doctor.

CALL YOUR CHILD'S DOCTOR NOW

POSSIBLE CAUSE Your child has had a seizure, which may be due to epilepsy.

ACTION If the child has not had a seizure before, your child's doctor will examine him or her and may arrange for an EEG test to record the electrical activity in the brain. Epilepsy will not be diagnosed until the child has had two or more seizures. If your child does have epilepsy, he or she may be prescribed drug treatment with *anticonvulsants* to prevent further attacks.

Did any of the following apply?
• Hot or airless conditions
• Prolonged standing
• Lack of food in recent hours
• Stress or anxiety
— YES →

NO ↓

SEE YOUR CHILD'S DOCTOR WITHIN 24 HOURS IF YOU ARE UNABLE TO MAKE A DIAGNOSIS FROM THIS CHART.

POSSIBLE CAUSE AND ACTION Your child probably fainted due to a temporary reduction in the amount of blood reaching the brain. Fainting occurs most often in early puberty but can occur at any age; it is rarely a cause for concern. If your child feels faint again, try self-help measures for dealing with faintness (opposite). A child who has frequent fainting attacks should be seen by a doctor, who may do tests to find out if he or she has anemia.

CALL YOUR CHILD'S DOCTOR NOW

POSSIBLE CAUSE Your child may have had a febrile convulsion (*see* FEBRILE CONVULSIONS IN BABIES AND CHILDREN, p.55). These seizures are often brought on by an infection that causes a high temperature. Although frightening, the seizures are not usually serious.

ACTION While waiting for medical help, take steps to reduce your child's temperature (*see* BRINGING DOWN A FEVER, p.77). Your child's doctor will examine your child and try to find a cause for the fever. In some cases, your child may need to be admitted to the hospital.

Continued on next page

Continued from previous page

Does your child have episodes in which he or she seems unaware of the surroundings for a few moments? **YES** ▸

NO

Is your child suffering from any of the following?
• The sensation that everything is spinning
• Loss of balance
• Nausea or vomiting **YES** ▸

NO

Does your child feel unsteady or faint? **YES** ▸

NO

SEE YOUR CHILD'S DOCTOR WITHIN 24 HOURS IF YOU ARE UNABLE TO MAKE A DIAGNOSIS FROM THIS CHART.

Is your child being treated for diabetes? **YES** ▸

NO

POSSIBLE CAUSE AND ACTION Feeling faint is not uncommon in children, especially if they are in a stuffy atmosphere, hungry, or anxious, and is rarely a cause for concern. Follow self-help measures for dealing with faintness (above). Consult your child's doctor if your child has frequent fainting attacks; the doctor may need to determine whether your child has anemia.

SELF-HELP Dealing with faintness

If your child suddenly turns pale, complains that his or her vision is closing in, and/or appears confused, he or she may be feeling faint. This condition is more likely if the atmosphere is hot or stuffy, if your child has not eaten, if he or she has been standing for a long time, or is particularly stressed or anxious. Your child should lie down with his or her feet raised to improve the blood flow to the brain. Make sure that plenty of fresh air is available, and loosen the child's clothes, if necessary. If you are sure that your child is fully conscious, offer him or her a sweet drink in order to raise the blood sugar level. If your child loses consciousness and does not regain it within 3 minutes, call an ambulance and administer first aid (*see* UNCONSCIOUSNESS, p.300).

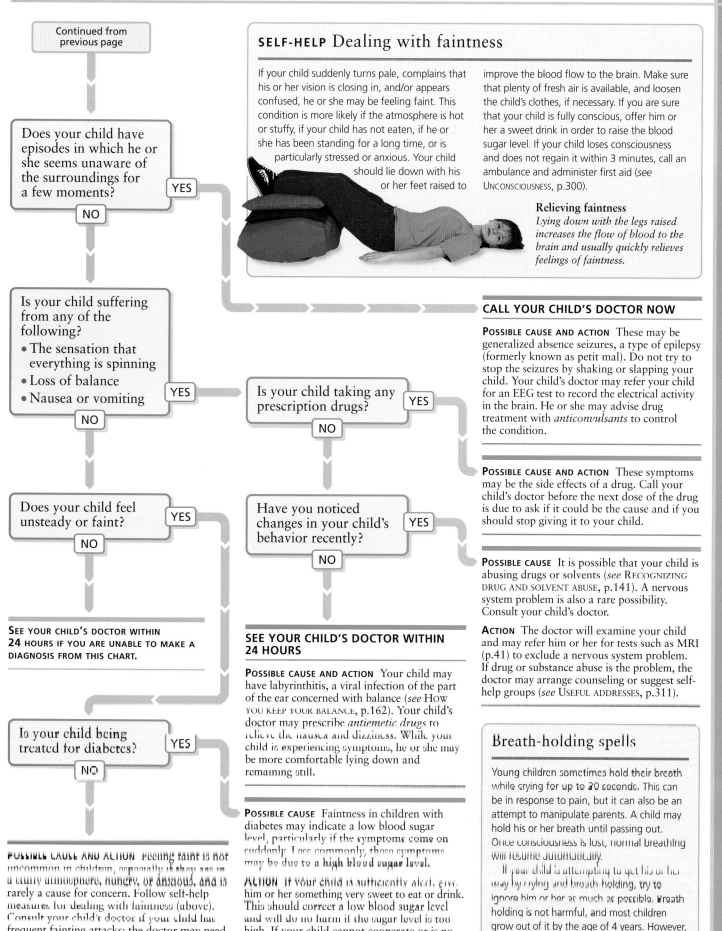

Relieving faintness
Lying down with the legs raised increases the flow of blood to the brain and usually quickly relieves feelings of faintness.

Is your child taking any prescription drugs? **YES** ▸

NO

Have you noticed changes in your child's behavior recently? **YES** ▸

NO

SEE YOUR CHILD'S DOCTOR WITHIN 24 HOURS

POSSIBLE CAUSE AND ACTION Your child may have labyrinthitis, a viral infection of the part of the ear concerned with balance (*see* HOW YOU KEEP YOUR BALANCE, p.162). Your child's doctor may prescribe *antiemetic drugs* to relieve the nausea and dizziness. While your child is experiencing symptoms, he or she may be more comfortable lying down and remaining still.

POSSIBLE CAUSE Faintness in children with diabetes may indicate a low blood sugar level, particularly if the symptoms come on suddenly. Less commonly, these symptoms may be due to a high blood sugar level.

ACTION If your child is sufficiently alert, give him or her something very sweet to eat or drink. This should correct a low blood sugar level and will do no harm if the sugar level is too high. If your child cannot cooperate or is no better within 10 minutes, call a doctor at once.

CALL YOUR CHILD'S DOCTOR NOW

POSSIBLE CAUSE AND ACTION These may be generalized absence seizures, a type of epilepsy (formerly known as petit mal). Do not try to stop the seizures by shaking or slapping your child. Your child's doctor may refer your child for an EEG test to record the electrical activity in the brain. He or she may advise drug treatment with *anticonvulsants* to control the condition.

POSSIBLE CAUSE AND ACTION These symptoms may be the side effects of a drug. Call your child's doctor before the next dose of the drug is due to ask if it could be the cause and if you should stop giving it to your child.

POSSIBLE CAUSE It is possible that your child is abusing drugs or solvents (*see* RECOGNIZING DRUG AND SOLVENT ABUSE, p.141). A nervous system problem is also a rare possibility. Consult your child's doctor.

ACTION The doctor will examine your child and may refer him or her for tests such as MRI (p.41) to exclude a nervous system problem. If drug or substance abuse is the problem, the doctor may arrange counseling or suggest self-help groups (*see* USEFUL ADDRESSES, p.311).

Breath-holding spells

Young children sometimes hold their breath while crying for up to 30 seconds. This can be in response to pain, but it can also be an attempt to manipulate parents. A child may hold his or her breath until passing out. Once consciousness is lost, normal breathing will resume automatically.

If your child is attempting to get his or her way by crying and breath-holding, try to ignore him or her as much as possible. Breath holding is not harmful, and most children grow out of it by the age of 4 years. However, if you are worried, consult your child's doctor.

21 Headache

Headaches are a very common complaint. By the age of 7, 40 percent of children have had a headache, and this figure rises to 75 percent by the age of 15. Parents may worry that the pain is due to a serious condition, such as meningitis or a brain tumor. However, these conditions are extremely rare. Headaches often occur on their own but may accompany any infection that causes a fever. They can also be a symptom of a number of relatively minor disorders. Consult this chart if your child complains of a headache with or without other symptoms. Always consult your child's doctor if a headache is severe, persistent, or recurs frequently, or if this is the first time that your child has had a particular type of headache.

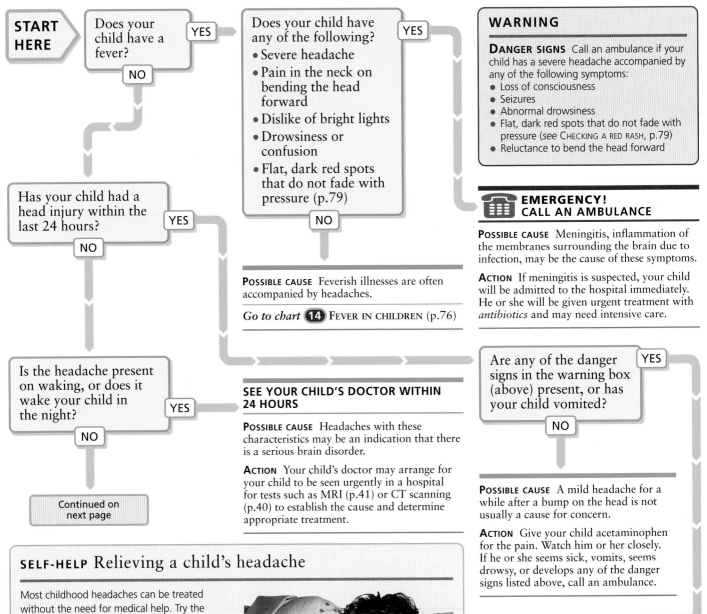

START HERE

Does your child have a fever? YES / NO

Does your child have any of the following?
- Severe headache
- Pain in the neck on bending the head forward
- Dislike of bright lights
- Drowsiness or confusion
- Flat, dark red spots that do not fade with pressure (p.79)

YES / NO

Has your child had a head injury within the last 24 hours? YES / NO

Is the headache present on waking, or does it wake your child in the night? YES / NO

Continued on next page

POSSIBLE CAUSE Feverish illnesses are often accompanied by headaches.

Go to chart **14** FEVER IN CHILDREN (p.76)

SEE YOUR CHILD'S DOCTOR WITHIN 24 HOURS

POSSIBLE CAUSE Headaches with these characteristics may be an indication that there is a serious brain disorder.

ACTION Your child's doctor may arrange for your child to be seen urgently in a hospital for tests such as MRI (p.41) or CT scanning (p.40) to establish the cause and determine appropriate treatment.

WARNING

DANGER SIGNS Call an ambulance if your child has a severe headache accompanied by any of the following symptoms:
- Loss of consciousness
- Seizures
- Abnormal drowsiness
- Flat, dark red spots that do not fade with pressure (*see* CHECKING A RED RASH, p.79)
- Reluctance to bend the head forward

EMERGENCY! CALL AN AMBULANCE

POSSIBLE CAUSE Meningitis, inflammation of the membranes surrounding the brain due to infection, may be the cause of these symptoms.

ACTION If meningitis is suspected, your child will be admitted to the hospital immediately. He or she will be given urgent treatment with *antibiotics* and may need intensive care.

Are any of the danger signs in the warning box (above) present, or has your child vomited? YES / NO

POSSIBLE CAUSE A mild headache for a while after a bump on the head is not usually a cause for concern.

ACTION Give your child acetaminophen for the pain. Watch him or her closely. If he or she seems sick, vomits, seems drowsy, or develops any of the danger signs listed above, call an ambulance.

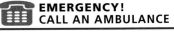

EMERGENCY! CALL AN AMBULANCE

POSSIBLE CAUSE Your child's head injury may have resulted in damage to the brain.

ACTION Once in the hospital, your child will be observed closely and may have tests such as CT scanning (p.40) to determine the treatment.

SELF-HELP Relieving a child's headache

Most childhood headaches can be treated without the need for medical help. Try the following self-help measures to relieve the pain.
- Give liquid acetaminophen.
- Encourage your child to rest in a cool, quiet, dimly lit room. He or she may want to go to sleep for a while.
- If your child is hungry, offer him or her a snack, such as a cookie and a drink of milk.
If the headache persists for more than 4 hours, if your child seems very ill, or if other symptoms develop, call your child's doctor.

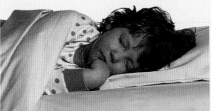

Headache relief
Encouraging a child to have a nap or a rest, after first taking an analgesic, *will often help relieve his or her headache.*

Continued from previous page

Does your child have recurrent headaches with or preceded by any of the following?
- Nausea or vomiting
- Abdominal pain
- Seeing flashing lights
- Pale appearance

YES → **Is your child completely well between attacks?**

YES → **POSSIBLE CAUSE** A severe headache associated with these symptoms may be a migraine, particularly if other members of the family also suffer from migraines. Consult your child's doctor.

ACTION The doctor will probably examine your child to exclude other possible causes.. Symptoms can often be eased by self-help measures, such as taking an *analgesic* and an *antiemetic* (drug that relieves nausea), drinking plenty of fluids, and resting in a darkened room. You should also try to discover whether there are any specific triggers, such as a food or an activity (*see* REDUCING THE FREQUENCY OF MIGRAINE, p.159).

NO → **CALL YOUR CHILD'S DOCTOR NOW**

POSSIBLE CAUSE If your child is not well between headaches or his or her performance at school has worsened recently, it may be an indication of a serious brain disorder that needs urgent investigation.

ACTION Your child's doctor will examine your child and may arrange for him or her to be seen urgently in the hospital for tests such as MRI (p.41) or CT scanning (p.40) in order to establish the cause.

NO

Do headaches occur mainly after reading or using a computer?

YES → **POSSIBLE CAUSE** Previously unrecognized eyesight problems may sometimes cause a child to develop a headache after activities such as these. Take your child to an ophthalmologist for an eyesight test.

ACTION The ophthalmologist will carry out a full vision test and, if a vision problem is found, will prescribe appropriate glasses for your child. If vision is normal, he or she will refer your child to the doctor, who will try to establish a cause for the headaches.

NO

Do either of the following describe your child's headache?
- Felt mainly in the forehead and face or teeth
- Worse when bending forward

YES → **POSSIBLE CAUSE** Sinusitis (inflammation of the membranes lining the air spaces in the skull) may be the cause of this type of headache, especially if your child recently had a cold or a runny or blocked nose.

ACTION Give your child acetaminophen for the pain. Steam inhalation (*see* TREATING A CHILD WITH A COLD, p.106) may also help. If your child is no better after 2 days, see your child's doctor within 24 hours; your child may need *antibiotics*.

NO

Could your child be anxious or under stress at home or at school?

YES → **POSSIBLE CAUSE** Anxiety is one of the most common causes of headaches in children. Tension headaches ususally worsen over the course of the day.

ACTION Discuss your child's problems and worries with him or her, and see if you can identify a pattern to the headaches. Approach teachers for further information. Consult your child's doctor if you and your child cannot sort out the problem or if the headaches are frequent.

NO

Is your child taking any prescription drugs?

YES → **POSSIBLE CAUSE AND ACTION** Certain drugs can cause headaches as a side effect. Consult your child's doctor. Meanwhile, your child should not stop taking the prescribed drugs.

NO

Are your child's headaches frequent, are they becoming more frequent, or has the nature of the headaches changed?

YES → **POSSIBLE CAUSE AND ACTION** You should bring any frequent or unusual headaches to the attention of your child's doctor. They are unlikely to be serious, but the doctor will want to rule out the possibility of an underlying disorder.

NO → CONSULT YOUR CHILD'S DOCTOR IF YOU ARE UNABLE TO MAKE A DIAGNOSIS FROM THIS CHART. IF THE HEADACHE IS SEVERE, CALL THE DOCTOR NOW.

22 Confusion and/or drowsiness

Children who are confused may talk nonsense, appear dazed or agitated, or see and hear things that are not real. This is a serious symptom that requires immediate medical attention. Drowsiness may be the result of a lack of sleep or a minor illness, or it may be a symptom of a serious disease, such as meningitis. Consult this chart if your child appears confused or if he or she suddenly becomes unusually sleepy or unresponsive or is difficult to rouse from sleep.

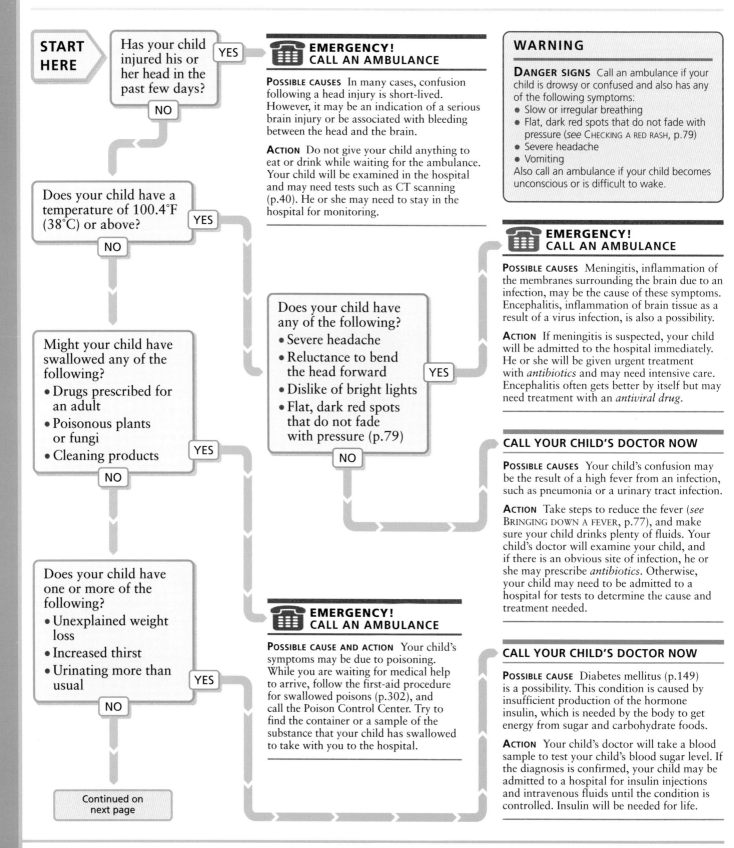

START HERE

Has your child injured his or her head in the past few days? — YES

NO

EMERGENCY! CALL AN AMBULANCE

POSSIBLE CAUSES In many cases, confusion following a head injury is short-lived. However, it may be an indication of a serious brain injury or be associated with bleeding between the head and the brain.

ACTION Do not give your child anything to eat or drink while waiting for the ambulance. Your child will be examined in the hospital and may need tests such as CT scanning (p.40). He or she may need to stay in the hospital for monitoring.

WARNING

DANGER SIGNS Call an ambulance if your child is drowsy or confused and also has any of the following symptoms:
- Slow or irregular breathing
- Flat, dark red spots that do not fade with pressure (*see* CHECKING A RED RASH, p.79)
- Severe headache
- Vomiting

Also call an ambulance if your child becomes unconscious or is difficult to wake.

Does your child have a temperature of 100.4°F (38°C) or above? — YES

NO

Does your child have any of the following?
- Severe headache
- Reluctance to bend the head forward
- Dislike of bright lights
- Flat, dark red spots that do not fade with pressure (p.79)

— YES

NO

EMERGENCY! CALL AN AMBULANCE

POSSIBLE CAUSES Meningitis, inflammation of the membranes surrounding the brain due to an infection, may be the cause of these symptoms. Encephalitis, inflammation of brain tissue as a result of a virus infection, is also a possibility.

ACTION If meningitis is suspected, your child will be admitted to the hospital immediately. He or she will be given urgent treatment with *antibiotics* and may need intensive care. Encephalitis often gets better by itself but may need treatment with an *antiviral drug*.

CALL YOUR CHILD'S DOCTOR NOW

POSSIBLE CAUSES Your child's confusion may be the result of a high fever from an infection, such as pneumonia or a urinary tract infection.

ACTION Take steps to reduce the fever (*see* BRINGING DOWN A FEVER, p.77), and make sure your child drinks plenty of fluids. Your child's doctor will examine your child, and if there is an obvious site of infection, he or she may prescribe *antibiotics*. Otherwise, your child may need to be admitted to a hospital for tests to determine the cause and treatment needed.

Might your child have swallowed any of the following?
- Drugs prescribed for an adult
- Poisonous plants or fungi
- Cleaning products

— YES

NO

EMERGENCY! CALL AN AMBULANCE

POSSIBLE CAUSE AND ACTION Your child's symptoms may be due to poisoning. While you are waiting for medical help to arrive, follow the first-aid procedure for swallowed poisons (p.302), and call the Poison Control Center. Try to find the container or a sample of the substance that your child has swallowed to take with you to the hospital.

Does your child have one or more of the following?
- Unexplained weight loss
- Increased thirst
- Urinating more than usual

— YES

NO

CALL YOUR CHILD'S DOCTOR NOW

POSSIBLE CAUSE Diabetes mellitus (p.149) is a possibility. This condition is caused by insufficient production of the hormone insulin, which is needed by the body to get energy from sugar and carbohydrate foods.

ACTION Your child's doctor will take a blood sample to test your child's blood sugar level. If the diagnosis is confirmed, your child may be admitted to a hospital for insulin injections and intravenous fluids until the condition is controlled. Insulin will be needed for life.

Continued on next page

Continued from previous page

Is your child being treated for diabetes? **YES**

NO

POSSIBLE CAUSES Confusion or drowsiness in children with diabetes may indicate a low blood sugar level, particularly if the symptoms have come on suddenly. Less commonly, these symptoms may be the result of a high blood sugar level and may have developed gradually.

ACTION If your child is sufficiently alert, give him or her something very sweet to eat or drink. This should correct a low blood sugar level and will do no harm if the sugar level is too high. If your child cannot cooperate or is no better within 10 minutes, call your child's doctor at once. However, you should call an ambulance if your child becomes unconscious.

Is there evidence that your child has had a seizure, for example, has your child done either of the following?
• Bitten his or her tongue
• Wet him- or herself
YES

NO

POSSIBLE CAUSE AND ACTION If your child has had an epileptic seizure, it may have left him or her drowsy or confused. If your child has been diagnosed as having epilepsy, consult your child's doctor because your child's treatment may need adjusting. However, you should call the doctor immediately if your child has not previously been diagnosed as having epilepsy: he or she needs to be assessed promptly.

Has your child had diarrhea, with or without vomiting, in the past 24 hours? **YES**

NO

CALL YOUR CHILD'S DOCTOR NOW

POSSIBLE CAUSE Your child's symptoms may be due to dehydration.

ACTION Your child's doctor will examine your child to assess how severely dehydrated he or she is. In most cases, giving your child fluids at home will treat the dehydration and prevent it worsening (*see* PREVENTING DEHYDRATION IN CHILDREN, p.123). However, if your child is very ill or unable to drink sufficient fluids to treat the dehydration, he or she may need to be admitted to the hospital.

Has your child been exposed to hot sunshine or high temperatures recently? **YES**

NO

☎ EMERGENCY! CALL AN AMBULANCE

POSSIBLE CAUSE Your child's symptoms may be due to heatstroke, in which a high temperature and dehydration can cause confusion and drowsiness.

ACTION While waiting for help, lay your child in a cool place and remove all his or her outer clothing. Sponge him or her with tepid water. If your child is able to cooperate, offer him or her cool drinks.

Is your child taking any prescription drugs or over-the-counter drugs? **YES**

NO

CALL YOUR CHILD'S DOCTOR NOW

POSSIBLE CAUSE AND ACTION Drowsiness or confusion may be a side effect of some drugs, including *antihistamines* and *anticonvulsants*. If your child is taking a prescribed drug, ask your child's doctor's advice before the next dose is due. Your child should stop taking any over-the-counter drugs.

Could your child have been drinking alcohol? **YES**

NO

POSSIBLE CAUSE Your child may be intoxicated or have alcohol poisoning.

ACTION Encourage your child to drink plenty of water, and wait for the effects to wear off. If your child becomes unconscious, call an ambulance.

Could your child be using recreational drugs or inhaling solvents? **YES**

NO

POSSIBLE CAUSE Drug or solvent abuse may cause drowsiness or confusion.

ACTION Watch your child carefully while he or she is confused or drowsy. If your child becomes unconscious, call an ambulance. While waiting for help, follow the first aid procedure for unconsciousness (p.300). Delay discussing the problem with your child until he or she is well enough to understand. If you think your child is becoming dependent on drugs, consult your child's doctor. Advice and support is also available from many self-help groups (*see* USEFUL ADDRESSES, p.311).

CALL YOUR CHILD'S DOCTOR NOW IF YOUR CHILD IS DROWSY OR CONFUSED AND YOU ARE UNABLE TO MAKE A DIAGNOSIS FROM THIS CHART.

23 Clumsiness

Children vary greatly in their levels of manual dexterity, physical coordination, and agility. Some children naturally acquire these skills later than others. They have difficulty in carrying out delicate tasks, such as tying shoelaces, and may often accidentally knock things over. Such clumsiness is unlikely to be a sign of an underlying disease, although poor vision can be an unrecognized cause. Severe clumsiness that has come on suddenly or that follows a head injury may result from a serious problem with the nervous system and needs urgent medical attention.

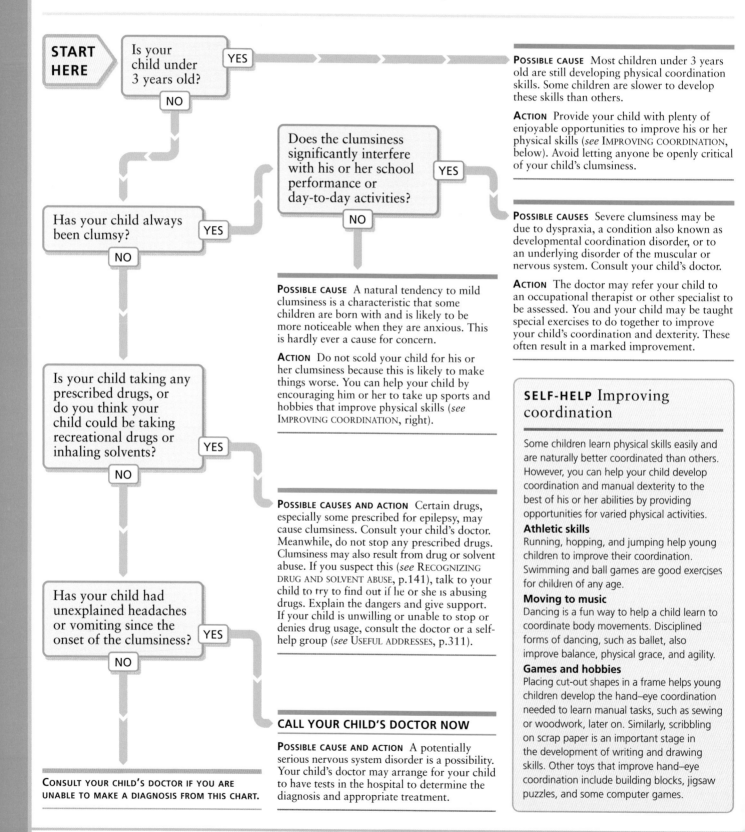

START HERE

Is your child under 3 years old? — YES

POSSIBLE CAUSE Most children under 3 years old are still developing physical coordination skills. Some children are slower to develop these skills than others.

ACTION Provide your child with plenty of enjoyable opportunities to improve his or her physical skills (see IMPROVING COORDINATION, below). Avoid letting anyone be openly critical of your child's clumsiness.

NO

Has your child always been clumsy? — YES

Does the clumsiness significantly interfere with his or her school performance or day-to-day activities? — YES

POSSIBLE CAUSES Severe clumsiness may be due to dyspraxia, a condition also known as developmental coordination disorder, or to an underlying disorder of the muscular or nervous system. Consult your child's doctor.

ACTION The doctor may refer your child to an occupational therapist or other specialist to be assessed. You and your child may be taught special exercises to do together to improve your child's coordination and dexterity. These often result in a marked improvement.

NO

NO

POSSIBLE CAUSE A natural tendency to mild clumsiness is a characteristic that some children are born with and is likely to be more noticeable when they are anxious. This is hardly ever a cause for concern.

ACTION Do not scold your child for his or her clumsiness because this is likely to make things worse. You can help your child by encouraging him or her to take up sports and hobbies that improve physical skills (see IMPROVING COORDINATION, right).

Is your child taking any prescribed drugs, or do you think your child could be taking recreational drugs or inhaling solvents? — YES

NO

POSSIBLE CAUSES AND ACTION Certain drugs, especially some prescribed for epilepsy, may cause clumsiness. Consult your child's doctor. Meanwhile, do not stop any prescribed drugs. Clumsiness may also result from drug or solvent abuse. If you suspect this (see RECOGNIZING DRUG AND SOLVENT ABUSE, p.141), talk to your child to try to find out if he or she is abusing drugs. Explain the dangers and give support. If your child is unwilling or unable to stop or denies drug usage, consult the doctor or a self-help group (see USEFUL ADDRESSES, p.311).

Has your child had unexplained headaches or vomiting since the onset of the clumsiness? — YES

NO

CALL YOUR CHILD'S DOCTOR NOW

POSSIBLE CAUSE AND ACTION A potentially serious nervous system disorder is a possibility. Your child's doctor may arrange for your child to have tests in the hospital to determine the diagnosis and appropriate treatment.

CONSULT YOUR CHILD'S DOCTOR IF YOU ARE UNABLE TO MAKE A DIAGNOSIS FROM THIS CHART.

SELF-HELP Improving coordination

Some children learn physical skills easily and are naturally better coordinated than others. However, you can help your child develop coordination and manual dexterity to the best of his or her abilities by providing opportunities for varied physical activities.

Athletic skills
Running, hopping, and jumping help young children to improve their coordination. Swimming and ball games are good exercises for children of any age.

Moving to music
Dancing is a fun way to help a child learn to coordinate body movements. Disciplined forms of dancing, such as ballet, also improve balance, physical grace, and agility.

Games and hobbies
Placing cut-out shapes in a frame helps young children develop the hand–eye coordination needed to learn manual tasks, such as sewing or woodwork, later on. Similarly, scribbling on scrap paper is an important stage in the development of writing and drawing skills. Other toys that improve hand–eye coordination include building blocks, jigsaw puzzles, and some computer games.

24 Speech difficulties

Consult this chart if your child has any problem with his or her speech, such as a delay in starting to talk, lack of clarity, defects in pronunciation, or stammering. Such difficulties often improve with time, but in most cases it is wise to

seek the advice of your child's doctor. If not addressed early, speech difficulties may cause behavior and school problems. A speech therapist will usually be able to improve your child's ability to communicate effectively.

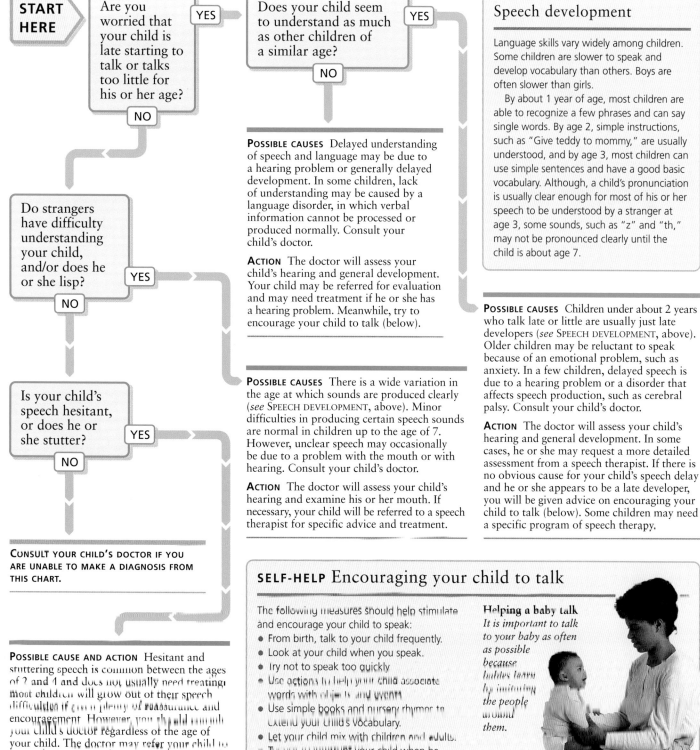

START HERE

Are you worried that your child is late starting to talk or talks too little for his or her age? — YES → **Does your child seem to understand as much as other children of a similar age?** — YES →

NO ↓ (from first box)

NO ↓ (from understand box)

POSSIBLE CAUSES Delayed understanding of speech and language may be due to a hearing problem or generally delayed development. In some children, lack of understanding may be caused by a language disorder, in which verbal information cannot be processed or produced normally. Consult your child's doctor.

ACTION The doctor will assess your child's hearing and general development. Your child may be referred for evaluation and may need treatment if he or she has a hearing problem. Meanwhile, try to encourage your child to talk (below).

Do strangers have difficulty understanding your child, and/or does he or she lisp? — YES →

NO ↓

POSSIBLE CAUSES There is a wide variation in the age at which sounds are produced clearly (*see* SPEECH DEVELOPMENT, above). Minor difficulties in producing certain speech sounds are normal in children up to the age of 7. However, unclear speech may occasionally be due to a problem with the mouth or with hearing. Consult your child's doctor.

ACTION The doctor will assess your child's hearing and examine his or her mouth. If necessary, your child will be referred to a speech therapist for specific advice and treatment.

Is your child's speech hesitant, or does he or she stutter? — YES →

NO ↓

CONSULT YOUR CHILD'S DOCTOR IF YOU ARE UNABLE TO MAKE A DIAGNOSIS FROM THIS CHART.

POSSIBLE CAUSE AND ACTION Hesitant and stuttering speech is common between the ages of 2 and 4 and does not usually need treating; most children will grow out of their speech difficulties if given plenty of reassurance and encouragement. However, you should consult your child's doctor regardless of the age of your child. The doctor may refer your child to a speech therapist to learn strategies that will help improve his or her speech.

Speech development

Language skills vary widely among children. Some children are slower to speak and develop vocabulary than others. Boys are often slower than girls.

By about 1 year of age, most children are able to recognize a few phrases and can say single words. By age 2, simple instructions, such as "Give teddy to mommy," are usually understood, and by age 3, most children can use simple sentences and have a good basic vocabulary. Although, a child's pronunciation is usually clear enough for most of his or her speech to be understood by a stranger at age 3, some sounds, such as "z" and "th," may not be pronounced clearly until the child is about age 7.

POSSIBLE CAUSES Children under about 2 years who talk late or little are usually just late developers (*see* SPEECH DEVELOPMENT, above). Older children may be reluctant to speak because of an emotional problem, such as anxiety. In a few children, delayed speech is due to a hearing problem or a disorder that affects speech production, such as cerebral palsy. Consult your child's doctor.

ACTION The doctor will assess your child's hearing and general development. In some cases, he or she may request a more detailed assessment from a speech therapist. If there is no obvious cause for your child's speech delay and he or she appears to be a late developer, you will be given advice on encouraging your child to talk (below). Some children may need a specific program of speech therapy.

SELF-HELP Encouraging your child to talk

The following measures should help stimulate and encourage your child to speak:
● From birth, talk to your child frequently.
● Look at your child when you speak.
● Try not to speak too quickly.
● Use actions to help your child associate words with objects and events.
● Use simple books and nursery rhymes to extend your child's vocabulary.
● Let your child mix with children and adults.
● Try not to interrupt your child when he or she is speaking.

Helping a baby talk
It is important to talk to your baby as often as possible because babies learn by imitating the people around them.

25 Behavior problems

Perception of what constitutes a behavior problem varies widely between parents. At some stage, most children will behave in a way that causes their parents concern, even if it is by doing something as minor as nail-biting (*see* HABITUAL

BEHAVIOR, opposite). However, most children outgrow these problems. This chart covers some of the more common or serious behavior problems that parents have to cope with. It will help you decide whether to consult your child's doctor.

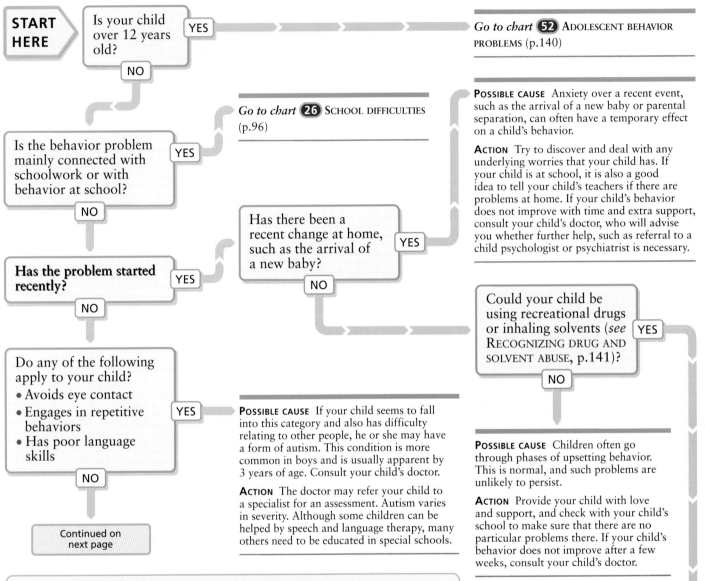

START HERE → Is your child over 12 years old? — **YES** → *Go to chart* **52** ADOLESCENT BEHAVIOR PROBLEMS (p.140)

NO ↓

Is the behavior problem mainly connected with schoolwork or with behavior at school? — **YES** → *Go to chart* **26** SCHOOL DIFFICULTIES (p.96)

NO ↓

Has the problem started recently? — **YES** → Has there been a recent change at home, such as the arrival of a new baby? — **YES** → **POSSIBLE CAUSE** Anxiety over a recent event, such as the arrival of a new baby or parental separation, can often have a temporary effect on a child's behavior.

ACTION Try to discover and deal with any underlying worries that your child has. If your child is at school, it is also a good idea to tell your child's teachers if there are problems at home. If your child's behavior does not improve with time and extra support, consult your child's doctor, who will advise you whether further help, such as referral to a child psychologist or psychiatrist is necessary.

NO (from recent change) ↓

NO (Has the problem started recently) ↓

Do any of the following apply to your child?
• Avoids eye contact
• Engages in repetitive behaviors
• Has poor language skills — **YES** → **POSSIBLE CAUSE** If your child seems to fall into this category and also has difficulty relating to other people, he or she may have a form of autism. This condition is more common in boys and is usually apparent by 3 years of age. Consult your child's doctor.

ACTION The doctor may refer your child to a specialist for an assessment. Autism varies in severity. Although some children can be helped by speech and language therapy, many others need to be educated in special schools.

NO ↓

Continued on next page

Could your child be using recreational drugs or inhaling solvents (*see* RECOGNIZING DRUG AND SOLVENT ABUSE, p.141)? — **YES** → **POSSIBLE CAUSE** Drug or substance abuse often results in behavior problems.

ACTION Talk to your child to try to find out whether there is an underlying problem. Try not to get aggressive or angry, but provide him or her with plenty of love. Giving your child support may provide him or her with the self-confidence to stop. If you think your child is becoming dependent on drugs, consult your child's doctor. Advice and support are also available from many self-help groups (*see* USEFUL ADDRESSES, p.311).

NO ↓

POSSIBLE CAUSE Children often go through phases of upsetting behavior. This is normal, and such problems are unlikely to persist.

ACTION Provide your child with love and support, and check with your child's school to make sure that there are no particular problems there. If your child's behavior does not improve after a few weeks, consult your child's doctor.

SELF-HELP Coping with the "terrible twos"

The period around the age of two years is a time during which children are beginning to appreciate that they have a separate identity and are able to influence their environment. It is often a time of alternating moods. Your child may have periods of self-assertion, during which he or she has violent temper tantrums if his or her wishes are frustrated. These may alternate with periods when he or she feels insecure and refuses to be separated from you. Such behavior can make the "terrible twos" a very trying time for parents.

If your child has temper tantrums, try to keep calm and to ignore the behavior, unless he or she could be injured. Also try to ignore other people who appear to be disapproving. If you are upset by the tantrums, it is better to leave the room than to show signs of distress yourself. Seek support from other parents of similar-aged children.

Your child will grow out of this phase, but, in the meantime, if you feel unable to cope with his or her behavior, consult your child's doctor for advice and support.

Continued from
previous page

Has your child become
unusually withdrawn
and lost interest in
activities that he or she
previously enjoyed? **YES**

NO

Is your child unruly,
noisy, and disobedient? **YES**

NO

CONSULT YOUR CHILD'S DOCTOR IF YOU ARE
UNABLE TO FIND AN EXPLANATION FOR YOUR
CHILD'S BEHAVIOR ON THIS CHART AND
YOUR CHILD CONTINUES TO BEHAVE IN A
WAY THAT WORRIES YOU.

Attention deficit
hyperactivity disorder

Young children are normally very active.
However, a child who is excessively restless,
impulsive, and unable to concentrate may
have attention deficit hyperactivity disorder
(ADHD). Children with ADHD may be
destructive, irritable, and aggressive and may
also have difficulty making friends. Such
behavior is very hard to deal with and
requires patience and understanding. Children
with ADHD often have low self-esteem
because of frequent scolding or criticism

If you suspect that your child may have
ADHD, consult your child's doctor, who will
assess your child's behavior and may refer
him or her to a child psychologist or child
psychiatrist. You may be taught various
techniques to improve your child's behavior,
and your child may be given drugs that will
help calm him or her. Your child may also
benefit from being taught in small groups.
Although the disorder often continues
through adolescence, behavioral problems
may become less severe if the treatment is
started early enough.

Habitual behavior

Childhood habits, such as nail-biting, are
common and rarely do any serious harm. They
may provide comfort from stress or be a means
of expressing emotion, such as anger. Rarely,
habits such as breath-holding attacks (p.87)
may be used to manipulate parents.

About one-third of children bite their nails, a
habit that may persist into adulthood. Thumb-
sucking is common in children under 3. Some
may continue up to the age of 6 or 7, when
they should be persuaded to stop, to keep the
adult teeth from being pushed out of position.

Children are often unaware of habitual
behavior. Draw your child's attention to it
when it occurs, but do not get angry. If you
are worried, consult your child's doctor.

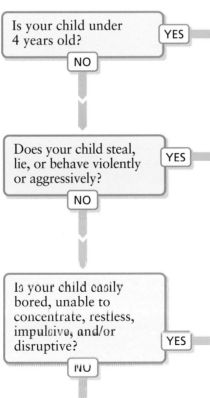

Twirling the hair
*Children of all ages
may play with their
hair, often unaware
that they are doing
so. In some cases,
this can lead
to hair loss.*

POSSIBLE CAUSES Both depression and
anxiety can cause these symptoms.

ACTION Talk to your child to see if there
is a reason for his or her behavior. Offer
support and encouragement, and try to
remove or reduce any sources of stress
that may be contributing. If your child's
symptoms persist for more than 2 weeks
or worsen, consult your child's doctor.

POSSIBLE CAUSE It is normal for small children
to test the rules and disobey their parents.
Many young children also go through a
period of particularly difficult behavior
known as the "terrible twos."

ACTION All children grow out of this
behavior. Meanwhile, follow the advice for
coping with the "terrible twos" (opposite). If,
at any stage, you feel that you cannot cope,
consult your child's doctor.

Is your child under
4 years old? **YES**

NO

POSSIBLE CAUSE Children are often rebellious.
However, if your child is persistently antisocial,
disruptive, or violent, he or she may have a
condition known as a conduct disorder.
Consult your child's doctor.

ACTION The doctor may refer your child to a
specialist for assessment. Child psychotherapy
or family therapy may be needed. However,
long-standing behavior problems may be
difficult to change.

Does your child steal,
lie, or behave violently
or aggressively? **YES**

NO

Is your child easily
bored, unable to
concentrate, restless,
impulsive, and/or
disruptive? **YES**

NO

POSSIBLE CAUSE Although this type of
behavior is normal in small children, school-
age children, particularly boys, who are
constantly active and disruptive may have
attention deficit hyperactivity disorder (left).
Consult your child's doctor.

ACTION The doctor will probably refer your
child to a specialist to confirm the diagnosis.
Children with this condition need extra
support and help both at home and in school,
and some also need drug treatment.

CONSULT YOUR CHILD'S DOCTOR IF YOU ARE
UNABLE TO FIND AN EXPLANATION FOR YOUR
CHILD'S BEHAVIOR ON THIS CHART AND
YOUR CHILD CONTINUES TO BEHAVE IN A WAY
THAT WORRIES YOU.

26 School difficulties

Difficulties at school fall into two main groups: those related mainly to learning, whether a specific subject or academic work in general; and those that are concerned with behavior, including classroom behavior as well as reluctance to go to school. Consult this chart if your child has any such difficulties, which may be the result of emotional problems, physical disorders, or social factors, or which may arise from a general developmental problem. Discussion with school staff usually helps the situation. Your child's doctor and the school medical services may also be able to help.

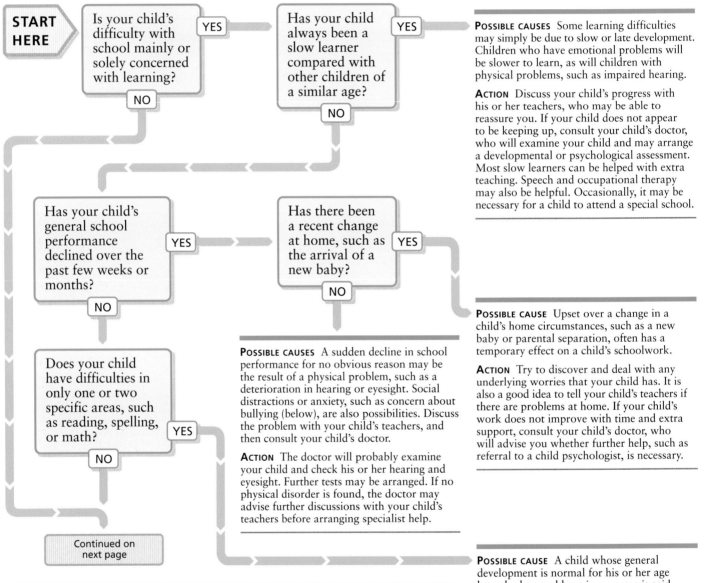

START HERE

Is your child's difficulty with school mainly or solely concerned with learning? → **YES** → Has your child always been a slow learner compared with other children of a similar age? → **YES**

NO ↓ (from first box)

NO ↓ (from second box)

POSSIBLE CAUSES Some learning difficulties may simply be due to slow or late development. Children who have emotional problems will be slower to learn, as will children with physical problems, such as impaired hearing.

ACTION Discuss your child's progress with his or her teachers, who may be able to reassure you. If your child does not appear to be keeping up, consult your child's doctor, who will examine your child and may arrange a developmental or psychological assessment. Most slow learners can be helped with extra teaching. Speech and occupational therapy may also be helpful. Occasionally, it may be necessary for a child to attend a special school.

Has your child's general school performance declined over the past few weeks or months? → **YES** → Has there been a recent change at home, such as the arrival of a new baby? → **YES**

NO ↓ (general school performance)

NO ↓ (recent change at home)

POSSIBLE CAUSE Upset over a change in a child's home circumstances, such as a new baby or parental separation, often has a temporary effect on a child's schoolwork.

ACTION Try to discover and deal with any underlying worries that your child has. It is also a good idea to tell your child's teachers if there are problems at home. If your child's work does not improve with time and extra support, consult your child's doctor, who will advise you whether further help, such as referral to a child psychologist, is necessary.

Does your child have difficulties in only one or two specific areas, such as reading, spelling, or math? → **YES**

NO ↓

POSSIBLE CAUSES A sudden decline in school performance for no obvious reason may be the result of a physical problem, such as a deterioration in hearing or eyesight. Social distractions or anxiety, such as concern about bullying (below), are also possibilities. Discuss the problem with your child's teachers, and then consult your child's doctor.

ACTION The doctor will probably examine your child and check his or her hearing and eyesight. Further tests may be arranged. If no physical disorder is found, the doctor may advise further discussions with your child's teachers before arranging specialist help.

Continued on next page

POSSIBLE CAUSE A child whose general development is normal for his or her age but who has problems in one area is said to have a specific learning difficulty. For example, difficulty in reading and writing is known as dyslexia (opposite). Discuss the problem with your child's teachers initially, and consult your child's doctor.

ACTION The doctor will probably examine your child to make sure that a physical problem, such as poor eyesight or an unrecognized illness, is not contributing to your child's difficulties. The doctor may contact the school medical services. Work with your child's school to encourage your child as much as possible. In some cases, extra support in school may be necessary.

Bullying

Bullying can take many forms. In addition to physical violence, it includes teasing, name-calling, spreading unpleasant stories, and excluding children from groups. Bullying is especially common in grade school.

A child who is being bullied is singled out for attention by the bully and may become very unhappy and insecure. He or she may not want to go to school, and his or her schoolwork may suffer. If your child is being bullied, it is vitally important that you reassure him or her that the bullying is not his or her fault. Build up your child's self-esteem, and talk to his or her school. Schools should have a policy on bullying.

The bully needs help, too. In many cases, bullying is an expression of an underlying problem such as a need for attention. If your child is a bully, it is important that you make it clear that this behavior is unacceptable and harmful, while also trying to find the cause.

Continued from previous page

Has your child been playing hooky? **YES** → Do any of the following apply to your child?
- He or she often comes home with unexplained bruises or cuts.
- Money or belongings are frequently "lost" at school.
- He or she comes home with broken belongings.

YES → **POSSIBLE CAUSE** Truancy combined with other antisocial behaviors, such as stealing, is more common in adolescents. In some cases, it is due to bullying (opposite) or the influence of friends. Talk to your child's teachers and doctor.

ACTION If problems persist despite intervention at school, it may be necessary to refer your child to a child psychologist. Long-standing behavior problems may be difficult to change.

NO (Has your child been playing hooky?)

NO (Do any of the following apply to your child?)

POSSIBLE CAUSE This type of problem may be due to bullying, even if your child is initially reluctant to admit it (*see* BULLYING, opposite).

ACTION Talk to your child about the situation, and speak to his or her teachers. Bullying or other violence at school should be taken very seriously. Your child's school should have a policy for dealing with bullying, and you can help by building up your child's confidence.

Has your child become reluctant to go to school? **YES** → Does your child resist all attempts to get him or her to school? **YES** →

NO (Has your child become reluctant)

NO (Does your child resist all attempts)

POSSIBLE CAUSES Dislike of school may be caused by a variety of factors. For example, children starting a new school may be anxious. Your child may be having difficulties with work at school or be afraid of certain teachers or pupils. If not tackled, a dislike of school may progress into a refusal to attend school.

ACTION Try to find out the cause of the problem, and discuss your child's feelings with his or her teachers so that they can watch out for signs of bullying (opposite). Do not keep your child at home. Depending on the cause of the problem, it may be necessary for your child to receive extra teaching or help from a child psychologist.

POSSIBLE CAUSES School refusal may be a sign that something is seriously wrong. There may be a problem at school, such as bullying (opposite), or a failure of the school to meet the child's needs. Occasionally, refusal to go to school is caused by anxiety at home or, in a young child, by anxiety over separation from his or her parents.

ACTION Try to discover the underlying cause of your child's refusal to go to school so that it can be dealt with, and make every effort to ensure that your child attends school. Discuss the problem with your child's teachers. If the situation does not improve, consult your child's doctor. He or she may recommend that you seek help for your child from a child psychologist.

Have teachers complained about your child's behavior at school? **YES** →

NO

SCHOOL DIFFICULTIES THAT HAVE NOT BEEN DESCRIBED ON THIS CHART SHOULD BE DISCUSSED WITH YOUR CHILD'S TEACHERS. YOUR CHILD'S DOCTOR MAY ALSO HAVE HELPFUL ADVICE IN SOME CASES.

Is your child easily bored, unable to concentrate, restless, impulsive, and/or disruptive? **YES** →

NO

POSSIBLE CAUSE Although this type of behavior is normal in small children, school-age children who are constantly active and disruptive may have attention deficit hyperactivity disorder (p.95). Consult your child's doctor.

ACTION The doctor will probably refer your child to a specialist to confirm the diagnosis. Children with this condition need extra support at home and in school, and some need drug treatment.

Dyslexia

Dyslexia means difficulty with words. Early signs include difficulty learning to read, write, and spell. Dyslexia is not linked to low intelligence. If you think your child may be dyslexic, talk to your child's doctor and teachers. They should be able to arrange for a formal assessment of your child and subsequent support (*see also* USEFUL ADDRESSES, p.[illegible]).

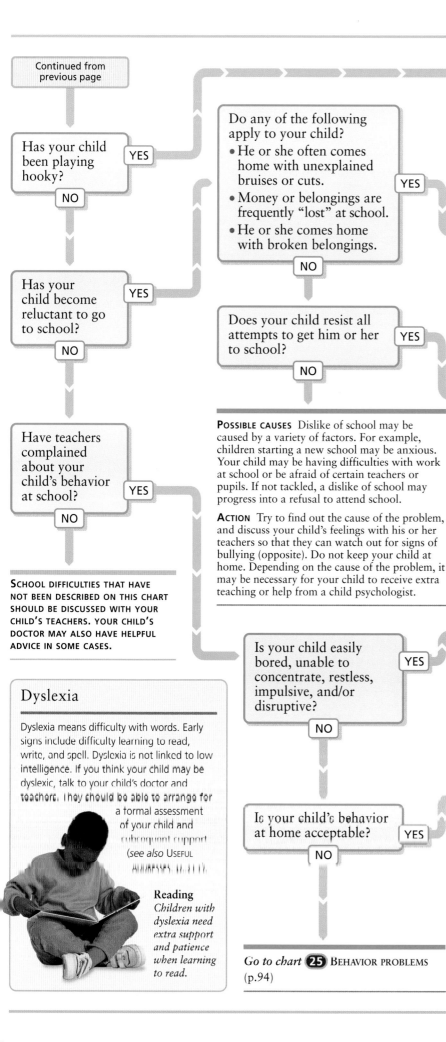

Reading
Children with dyslexia need extra support and patience when learning to read.

Is your child's behavior at home acceptable? **YES** →

NO

POSSIBLE CAUSES Bad behavior that is confined to school can be due to a number of problems. Schoolwork may be too easy, leading to boredom, or it may be too difficult, possibly because of an unrecognized learning difficulty, resulting in loss of interest. Bad behavior may also be the result of rejecting authority. In some cases, poor behavior at school may be due to bullying (opposite).

ACTION Talk to your child to try to uncover the cause of the problem. It is also wise to discuss the problem with your child's teachers. Adjustments may need to be made to your child's schoolwork so that it meets his or her needs more closely. In some cases, help from a child psychologist may be arranged by your child's doctor.

Go to chart **25** BEHAVIOR PROBLEMS (p.94)

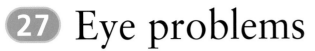 27 Eye problems

For blurred vision in children, see chart 28, DISTURBED OR
IMPAIRED VISION **(p.100).**
This chart deals with pain, itching, redness, and/or discharge
from one or both eyes. In children, such symptoms are most
commonly the result of infection or local irritation. In most

cases, it is reasonable to treat these problems at home
initially. Always seek immediate medical advice about injury
to the eye or for any foreign body in the eye that cannot be
removed by simple self-help measures. You should also seek
medical help if home treatment is not effective.

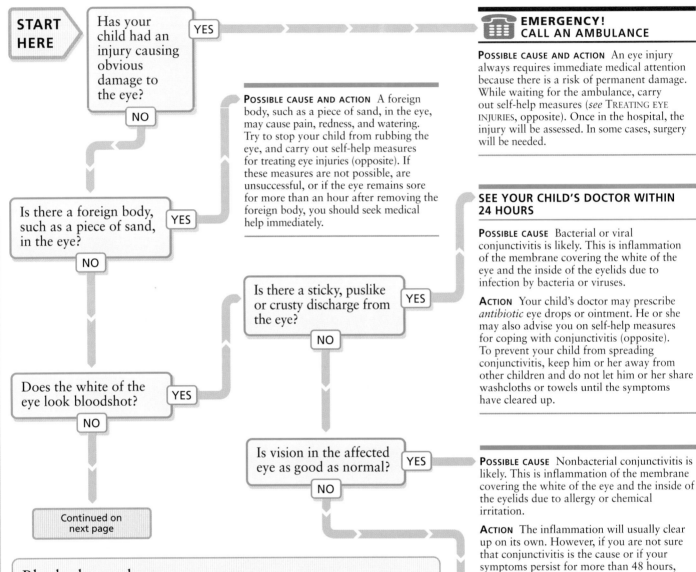

START HERE

Has your child had an injury causing obvious damage to the eye? — YES

EMERGENCY! CALL AN AMBULANCE

POSSIBLE CAUSE AND ACTION An eye injury always requires immediate medical attention because there is a risk of permanent damage. While waiting for the ambulance, carry out self-help measures (*see* TREATING EYE INJURIES, opposite). Once in the hospital, the injury will be assessed. In some cases, surgery will be needed.

NO

Is there a foreign body, such as a piece of sand, in the eye? — YES

POSSIBLE CAUSE AND ACTION A foreign body, such as a piece of sand, in the eye, may cause pain, redness, and watering. Try to stop your child from rubbing the eye, and carry out self-help measures for treating eye injuries (opposite). If these measures are not possible, are unsuccessful, or if the eye remains sore for more than an hour after removing the foreign body, you should seek medical help immediately.

NO

Is there a sticky, puslike or crusty discharge from the eye? — YES

SEE YOUR CHILD'S DOCTOR WITHIN 24 HOURS

POSSIBLE CAUSE Bacterial or viral conjunctivitis is likely. This is inflammation of the membrane covering the white of the eye and the inside of the eyelids due to infection by bacteria or viruses.

ACTION Your child's doctor may prescribe *antibiotic* eye drops or ointment. He or she may also advise you on self-help measures for coping with conjunctivitis (opposite). To prevent your child from spreading conjunctivitis, keep him or her away from other children and do not let him or her share washcloths or towels until the symptoms have cleared up.

NO

Does the white of the eye look bloodshot? — YES

Is vision in the affected eye as good as normal? — YES

POSSIBLE CAUSE Nonbacterial conjunctivitis is likely. This is inflammation of the membrane covering the white of the eye and the inside of the eyelids due to allergy or chemical irritation.

ACTION The inflammation will usually clear up on its own. However, if you are not sure that conjunctivitis is the cause or if your symptoms persist for more than 48 hours, you should consult your child's doctor.

NO

NO

Continued on next page

CALL YOUR CHILD'S DOCTOR NOW

POSSIBLE CAUSE Iritis, inflammation of the colored part of the eye, is a possibility.

ACTION Your child's doctor will refer your child to a specialist for a detailed eye examination and for other tests to look for disorders that sometimes occur with iritis, such as arthritis. Iritis needs immediate treatment with *corticosteroid* eye drops or pills to prevent permanent damage to vision.

Blocked tear duct

Tears are produced continuously to clean and moisturize the front of the eye. Excess tears drain away through the tear ducts. These are narrow passages that lead from the inner corner of the lower eyelid to the inside of the nose. If a tear duct becomes blocked, tears cannot drain away normally and the eye waters.

Blocked tear ducts are common in babies. One or both tear ducts may be blocked at birth. This is not a cause for concern because in most cases the ducts open

naturally by the time a child is 1 year old. Massage may help unblock and open a tear duct. Wash your hands thoroughly, and use a forefinger to massage the skin just below the inner corner of the eye in a gentle circular motion. Repeat the massage three or four times a day for 1 or 2 weeks. If a blocked tear duct has not opened by the age of 1 year, the doctor may refer your child to a specialist for treatment. The duct may have to be opened with a thin probe under a general anesthetic.

Continued from previous page

Are only the eyelids red and itchy?

NO / YES

YES →

POSSIBLE CAUSE Blepharitis, inflammation of the lid margins, is a likely cause of itchy, scaly eyelids. This condition is often associated with dandruff. Allergic conjunctivitis is also a possibility. Consult your child's doctor.

ACTION The doctor may prescribe an ointment that should be applied to the eyelids. Treating the scalp with an over-the-counter anti-dandruff shampoo may also result in an improvement in the eyelids. Antihistamine medications or eyedrops may be given for allergic eye symptoms.

Is there a red lump on one eyelid?

NO / YES

YES →

POSSIBLE CAUSE A stye, a boil-like infection at the root of an eyelash, is likely.

ACTION A stye will usually clear up within a week without special treatment. It will either burst, releasing pus, or gradually disappear. If pus is released, use a clean piece of cotton moistened with warm water to clear away the discharge, wiping toward the outer side of the eye. To prevent infection from spreading, try to discourage your child from touching the affected eye. Consult your doctor if a stye fails to heal within a week or if styes recur often.

Do one or both eyes water continuously?

NO / YES

Is your child less than 1 year old?

NO / YES

CONSULT YOUR CHILD'S DOCTOR IF YOU ARE UNABLE TO MAKE A DIAGNOSIS FROM THIS CHART.

CONSULT YOUR CHILD'S DOCTOR IF YOU ARE UNABLE TO MAKE A DIAGNOSIS FROM THIS CHART.

SELF-HELP Coping with conjunctivitis

A common cause of conjunctivitis in children is a bacterial or viral infection, which is easily spread. If your child has conjunctivitis, you should try to stop him or her from touching the affected eye. Remove the discharge from your child's eye with warm water and cotton as often as necessary. Keep your child away from other children until his or her symptoms have cleared up. You can help prevent other family members from catching conjunctivitis by having a separate towel and washcloth for your child.

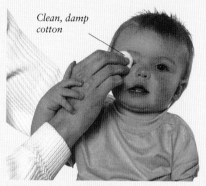

Clean, damp cotton

Cleaning your child's eye
Gently wipe from the inside to the outer edge of the eye. Use a clean piece of damp cotton each time.

POSSIBLE CAUSE A blocked tear duct may be causing your baby's symptoms. This condition is common in babies and usually corrects itself without treatment by the end of the first year.

ACTION You may be able to help open a blocked duct by gentle massage (see BLOCKED TEAR DUCT, opposite). In rare cases, the duct does not open and an operation is needed.

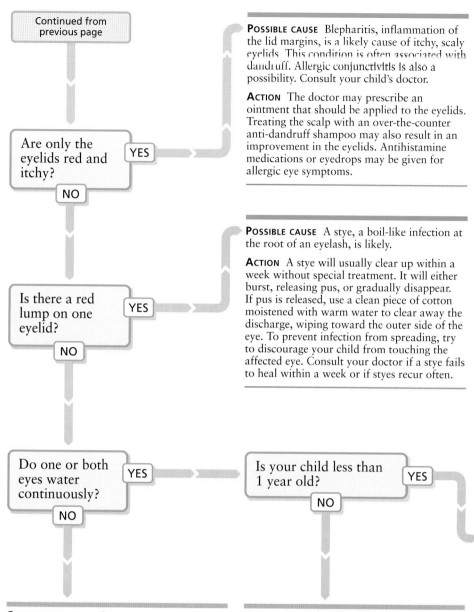

SELF-HELP Treating eye injuries

You should seek prompt medical attention for a blow to the eye or an eye wound. If there is a visible wound, lay the victim down with his or her head elevated and place a pad of clean, non-fluffy material gently over the eye. Do not press down on it. Keep the victim as still as possible while you are waiting for medical help to arrive.

A foreign body floating on the white of the eye is usually easily removed (right). However, if it is embedded in the eye or rests on the colored part of the eye, do not attempt to remove it. Take the person to the hospital.

If chemicals have splashed into someone's eye, immediate self-help treatment (far right) can help minimize damage to the eye, but this must be followed by treatment in the hospital.

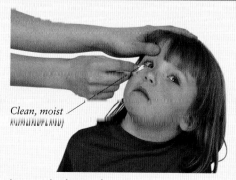

Clean, moist handkerchief

Foreign bodies in the eye
Gently ease the eyelid away from the eye. Lift the foreign body off the surface of the eye using the corner of a clean, moist handkerchief.

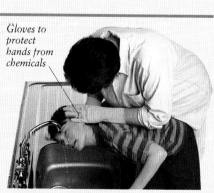

Gloves to protect hands from chemicals

Chemicals in the eye
Gently run cold water over the eye for 10 minutes. Keep the unaffected eye uppermost to keep chemicals from being washed into it.

28 Disturbed or impaired vision

Serious defects in a child's vision are usually picked up during a routine eye test. However, you may suspect that your child has an undetected problem with his or her eyesight if he or she squints or always holds books very close to the face. When your child begins school, a teacher may notice that he or she performs less well sitting at the back of the classroom, where it may be difficult to see the board. Consult your ophthalmologist if you suspect a problem with your child's eyesight. If your child develops a sudden problem with his or her vision, he or she should receive urgent medical assessment. Fortunately, disorders causing a sudden disturbance of vision are rare in childhood.

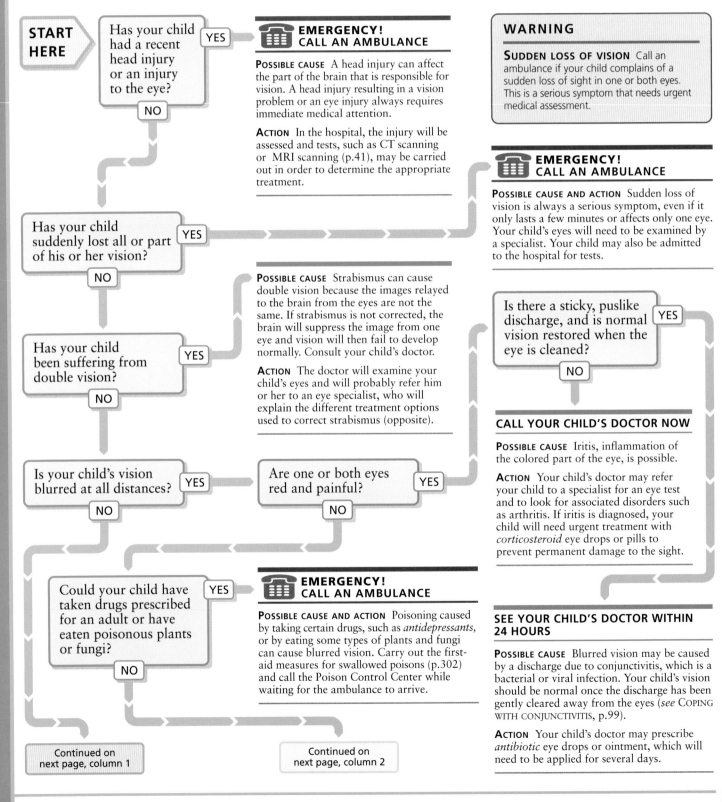

START HERE

Has your child had a recent head injury or an injury to the eye? — YES →

☎ EMERGENCY! CALL AN AMBULANCE

POSSIBLE CAUSE A head injury can affect the part of the brain that is responsible for vision. A head injury resulting in a vision problem or an eye injury always requires immediate medical attention.

ACTION In the hospital, the injury will be assessed and tests, such as CT scanning or MRI scanning (p.41), may be carried out in order to determine the appropriate treatment.

WARNING

SUDDEN LOSS OF VISION Call an ambulance if your child complains of a sudden loss of sight in one or both eyes. This is a serious symptom that needs urgent medical assessment.

— NO ↓

Has your child suddenly lost all or part of his or her vision? — YES →

☎ EMERGENCY! CALL AN AMBULANCE

POSSIBLE CAUSE AND ACTION Sudden loss of vision is always a serious symptom, even if it only lasts a few minutes or affects only one eye. Your child's eyes will need to be examined by a specialist. Your child may also be admitted to the hospital for tests.

— NO ↓

Has your child been suffering from double vision? — YES →

POSSIBLE CAUSE Strabismus can cause double vision because the images relayed to the brain from the eyes are not the same. If strabismus is not corrected, the brain will suppress the image from one eye and vision will then fail to develop normally. Consult your child's doctor.

ACTION The doctor will examine your child's eyes and will probably refer him or her to an eye specialist, who will explain the different treatment options used to correct strabismus (opposite).

Is there a sticky, puslike discharge, and is normal vision restored when the eye is cleaned? — YES →

— NO ↓

CALL YOUR CHILD'S DOCTOR NOW

POSSIBLE CAUSE Iritis, inflammation of the colored part of the eye, is possible.

ACTION Your child's doctor may refer your child to a specialist for an eye test and to look for associated disorders such as arthritis. If iritis is diagnosed, your child will need urgent treatment with *corticosteroid* eye drops or pills to prevent permanent damage to the sight.

— NO ↓

Is your child's vision blurred at all distances? — YES →

Are one or both eyes red and painful? — YES →

— NO ↓   — NO ↓

Could your child have taken drugs prescribed for an adult or have eaten poisonous plants or fungi? — YES →

☎ EMERGENCY! CALL AN AMBULANCE

POSSIBLE CAUSE AND ACTION Poisoning caused by taking certain drugs, such as *antidepressants*, or by eating some types of plants and fungi can cause blurred vision. Carry out the first-aid measures for swallowed poisons (p.302) and call the Poison Control Center while waiting for the ambulance to arrive.

SEE YOUR CHILD'S DOCTOR WITHIN 24 HOURS

POSSIBLE CAUSE Blurred vision may be caused by a discharge due to conjunctivitis, which is a bacterial or viral infection. Your child's vision should be normal once the discharge has been gently cleared away from the eyes (see COPING WITH CONJUNCTIVITIS, p.99).

ACTION Your child's doctor may prescribe *antibiotic* eye drops or ointment, which will need to be applied for several days.

— NO ↓

Continued on next page, column 1

Continued on next page, column 2

Continued from previous page, column 1

Continued from previous page, column 2

Is your child taking any prescribed drugs? **YES**

NO

Does your child have difficulty seeing either near or distant objects? **YES**

NO

POSSIBLE CAUSE A severe focusing disorder may cause blurred vision at all distances. Consult your child's doctor.

ACTION The doctor will examine your child's eyes and will probably recommend that your child receives a complete vision assessment from an ophthalmologist. Depending on the results, your child may need glasses and/or referral to a specialist for further treatment.

POSSIBLE CAUSE Fargsightedness (difficulty seeing close objects) or nearsightedness (difficulty seeing distant objects) is likely. Consult an ophthalmologist.

ACTION The ophthalmologist will examine your child's eyes and check his or her vision (*see* VISION TESTING IN CHILDREN, below). Your child may need to wear glasses.

Has your child been seeing flashing lights or floating spots? **YES**

NO

Has this happened in the past, and has a severe headache followed? **YES**

NO

Strabismus

Strabismus is a condition in which only one eye looks directly at the object being viewed. It is common in babies until the age of 3 months, when their eye muscles and vision improve. In children over 3 months it may be due to an imbalance in the eye muscles or near- or farsightedness in one eye. The brain receives different images, which may cause double vision or lead to the stronger eye being used in preference to the weaker one, so that they do not work together.

If your child is near- or farsighted, he or she may need to wear glasses, which will also correct strabismus. A patch worn over the good eye for 1–2 hours a day will ensure that the weaker eye is used. Occasionally, surgery on the eye muscles may be needed.

If strabismus is not treated in childhood, the vision centers in the brain will fail to develop normally. Treatment later in life will not be able to improve vision.

POSSIBLE CAUSE AND ACTION Certain drugs can cause blurred vision as a side effect. Call your child's doctor to ask whether you should stop giving the prescribed drug.

POSSIBLE CAUSE Migraine, recurrent severe headaches, may begin in childhood. This is especially likely if the condition affects one or both parents. Consult your child's doctor.

ACTION If migraine is diagnosed, the doctor may prescribe *analgesics* for your child to take during attacks. Try self-help measures for relieving a child's headache (p.88) and for reducing the frequency of migraine (p.159).

SEE YOUR CHILD'S DOCTOR WITHIN 24 HOURS IF YOUR CHILD HAS A VISION PROBLEM AND YOU ARE UNABLE TO MAKE A DIAGNOSIS FROM THIS CHART.

SEE YOUR CHILD'S DOCTOR WITHIN 24 HOURS IF YOUR CHILD HAS A VISION PROBLEM AND YOU ARE UNABLE TO MAKE A DIAGNOSIS FROM THIS CHART.

Vision testing in children

Simple vision tests are routinely carried out in babies as part of their developmental checks. Further tests may be recommended if a problem is suspected. Vision tests for babies and children vary depending on their age. In infants, eye drops are given to dilate the pupil. A beam of light is then shone into each eye in turn using an instrument called a retinoscope. The effect at different lenses on the beam of light determines whether vision is normal. Older children are often tested by being asked to identify letters on cards held at a distance. Each eye is tested separately.

At all ages, a vision test also includes careful examination of the retina, which is the light-sensitive membrane at the back of the eye.

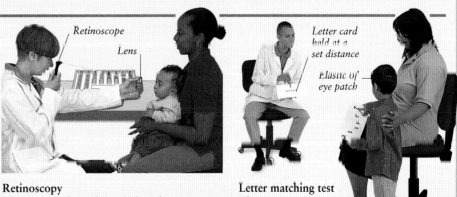

Retinoscopy
The test is performed in a darkened room. An instrument called a retinoscope is used to shine a beam of light through a lens into each of the child's eyes in turn.

Letter matching test
The tester points to a letter and asks the child to identify a matching letter.

29 Painful or irritated ear

For hearing problems in children, see chart 30, HEARING PROBLEMS (p.104).

Earache is common in children and can be very distressing. In most cases, earache is caused by an infection spreading from the back of the throat to the ear (*see* STRUCTURE OF THE EAR IN CHILDREN, opposite). Fortunately, such ear infections become less common as children grow up. A child who is not old enough to tell you that he or she has an earache may wake unexpectedly in the night and may cry inconsolably, shriek loudly, or pull at the affected ear.

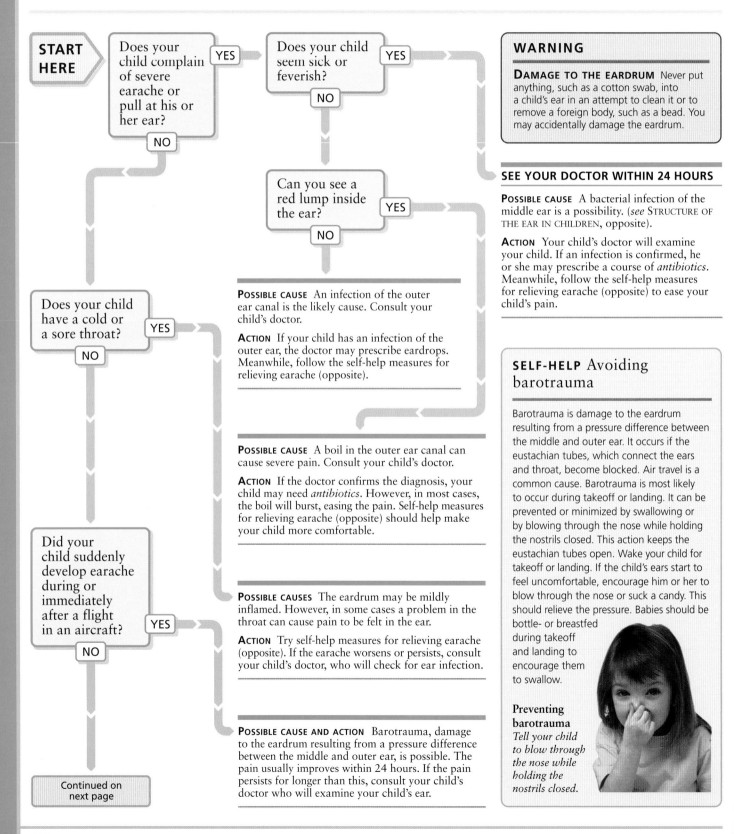

START HERE

Does your child complain of severe earache or pull at his or her ear? — YES / NO

Does your child seem sick or feverish? — YES / NO

Can you see a red lump inside the ear? — YES / NO

Does your child have a cold or a sore throat? — YES / NO

Did your child suddenly develop earache during or immediately after a flight in an aircraft? — YES / NO

Continued on next page

WARNING

DAMAGE TO THE EARDRUM Never put anything, such as a cotton swab, into a child's ear in an attempt to clean it or to remove a foreign body, such as a bead. You may accidentally damage the eardrum.

SEE YOUR DOCTOR WITHIN 24 HOURS

POSSIBLE CAUSE A bacterial infection of the middle ear is a possibility. (*see* STRUCTURE OF THE EAR IN CHILDREN, opposite).

ACTION Your child's doctor will examine your child. If an infection is confirmed, he or she may prescribe a course of *antibiotics*. Meanwhile, follow the self-help measures for relieving earache (opposite) to ease your child's pain.

POSSIBLE CAUSE An infection of the outer ear canal is the likely cause. Consult your child's doctor.

ACTION If your child has an infection of the outer ear, the doctor may prescribe eardrops. Meanwhile, follow the self-help measures for relieving earache (opposite).

POSSIBLE CAUSE A boil in the outer ear canal can cause severe pain. Consult your child's doctor.

ACTION If the doctor confirms the diagnosis, your child may need *antibiotics*. However, in most cases, the boil will burst, easing the pain. Self-help measures for relieving earache (opposite) should help make your child more comfortable.

POSSIBLE CAUSES The eardrum may be mildly inflamed. However, in some cases a problem in the throat can cause pain to be felt in the ear.

ACTION Try self-help measures for relieving earache (opposite). If the earache worsens or persists, consult your child's doctor, who will check for ear infection.

POSSIBLE CAUSE AND ACTION Barotrauma, damage to the eardrum resulting from a pressure difference between the middle and outer ear, is possible. The pain usually improves within 24 hours. If the pain persists for longer than this, consult your child's doctor who will examine your child's ear.

SELF-HELP Avoiding barotrauma

Barotrauma is damage to the eardrum resulting from a pressure difference between the middle and outer ear. It occurs if the eustachian tubes, which connect the ears and throat, become blocked. Air travel is a common cause. Barotrauma is most likely to occur during takeoff or landing. It can be prevented or minimized by swallowing or by blowing through the nose while holding the nostrils closed. This action keeps the eustachian tubes open. Wake your child for takeoff or landing. If the child's ears start to feel uncomfortable, encourage him or her to blow through the nose or suck a candy. This should relieve the pressure. Babies should be bottle- or breastfed during takeoff and landing to encourage them to swallow.

Preventing barotrauma
Tell your child to blow through the nose while holding the nostrils closed.

Continued from
previous page

Is there a
discharge from
the affected ear?

YES

NO

Does your child
have itching
or irritation
inside the ear?

YES

NO

CONSULT YOUR CHILD'S DOCTOR IF YOU ARE UNABLE TO MAKE A DIAGNOSIS FROM THIS CHART.

Is the skin
around the
child's ear red
and inflamed?

YES

NO

POSSIBLE CAUSES Your child may have pushed a small object, such as a bead or small piece of food, into his or her ear. Alternatively, an insect may have flown or crawled into the ear. Consult your child's doctor.

ACTION The doctor will examine your child's ear. If there is an insect or any other foreign body in the ear canal, it may be possible for the doctor to wash it out. If the doctor cannot remove it, he or she will refer your child to a specialist to have it removed.

Structure of the ear in children

From the outside, children's ears look much the same as those of adults. However, the eustachian tube, which connects the middle ear to the back of the throat, is shorter and more horizontal than in adults, allowing infections to reach the middle ear more easily. In addition, the adenoids (see TONSILS AND ADENOIDS, p.107), lymphatic tissue that lie close to the back of the throat, tend to be larger in children; they can readily block the eustachian tubes, preventing drainage and increasing the risk of infection.

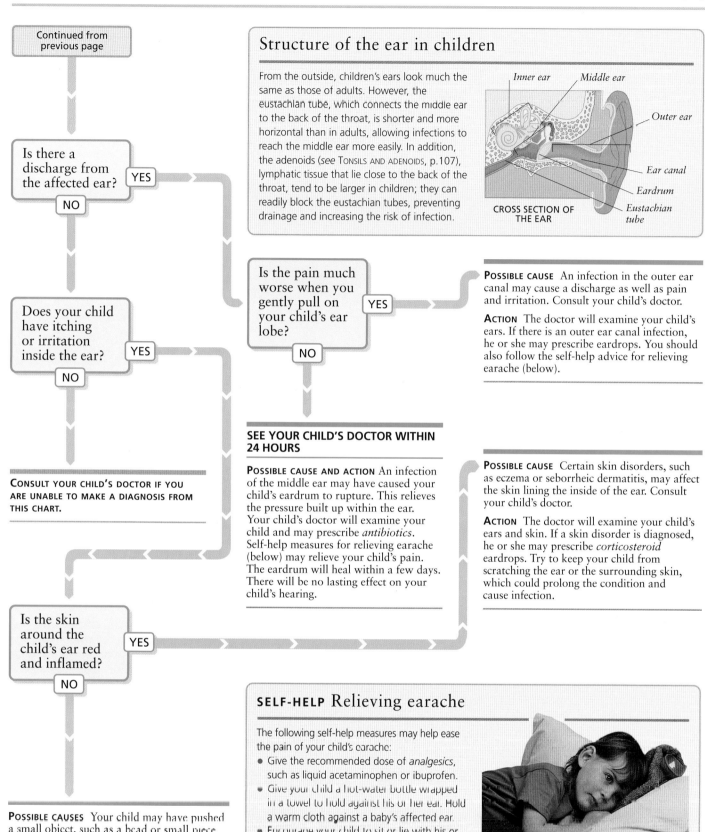

CROSS SECTION OF
THE EAR

Inner ear Middle ear

Outer ear

Ear canal

Eardrum

Eustachian
tube

Is the pain much
worse when you
gently pull on
your child's ear
lobe?

YES

NO

SEE YOUR CHILD'S DOCTOR WITHIN 24 HOURS

POSSIBLE CAUSE AND ACTION An infection of the middle ear may have caused your child's eardrum to rupture. This relieves the pressure built up within the ear. Your child's doctor will examine your child and may prescribe *antibiotics*. Self-help measures for relieving earache (below) may relieve your child's pain. The eardrum will heal within a few days. There will be no lasting effect on your child's hearing.

POSSIBLE CAUSE An infection in the outer ear canal may cause a discharge as well as pain and irritation. Consult your child's doctor.

ACTION The doctor will examine your child's ears. If there is an outer ear canal infection, he or she may prescribe eardrops. You should also follow the self-help advice for relieving earache (below).

POSSIBLE CAUSE Certain skin disorders, such as eczema or seborrheic dermatitis, may affect the skin lining the inside of the ear. Consult your child's doctor.

ACTION The doctor will examine your child's ears and skin. If a skin disorder is diagnosed, he or she may prescribe *corticosteroid* eardrops. Try to keep your child from scratching the ear or the surrounding skin, which could prolong the condition and cause infection.

SELF-HELP Relieving earache

The following self-help measures may help ease the pain of your child's earache:
- Give the recommended dose of *analgesics*, such as liquid acetaminophen or ibuprofen.
- Give your child a hot-water bottle wrapped in a towel to hold against his or her ear. Hold a warm cloth against a baby's affected ear.
- Encourage your child to sit or lie with his or her head raised on pillows (lying flat may worsen the pain). Resting the affected ear facing downward will allow any discharge to drain out.

Do not put eardrops or olive oil into your child's ear unless advised otherwise by your child's doctor. Do not put cotton in the ear: this could prevent a discharge from draining out.

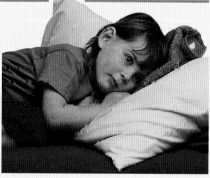

Easing earache
Resting the ear against a covered hot-water bottle with the head slightly raised may help to ease the pain of earache.

30 Hearing problems

Hearing problems are often not noticed in a child. If your child always needs to have the television or radio on louder than you think necessary or there is a sudden deterioration in your child's school performance, a hearing problem may be the cause. Hearing problems in babies are often detected at routine developmental checks by your child's doctor, but you may be the first to notice that your baby is not responding to sounds or learning to speak as quickly as you think he or she should. This should always be brought to the doctor's attention.

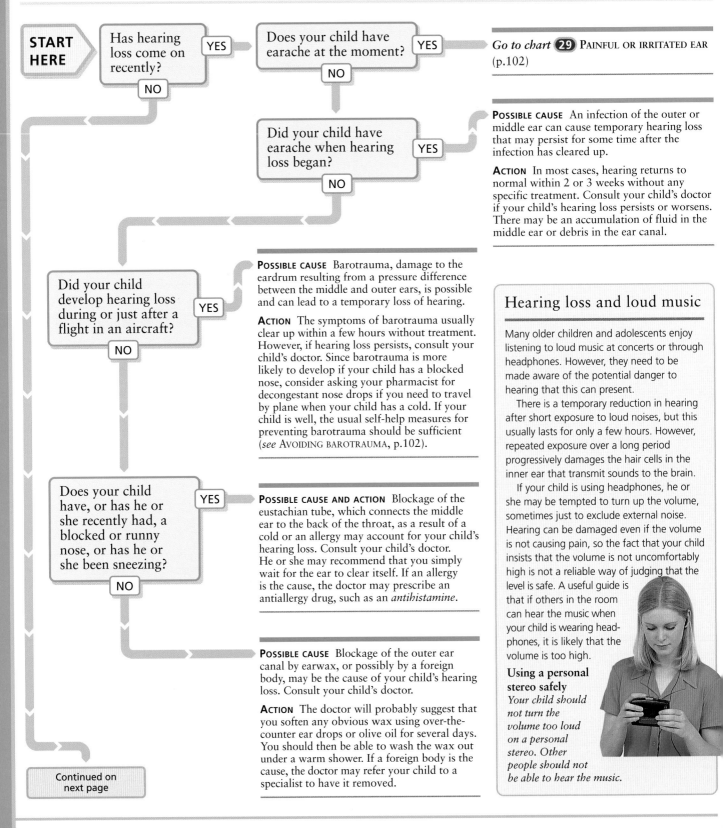

START HERE → **Has hearing loss come on recently?**

YES → **Does your child have earache at the moment?**

YES → *Go to chart* 29 PAINFUL OR IRRITATED EAR (p.102)

NO (from "Does your child have earache at the moment?") → **Did your child have earache when hearing loss began?**

YES → **POSSIBLE CAUSE** An infection of the outer or middle ear can cause temporary hearing loss that may persist for some time after the infection has cleared up.

ACTION In most cases, hearing returns to normal within 2 or 3 weeks without any specific treatment. Consult your child's doctor if your child's hearing loss persists or worsens. There may be an accumulation of fluid in the middle ear or debris in the ear canal.

NO (from "Has hearing loss come on recently?") continues down.

Did your child develop hearing loss during or just after a flight in an aircraft?

YES → **POSSIBLE CAUSE** Barotrauma, damage to the eardrum resulting from a pressure difference between the middle and outer ears, is possible and can lead to a temporary loss of hearing.

ACTION The symptoms of barotrauma usually clear up within a few hours without treatment. However, if hearing loss persists, consult your child's doctor. Since barotrauma is more likely to develop if your child has a blocked nose, consider asking your pharmacist for decongestant nose drops if you need to travel by plane when your child has a cold. If your child is well, the usual self-help measures for preventing barotrauma should be sufficient (*see* AVOIDING BAROTRAUMA, p.102).

NO → **Does your child have, or has he or she recently had, a blocked or runny nose, or has he or she been sneezing?**

YES → **POSSIBLE CAUSE AND ACTION** Blockage of the eustachian tube, which connects the middle ear to the back of the throat, as a result of a cold or an allergy may account for your child's hearing loss. Consult your child's doctor. He or she may recommend that you simply wait for the ear to clear itself. If an allergy is the cause, the doctor may prescribe an antiallergy drug, such as an *antihistamine*.

NO → **POSSIBLE CAUSE** Blockage of the outer ear canal by earwax, or possibly by a foreign body, may be the cause of your child's hearing loss. Consult your child's doctor.

ACTION The doctor will probably suggest that you soften any obvious wax using over-the-counter ear drops or olive oil for several days. You should then be able to wash the wax out under a warm shower. If a foreign body is the cause, the doctor may refer your child to a specialist to have it removed.

Continued on next page

Hearing loss and loud music

Many older children and adolescents enjoy listening to loud music at concerts or through headphones. However, they need to be made aware of the potential danger to hearing that this can present.

There is a temporary reduction in hearing after short exposure to loud noises, but this usually lasts for only a few hours. However, repeated exposure over a long period progressively damages the hair cells in the inner ear that transmit sounds to the brain.

If your child is using headphones, he or she may be tempted to turn up the volume, sometimes just to exclude external noise. Hearing can be damaged even if the volume is not causing pain, so the fact that your child insists that the volume is not uncomfortably high is not a reliable way of judging that the level is safe. A useful guide is that if others in the room can hear the music when your child is wearing headphones, it is likely that the volume is too high.

Using a personal stereo safely
Your child should not turn the volume too loud on a personal stereo. Other people should not be able to hear the music.

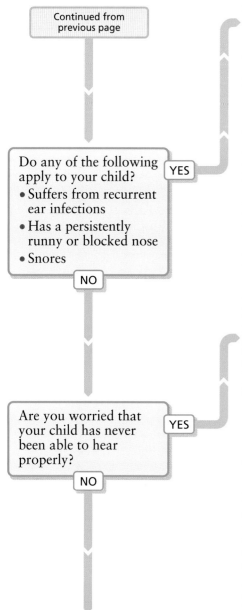

Continued from previous page

Do any of the following apply to your child?
• Suffers from recurrent ear infections
• Has a persistently runny or blocked nose
• Snores

YES → NO

Are you worried that your child has never been able to hear properly?

YES → NO

CONSULT YOUR CHILD'S DOCTOR IF YOU ARE UNABLE TO MAKE A DIAGNOSIS FROM THIS CHART.

POSSIBLE CAUSES Your child may have otitis media with effusion, in which fluid builds up in the middle ear, causing hearing problems. This condition may be due to an allergy or to persistently enlarged adenoids blocking the eustachian tube, which connects the middle ear and the back of the throat (*see* STRUCTURE OF THE EAR IN CHILDREN, p.103).

ACTION your child's doctor will probably arrange for hearing tests, including tympanometry (*see* HEARING TESTS IN CHILDHOOD, below), to confirm the diagnosis. He or she may suggest antiallergy drugs such as *antihistamines*. If the fluid persists, the doctor may recommend surgical removal of the adenoids and/or the insertion of a tiny tube through the eardrum to drain the fluid (*see* TREATING OTITIS MEDIA WITH EFFUSION, right). In most cases, normal hearing is restored.

During pregnancy, did you come into contact with someone who had rubella (German measles) or did you have a fever and rash?

YES → NO

POSSIBLE CAUSE Your child may have an inherited hearing problem, possibly due to abnormal development of the inner ear or the nerve that transmits sounds to the brain. This type of hearing problem is most likely if there is a family history of such abnormalities. Consult your child's doctor.

ACTION The doctor will probably arrange for your child to have hearing tests (below). If your child is found to have a problem with hearing, he or she will need additional help with language development at school and home.

Treating otitis media with effusion

In otitis media with effusion, fluid builds up in the middle ear, resulting in reduced hearing. The condition may be treated surgically by inserting a tiny plastic tube, a tympanostomy tube, through the eardrum. The tube allows air into the middle ear and fluid to drain away. The tube is left in place and usually falls out after 6–18 months. The eardrum then heals. The operation to insert a tube is usually performed under general anesthesia as day surgery and rarely needs to be repeated.

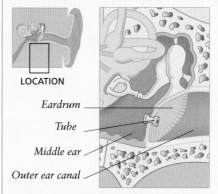

LOCATION

Eardrum
Tube
Middle ear
Outer ear canal

Tympanostomy tube in place
The tube inserted into the eardrum provides a channel between the middle and outer ear, allowing air to circulate normally in the ear, which improves hearing.

POSSIBLE CAUSE Exposure of the unborn child to rubella and certain other infections can damage hearing. Consult your child's doctor.

ACTION The doctor will arrange for your child to have hearing tests (below) and may refer him or her to a specialist for assessment.

Hearing tests in childhood

Tests to assess hearing are performed throughout childhood as part of routine developmental screening; the type of test depends on the age of the child. Newborn babies can be assessed using tests such as otoacoustic emission, in which a sound is played into the ear and an earpiece measures the resulting echo from the inner ear. Speech discrimination tests can be used to detect hearing loss in young children who have a simple vocabulary. For example, in the McCormick toy discrimination test, the child is shown various toys and is asked to identify pairs of toys that have similar sounding names, such as tree and key. Tympanometry (p.190) is

a test that is also used for adults. It measures movement of the eardrum in response to sound and is useful in detecting a buildup of fluid in the middle ear. By age 4, most children are able to cooperate with a simple form of audiometry (p.190), which measures how loud sounds of various frequencies need to be for the child to hear them.

The McCormick test
The doctor prevents the child from lip-reading by covering his or her mouth and then asks the child to identify various toys.

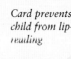

Card prevents child from lip-reading

Child selects toy

31 Runny or blocked nose

A runny nose can be irritating for a child, and a blocked nose can be distressing for a baby because it makes feeding difficult, but neither symptom on its own is likely to be a sign of serious disease. All children have a runny or blocked nose from time to time (often accompanied by sneezing), and, in most cases, a common cold is responsible. If your child gets a nosebleed from picking or blowing a blocked nose, follow the treatment advice for nosebleeds (p.194).

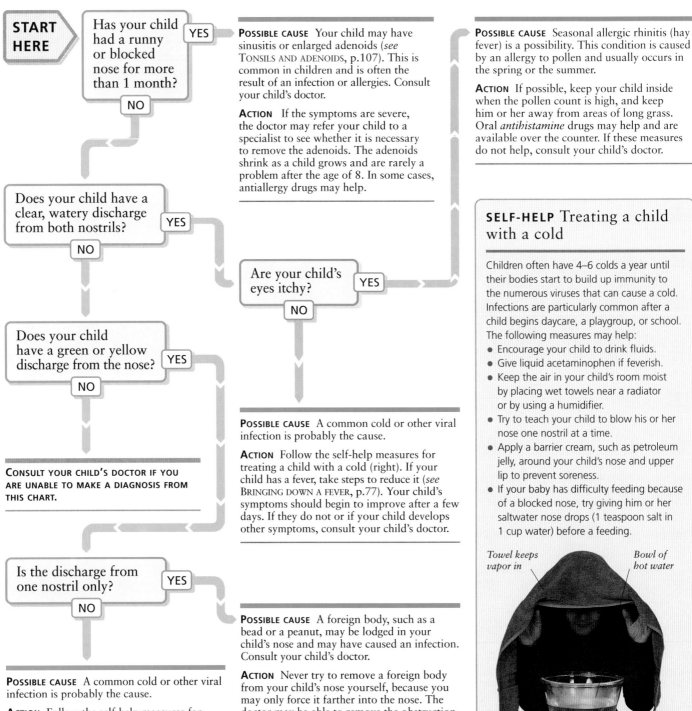

START HERE

Has your child had a runny or blocked nose for more than 1 month?
YES → **POSSIBLE CAUSE** Your child may have sinusitis or enlarged adenoids (*see* TONSILS AND ADENOIDS, p.107). This is common in children and is often the result of an infection or allergies. Consult your child's doctor.

ACTION If the symptoms are severe, the doctor may refer your child to a specialist to see whether it is necessary to remove the adenoids. The adenoids shrink as a child grows and are rarely a problem after the age of 8. In some cases, antiallergy drugs may help.

NO ↓

Does your child have a clear, watery discharge from both nostrils?
YES →

NO ↓

Are your child's eyes itchy?
YES → **POSSIBLE CAUSE** Seasonal allergic rhinitis (hay fever) is a possibility. This condition is caused by an allergy to pollen and usually occurs in the spring or the summer.

ACTION If possible, keep your child inside when the pollen count is high, and keep him or her away from areas of long grass. Oral *antihistamine* drugs may help and are available over the counter. If these measures do not help, consult your child's doctor.

NO ↓

POSSIBLE CAUSE A common cold or other viral infection is probably the cause.

ACTION Follow the self-help measures for treating a child with a cold (right). If your child has a fever, take steps to reduce it (*see* BRINGING DOWN A FEVER, p.77). Your child's symptoms should begin to improve after a few days. If they do not or if your child develops other symptoms, consult your child's doctor.

Does your child have a green or yellow discharge from the nose?
YES →

NO ↓

CONSULT YOUR CHILD'S DOCTOR IF YOU ARE UNABLE TO MAKE A DIAGNOSIS FROM THIS CHART.

Is the discharge from one nostril only?
YES → **POSSIBLE CAUSE** A foreign body, such as a bead or a peanut, may be lodged in your child's nose and may have caused an infection. Consult your child's doctor.

ACTION Never try to remove a foreign body from your child's nose yourself, because you may only force it farther into the nose. The doctor may be able to remove the obstruction. However, if the foreign body is difficult to reach, your child may need to be admitted to the hospital for a minor operation under general anesthetic to remove it. The infection should then clear up by itself, but in some cases *antibiotics* are needed to treat it.

NO ↓

POSSIBLE CAUSE A common cold or other viral infection is probably the cause.

ACTION Follow the self-help measures for treating a child with a cold (right). If your child has a fever, take steps to reduce it (*see* BRINGING DOWN A FEVER, p.77). Your child's symptoms should begin to improve after a few days. If they do not or if your child develops other symptoms, consult your child's doctor.

SELF-HELP Treating a child with a cold

Children often have 4–6 colds a year until their bodies start to build up immunity to the numerous viruses that can cause a cold. Infections are particularly common after a child begins daycare, a playgroup, or school. The following measures may help:

- Encourage your child to drink fluids.
- Give liquid acetaminophen if feverish.
- Keep the air in your child's room moist by placing wet towels near a radiator or by using a humidifier.
- Try to teach your child to blow his or her nose one nostril at a time.
- Apply a barrier cream, such as petroleum jelly, around your child's nose and upper lip to prevent soreness.
- If your baby has difficulty feeding because of a blocked nose, try giving him or her saltwater nose drops (1 teaspoon salt in 1 cup water) before a feeding.

Towel keeps vapor in   *Bowl of hot water*

Relieving congestion
Inhaling steam from a bowl of hot, but not boiling, water can help clear a blocked nose. Children should always be supervised.

32 Sore throat

Sore throats are common in childhood. An older child will usually tell you if his or her throat hurts. In a baby or a young child, the first sign you may have that something is wrong may be a reluctance to eat because of the pain caused by swallowing. Most sore throats are the result of minor viral infections that clear up within 2–3 days without the need for medical treatment. In a few cases, however, *antibiotics* may be needed to treat a bacterial infection.

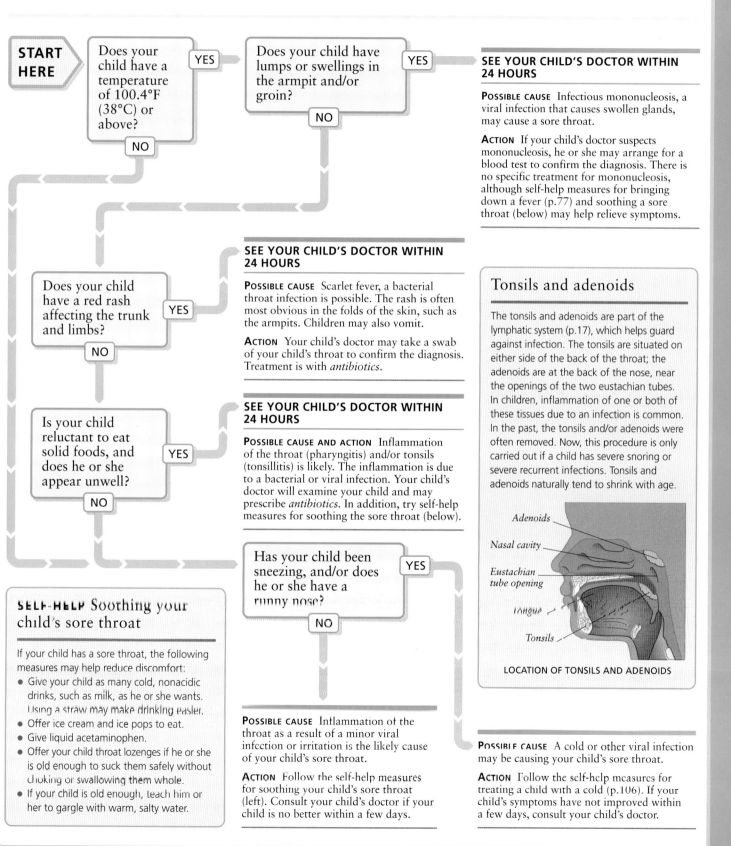

START HERE → Does your child have a temperature of 100.4°F (38°C) or above? — YES → Does your child have lumps or swellings in the armpit and/or groin? — YES →

SEE YOUR CHILD'S DOCTOR WITHIN 24 HOURS

POSSIBLE CAUSE Infectious mononucleosis, a viral infection that causes swollen glands, may cause a sore throat.

ACTION If your child's doctor suspects mononucleosis, he or she may arrange for a blood test to confirm the diagnosis. There is no specific treatment for mononucleosis, although self-help measures for bringing down a fever (p.77) and soothing a sore throat (below) may help relieve symptoms.

Does your child have a temperature... — NO

Does your child have lumps or swellings... — NO

Does your child have a red rash affecting the trunk and limbs? — YES →

SEE YOUR CHILD'S DOCTOR WITHIN 24 HOURS

POSSIBLE CAUSE Scarlet fever, a bacterial throat infection is possible. The rash is often most obvious in the folds of the skin, such as the armpits. Children may also vomit.

ACTION Your child's doctor may take a swab of your child's throat to confirm the diagnosis. Treatment is with *antibiotics*.

Does your child have a red rash... — NO

Is your child reluctant to eat solid foods, and does he or she appear unwell? — YES →

SEE YOUR CHILD'S DOCTOR WITHIN 24 HOURS

POSSIBLE CAUSE AND ACTION Inflammation of the throat (pharyngitis) and/or tonsils (tonsillitis) is likely. The inflammation is due to a bacterial or viral infection. Your child's doctor will examine your child and may prescribe *antibiotics*. In addition, try self-help measures for soothing the sore throat (below).

Is your child reluctant to eat... — NO

Has your child been sneezing, and/or does he or she have a runny nose? — YES →

POSSIBLE CAUSE A cold or other viral infection may be causing your child's sore throat.

ACTION Follow the self-help measures for treating a child with a cold (p.106). If your child's symptoms have not improved within a few days, consult your child's doctor.

Has your child been sneezing... — NO

POSSIBLE CAUSE Inflammation of the throat as a result of a minor viral infection or irritation is the likely cause of your child's sore throat.

ACTION Follow the self-help measures for soothing your child's sore throat (left). Consult your child's doctor if your child is no better in a few days.

SELF-HELP Soothing your child's sore throat

If your child has a sore throat, the following measures may help reduce discomfort:
- Give your child as many cold, nonacidic drinks, such as milk, as he or she wants. Using a straw may make drinking easier.
- Offer ice cream and ice pops to eat.
- Give liquid acetaminophen.
- Offer your child throat lozenges if he or she is old enough to suck them safely without choking or swallowing them whole.
- If your child is old enough, teach him or her to gargle with warm, salty water.

Tonsils and adenoids

The tonsils and adenoids are part of the lymphatic system (p.17), which helps guard against infection. The tonsils are situated on either side of the back of the throat; the adenoids are at the back of the nose, near the openings of the two eustachian tubes. In children, inflammation of one or both of these tissues due to an infection is common. In the past, the tonsils and/or adenoids were often removed. Now, this procedure is only carried out if a child has severe snoring or severe recurrent infections. Tonsils and adenoids naturally tend to shrink with age.

Adenoids
Nasal cavity
Eustachian tube opening
Tongue
Tonsils

LOCATION OF TONSILS AND ADENOIDS

33 Coughing

Coughing is a normal protective reaction to irritation of the throat or lungs. In babies under 6 months, coughs are unusual and can be a sign of a serious lung infection if the child is also unwell. In older children, the vast majority of coughs are due to minor infections of the throat or upper airways, such as colds. A runny nose can cause a cough, particularly at night as fluid drips down the back of the throat and causes irritation. A cough at night, even if it is not accompanied by wheezing, can be a symptom of asthma; you should consult your child's doctor if you are concerned.

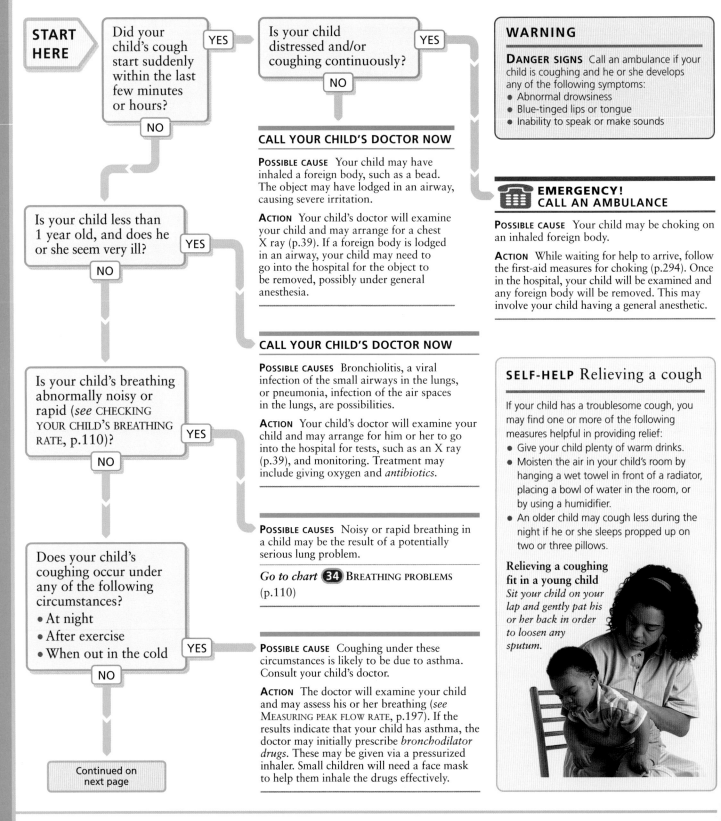

START HERE

Did your child's cough start suddenly within the last few minutes or hours?
— YES →
— NO ↓

Is your child distressed and/or coughing continuously?
— YES →
— NO ↓

Is your child less than 1 year old, and does he or she seem very ill?
— YES →
— NO ↓

Is your child's breathing abnormally noisy or rapid (see CHECKING YOUR CHILD'S BREATHING RATE, p.110)?
— YES →
— NO ↓

Does your child's coughing occur under any of the following circumstances?
- At night
- After exercise
- When out in the cold
— YES →
— NO ↓

Continued on next page

CALL YOUR CHILD'S DOCTOR NOW

POSSIBLE CAUSE Your child may have inhaled a foreign body, such as a bead. The object may have lodged in an airway, causing severe irritation.

ACTION Your child's doctor will examine your child and may arrange for a chest X ray (p.39). If a foreign body is lodged in an airway, your child may need to go into the hospital for the object to be removed, possibly under general anesthesia.

CALL YOUR CHILD'S DOCTOR NOW

POSSIBLE CAUSES Bronchiolitis, a viral infection of the small airways in the lungs, or pneumonia, infection of the air spaces in the lungs, are possibilities.

ACTION Your child's doctor will examine your child and may arrange for him or her to go into the hospital for tests, such as an X ray (p.39), and monitoring. Treatment may include giving oxygen and *antibiotics*.

POSSIBLE CAUSES Noisy or rapid breathing in a child may be the result of a potentially serious lung problem.

Go to chart **34** BREATHING PROBLEMS (p.110)

POSSIBLE CAUSE Coughing under these circumstances is likely to be due to asthma. Consult your child's doctor.

ACTION The doctor will examine your child and may assess his or her breathing (*see* MEASURING PEAK FLOW RATE, p.197). If the results indicate that your child has asthma, the doctor may initially prescribe *bronchodilator drugs*. These may be given via a pressurized inhaler. Small children will need a face mask to help them inhale the drugs effectively.

WARNING

DANGER SIGNS Call an ambulance if your child is coughing and he or she develops any of the following symptoms:
- Abnormal drowsiness
- Blue-tinged lips or tongue
- Inability to speak or make sounds

☎ EMERGENCY! CALL AN AMBULANCE

POSSIBLE CAUSE Your child may be choking on an inhaled foreign body.

ACTION While waiting for help to arrive, follow the first-aid measures for choking (p.294). Once in the hospital, your child will be examined and any foreign body will be removed. This may involve your child having a general anesthetic.

SELF-HELP Relieving a cough

If your child has a troublesome cough, you may find one or more of the following measures helpful in providing relief:
- Give your child plenty of warm drinks.
- Moisten the air in your child's room by hanging a wet towel in front of a radiator, placing a bowl of water in the room, or by using a humidifier.
- An older child may cough less during the night if he or she sleeps propped up on two or three pillows.

Relieving a coughing fit in a young child
Sit your child on your lap and gently pat his or her back in order to loosen any sputum.

Continued from previous page

Has your child been immunized against pertussis? **YES**

NO

POSSIBLE CAUSE Even though your child has been immunized, a mild attack of pertussis (whooping cough), an infectious disease that causes bouts of coughing, may be the cause. The infection is much less serious in children who have been immunized than in those who have not. Consult your child's doctor.

ACTION The doctor will probably prescribe *antibiotics* for your child to reduce the chance of him or her passing the infection on to others. Coughing may persist for several weeks, but symptoms are rarely severe enough for the child to need hospital admission.

Does your child have bouts of uncontrollable coughing followed by a noisy intake of breath, and/or is coughing often followed by vomiting? **YES**

NO

SEE YOUR CHILD'S DOCTOR WITHIN 24 HOURS

POSSIBLE CAUSE Your child may have pertussis (whooping cough), an infectious disease that causes bouts of severe, uncontrollable coughing.

ACTION Your child's doctor will probably prescribe *antibiotics* to reduce the chance of your child passing the infection on to others. If the condition is severe, the doctor may send your child to the hospital for treatment. Episodes of coughing may persist for several months.

POSSIBLE CAUSES Your child may have enlarged tonsils or adenoids (p.107), which can block the airway. Consult your child's doctor.

ACTION The doctor will examine your child and may arrange for hearing tests (p.105) or refer your child to a specialist. In some cases, removal of the tonsils and/or adenoids is advised, although symptoms often improve as the child grows up. Adenoids rarely cause a problem in children over 8 years.

Does your child always have a runny nose? **YES**

NO

Does your child have any of the following?
• Frequent ear infections
• Nasal speech
• Snoring
• Poor hearing
YES

NO

POSSIBLE CAUSE Perennial allergic rhinitis may be the cause. In this condition, an allergic reaction to substances such as house dust, animal fur, or mold spores causes symptoms all year round.

ACTION If you think you know the trigger for your child's allergy, try to limit his or her contact with it. *Antihistamines*, some of which are available over the counter, may provide relief. If these do not help, consult your child's doctor, who may prescribe alternative drug treatment.

Does your child have a temperature of 100.4°F (38°C) or above and/or a runny nose? **YES**

NO

POSSIBLE CAUSES A common cold or other viral infection is a possibility.

ACTION Take steps to lower your child's temperature (*see* BRINGING DOWN A FEVER, p.77), and follow the self-help measures for treating a child with a cold (p.106) and relieving a cough (opposite). If your child develops a rash or is no better within 2 days, consult your child's doctor.

Does anyone in the home smoke, or could your child have been smoking? **YES**

NO

POSSIBLE CAUSE AND ACTION A smoky atmosphere and smoking itself will irritate a child's throat and lungs, causing a persistent cough. If your child has begun to smoke, you should persuade him or her to stop. The longer he or she smokes, the more difficult it will be to give up. If family members continue to smoke, they should avoid smoking in the home.

CONSULT YOUR CHILD'S DOCTOR IF YOU ARE UNABLE TO MAKE A DIAGNOSIS FROM THIS CHART.

34 Breathing problems

Breathing problems in children include excessively noisy or fast breathing and shortness of breath. Although rapid or noisy breathing is usually obvious, shortness of breath may be less noticeable because a child may simply avoid activities that make him or her breathless. Any child who starts to wheeze needs to be seen by a doctor, and a child with severe difficulty in breathing needs urgent attention. Breathing problems that occur suddenly also need immediate attention.

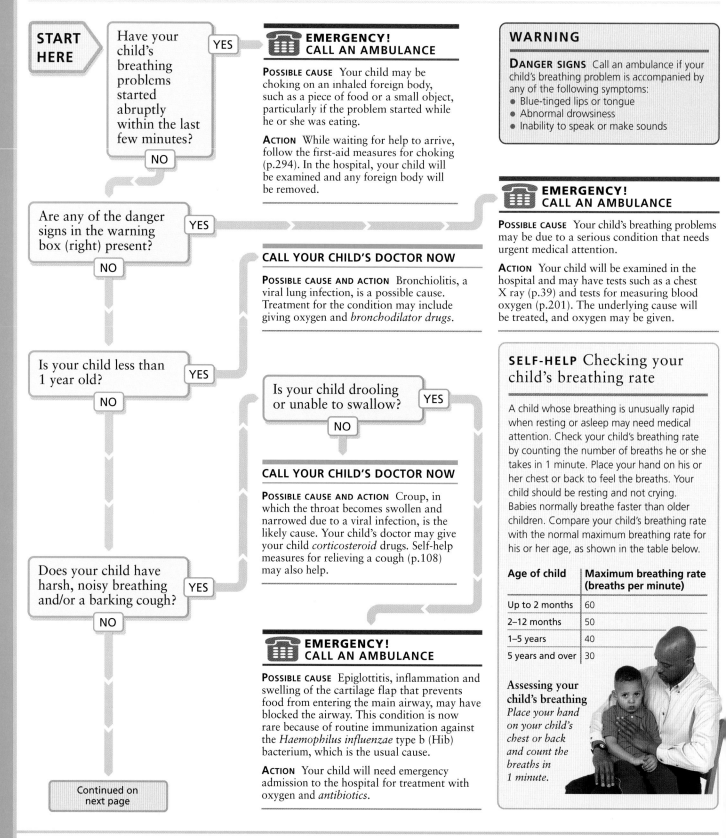

START HERE

Have your child's breathing problems started abruptly within the last few minutes? — YES →

☎ EMERGENCY! CALL AN AMBULANCE

POSSIBLE CAUSE Your child may be choking on an inhaled foreign body, such as a piece of food or a small object, particularly if the problem started while he or she was eating.

ACTION While waiting for help to arrive, follow the first-aid measures for choking (p.294). In the hospital, your child will be examined and any foreign body will be removed.

NO ↓

Are any of the danger signs in the warning box (right) present? — YES →

NO ↓

CALL YOUR CHILD'S DOCTOR NOW

POSSIBLE CAUSE AND ACTION Bronchiolitis, a viral lung infection, is a possible cause. Treatment for the condition may include giving oxygen and *bronchodilator drugs*.

Is your child less than 1 year old? — YES →

NO ↓

Is your child drooling or unable to swallow? — YES →

NO ↓

CALL YOUR CHILD'S DOCTOR NOW

POSSIBLE CAUSE AND ACTION Croup, in which the throat becomes swollen and narrowed due to a viral infection, is the likely cause. Your child's doctor may give your child *corticosteroid* drugs. Self-help measures for relieving a cough (p.108) may also help.

Does your child have harsh, noisy breathing and/or a barking cough? — YES →

NO ↓

☎ EMERGENCY! CALL AN AMBULANCE

POSSIBLE CAUSE Epiglottitis, inflammation and swelling of the cartilage flap that prevents food from entering the main airway, may have blocked the airway. This condition is now rare because of routine immunization against the *Haemophilus influenzae* type b (Hib) bacterium, which is the usual cause.

ACTION Your child will need emergency admission to the hospital for treatment with oxygen and *antibiotics*.

Continued on next page

WARNING

DANGER SIGNS Call an ambulance if your child's breathing problem is accompanied by any of the following symptoms:
- Blue-tinged lips or tongue
- Abnormal drowsiness
- Inability to speak or make sounds

☎ EMERGENCY! CALL AN AMBULANCE

POSSIBLE CAUSE Your child's breathing problems may be due to a serious condition that needs urgent medical attention.

ACTION Your child will be examined in the hospital and may have tests such as a chest X ray (p.39) and tests for measuring blood oxygen (p.201). The underlying cause will be treated, and oxygen may be given.

SELF-HELP Checking your child's breathing rate

A child whose breathing is unusually rapid when resting or asleep may need medical attention. Check your child's breathing rate by counting the number of breaths he or she takes in 1 minute. Place your hand on his or her chest or back to feel the breaths. Your child should be resting and not crying. Babies normally breathe faster than older children. Compare your child's breathing rate with the normal maximum breathing rate for his or her age, as shown in the table below.

Age of child	Maximum breathing rate (breaths per minute)
Up to 2 months	60
2–12 months	50
1–5 years	40
5 years and over	30

Assessing your child's breathing
Place your hand on your child's chest or back and count the breaths in 1 minute.

SELF-HELP Easing breathing in an asthma attack

If your child is having severe difficulty in breathing, call an ambulance. While waiting for help to arrive, you should:
- Help your child sit upright, leaning forward slightly, with his or her forearms supported on a table or the back of a chair.
- Make sure any prescribed drugs for asthma have been taken according to the treatment plan.
- Try to stay calm and keep your child calm. Do not leave him or her alone. Try to keep other people from crowding around your child to prevent him or her from becoming more anxious.

Easing breathing
Sit your child upright with his or her arms supported. Do not leave your child alone.

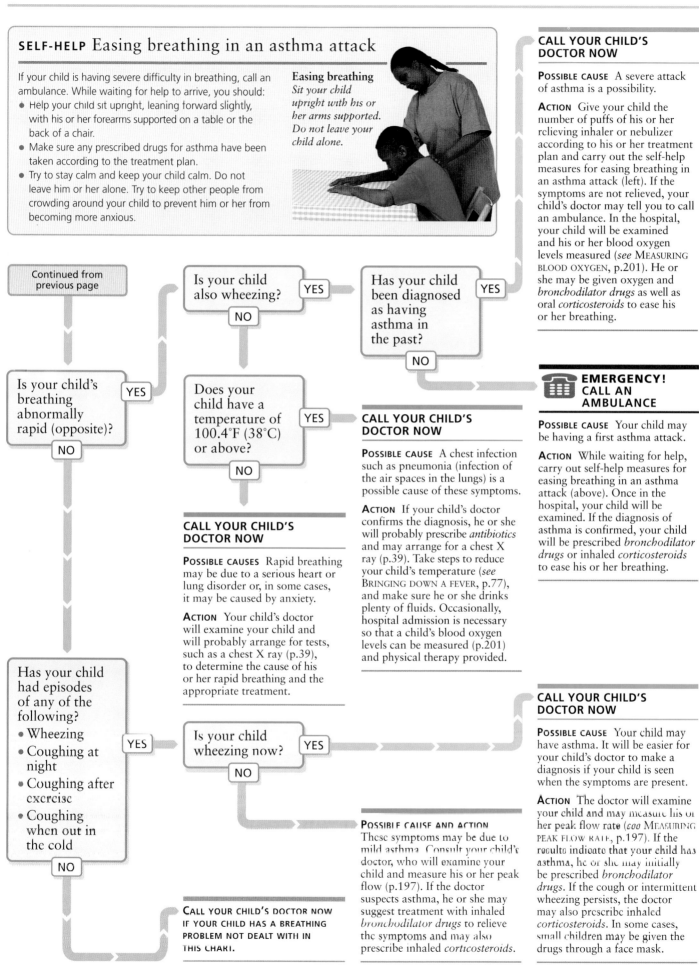

CALL YOUR CHILD'S DOCTOR NOW

POSSIBLE CAUSE A severe attack of asthma is a possibility.

ACTION Give your child the number of puffs of his or her relieving inhaler or nebulizer according to his or her treatment plan and carry out the self-help measures for easing breathing in an asthma attack (left). If the symptoms are not relieved, your child's doctor may tell you to call an ambulance. In the hospital, your child will be examined and his or her blood oxygen levels measured (*see* MEASURING BLOOD OXYGEN, p.201). He or she may be given oxygen and *bronchodilator drugs* as well as oral *corticosteroids* to ease his or her breathing.

Continued from previous page

Is your child also wheezing? YES

NO

Has your child been diagnosed as having asthma in the past? YES

NO

📞 EMERGENCY! CALL AN AMBULANCE

POSSIBLE CAUSE Your child may be having a first asthma attack.

ACTION While waiting for help, carry out self-help measures for easing breathing in an asthma attack (above). Once in the hospital, your child will be examined. If the diagnosis of asthma is confirmed, your child will be prescribed *bronchodilator drugs* or inhaled *corticosteroids* to ease his or her breathing.

Is your child's breathing abnormally rapid (opposite)? YES

NO

Does your child have a temperature of 100.4°F (38°C) or above? YES

NO

CALL YOUR CHILD'S DOCTOR NOW

POSSIBLE CAUSE A chest infection such as pneumonia (infection of the air spaces in the lungs) is a possible cause of these symptoms.

ACTION If your child's doctor confirms the diagnosis, he or she will probably prescribe *antibiotics* and may arrange for a chest X ray (p.39). Take steps to reduce your child's temperature (*see* BRINGING DOWN A FEVER, p.77), and make sure he or she drinks plenty of fluids. Occasionally, hospital admission is necessary so that a child's blood oxygen levels can be measured (p.201) and physical therapy provided.

CALL YOUR CHILD'S DOCTOR NOW

POSSIBLE CAUSES Rapid breathing may be due to a serious heart or lung disorder or, in some cases, it may be caused by anxiety.

ACTION Your child's doctor will examine your child and will probably arrange for tests, such as a chest X ray (p.39), to determine the cause of his or her rapid breathing and the appropriate treatment.

CALL YOUR CHILD'S DOCTOR NOW

POSSIBLE CAUSE Your child may have asthma. It will be easier for your child's doctor to make a diagnosis if your child is seen when the symptoms are present.

ACTION The doctor will examine your child and may measure his or her peak flow rate (*see* MEASURING PEAK FLOW RATE, p.197). If the results indicate that your child has asthma, he or she may initially be prescribed *bronchodilator drugs*. If the cough or intermittent wheezing persists, the doctor may also prescribe inhaled *corticosteroids*. In some cases, small children may be given the drugs through a face mask.

Has your child had episodes of any of the following?
- Wheezing
- Coughing at night
- Coughing after exercise
- Coughing when out in the cold

YES

NO

Is your child wheezing now? YES

NO

POSSIBLE CAUSE AND ACTION These symptoms may be due to mild asthma. Consult your child's doctor, who will examine your child and measure his or her peak flow (p.197). If the doctor suspects asthma, he or she may suggest treatment with inhaled *bronchodilator drugs* to relieve the symptoms and may also prescribe inhaled *corticosteroids*.

CALL YOUR CHILD'S DOCTOR NOW IF YOUR CHILD HAS A BREATHING PROBLEM NOT DEALT WITH IN THIS CHART.

35 Mouth problems

For problems specifically relating to the teeth, see chart 36, TEETH PROBLEMS (p.114).

Consult this chart if your child complains of a painful mouth or has sores in the mouth or on the tongue or lips. Since the lining of the mouth and the skin of the lips are thin and delicate, these areas are susceptible to minor injuries and infections. Younger children often pick up infections affecting the mouth and lips because they tend to put objects into their mouths. Allergies can cause swelling of the mouth or tongue, which can be serious (*see* WARNING, below).

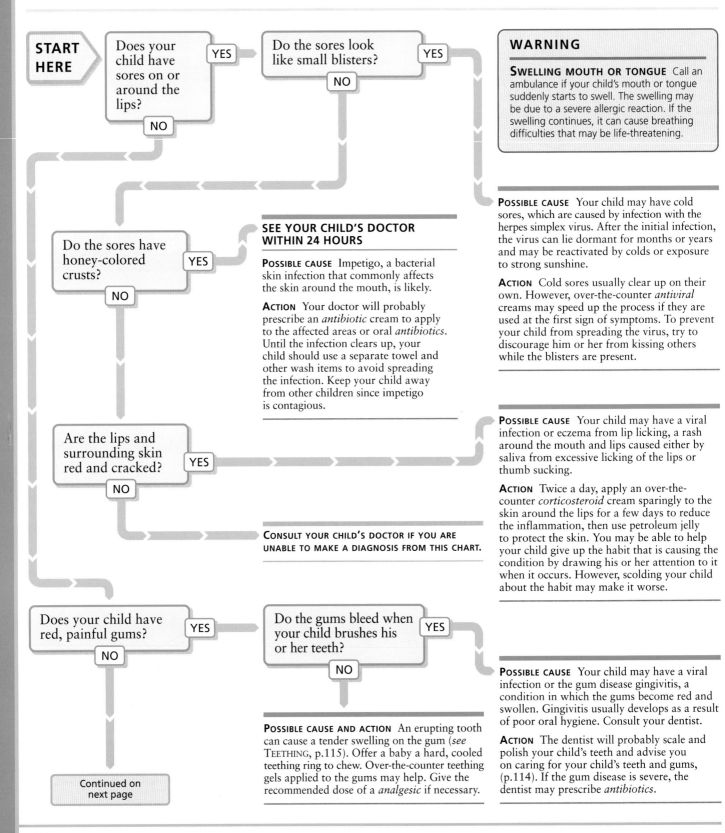

START HERE

Does your child have sores on or around the lips? — YES → **Do the sores look like small blisters?** — YES →

NO ↓ / NO ↓

WARNING

SWELLING MOUTH OR TONGUE Call an ambulance if your child's mouth or tongue suddenly starts to swell. The swelling may be due to a severe allergic reaction. If the swelling continues, it can cause breathing difficulties that may be life-threatening.

Do the sores have honey-colored crusts? — YES →

NO ↓

SEE YOUR CHILD'S DOCTOR WITHIN 24 HOURS

POSSIBLE CAUSE Impetigo, a bacterial skin infection that commonly affects the skin around the mouth, is likely.

ACTION Your doctor will probably prescribe an *antibiotic* cream to apply to the affected areas or oral *antibiotics*. Until the infection clears up, your child should use a separate towel and other wash items to avoid spreading the infection. Keep your child away from other children since impetigo is contagious.

POSSIBLE CAUSE Your child may have cold sores, which are caused by infection with the herpes simplex virus. After the initial infection, the virus can lie dormant for months or years and may be reactivated by colds or exposure to strong sunshine.

ACTION Cold sores usually clear up on their own. However, over-the-counter *antiviral* creams may speed up the process if they are used at the first sign of symptoms. To prevent your child from spreading the virus, try to discourage him or her from kissing others while the blisters are present.

Are the lips and surrounding skin red and cracked? — YES →

NO ↓

CONSULT YOUR CHILD'S DOCTOR IF YOU ARE UNABLE TO MAKE A DIAGNOSIS FROM THIS CHART.

POSSIBLE CAUSE Your child may have a viral infection or eczema from lip licking, a rash around the mouth and lips caused either by saliva from excessive licking of the lips or thumb sucking.

ACTION Twice a day, apply an over-the-counter *corticosteroid* cream sparingly to the skin around the lips for a few days to reduce the inflammation, then use petroleum jelly to protect the skin. You may be able to help your child give up the habit that is causing the condition by drawing his or her attention to it when it occurs. However, scolding your child about the habit may make it worse.

Does your child have red, painful gums? — YES → **Do the gums bleed when your child brushes his or her teeth?** — YES →

NO ↓ / NO ↓

POSSIBLE CAUSE AND ACTION An erupting tooth can cause a tender swelling on the gum (*see* TEETHING, p.115). Offer a baby a hard, cooled teething ring to chew. Over-the-counter teething gels applied to the gums may help. Give the recommended dose of a *analgesic* if necessary.

POSSIBLE CAUSE Your child may have a viral infection or the gum disease gingivitis, a condition in which the gums become red and swollen. Gingivitis usually develops as a result of poor oral hygiene. Consult your dentist.

ACTION The dentist will probably scale and polish your child's teeth and advise you on caring for your child's teeth and gums, (p.114). If the gum disease is severe, the dentist may prescribe *antibiotics*.

Continued on next page

Continued from previous page

Does your child have creamy yellow or white patches inside the mouth and/or on the tongue? — YES / NO

Does your child also have blisters on the palms of the hands and the soles of the feet? — YES / NO

Does your child have one or more shallow, gray, ulcerated patches or blisters in the mouth? — YES / NO

Does your child have a fever and/or seem generally ill? — YES / NO

Does your child have a sore area inside a cheek or on the side of the tongue? — YES / NO

SEE YOUR CHILD'S DOCTOR WITHIN 24 HOURS

POSSIBLE CAUSE Oral thrush, a fungal infection, is a possibility. This condition is most common in young babies or in older children whose immunity has been lowered by certain diseases or drug treatments.

ACTION Your child's doctor will probably prescribe *antifungal* medicine to clear up the infection. To prevent reinfection, sterilize any pacifiers, bottle nipples, and teething rings that your child uses.

POSSIBLE CAUSE Your child may have hand, foot, and mouth disease, a mild infection caused by a virus. The blisters on the hands and feet often appear approximately 48 hours after the ones in the mouth. Consult your child's doctor.

ACTION There is no specific treatment for this condition. If the blisters burst and form ulcers, encourage your child to rinse his or her mouth with a solution of bicarbonate of soda. Give your child the recommended dose of a *analgesic* if necessary (*see* RELIEVING A SORE MOUTH, below). Make sure your child drinks plenty of fluids (*see* ENCOURAGING YOUR CHILD TO DRINK, p.67).

POSSIBLE CAUSE Your child may have mouth ulcers. These often develop for no apparent reason but tend to recur in times of stress or at the site of a minor injury, such as damage from a toothbrush. Mouth ulcers can be painful but are not serious.

ACTION Rinsing the mouth with a solution of bicarbonate of soda may help relieve the pain (*see* RELIEVING A SORE MOUTH, below). Over-the-counter treatments can also relieve pain and may help the ulcers to heal. If an ulcer does not heal within 10 days or your child has several ulcers at the same time, consult your child's doctor.

SEE YOUR CHILD'S DOCTOR WITHIN 24 HOURS

POSSIBLE CAUSES The most likely cause is infection with the virus that causes cold sores. When babies or young children have a first infection with this virus they may be sick and have a very sore mouth. Similar symptoms can be due to other viruses or, in some cases, to prescription drugs.

ACTION If the child's mouth is so sore that he or she is unable to drink, your child's doctor may recommend hospital admission. In less severe cases, your doctor will recommend self-help measures (*see* RELIEVING A SORE MOUTH, below). If prescription drugs are thought to be the cause they will be stopped.

CONSULT YOUR CHILD'S DOCTOR IF YOU ARE UNABLE TO MAKE A DIAGNOSIS FROM THIS CHART.

POSSIBLE CAUSE AND ACTION A new or jagged tooth may cause enough friction to make your child's cheek or tongue sore. Take steps to relieve the pain (*see* RELIEVING A SORE MOUTH, right). If the sore persists or appears to be cause by a jagged tooth, consult your dentist, who may be able to smooth a rough edge.

SELF-HELP Relieving a sore mouth

The following self-help measures may help relieve the pain of a sore mouth:
- If necessary, give your child the appropriate dose of a *analgesic*, such as acetaminophen.
- If your child is old enough to cooperate, he or she should rinse the mouth hourly with ¼ teaspoon of bicarbonate of soda dissolved in 3½ fl.oz (100 ml) of warm water.
- Offer soft foods, such as ice cream.
- Serve drinks with drinking straws to keep liquids away from sores on the lips.
- Avoid very salty foods, and acidic foods and sour drinks, such as oranges or fruit juices
- Try to continue brushing your child's teeth twice daily, but take care near the sore areas.

Easy-to-eat foods
Soft foods are easy for a child with a sore mouth to eat. Ice cream is ideal because the coldness helps numb the mouth, relieving pain.

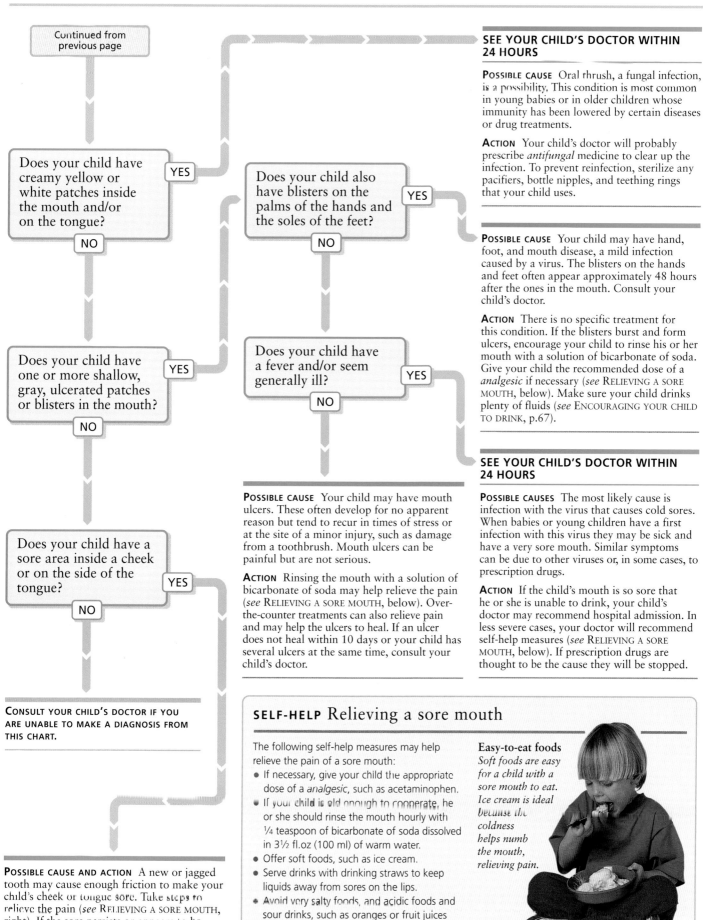

36 Teeth problems

Your child's teeth are constantly at risk of decay. Regular brushing can help prevent decay (*see* CARING FOR YOUR CHILD'S TEETH AND GUMS, below), which, if untreated, can spread to central parts of the tooth, causing serious damage. Your child should have regular dental checkups from about 3 years of age. If symptoms of decay, such as toothache, develop between

checkups, make an appointment with your dentist. In young children, pain associated with the teeth may be due to teething (opposite), which is usually no cause for concern. If your child has toothache or an accident needing urgent dental treatment and your dentist is unavailable, call the emergency department of a local hospital for advice.

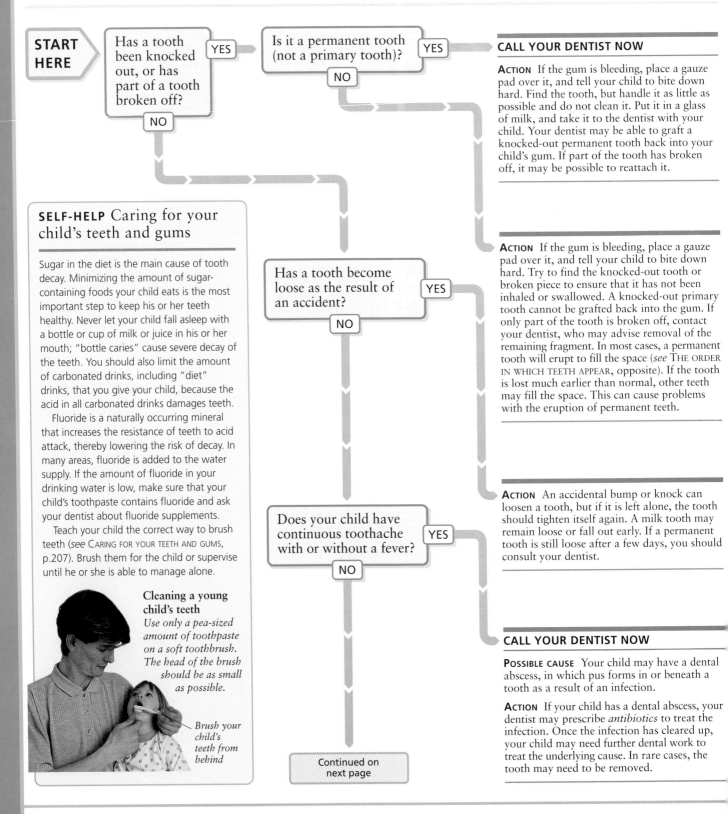

START HERE

Has a tooth been knocked out, or has part of a tooth broken off? — YES → **Is it a permanent tooth (not a primary tooth)?** — YES →

NO

NO

CALL YOUR DENTIST NOW

ACTION If the gum is bleeding, place a gauze pad over it, and tell your child to bite down hard. Find the tooth, but handle it as little as possible and do not clean it. Put it in a glass of milk, and take it to the dentist with your child. Your dentist may be able to graft a knocked-out permanent tooth back into your child's gum. If part of the tooth has broken off, it may be possible to reattach it.

Has a tooth become loose as the result of an accident? — YES →

NO

ACTION If the gum is bleeding, place a gauze pad over it, and tell your child to bite down hard. Try to find the knocked-out tooth or broken piece to ensure that it has not been inhaled or swallowed. A knocked-out primary tooth cannot be grafted back into the gum. If only part of the tooth is broken off, contact your dentist, who may advise removal of the remaining fragment. In most cases, a permanent tooth will erupt to fill the space (*see* THE ORDER IN WHICH TEETH APPEAR, opposite). If the tooth is lost much earlier than normal, other teeth may fill the space. This can cause problems with the eruption of permanent teeth.

Does your child have continuous toothache with or without a fever? — YES →

NO

ACTION An accidental bump or knock can loosen a tooth, but if it is left alone, the tooth should tighten itself again. A milk tooth may remain loose or fall out early. If a permanent tooth is still loose after a few days, you should consult your dentist.

CALL YOUR DENTIST NOW

POSSIBLE CAUSE Your child may have a dental abscess, in which pus forms in or beneath a tooth as a result of an infection.

ACTION If your child has a dental abscess, your dentist may prescribe *antibiotics* to treat the infection. Once the infection has cleared up, your child may need further dental work to treat the underlying cause. In rare cases, the tooth may need to be removed.

SELF-HELP Caring for your child's teeth and gums

Sugar in the diet is the main cause of tooth decay. Minimizing the amount of sugar-containing foods your child eats is the most important step to keep his or her teeth healthy. Never let your child fall asleep with a bottle or cup of milk or juice in his or her mouth; "bottle caries" cause severe decay of the teeth. You should also limit the amount of carbonated drinks, including "diet" drinks, that you give your child, because the acid in all carbonated drinks damages teeth.

Fluoride is a naturally occurring mineral that increases the resistance of teeth to acid attack, thereby lowering the risk of decay. In many areas, fluoride is added to the water supply. If the amount of fluoride in your drinking water is low, make sure that your child's toothpaste contains fluoride and ask your dentist about fluoride supplements.

Teach your child the correct way to brush teeth (*see* CARING FOR YOUR TEETH AND GUMS, p.207). Brush them for the child or supervise until he or she is able to manage alone.

Cleaning a young child's teeth
Use only a pea-sized amount of toothpaste on a soft toothbrush. The head of the brush should be as small as possible.

Brush your child's teeth from behind

Continued on next page

Continued from
previous page

**Does your child feel
pain in his or her teeth
when they are exposed
to hot or cold foods?** → YES

NO ↓

**Does your child feel
pain when he or she
bites on a tooth that
has been filled recently?** → YES

NO ↓

POSSIBLE CAUSE AND ACTION It is
quite common for a tooth to feel
uncomfortable for a while after a
filling has been put in, especially if
the filling is large. If the pain gets
worse or if your child is no better
within 48 hours, consult your
dentist, who will check the filling
and adjust it if necessary.

**Does your child have
pain in several of the
teeth in the upper jaw?** → YES

NO ↓

**Does your child have
tender gums behind the
back teeth?** → YES

NO ↓

CONSULT YOUR DENTIST IF YOU ARE UNABLE
TO MAKE A DIAGNOSIS FROM THIS CHART.

POSSIBLE CAUSE Your child's second molars
may be beginning to emerge (*see* THE ORDER
IN WHICH TEETH APPEAR, right). The gums
may become inflamed as the teeth erupt, but
this is usually short-lived.

ACTION If necessary, give your child the
recommended dose of a *analgesic*, such as
acetaminophen. Consult your dentist if
the pain is severe or if it is no better within
48 hours.

**Does the pain last only
a few seconds?** → YES

NO ↓

**SEE YOUR DENTIST WITHIN
24 HOURS**

POSSIBLE CAUSE Your child may have
decay deep within a tooth or in a crack
in a tooth. This is especially likely if your
child also has bouts of throbbing tooth
pain not brought on by food or drink.

ACTION Your dentist will examine your
child's teeth and may need to remove and
fill any decayed areas.

POSSIBLE CAUSE Aching in several
teeth can be a symptom of sinusitis
(inflammation of the membranes lining
the air spaces in the skull), especially if
your child has recently had a cold or a
runny or blocked nose.

ACTION Give your child acetaminophen
for the pain. Steam inhalation may help
(p.194). Consult your doctor if your
child's symptoms are no better within
48 hours; he or she may need treatment
with *antibiotics*.

Teething

The eruption of a tooth, particularly a molar,
can be uncomfortable and may make your
child irritable and restless. You may be able
to feel the emerging tooth if you run your
finger over the gum. A baby may have
flushed cheeks, be less willing to feed, and
may sleep poorly when teething. However,
you should not attribute other symptoms,
such as a fever or diarrhea, to teething.

Babies who are teething often seem to
like chewing on a cold, hard object, such as
a chilled teething ring. Over-the-counter
local anesthetic gels can be soothing if
gently applied to the affected gums. The
recommended dose of a *analgesic* can also
be given if necessary.

POSSIBLE CAUSE Teeth can become sensitive
to extremes of temperature if their protective
surfaces become thin or damaged. This may
be due to tooth decay. Consult your dentist.

ACTION Your dentist will examine your child's
teeth and treat any decay. If no abnormality is
found, he or she may advise that your child
brushes with a toothpaste for sensitive teeth and
rubs a small amount over the teeth afterward.

The order in which teeth appear

The ages at which teeth appear vary from child
to child. A few children have one or more teeth
at birth, while others still have none at a year
old. There are 20 teeth in the first, or primary,
set. The sequence in which they erupt is more
important than the age of eruption. By the age
of 13, the primary teeth have usually fallen out
and most of the 32 permanent, or adult, teeth
have erupted. In some people, the third molars,
known as the wisdom teeth, never appear.

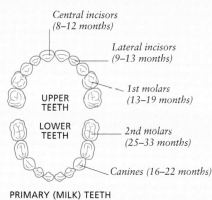

*Central incisors
(8–12 months)*

*Lateral incisors
(9–13 months)*

1st molars
(13–19 months)

UPPER
TEETH

LOWER
TEETH

2nd molars
(25–33 months)

Canines (16–22 months)

PRIMARY (MILK) TEETH

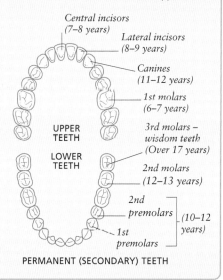

*Central incisors
(7–8 years)*

*Lateral incisors
(8–9 years)*

Canines
(11–12 years)

1st molars
(6–7 years)

UPPER
TEETH

LOWER
TEETH

3rd molars –
wisdom teeth
(Over 17 years)

2nd molars
(12–13 years)

2nd
premolars
} (10–12
years)

1st
premolars

PERMANENT (SECONDARY) TEETH

The ages at which teeth appear
*The figures in brackets indicate the average ages
at which the teeth erupt. However, neither early
nor late eruption is a cause for concern.*

37 Eating problems

For children under 1 year, see chart 6, FEEDING PROBLEMS (p.60).
The appetites of children are more closely governed by their
body's energy requirements than are the appetites of adults.
Most children alternate between active periods, during
which they have large appetites, and inactive periods, when
they eat much less. In addition, when children are growing
rapidly, their appetites will be larger than usual. Some
children naturally burn up less energy than others and have

smaller appetites. Such variations in appetite are normal and
are not a problem as long as your child seems well and is
growing normally. Some children may refuse to eat to gain
their parents' attention or control. This is relatively common
in young children; however, they usually grow out of it. In
older children and adolescents, a refusal to eat may be a
symptom of the potentially life-threatening disorder
anorexia nervosa (*see* EATING DISORDERS, p.139).

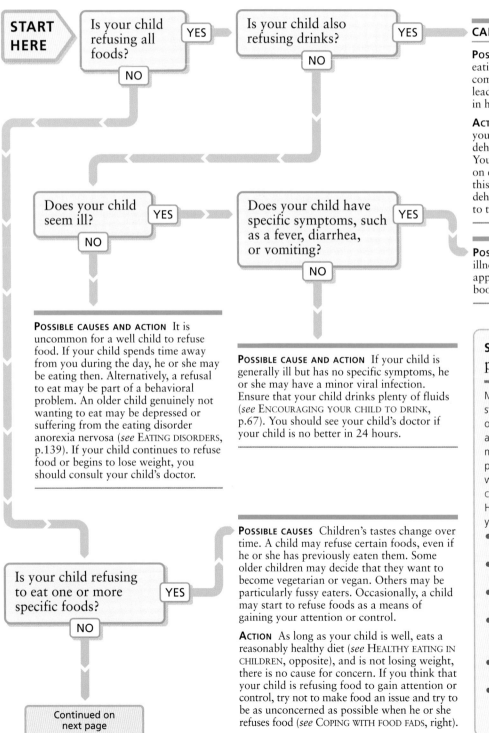

START HERE

Is your child refusing all foods? — YES → **Is your child also refusing drinks?** — YES →

NO

NO

CALL YOUR CHILD'S DOCTOR NOW

POSSIBLE CAUSES A child can go without
eating very much for several days and not
come to any harm, but refusal to drink can
lead to dehydration more rapidly, particularly
in hot weather or if the child has a fever.

ACTION Your child's doctor will examine
your child to ensure that he or she is not
dehydrated and look for an underlying cause.
Your doctor will probably give you advice
on encouraging your child to drink (p.67). If
this is not successful or if your child is already
dehydrated, he or she may need to be admitted
to the hospital.

Does your child seem ill? — YES → **Does your child have specific symptoms, such as a fever, diarrhea, or vomiting?** — YES →

NO

NO

POSSIBLE CAUSE AND ACTION An underlying
illness can often cause a temporary loss of
appetite. Consult the relevant chart in this
book and follow the advice given.

POSSIBLE CAUSES AND ACTION It is
uncommon for a well child to refuse
food. If your child spends time away
from you during the day, he or she may
be eating then. Alternatively, a refusal
to eat may be part of a behavioral
problem. An older child genuinely not
wanting to eat may be depressed or
suffering from the eating disorder
anorexia nervosa (*see* EATING DISORDERS,
p.139). If your child continues to refuse
food or begins to lose weight, you
should consult your child's doctor.

POSSIBLE CAUSE AND ACTION If your child is
generally ill but has no specific symptoms, he
or she may have a minor viral infection.
Ensure that your child drinks plenty of fluids
(*see* ENCOURAGING YOUR CHILD TO DRINK,
p.67). You should see your child's doctor if
your child is no better in 24 hours.

SELF-HELP Coping with picky eaters

Most children become picky eaters at some
stage. Sometimes a child will refuse only one
or two foods or will accept foods only if they
are prepared in a particular way. The child
may claim to dislike foods that he or she
previously enjoyed. As long as your child is
well and is growing normally (*see* GROWTH
CHARTS, p.26), there is no need for concern.
However, there are some self-help measures
you can take to encourage your child to eat:
- Keep mealtimes relaxed. Do not insist that
  your child eat everything on his or her plate.
- Serve small portions, giving second
  helpings if requested.
- Do not give your child snacks and
  numerous drinks between meals.
- Do not persist in offering rejected foods.
  Keep them off the menu for a week or
  two, then try again.
- Avoid distractions, such as toys or
  television, during mealtimes.
- Be imaginative when preparing food; for
  example, cut it into decorative shapes or
  create pictures on the plate.

Is your child refusing to eat one or more specific foods? — YES →

NO

POSSIBLE CAUSES Children's tastes change over
time. A child may refuse certain foods, even if
he or she has previously eaten them. Some
older children may decide that they want to
become vegetarian or vegan. Others may be
particularly fussy eaters. Occasionally, a child
may start to refuse foods as a means of
gaining your attention or control.

ACTION As long as your child is well, eats a
reasonably healthy diet (*see* HEALTHY EATING IN
CHILDREN, opposite), and is not losing weight,
there is no cause for concern. If you think that
your child is refusing food to gain attention or
control, try not to make food an issue and try to
be as unconcerned as possible when he or she
refuses food (*see* COPING WITH FOOD FADS, right).

Continued on next page

Continued from
previous page

Has your child been eating less than you think is appropriate for longer than 3 months? — **NO** / **YES**

Are your child's height and weight within the normal range for his or her age (*see* GROWTH CHARTS, p.26)? — **NO** / **YES**

POSSIBLE CAUSE Your child's appetite may be reduced if he or she is in a phase of slow growth or is getting less exercise than previously.

ACTION As long as your child seems well and happy and is not losing weight, there is no cause for concern. However, if your child begins to lose weight or fails to grow normally, you should consult your child's doctor.

Is your child over 12 years old? — **NO** / **YES**

POSSIBLE CAUSES Your child may have an underlying illness such as an intestinal disorder that is causing a loss of appetite and poor growth. However, dieting or the eating disorder anorexia nervosa (*see* EATING DISORDERS, p.139) need to be considered. Consult your child's doctor.

ACTION The doctor will examine your child and may arrange for tests to exclude an underlying disorder. If it is appropriate, an assessment by a psychiatrist may be suggested.

Does your child refuse to eat when at home but eat well at school or other people's homes? — **NO** / **YES**

POSSIBLE CAUSES AND ACTION When away from home, it is quite common for peer pressure to lead a child to eat foods he or she would not normally eat. Alternatively, a child may refuse to eat at home as a means of gaining your attention. Try not to make food an issue, and show as little concern as possible when your child refuses food. Follow self-help measures for coping with picky eaters (opposite).

POSSIBLE CAUSES Your child may have an underlying illness such as an intestinal disorder that is causing a loss of appetite and poor growth. The eating disorder anorexia nervosa (*see* EATING DISORDERS, p.139) may develop in children under 12 years of age but is not common. Consult your child's doctor.

ACTION The doctor will examine your child and may arrange for tests to look for an underlying illness and determine the appropriate treatment. If it is appropriate, an assessment by a psychiatrist may be suggested.

Is your child taking any prescribed drugs? — **NO** / **YES**

POSSIBLE CAUSE AND ACTION Certain drugs can interfere with appetite, in some cases by causing mild nausea as a side effect. Consult your child's doctor. Meanwhile, do not stop your child's prescribed drugs.

Has there been a recent change or upset at home or at school? — **NO** / **YES**

CONSULT YOUR CHILD'S DOCTOR IF YOU ARE UNABLE TO MAKE A DIAGNOSIS FROM THIS CHART.

POSSIBLE CAUSE Your child may be anxious or upset about a recent event. This can often lead to a loss of appetite.

ACTION Try to discover and deal with any underlying worries your child might have. It may help to talk to your child's teachers in case there are problems at school that you are unaware of. If your child's appetite does not improve or if he or she seems unwell, consult your child's doctor.

Healthy eating in children

Relative to their size, children need to eat more food than adults because they need fuel for growth and are more active. Over the age of 5, children should eat carbohydrates, proteins, and fats in the same proportions as adults: carbohydrates should make up roughly half of the diet; fats, just over a third; and proteins, the remainder. Children under 5 need more fats, because fats are high in calories and are important for the development of nerves. Children under 2 should have whole milk, rather than low-fat. A varied diet that includes fruit, vegetables, meats, dairy products, and carbohydrates such as bread will provide your child with the nutrients he or she needs (*see* A HEALTHY DIET, p.28).

On the whole, fresh foods are better than processed. If you often buy convenience foods because of the pressures of time, provide a balance with plenty of fresh fruit and vegetables. Give your child healthy snacks, such as granola bars, yogurts, and dried fruit, but introduce healthier foods into your child's diet gradually. Keep fried and sugary foods to a minimum. Do not give your child tea or coffee or put salt on his or her meals. If you establish sensible eating habits now, your child will be less likely to become overweight or suffer from diet-related health problems in later life.

Healthy meals
Encourage your child to enjoy healthy eating by providing a range of tasty, nutritious meals.

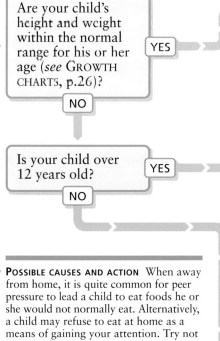

38 Vomiting in children

For children under 1 year, see chart 4, VOMITING IN BABIES **(p.56).**
When a child vomits only once, this is usually caused by overeating or an emotional upset and is rarely due to a serious disorder. Repeated vomiting is most likely to be due to an infection of the digestive tract. Infections elsewhere in the body, such as in the urinary tract, can also cause vomiting in children, but there will usually be other symptoms as well. Rarely, vomiting can be a symptom of a serious condition needing urgent treatment. If your child is vomiting, make sure he or she drinks plenty of fluids to avoid dehydration (*see* PREVENTING DEHYDRATION IN CHILDREN, p.123).

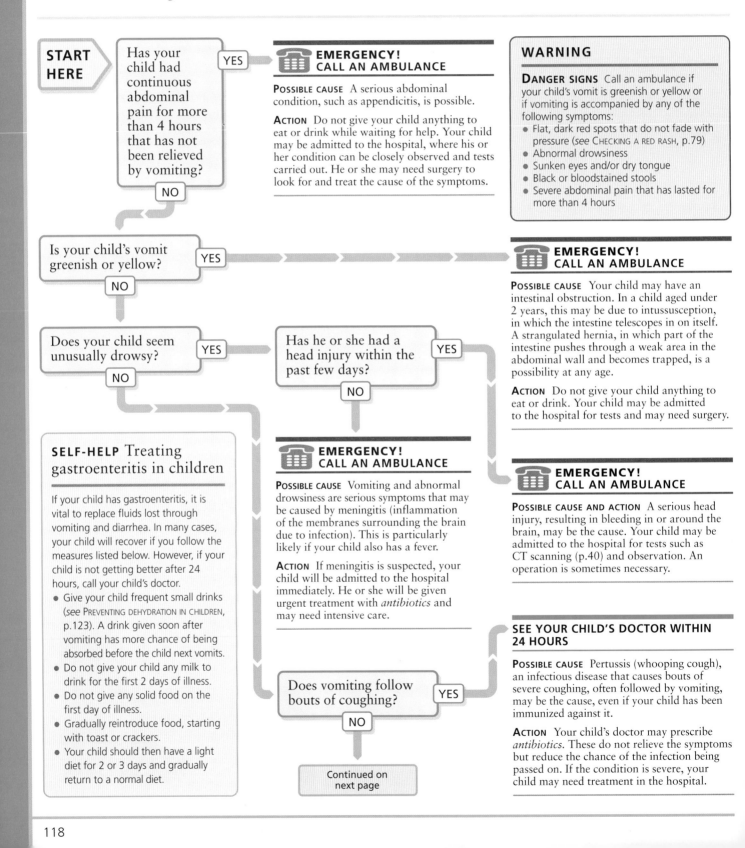

START HERE

Has your child had continuous abdominal pain for more than 4 hours that has not been relieved by vomiting? — YES →

EMERGENCY! CALL AN AMBULANCE

POSSIBLE CAUSE A serious abdominal condition, such as appendicitis, is possible.

ACTION Do not give your child anything to eat or drink while waiting for help. Your child may be admitted to the hospital, where his or her condition can be closely observed and tests carried out. He or she may need surgery to look for and treat the cause of the symptoms.

NO ↓

Is your child's vomit greenish or yellow? — YES →

NO ↓

Does your child seem unusually drowsy? — YES → **Has he or she had a head injury within the past few days?** — YES →

NO ↓   NO ↓

WARNING

DANGER SIGNS Call an ambulance if your child's vomit is greenish or yellow or if vomiting is accompanied by any of the following symptoms:
- Flat, dark red spots that do not fade with pressure (*see* CHECKING A RED RASH, p.79)
- Abnormal drowsiness
- Sunken eyes and/or dry tongue
- Black or bloodstained stools
- Severe abdominal pain that has lasted for more than 4 hours

---

EMERGENCY! CALL AN AMBULANCE

POSSIBLE CAUSE Your child may have an intestinal obstruction. In a child aged under 2 years, this may be due to intussusception, in which the intestine telescopes in on itself. A strangulated hernia, in which part of the intestine pushes through a weak area in the abdominal wall and becomes trapped, is a possibility at any age.

ACTION Do not give your child anything to eat or drink. Your child may be admitted to the hospital for tests and may need surgery.

EMERGENCY! CALL AN AMBULANCE

POSSIBLE CAUSE AND ACTION A serious head injury, resulting in bleeding in or around the brain, may be the cause. Your child may be admitted to the hospital for tests such as CT scanning (p.40) and observation. An operation is sometimes necessary.

SELF-HELP Treating gastroenteritis in children

If your child has gastroenteritis, it is vital to replace fluids lost through vomiting and diarrhea. In many cases, your child will recover if you follow the measures listed below. However, if your child is not getting better after 24 hours, call your child's doctor.
- Give your child frequent small drinks (*see* PREVENTING DEHYDRATION IN CHILDREN, p.123). A drink given soon after vomiting has more chance of being absorbed before the child next vomits.
- Do not give your child any milk to drink for the first 2 days of illness.
- Do not give any solid food on the first day of illness.
- Gradually reintroduce food, starting with toast or crackers.
- Your child should then have a light diet for 2 or 3 days and gradually return to a normal diet.

EMERGENCY! CALL AN AMBULANCE

POSSIBLE CAUSE Vomiting and abnormal drowsiness are serious symptoms that may be caused by meningitis (inflammation of the membranes surrounding the brain due to infection). This is particularly likely if your child also has a fever.

ACTION If meningitis is suspected, your child will be admitted to the hospital immediately. He or she will be given urgent treatment with *antibiotics* and may need intensive care.

Does vomiting follow bouts of coughing? — YES →

NO ↓

Continued on next page

SEE YOUR CHILD'S DOCTOR WITHIN 24 HOURS

POSSIBLE CAUSE Pertussis (whooping cough), an infectious disease that causes bouts of severe coughing, often followed by vomiting, may be the cause, even if your child has been immunized against it.

ACTION Your child's doctor may prescribe *antibiotics*. These do not relieve the symptoms but reduce the chance of the infection being passed on. If the condition is severe, your child may need treatment in the hospital.

Continued from previous page

Does your child have diarrhea? — YES

NO ↓

POSSIBLE CAUSE Gastroenteritis, inflammation of the digestive tract, usually due to a viral infection, is the most likely cause and may be associated with abdominal pain.

ACTION Follow the self-help measures for preventing dehydration in children (p.123) and treating gastroenteritis in children (opposite). If your child has not started to recover after 24 hours or if he or she develops further symptoms, call your child's doctor.

Does your child have two or more of the following symptoms?
- Unexplained loss of weight
- Increased thirst
- Urinating more than usual
- Excessive fatigue

— YES

NO ↓

CALL YOUR CHILD'S DOCTOR NOW

POSSIBLE CAUSE These symptoms may be due to diabetes mellitus. This condition is caused by insufficient production of the hormone insulin, which is needed by the body to get energy from sugar and carbohydrate foods.

ACTION Your child's doctor may take a blood or urine sample to check your child's blood sugar level. If the diagnosis is confirmed and your child is vomiting, he or she will probably need to be admitted to the hospital. Your child will probably need insulin injections for life and will be taught how to inject the insulin and monitor his or her blood sugar level. The doctor will also advise you on your child's diet and lifestyle (see DIABETES MELLITUS, p.149).

Does your child have two or more of the following symptoms?
- Fever
- Pain on urinating
- Bedwetting or daytime wetting after being dry
- Offensive-smelling or cloudy urine

— YES

NO →

Is your child passing pale stools and unusually dark urine, and/or are your child's skin and whites of the eyes yellow? — YES

NO ↓

Was your child very excited or upset just before vomiting? — YES

NO ↓

POSSIBLE CAUSE Vomiting when excited or before stressful events, such as the first day at school, is common in children.

ACTION Be sympathetic: the vomiting will have made your child feel even worse. Talk to your child about his or her feelings, and help him or her to find ways of coping with stressful situations. If your child is at school, his or her teachers may also be able to help.

Does your child regularly vomit during or soon after traveling? — YES

NO ↓

POSSIBLE CAUSE Motion sickness is the probable cause of your child's vomiting. The condition tends to run in families.

ACTION When your child travels, follow self-help measures for coping with motion sickness (above). Most children become less susceptible to motion sickness as they grow older.

AN OCCASIONAL BOUT OF VOMITING IS COMMON DURING CHILDHOOD AND MAY OFTEN HAVE NO OBVIOUS PHYSICAL CAUSE. HOWEVER, IF YOU ARE CONCERNED OR THE VOMITING IS RECURRENT, CONSULT YOUR CHILD'S DOCTOR.

SELF-HELP Coping with motion sickness

If your child suffers from motion sickness, some of the following suggestions may help:
- Give only light meals or snacks before and during your trip.
- Try to travel at night to encourage your child to sleep through the trip.
- Keep a car window open.
- Discourage your child from reading during your trip.
- Provide plenty of distractions, such as tapes of stories and songs.
- Try giving your child an over-the-counter motion sickness remedy before the trip. Your pharmacist can advise you.
- Be prepared. For example, bring a change of clothes for your child.

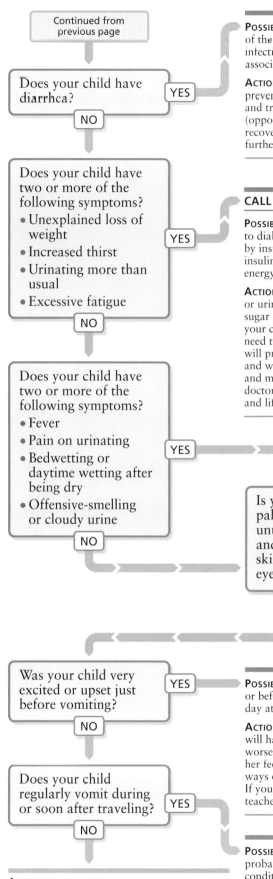

Looking out of the window
If your child suffers from motion sickness, games that encourage him or her to look out the window may help.

SEE YOUR CHILD'S DOCTOR WITHIN 24 HOURS

POSSIBLE CAUSE Your child's symptoms may be due to a urinary tract infection (p.126).

ACTION Your child's doctor will test a sample of your child's urine. If the diagnosis is confirmed, a urine sample will be sent to a laboratory for analysis, and your child will be prescribed *antibiotics*. In some cases, further tests, such as ultrasound scanning (see INVESTIGATING THE URINARY TRACT IN CHILDREN, p.127), may be needed to look for any associated problems.

SEE YOUR CHILD'S DOCTOR WITHIN 24 HOURS

POSSIBLE CAUSE Your child may have a liver problem such as hepatitis, in which a viral infection causes inflammation of liver cells.

ACTION Your child's doctor will arrange for a blood test to confirm the diagnosis. He or she may also refer your child to the hospital for further tests. To prevent the infection from spreading within the family, keep your child's eating utensils and towels separate. The doctor may recommend that other members of the family are immunized against the disease.

39 Abdominal pain

In, most cases, abdominal pain is short-lived and disappears on its own without treatment. However, in some cases, there may be a serious physical cause, such as appendicitis, that needs urgent medical attention. It can be difficult to decide whether abdominal pain in a child, particularly a young child, needs medical attention or whether to wait and see. If your child has a stomachache or if his or her behavior causes you to suspect abdominal pain, consult this chart for advice.

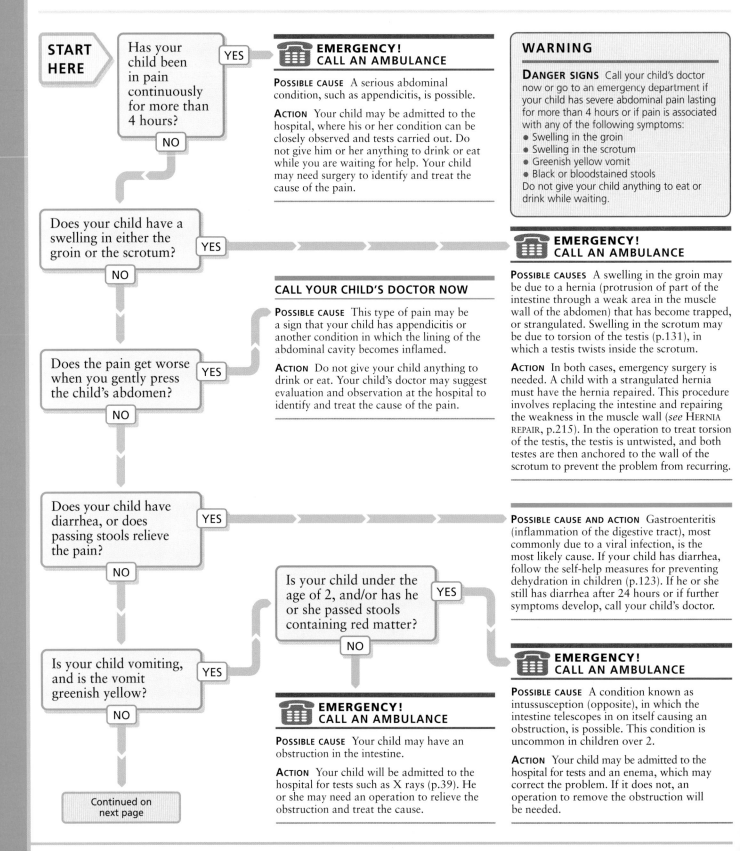

START HERE

Has your child been in pain continuously for more than 4 hours?

YES →

EMERGENCY! CALL AN AMBULANCE

POSSIBLE CAUSE A serious abdominal condition, such as appendicitis, is possible.

ACTION Your child may be admitted to the hospital, where his or her condition can be closely observed and tests carried out. Do not give him or her anything to drink or eat while you are waiting for help. Your child may need surgery to identify and treat the cause of the pain.

NO

WARNING

DANGER SIGNS Call your child's doctor now or go to an emergency department if your child has severe abdominal pain lasting for more than 4 hours or if pain is associated with any of the following symptoms:
- Swelling in the groin
- Swelling in the scrotum
- Greenish yellow vomit
- Black or bloodstained stools

Do not give your child anything to eat or drink while waiting.

Does your child have a swelling in either the groin or the scrotum?

YES →

EMERGENCY! CALL AN AMBULANCE

POSSIBLE CAUSES A swelling in the groin may be due to a hernia (protrusion of part of the intestine through a weak area in the muscle wall of the abdomen) that has become trapped, or strangulated. Swelling in the scrotum may be due to torsion of the testis (p.131), in which a testis twists inside the scrotum.

ACTION In both cases, emergency surgery is needed. A child with a strangulated hernia must have the hernia repaired. This procedure involves replacing the intestine and repairing the weakness in the muscle wall (*see* HERNIA REPAIR, p.215). In the operation to treat torsion of the testis, the testis is untwisted, and both testes are then anchored to the wall of the scrotum to prevent the problem from recurring.

NO

Does the pain get worse when you gently press the child's abdomen?

YES →

CALL YOUR CHILD'S DOCTOR NOW

POSSIBLE CAUSE This type of pain may be a sign that your child has appendicitis or another condition in which the lining of the abdominal cavity becomes inflamed.

ACTION Do not give your child anything to drink or eat. Your child's doctor may suggest evaluation and observation at the hospital to identify and treat the cause of the pain.

NO

Does your child have diarrhea, or does passing stools relieve the pain?

YES →

POSSIBLE CAUSE AND ACTION Gastroenteritis (inflammation of the digestive tract), most commonly due to a viral infection, is the most likely cause. If your child has diarrhea, follow the self-help measures for preventing dehydration in children (p.123). If he or she still has diarrhea after 24 hours or if further symptoms develop, call your child's doctor.

NO

Is your child under the age of 2, and/or has he or she passed stools containing red matter?

YES →

EMERGENCY! CALL AN AMBULANCE

POSSIBLE CAUSE A condition known as intussusception (opposite), in which the intestine telescopes in on itself causing an obstruction, is possible. This condition is uncommon in children over 2.

ACTION Your child may be admitted to the hospital for tests and an enema, which may correct the problem. If it does not, an operation to remove the obstruction will be needed.

NO

Is your child vomiting, and is the vomit greenish yellow?

YES →

EMERGENCY! CALL AN AMBULANCE

POSSIBLE CAUSE Your child may have an obstruction in the intestine.

ACTION Your child will be admitted to the hospital for tests such as X rays (p.39). He or she may need an operation to relieve the obstruction and treat the cause.

NO

Continued on next page

Continued from previous page

Does your child also have a sore throat, a cough, or a runny nose? **YES**

NO

Does your child have any of the following?
- Pain on urinating
- Frequent urinating
- Bedwetting or daytime wetting after being dry
- Offensive-smelling or cloudy urine
- Fever

YES

NO

Has your child had repeated episodes of abdominal pain? **YES**

NO

SEE YOUR CHILD'S DOCTOR IF THE PAIN PERSISTS FOR MORE THAN 24 HOURS AND YOU ARE UNABLE TO MAKE A DIAGNOSIS FROM THIS CHART.

SELF-HELP Relieving abdominal pain

The following measures may help relieve mild abdominal pain in a child:
- Let your child hold a wrapped hot-water bottle against the abdomen.
- Give your child only water to drink and nothing to eat while he or she is in pain.

If the pain worsens or is still present the next day, call your child's doctor. Call an ambulance if severe pains lasts more than 4 hours.

Covered hot-water bottle

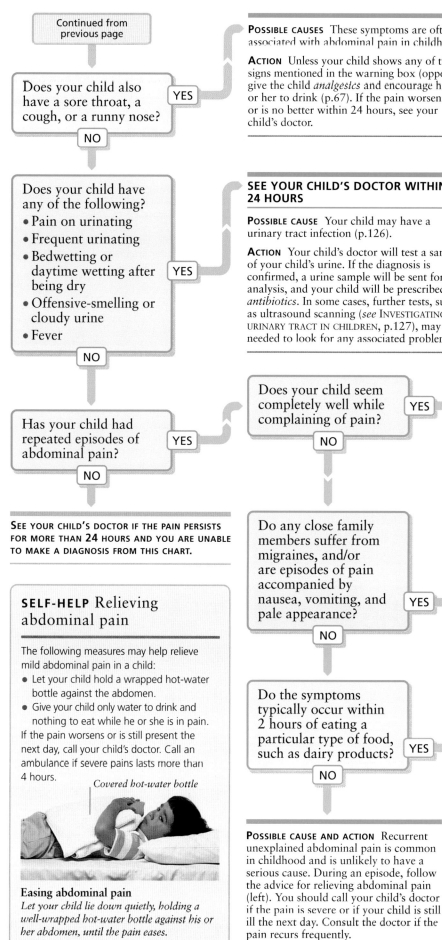

Easing abdominal pain
Let your child lie down quietly, holding a well-wrapped hot-water bottle against his or her abdomen, until the pain eases.

POSSIBLE CAUSES These symptoms are often associated with abdominal pain in childhood.

ACTION Unless your child shows any of the signs mentioned in the warning box (opposite), give the child *analgesics* and encourage him or her to drink (p.67). If the pain worsens or is no better within 24 hours, see your child's doctor.

SEE YOUR CHILD'S DOCTOR WITHIN 24 HOURS

POSSIBLE CAUSE Your child may have a urinary tract infection (p.126).

ACTION Your child's doctor will test a sample of your child's urine. If the diagnosis is confirmed, a urine sample will be sent for analysis, and your child will be prescribed *antibiotics*. In some cases, further tests, such as ultrasound scanning (*see* INVESTIGATING THE URINARY TRACT IN CHILDREN, p.127), may be needed to look for any associated problems.

Does your child seem completely well while complaining of pain? **YES**

NO

Do any close family members suffer from migraines, and/or are episodes of pain accompanied by nausea, vomiting, and pale appearance? **YES**

NO

Do the symptoms typically occur within 2 hours of eating a particular type of food, such as dairy products? **YES**

NO

POSSIBLE CAUSE AND ACTION Recurrent unexplained abdominal pain is common in childhood and is unlikely to have a serious cause. During an episode, follow the advice for relieving abdominal pain (left). You should call your child's doctor if the pain is severe or if your child is still ill the next day. Consult the doctor if the pain recurs frequently.

Intussusception

In intussusception, part of the intestine telescopes into itself, causing an obstruction. The cause is unknown, but it may occur during viral infections. If your child's doctor suspects that your child has intussusception, your child will be admitted to the hospital and may be given intravenous fluids. An enema will probably be given to confirm the diagnosis. This may also correct the problem by forcing the intestine back into position. If the enema does not help, emergency surgery may be needed to relieve the obstruction and remove any damaged intestine.

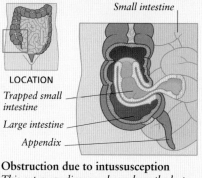

LOCATION

Small intestine

Trapped small intestine

Large intestine

Appendix

Obstruction due to intussusception
This cut-away diagram shows how the last part of the small intestine pushes into part of the large intestine to cause an obstruction.

POSSIBLE CAUSE AND ACTION The episodes of pain may be an expression of anxiety or stress. Talk to your child to try to find out if anything is worrying him or her. Call your child's doctor if other symptoms develop, if the pain is severe, or if your child still has abdominal pain the next day.

POSSIBLE CAUSE Your child may have migraine. In children under age 8, the symptoms often include recurrent episodes of abdominal pain instead of the one-sided headaches that are typical of migraine in older children and adults. Consult your child's doctor.

ACTION The doctor will examine your child and may arrange for tests such as a urine test (p.38) to exclude other disorders. Taking *analgesics* should help to relieve the symptoms.

POSSIBLE CAUSE Your child may have a food intolerance, such as lactose intolerance (p.122), in which symptoms such as abdominal pain, vomiting, and/or diarrhea occur whenever a particular food is eaten. Consult your child's doctor.

ACTION The doctor may suggest excluding possible problem foods or food groups from your child's diet for a trial period. If you need to exclude a food permanently from the diet, you may be referred to a dietician for advice.

40 Diarrhea in children

For children under 1 year, see chart 5, DIARRHEA IN BABIES **(p.58).**
Diarrhea is the frequent passing of abnormally loose or watery stools. While diarrhea can be serious in babies, in older children, it is unlikely to be a cause for concern.

The most common cause of diarrhea in children is a viral infection of the digestive tract. In most cases, drug treatment is inappropriate; avoiding food, so that the intestines are rested, and drinking plenty of fluids (*see* PREVENTING DEHYDRATION IN CHILDREN, opposite) is the best course of action.

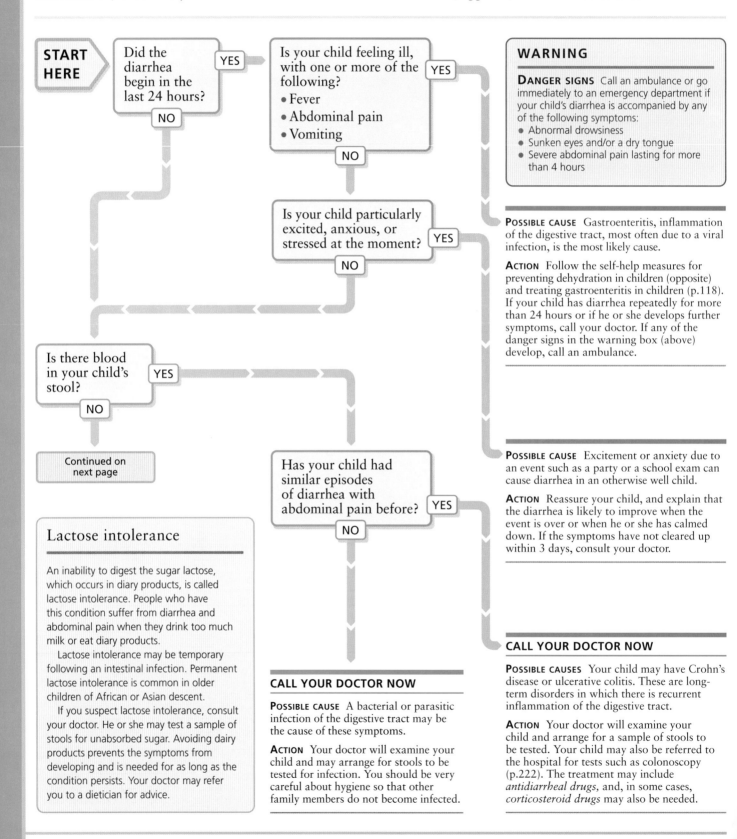

START HERE

Did the diarrhea begin in the last 24 hours? **YES** / **NO**

Is your child feeling ill, with one or more of the following?
• Fever
• Abdominal pain
• Vomiting
YES / **NO**

Is your child particularly excited, anxious, or stressed at the moment? **YES** / **NO**

Is there blood in your child's stool? **YES** / **NO**

Has your child had similar episodes of diarrhea with abdominal pain before? **YES** / **NO**

Continued on next page

WARNING

DANGER SIGNS Call an ambulance or go immediately to an emergency department if your child's diarrhea is accompanied by any of the following symptoms:
• Abnormal drowsiness
• Sunken eyes and/or a dry tongue
• Severe abdominal pain lasting for more than 4 hours

POSSIBLE CAUSE Gastroenteritis, inflammation of the digestive tract, most often due to a viral infection, is the most likely cause.

ACTION Follow the self-help measures for preventing dehydration in children (opposite) and treating gastroenteritis in children (p.118). If your child has diarrhea repeatedly for more than 24 hours or if he or she develops further symptoms, call your doctor. If any of the danger signs in the warning box (above) develop, call an ambulance.

POSSIBLE CAUSE Excitement or anxiety due to an event such as a party or a school exam can cause diarrhea in an otherwise well child.

ACTION Reassure your child, and explain that the diarrhea is likely to improve when the event is over or when he or she has calmed down. If the symptoms have not cleared up within 3 days, consult your doctor.

Lactose intolerance

An inability to digest the sugar lactose, which occurs in diary products, is called lactose intolerance. People who have this condition suffer from diarrhea and abdominal pain when they drink too much milk or eat diary products.

Lactose intolerance may be temporary following an intestinal infection. Permanent lactose intolerance is common in older children of African or Asian descent.

If you suspect lactose intolerance, consult your doctor. He or she may test a sample of stools for unabsorbed sugar. Avoiding dairy products prevents the symptoms from developing and is needed for as long as the condition persists. Your doctor may refer you to a dietician for advice.

CALL YOUR DOCTOR NOW

POSSIBLE CAUSE A bacterial or parasitic infection of the digestive tract may be the cause of these symptoms.

ACTION Your doctor will examine your child and may arrange for stools to be tested for infection. You should be very careful about hygiene so that other family members do not become infected.

CALL YOUR DOCTOR NOW

POSSIBLE CAUSES Your child may have Crohn's disease or ulcerative colitis. These are long-term disorders in which there is recurrent inflammation of the digestive tract.

ACTION Your doctor will examine your child and arrange for a sample of stools to be tested. Your child may also be referred to the hospital for tests such as colonoscopy (p.222). The treatment may include *antidiarrheal drugs,* and, in some cases, *corticosteroid drugs* may also be needed.

Continued from previous page

Does the diarrhea occur after your child has milk or other dairy products? — YES →

POSSIBLE CAUSE Lactose intolerance (opposite), in which the body cannot digest lactose, the natural sugar found in milk, may be the cause. This condition is usually temporary. Consult your doctor.

ACTION If your doctor suspects lactose intolerance, he or she will probably arrange for a sample of your child's stools to be tested to detect undigested sugars. If your child is lactose intolerant, you will need advice from a dietitian on a lactose-free diet.

NO ↓

Is your child taking any prescription drugs? — YES →

POSSIBLE CAUSE AND ACTION Certain drugs, such as *antibiotics*, can cause diarrhea. Call your doctor before the next dose of the drug is due to ask if it could be the cause and if you should stop giving it to your child.

NO ↓

Has the diarrhea followed a period of constipation, and have you noticed any soiling of your child's underclothes? — YES →

POSSIBLE CAUSE Your child may have chronic constipation blocking the rectum. The soiling is due to the overflow of liquid stools past the blockage. Consult your doctor.

ACTION Your doctor may initially prescribe a *laxative* to clear the blockage. He or she will probably also recommend adding extra fiber-rich foods to your child's diet (*see* AVOIDING CONSTIPATION, p.124). If your doctor suspects that the condition is caused by an underlying physical or behavioral problem, he or she may refer your child to a specialist.

NO ↓

Are your child's height and weight within the normal range for his or her age (*see* GROWTH CHARTS, p.26)? — YES →

Is your child under 3 years, and does the diarrhea contain any recognizable pieces of food? — YES →

NO ↓ (height/weight)   **NO** ↓ (under 3 years)

Is your child passing pale, bulky stools? — YES →

POSSIBLE CAUSE An inability to absorb nutrients from food due to a disorder such as cystic fibrosis (p.73) or celiac disease, in which the intestine is damaged by a gluten allergy, may be the cause.

ACTION Your doctor will examine your child and will probably arrange for initial tests. Treatment depends on the cause but may include drugs to aid digestion or a special diet with vitamin and mineral supplements. If cystic fibrosis is suspected, your child may be referred to a specialist for further tests.

NO ↓

GIVE YOUR CHILD PLENTY OF FLUIDS, AND SEE YOUR DOCTOR WITHIN 24 HOURS.

POSSIBLE CAUSE AND ACTION Toddler diarrhea, a common condition in which a young child fails to digest food properly, is likely. This may be due partly to your child not being able to chew his or her food enough. It is not a danger to health; however, you should consult your doctor so that he or she can make sure an infection is not the cause.

POSSIBLE CAUSE AND ACTION Some children routinely produce soft stools that can be mistaken for diarrhea. If you are not sure whether or not your child's stools are normal, consult your doctor for advice.

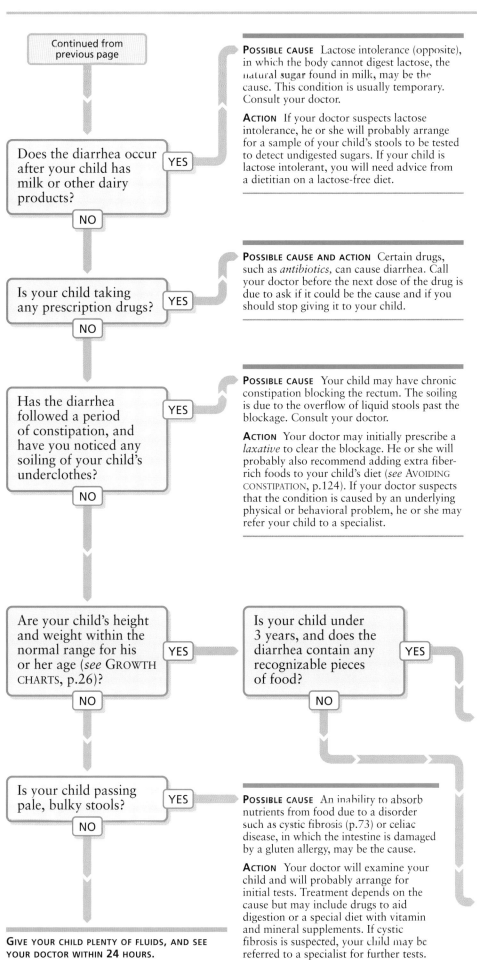

SELF-HELP Preventing dehydration in children

If your child has diarrhea, vomiting, and/or a fever, it is important to give him or her plenty of fluids to prevent or treat dehydration, a potentially life-threatening condition.

The most suitable fluid to give your child is oral rehydrating solution, which can be bought over the counter. These solutions contain sodium, potassium, and glucose as well as water. You can also give your child diluted, unsweetened fruit juice as an alternative to the rehydrating solution, but avoid giving him or her milk.

While the symptoms last, offer your child drinks at frequent intervals. He or she should drink 4–7 cups (1–1½ liters) of fluid per day. If your child vomits, give him or her a drink soon afterward to replace the lost fluid.

If your child still has diarrhea after 24 hours, call your doctor.

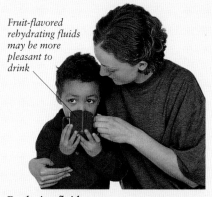

Fruit-flavored rehydrating fluids may be more pleasant to drink

Replacing fluids
Encourage your child to sip rehydrating solution or diluted fruit juice at least once an hour while symptoms last. He or she should also drink soon after vomiting.

41 Constipation

Consult this chart if your child is not having regular bowel movements or if he or she is passing very hard or pelletlike stools. There is a wide variation in the normal frequency with which children move their bowels. Some children have a bowel movement several times a day; others have one every 2 or 3 days. Both of these extremes are normal as long as the child is otherwise well and the stools are not hard or painful to pass. It is also normal for babies and toddlers to strain and turn bright red in the face when passing a normal, soft stools, although parents sometimes mistake this as a sign that their child is constipated. Minor changes to a child's usual bowel habit are often caused by a change in diet or in the daily routine, an illness, dehydration (especially in hot weather), or emotional stress.

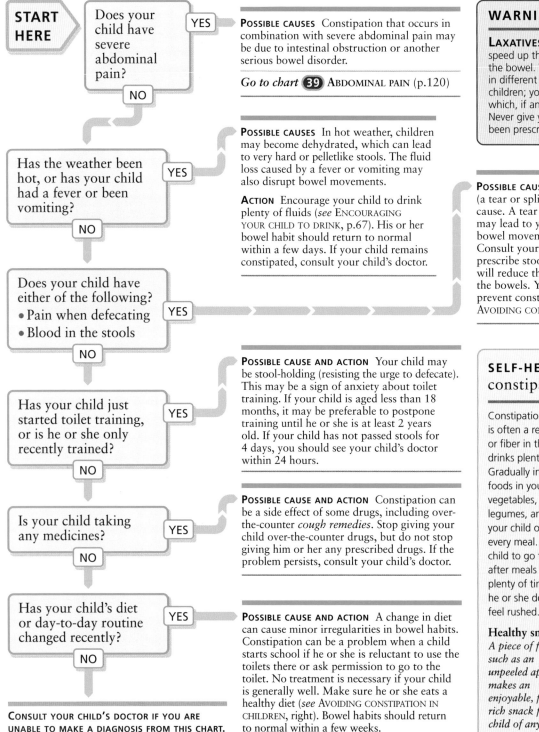

START HERE

Does your child have severe abdominal pain? — **YES**

POSSIBLE CAUSES Constipation that occurs in combination with severe abdominal pain may be due to intestinal obstruction or another serious bowel disorder.

Go to chart **39** ABDOMINAL PAIN (p.120)

NO

Has the weather been hot, or has your child had a fever or been vomiting? — **YES**

POSSIBLE CAUSES In hot weather, children may become dehydrated, which can lead to very hard or pelletlike stools. The fluid loss caused by a fever or vomiting may also disrupt bowel movements.

ACTION Encourage your child to drink plenty of fluids (*see* ENCOURAGING YOUR CHILD TO DRINK, p.67). His or her bowel habit should return to normal within a few days. If your child remains constipated, consult your child's doctor.

NO

Does your child have either of the following?
• **Pain when defecating**
• **Blood in the stools** — **YES**

POSSIBLE CAUSE AND ACTION An anal fissure (a tear or split inside the anus) is a possible cause. A tear makes defecation painful, which may lead to your child being afraid to have a bowel movement for fear of further pain. Consult your child's doctor, who will probably prescribe stool-softeners for your child. These will reduce the pain associated with opening the bowels. You should also take steps to prevent constipation from recurring (*see* AVOIDING CONSTIPATION IN CHILDREN, below).

NO

Has your child just started toilet training, or is he or she only recently trained? — **YES**

POSSIBLE CAUSE AND ACTION Your child may be stool-holding (resisting the urge to defecate). This may be a sign of anxiety about toilet training. If your child is aged less than 18 months, it may be preferable to postpone training until he or she is at least 2 years old. If your child has not passed stools for 4 days, you should see your child's doctor within 24 hours.

NO

Is your child taking any medicines? — **YES**

POSSIBLE CAUSE AND ACTION Constipation can be a side effect of some drugs, including over-the-counter *cough remedies*. Stop giving your child over-the-counter drugs, but do not stop giving him or her any prescribed drugs. If the problem persists, consult your child's doctor.

NO

Has your child's diet or day-to-day routine changed recently? — **YES**

POSSIBLE CAUSE AND ACTION A change in diet can cause minor irregularities in bowel habits. Constipation can be a problem when a child starts school if he or she is reluctant to use the toilets there or ask permission to go to the toilet. No treatment is necessary if your child is generally well. Make sure he or she eats a healthy diet (*see* AVOIDING CONSTIPATION IN CHILDREN, right). Bowel habits should return to normal within a few weeks.

NO

CONSULT YOUR CHILD'S DOCTOR IF YOU ARE UNABLE TO MAKE A DIAGNOSIS FROM THIS CHART.

WARNING

LAXATIVES *Laxatives* are medicines that speed up the movement of stools through the bowel. There are several types that work in different ways. Some are not suitable for children; your child's doctor should decide which, if any, is appropriate for your child. Never give your child a laxative unless it has been prescribed or suggested by the doctor.

SELF-HELP Avoiding constipation in children

Constipation in children aged over 6 months is often a result of a lack of sufficient fluids or fiber in the diet. Make sure your child drinks plenty of fluids throughout the day. Gradually increase the amount of fiber-rich foods in your child's diet; these include fruits, vegetables, wholegrain cereals, beans and legumes, and wholegrain bread. Try to give your child one or more of these foods at every meal. Encourage your child to go to the toilet after meals and allow plenty of time so that he or she does not feel rushed.

Healthy snacks
A piece of fruit, such as an unpeeled apple, makes an enjoyable, fiber-rich snack for a child of any age.

42 Abnormal-looking stools

For hard or pelletlike stools, see chart 41, CONSTIPATION (p.124). For runny stools in a child under 1 year, see chart 5, DIARRHEA IN BABIES (p.58); for a child over 1 year, see chart 40, DIARRHEA IN CHILDREN (p.122).
It is normal for stools to vary slightly in their color, smell, or consistency. Consult this chart only if there is a marked change in the appearance of your child's stools. Sudden differences are almost always caused by something your child has eaten, and the change should only last a few days. However, there may be an underlying disorder causing the problem. If the stools still look abnormal in 48 hours or if they are accompanied by other symptoms such as abdominal pain, you should consult your child's doctor, taking a sample of the stools in a clean container for him or her to examine.

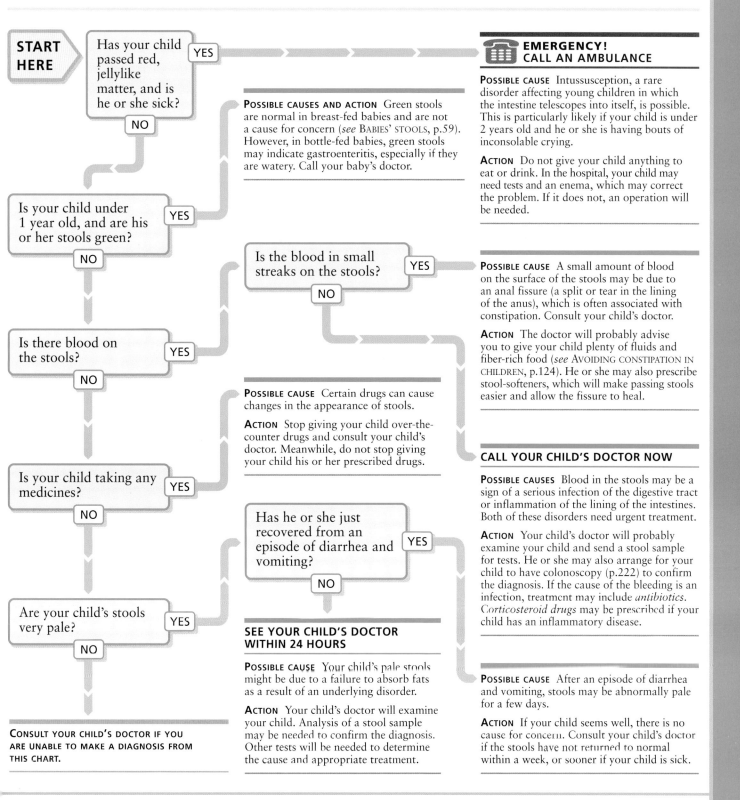

START HERE

Has your child passed red, jellylike matter, and is he or she sick? YES / NO

Is your child under 1 year old, and are his or her stools green? YES / NO

Is there blood on the stools? YES / NO

Is your child taking any medicines? YES / NO

Are your child's stools very pale? YES / NO

CONSULT YOUR CHILD'S DOCTOR IF YOU ARE UNABLE TO MAKE A DIAGNOSIS FROM THIS CHART.

POSSIBLE CAUSES AND ACTION Green stools are normal in breast-fed babies and are not a cause for concern (*see* BABIES' STOOLS, p.59). However, in bottle-fed babies, green stools may indicate gastroenteritis, especially if they are watery. Call your baby's doctor.

Is the blood in small streaks on the stools? YES / NO

POSSIBLE CAUSE Certain drugs can cause changes in the appearance of stools.

ACTION Stop giving your child over-the-counter drugs and consult your child's doctor. Meanwhile, do not stop giving your child his or her prescribed drugs.

Has he or she just recovered from an episode of diarrhea and vomiting? YES / NO

SEE YOUR CHILD'S DOCTOR WITHIN 24 HOURS

POSSIBLE CAUSE Your child's pale stools might be due to a failure to absorb fats as a result of an underlying disorder.

ACTION Your child's doctor will examine your child. Analysis of a stool sample may be needed to confirm the diagnosis. Other tests will be needed to determine the cause and appropriate treatment.

EMERGENCY! CALL AN AMBULANCE

POSSIBLE CAUSE Intussusception, a rare disorder affecting young children in which the intestine telescopes into itself, is possible. This is particularly likely if your child is under 2 years old and he or she is having bouts of inconsolable crying.

ACTION Do not give your child anything to eat or drink. In the hospital, your child may need tests and an enema, which may correct the problem. If it does not, an operation will be needed.

POSSIBLE CAUSE A small amount of blood on the surface of the stools may be due to an anal fissure (a split or tear in the lining of the anus), which is often associated with constipation. Consult your child's doctor.

ACTION The doctor will probably advise you to give your child plenty of fluids and fiber-rich food (*see* AVOIDING CONSTIPATION IN CHILDREN, p.124). He or she may also prescribe stool-softeners, which will make passing stools easier and allow the fissure to heal.

CALL YOUR CHILD'S DOCTOR NOW

POSSIBLE CAUSES Blood in the stools may be a sign of a serious infection of the digestive tract or inflammation of the lining of the intestines. Both of these disorders need urgent treatment.

ACTION Your child's doctor will probably examine your child and send a stool sample for tests. He or she may also arrange for your child to have colonoscopy (p.222) to confirm the diagnosis. If the cause of the bleeding is an infection, treatment may include *antibiotics*. *Corticosteroid drugs* may be prescribed if your child has an inflammatory disease.

POSSIBLE CAUSE After an episode of diarrhea and vomiting, stools may be abnormally pale for a few days.

ACTION If your child seems well, there is no cause for concern. Consult your child's doctor if the stools have not returned to normal within a week, or sooner if your child is sick.

43 Urinary problems

For problems with bladder control, see chart 44, TOILET-TRAINING PROBLEMS *(p.128).*

Most children urinate more frequently than adults because children have smaller bladders and less well-developed muscular control. Urinary problems, such as urinary tract infections, are common in children and especially in girls. Symptoms of urinary problems in children include pain on urinating, needing to urinate more often than usual, cloudy urine, or unpleasant-smelling urine. Occasionally, unexplained vomiting and fever may be due to a urinary tract infection. In some children, urinary tract infections are associated with reflux, in which urine flows back toward the kidneys when the bladder is emptied. Urinary problems in a child should always be assessed promptly by your child's doctor.

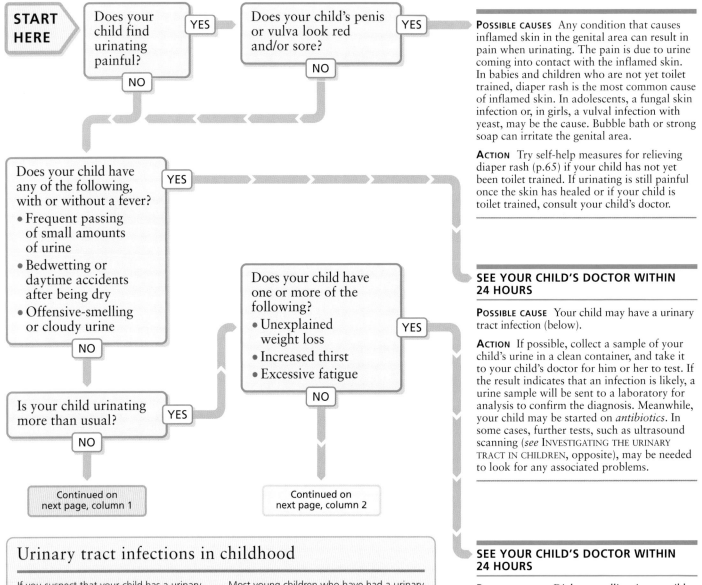

START HERE

Does your child find urinating painful? — YES → **Does your child's penis or vulva look red and/or sore?** — YES →

NO ↓ / NO ↓

POSSIBLE CAUSES Any condition that causes inflamed skin in the genital area can result in pain when urinating. The pain is due to urine coming into contact with the inflamed skin. In babies and children who are not yet toilet trained, diaper rash is the most common cause of inflamed skin. In adolescents, a fungal skin infection or, in girls, a vulval infection with yeast, may be the cause. Bubble bath or strong soap can irritate the genital area.

ACTION Try self-help measures for relieving diaper rash (p.65) if your child has not yet been toilet trained. If urinating is still painful once the skin has healed or if your child is toilet trained, consult your child's doctor.

Does your child have any of the following, with or without a fever?
• Frequent passing of small amounts of urine
• Bedwetting or daytime accidents after being dry
• Offensive-smelling or cloudy urine

— YES →

NO ↓

Is your child urinating more than usual? — YES →

NO ↓

Does your child have one or more of the following?
• Unexplained weight loss
• Increased thirst
• Excessive fatigue

— YES →

NO ↓

Continued on next page, column 1

Continued on next page, column 2

SEE YOUR CHILD'S DOCTOR WITHIN 24 HOURS

POSSIBLE CAUSE Your child may have a urinary tract infection (below).

ACTION If possible, collect a sample of your child's urine in a clean container, and take it to your child's doctor for him or her to test. If the result indicates that an infection is likely, a urine sample will be sent to a laboratory for analysis to confirm the diagnosis. Meanwhile, your child may be started on *antibiotics*. In some cases, further tests, such as ultrasound scanning (*see* INVESTIGATING THE URINARY TRACT IN CHILDREN, opposite), may be needed to look for any associated problems.

SEE YOUR CHILD'S DOCTOR WITHIN 24 HOURS

POSSIBLE CAUSE Diabetes mellitus is a possible cause of these symptoms. It is caused by insufficient production of the hormone insulin, which is needed by the body to get energy from sugar and carbohydrate foods.

ACTION Your child's doctor will take a blood or urine sample to check your child's sugar level. If the diagnosis of diabetes is confirmed, you will be given advice on your child's diet and lifestyle (*see* DIABETES MELLITUS, p.149). Your child will also need to have insulin injections for the rest of his or her life.

Urinary tract infections in childhood

If you suspect that your child has a urinary tract infection, it is important to bring it to your child's doctor's attention within 24 hours. Urinary tract infections can be more serious in children than in adults because they may be associated with reflux, in which urine flows back up the ureters toward the kidneys when the bladder is emptied. If untreated, reflux of infected urine can cause permanent scarring of the kidneys and impaired kidney function in later life.

Most young children who have had a urinary tract infection will need to have tests (*see* INVESTIGATING THE URINARY TRACT IN CHILDREN, opposite) to establish whether reflux is occurring and to assess kidney function. If your child is diagnosed as having reflux, he or she may be prescribed continuous, low-dose antibiotics to reduce the risk of subsequent infection and kidney damage. This treatment can often be discontinued by the time your child is 5 years old.

Continued from previous page, column 1

Continued from previous page, column 2

Is your child excited, anxious, or cold? **YES**

NO

POSSIBLE CAUSE AND ACTION It is normal to need to urinate more frequently in times of excitement or anxiety or when exposed to cold temperatures. If your child continues to urinate frequently after his or her situation returns to normal, consult your child's doctor.

Is your child an uncircumcised boy, and does his foreskin balloon when he urinates? **YES**

NO

CONSULT YOUR CHILD'S DOCTOR IF YOU ARE UNABLE TO MAKE A DIAGNOSIS FROM THIS CHART.

POSSIBLE CAUSE Your child may have phimosis, in which the opening in the foreskin is too small.

Go to chart **45** GENITAL PROBLEMS IN BOYS (p.130)

Is your child's urine discolored? **YES**

NO

POSSIBLE CAUSES AND ACTION Some foods, such as beets, and some drugs may change the color of your child's urine. Rarely, however, a change in urine color is a sign of liver or kidney disease or is due to blood in the urine. If you cannot identify a dietary cause for the change, consult your child's doctor, taking a urine sample with you. The doctor will test the urine for the presence of abnormal substances, including blood.

Does your child have problems with bladder control? **YES**

NO

Does your child regularly wet himself or herself during the day and/or at night? **YES**

NO

Go to chart **44** TOILET-TRAINING PROBLEMS (p.128)

CONSULT YOUR CHILD'S DOCTOR IF YOU ARE UNABLE TO MAKE A DIAGNOSIS FROM THIS CHART.

Is your child reluctant or unable to urinate? **YES**

NO

Investigating the urinary tract in children

If your child has had a urinary tract infection (*see* URINARY TRACT INFECTIONS IN CHILDHOOD, opposite), he or she will probably be referred for further tests to check kidney and bladder function and to exclude damage from urinary reflux, in which urine flows back toward the kidneys when the bladder is emptied.

Ultrasound scanning (p.41), a quick and painless procedure, is performed to check that the kidneys and bladder are of normal size.

In some cases, your child may also need DMSA scanning, a procedure that provides extra information on kidney functioning. A voiding cystourethragram (VCUG) may be ordered to diagnose urinary reflux. During the procedure, a very small amount of a radioactive substance called DMSA is given to the child by an intravenous injection. After the DMSA has passed into the urinary system, detailed images of the kidneys can be taken with a gamma camera and viewed on a computer monitor. The DMSA will be excreted in the urine and will be gone within 24 hours. It will not harm your child.

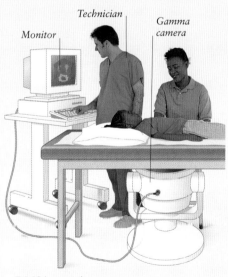

Monitor *Technician* *Gamma camera*

DMSA scanning
Your child will be scanned approximately 2 hours after an injection of DMSA. The gamma camera picks up radioactivity released by the kidneys and produces a picture on a monitor.

CONSULT YOUR CHILD'S DOCTOR IF YOU ARE UNABLE TO MAKE A DIAGNOSIS FROM THIS CHART.

CALL YOUR CHILD'S DOCTOR NOW

POSSIBLE CAUSES Local soreness or severe constipation are possible causes. In some cases, a urinary infection (opposite) may be causing pain on urinating, and your child may be reluctant to try to urinate again. A child who feels a strong urge to urinate but is unable to do so needs urgent medical help.

ACTION Your child's doctor will examine your child to try to establish the cause of the problem. He or she may suggest *analgesics* and suggest you encourage your child to urinate while in a warm bath. If this fails, your child may need hospital admission.

44 Toilet training problems

Most children gain full control over their bladder and bowel functions between the ages of 2 and 5 years. Few children have reliable control before the age of 2 years, and few have problems, apart from the occasional "accident," after the age of 5. However, the age at which an individual child masters the different skills of toilet training such as nighttime control varies widely. It is not known why some children learn later than others, but it is seldom due to an unwillingness to learn.

Changes in circumstances, such as a new baby in the family or starting school, may make a child anxious and delay toilet training. Children whose parents were late to learn may also be later in learning reliable control. Unless there is a physical problem, toilet training occurs naturally, and the process cannot be speeded up by pressure from parents. Consult this chart if you are concerned about your child's ability to control his or her bladder or bowels.

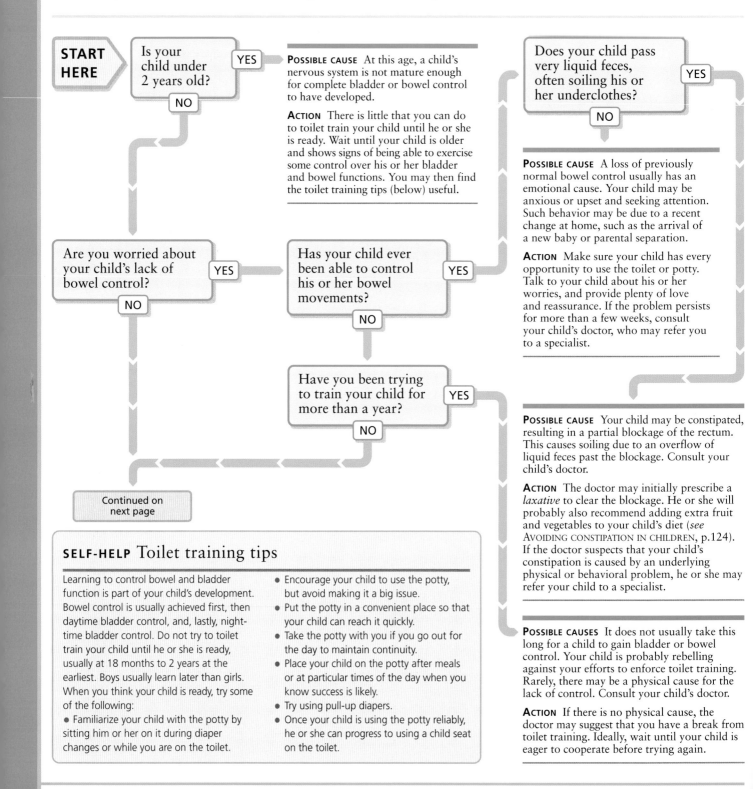

START HERE

Is your child under 2 years old? — YES

POSSIBLE CAUSE At this age, a child's nervous system is not mature enough for complete bladder or bowel control to have developed.

ACTION There is little that you can do to toilet train your child until he or she is ready. Wait until your child is older and shows signs of being able to exercise some control over his or her bladder and bowel functions. You may then find the toilet training tips (below) useful.

NO ↓

Are you worried about your child's lack of bowel control? — NO

Has your child ever been able to control his or her bowel movements? — YES

NO ↓

Have you been trying to train your child for more than a year? — YES

NO ↓

Continued on next page

Does your child pass very liquid feces, often soiling his or her underclothes? — YES

NO ↓

POSSIBLE CAUSE A loss of previously normal bowel control usually has an emotional cause. Your child may be anxious or upset and seeking attention. Such behavior may be due to a recent change at home, such as the arrival of a new baby or parental separation.

ACTION Make sure your child has every opportunity to use the toilet or potty. Talk to your child about his or her worries, and provide plenty of love and reassurance. If the problem persists for more than a few weeks, consult your child's doctor, who may refer you to a specialist.

POSSIBLE CAUSE Your child may be constipated, resulting in a partial blockage of the rectum. This causes soiling due to an overflow of liquid feces past the blockage. Consult your child's doctor.

ACTION The doctor may initially prescribe a *laxative* to clear the blockage. He or she will probably also recommend adding extra fruit and vegetables to your child's diet (*see* AVOIDING CONSTIPATION IN CHILDREN, p.124). If the doctor suspects that your child's constipation is caused by an underlying physical or behavioral problem, he or she may refer your child to a specialist.

POSSIBLE CAUSES It does not usually take this long for a child to gain bladder or bowel control. Your child is probably rebelling against your efforts to enforce toilet training. Rarely, there may be a physical cause for the lack of control. Consult your child's doctor.

ACTION If there is no physical cause, the doctor may suggest that you have a break from toilet training. Ideally, wait until your child is eager to cooperate before trying again.

SELF-HELP Toilet training tips

Learning to control bowel and bladder function is part of your child's development. Bowel control is usually achieved first, then daytime bladder control, and, lastly, nighttime bladder control. Do not try to toilet train your child until he or she is ready, usually at 18 months to 2 years at the earliest. Boys usually learn later than girls. When you think your child is ready, try some of the following:
● Familiarize your child with the potty by sitting him or her on it during diaper changes or while you are on the toilet.

● Encourage your child to use the potty, but avoid making it a big issue.
● Put the potty in a convenient place so that your child can reach it quickly.
● Take the potty with you if you go out for the day to maintain continuity.
● Place your child on the potty after meals or at particular times of the day when you know success is likely.
● Try using pull-up diapers.
● Once your child is using the potty reliably, he or she can progress to using a child seat on the toilet.

Continued from previous page

Are you worried about your child's lack of bladder control?

NO → **CONSULT YOUR CHILD'S DOCTOR IF YOU ARE UNABLE TO FIND A CAUSE FOR YOUR CHILD'S PROBLEM FROM THIS CHART.**

YES →

SELF-HELP Overcoming bedwetting

If your child regularly wets the bed, try to be patient. Reassure your child that you are not angry and that he or she will learn to stay dry through the night. Encourage him or her to use the toilet before going to bed, and perhaps also wake your child to use the toilet when you go to bed. A chart on which you award your child a star after each dry night may help, as may a pad-and-buzzer system. The pad, which can detect moisture, is laid under the bottom sheet. As soon as your child wets the bed, the buzzer sounds. The child will soon learn to wake before the buzzer goes off.

Pad and buzzer
The moisture-detecting pad is placed on an undersheet, and the bed is then made up as usual. The buzzer is placed on the bed or nearby.

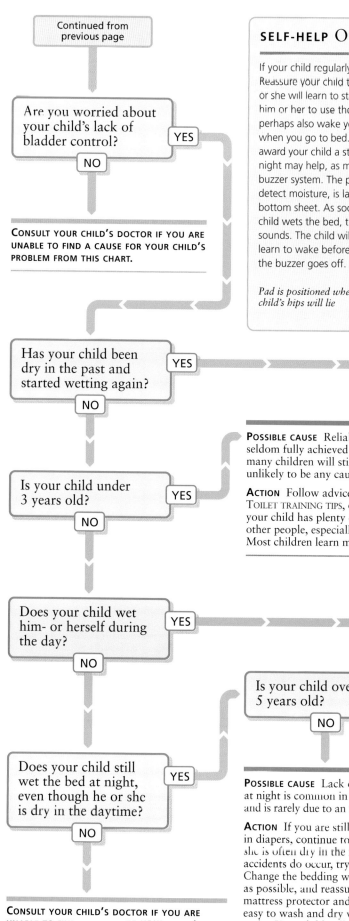

Buzzer

Pad is positioned where child's hips will lie

Has your child been dry in the past and started wetting again?

NO ↓

YES →

SEE YOUR CHILD'S DOCTOR WITHIN 24 HOURS

POSSIBLE CAUSES Your child may have a urinary tract infection (*see* URINARY TRACT INFECTIONS IN CHILDHOOD, p.126). Alternatively, an emotional problem may be the cause.

ACTION Your child's doctor will test a sample of your child's urine. If the result indicates that an infection is likely, a urine sample will be analyzed to confirm the diagnosis. Meanwhile, your child will be started on *antibiotics*. Further tests, such as ultrasound scanning (*see* INVESTIGATING THE URINARY TRACT IN CHILDREN, p.127), may be needed to look for any associated problems. If no infection is found, the doctor will discuss the possibility of an emotional upset with you and your child.

Is your child under 3 years old?

NO ↓

YES →

POSSIBLE CAUSE Reliable bladder control is seldom fully achieved before the age of 3, and many children will still be in diapers. There is unlikely to be any cause for concern.

ACTION Follow advice on toilet training (*see* TOILET TRAINING TIPS, opposite), and make sure your child has plenty of opportunities to see other people, especially children, use the toilet. Most children learn most quickly by imitation.

Does your child wet him- or herself during the day?

NO ↓

YES →

POSSIBLE CAUSES Lack of bladder control during the day is unlikely to have a medical cause in a child under 5, but in an older child, it may indicate a physical or emotional problem. Consult your child's doctor, whatever the age of your child.

ACTION The doctor will examine your child and may arrange for tests, including urine tests, to find an underlying cause. If no physical cause is found, follow advice on toilet training (*see* TOILET TRAINING TIPS, opposite). Children over 5 years may need to be referred to a specialist.

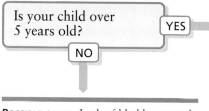

Is your child over 5 years old?

NO ↓

YES →

Does your child still wet the bed at night, even though he or she is dry in the daytime?

NO ↓

YES →

POSSIBLE CAUSE Lack of bladder control at night is common in children under 5 and is rarely due to an underlying disorder.

ACTION If you are still putting your child in diapers, continue to do so until he or she is often dry in the morning. When accidents do occur, try not to get angry. Change the bedding with as little fuss as possible, and reassure your child. A mattress protector and bedding that are easy to wash and dry will make coping easier. Your child will eventually achieve nighttime control.

POSSIBLE CAUSE About 1 in 6 children wet their beds at age 5, and 1 in 20 still wet their beds at age 10. Regular bedwetting rarely has a physical cause, even in an older child, and is particularly common if one or both parents were late to acquire nighttime bladder control.

ACTION Follow measures for overcoming bedwetting (above). If these do not help, consult your child's doctor, who may prescribe a course of drug treatment or drugs that can be used for events such as an overnight trip.

CONSULT YOUR CHILD'S DOCTOR IF YOU ARE UNABLE TO FIND A CAUSE FOR YOUR CHILD'S PROBLEM FROM THIS CHART.

45 Genital problems in boys

Consult this chart if your son develops a painful or swollen penis or a problem with his scrotum (the supportive bag that encloses the testes). Although most genital problems in boys are a result of minor infections, you should always consult your child's doctor promptly if your son develops a problem anywhere in the genital area. In some cases – for example, torsion of a testis – a delay in medical treatment can have serious consequences.

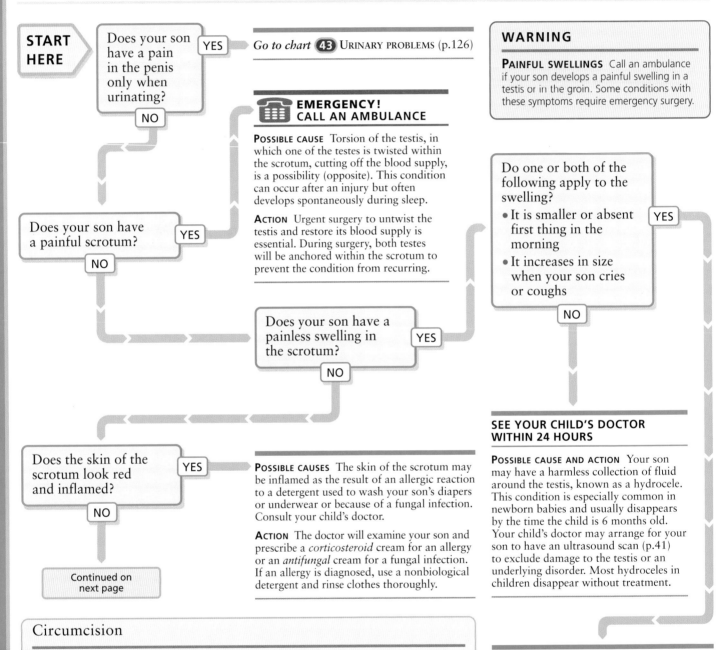

START HERE

Does your son have a pain in the penis only when urinating?
YES → *Go to chart* **43** URINARY PROBLEMS (p.126)
NO

Does your son have a painful scrotum?
YES →
NO

☎ EMERGENCY! CALL AN AMBULANCE

POSSIBLE CAUSE Torsion of the testis, in which one of the testes is twisted within the scrotum, cutting off the blood supply, is a possibility (opposite). This condition can occur after an injury but often develops spontaneously during sleep.

ACTION Urgent surgery to untwist the testis and restore its blood supply is essential. During surgery, both testes will be anchored within the scrotum to prevent the condition from recurring.

Does your son have a painless swelling in the scrotum?
YES →
NO

Do one or both of the following apply to the swelling?
- It is smaller or absent first thing in the morning
- It increases in size when your son cries or coughs
YES →
NO

Does the skin of the scrotum look red and inflamed?
YES →
NO

Continued on next page

POSSIBLE CAUSES The skin of the scrotum may be inflamed as the result of an allergic reaction to a detergent used to wash your son's diapers or underwear or because of a fungal infection. Consult your child's doctor.

ACTION The doctor will examine your son and prescribe a *corticosteroid* cream for an allergy or an *antifungal* cream for a fungal infection. If an allergy is diagnosed, use a nonbiological detergent and rinse clothes thoroughly.

WARNING

PAINFUL SWELLINGS Call an ambulance if your son develops a painful swelling in a testis or in the groin. Some conditions with these symptoms require emergency surgery.

SEE YOUR CHILD'S DOCTOR WITHIN 24 HOURS

POSSIBLE CAUSE AND ACTION Your son may have a harmless collection of fluid around the testis, known as a hydrocele. This condition is especially common in newborn babies and usually disappears by the time the child is 6 months old. Your child's doctor may arrange for your son to have an ultrasound scan (p.41) to exclude damage to the testis or an underlying disorder. Most hydroceles in children disappear without treatment.

SEE YOUR CHILD'S DOCTOR WITHIN 24 HOURS

POSSIBLE CAUSE Your son probably has a hernia, in which a loop of intestine bulges through a weak area in the abdominal wall. This condition is most common in babies.

ACTION Your child's doctor will examine your son. If the diagnosis is confirmed, the hernia should be repaired to prevent a loop of intestine becoming trapped. The operation is carried out under general anesthetic.

Circumcision

Circumcision is a surgical operation to remove the foreskin, which is the fold of skin that covers the tip of the penis. In some cases, circumcision may also be recommended if a boy's foreskin is too tight or if a boy has recurrent infections of the penis. In the past, circumcision was often performed routinely in childhood in the belief that it would improve hygiene, but this practice is no longer recommended.

In newborn boys, circumcision is most often carried out under local anesthetic, whereas, in older boys or in men, it is usually performed under general anesthesia.

During the operation, most of the foreskin is cut away. The remnant that remains is then stitched to the skin just behind the head of the penis, leaving the head uncovered. No dressing is needed while the wound heals. The stitches will either dissolve or fall out after a few days.

Continued from previous page

Does one or both of the testes appear to be absent from your son's scrotum? **YES**

NO

Torsion of the testis

Twisting (torsion) of the testis within the scrotum reduces or stops blood flow to the testis. It can affect males of any age but is most common in boys aged 12–18 years. The symptoms can start during sleep or following an injury and include pain in the scrotum, groin, and/or abdomen and redness and tenderness of the scrotum. There may be associated nausea and/or vomiting. Torsion of the testis requires urgent surgery, which must be carried out within 6 hours in order to prevent permanent damage to the testis. During surgery, the blood vessels are untwisted and then both of the testes are anchored to the scrotum to prevent recurrence.

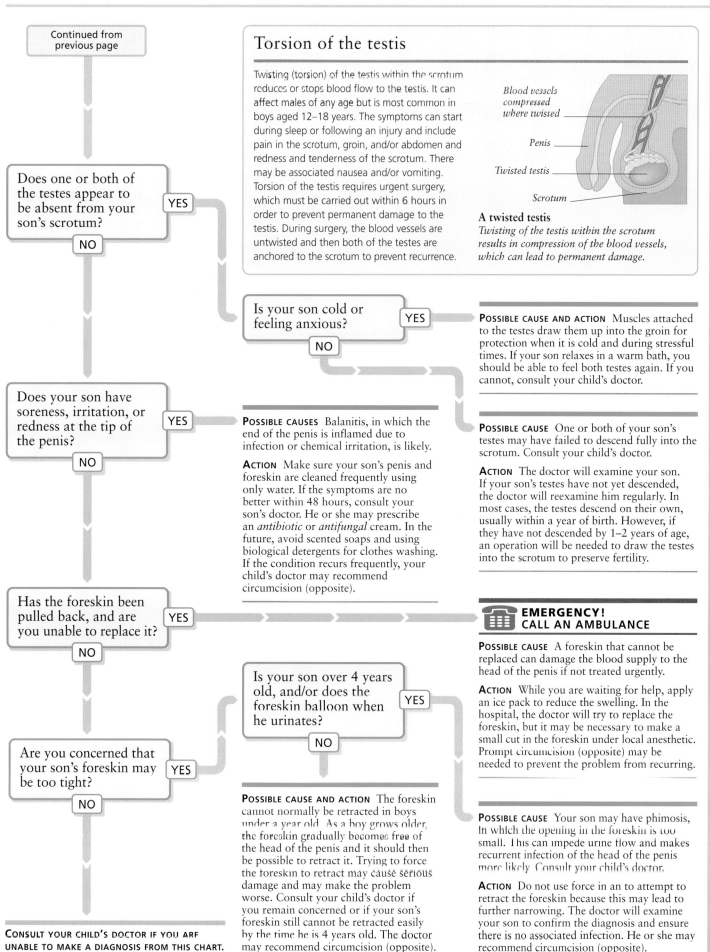

Blood vessels compressed where twisted

Penis

Twisted testis

Scrotum

A twisted testis
Twisting of the testis within the scrotum results in compression of the blood vessels, which can lead to permanent damage.

Is your son cold or feeling anxious? **YES**

NO

POSSIBLE CAUSE AND ACTION Muscles attached to the testes draw them up into the groin for protection when it is cold and during stressful times. If your son relaxes in a warm bath, you should be able to feel both testes again. If you cannot, consult your child's doctor.

Does your son have soreness, irritation, or redness at the tip of the penis? **YES**

NO

POSSIBLE CAUSES Balanitis, in which the end of the penis is inflamed due to infection or chemical irritation, is likely.

ACTION Make sure your son's penis and foreskin are cleaned frequently using only water. If the symptoms are no better within 48 hours, consult your son's doctor. He or she may prescribe an *antibiotic* or *antifungal* cream. In the future, avoid scented soaps and using biological detergents for clothes washing. If the condition recurs frequently, your child's doctor may recommend circumcision (opposite).

POSSIBLE CAUSE One or both of your son's testes may have failed to descend fully into the scrotum. Consult your child's doctor.

ACTION The doctor will examine your son. If your son's testes have not yet descended, the doctor will reexamine him regularly. In most cases, the testes descend on their own, usually within a year of birth. However, if they have not descended by 1–2 years of age, an operation will be needed to draw the testes into the scrotum to preserve fertility.

Has the foreskin been pulled back, and are you unable to replace it? **YES**

NO

☎ EMERGENCY! CALL AN AMBULANCE

POSSIBLE CAUSE A foreskin that cannot be replaced can damage the blood supply to the head of the penis if not treated urgently.

ACTION While you are waiting for help, apply an ice pack to reduce the swelling. In the hospital, the doctor will try to replace the foreskin, but it may be necessary to make a small cut in the foreskin under local anesthetic. Prompt circumcision (opposite) may be needed to prevent the problem from recurring.

Is your son over 4 years old, and/or does the foreskin balloon when he urinates? **YES**

NO

Are you concerned that your son's foreskin may be too tight? **YES**

NO

POSSIBLE CAUSE AND ACTION The foreskin cannot normally be retracted in boys under a year old. As a boy grows older, the foreskin gradually becomes free of the head of the penis and it should then be possible to retract it. Trying to force the foreskin to retract may cause serious damage and may make the problem worse. Consult your child's doctor if you remain concerned or if your son's foreskin still cannot be retracted easily by the time he is 4 years old. The doctor may recommend circumcision (opposite).

POSSIBLE CAUSE Your son may have phimosis, in which the opening in the foreskin is too small. This can impede urine flow and makes recurrent infection of the head of the penis more likely. Consult your child's doctor.

ACTION Do not use force in an to attempt to retract the foreskin because this may lead to further narrowing. The doctor will examine your son to confirm the diagnosis and ensure there is no associated infection. He or she may recommend circumcision (opposite).

CONSULT YOUR CHILD'S DOCTOR IF YOU ARE UNABLE TO MAKE A DIAGNOSIS FROM THIS CHART.

46 Genital problems in girls

The most common genital problems in young girls are itching, inflammation of the external genital area and, less commonly, an unusual discharge, sometimes with pain on urinating.

These symptoms may be caused by a minor infection or by irritation from toiletries or laundry products. Consult this chart if your daughter complains of any of these symptoms.

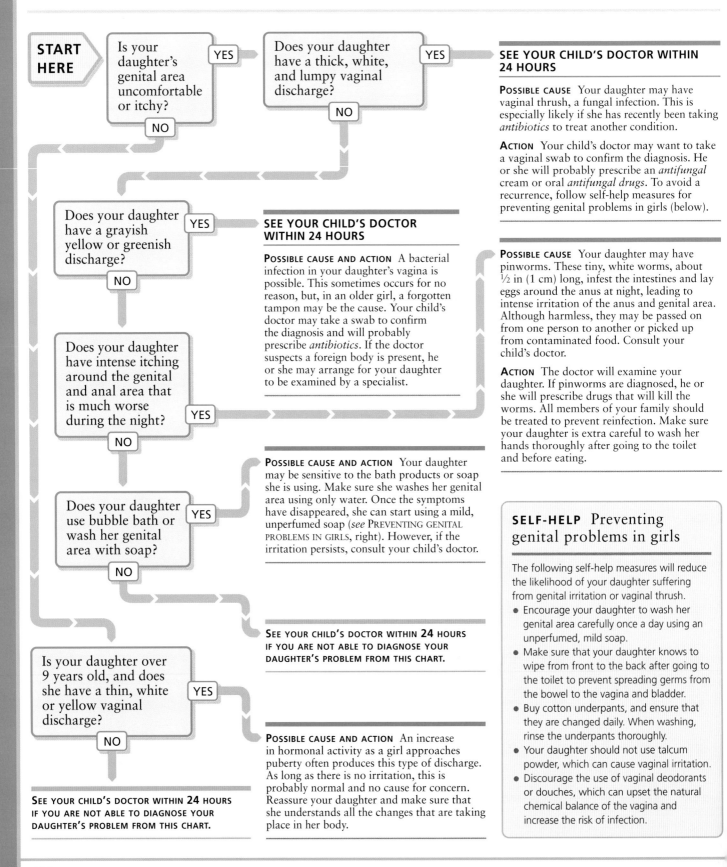

START HERE

Is your daughter's genital area uncomfortable or itchy? — **YES** → Does your daughter have a thick, white, and lumpy vaginal discharge? — **YES** →

NO ↓

NO ↓

SEE YOUR CHILD'S DOCTOR WITHIN 24 HOURS

POSSIBLE CAUSE Your daughter may have vaginal thrush, a fungal infection. This is especially likely if she has recently been taking *antibiotics* to treat another condition.

ACTION Your child's doctor may want to take a vaginal swab to confirm the diagnosis. He or she will probably prescribe an *antifungal* cream or oral *antifungal drugs*. To avoid a recurrence, follow self-help measures for preventing genital problems in girls (below).

Does your daughter have a grayish yellow or greenish discharge? — **YES** →

NO ↓

SEE YOUR CHILD'S DOCTOR WITHIN 24 HOURS

POSSIBLE CAUSE AND ACTION A bacterial infection in your daughter's vagina is possible. This sometimes occurs for no reason, but, in an older girl, a forgotten tampon may be the cause. Your child's doctor may take a swab to confirm the diagnosis and will probably prescribe *antibiotics*. If the doctor suspects a foreign body is present, he or she may arrange for your daughter to be examined by a specialist.

POSSIBLE CAUSE Your daughter may have pinworms. These tiny, white worms, about ½ in (1 cm) long, infest the intestines and lay eggs around the anus at night, leading to intense irritation of the anus and genital area. Although harmless, they may be passed on from one person to another or picked up from contaminated food. Consult your child's doctor.

ACTION The doctor will examine your daughter. If pinworms are diagnosed, he or she will prescribe drugs that will kill the worms. All members of your family should be treated to prevent reinfection. Make sure your daughter is extra careful to wash her hands thoroughly after going to the toilet and before eating.

Does your daughter have intense itching around the genital and anal area that is much worse during the night? — **YES** →

NO ↓

POSSIBLE CAUSE AND ACTION Your daughter may be sensitive to the bath products or soap she is using. Make sure she washes her genital area using only water. Once the symptoms have disappeared, she can start using a mild, unperfumed soap (*see* PREVENTING GENITAL PROBLEMS IN GIRLS, right). However, if the irritation persists, consult your child's doctor.

Does your daughter use bubble bath or wash her genital area with soap? — **YES** →

NO ↓

SEE YOUR CHILD'S DOCTOR WITHIN 24 HOURS IF YOU ARE NOT ABLE TO DIAGNOSE YOUR DAUGHTER'S PROBLEM FROM THIS CHART.

Is your daughter over 9 years old, and does she have a thin, white or yellow vaginal discharge? — **YES** →

NO ↓

POSSIBLE CAUSE AND ACTION An increase in hormonal activity as a girl approaches puberty often produces this type of discharge. As long as there is no irritation, this is probably normal and no cause for concern. Reassure your daughter and make sure that she understands all the changes that are taking place in her body.

SEE YOUR CHILD'S DOCTOR WITHIN 24 HOURS IF YOU ARE NOT ABLE TO DIAGNOSE YOUR DAUGHTER'S PROBLEM FROM THIS CHART.

SELF-HELP Preventing genital problems in girls

The following self-help measures will reduce the likelihood of your daughter suffering from genital irritation or vaginal thrush.

- Encourage your daughter to wash her genital area carefully once a day using an unperfumed, mild soap.
- Make sure that your daughter knows to wipe from front to the back after going to the toilet to prevent spreading germs from the bowel to the vagina and bladder.
- Buy cotton underpants, and ensure that they are changed daily. When washing, rinse the underpants thoroughly.
- Your daughter should not use talcum powder, which can cause vaginal irritation.
- Discourage the use of vaginal deodorants or douches, which can upset the natural chemical balance of the vagina and increase the risk of infection.

47 Painful arm or leg

Consult this chart if your child complains of arm or leg pain. Parents often attribute a recurrent ache in a child's limb to growing pains (below). However, minor injuries are a more likely cause. Sprains and strains are usually not serious, but a broken bone (fracture) needs immediate medical attention.

Cramps, another common cause of limb pain, can be relieved by self-help measures such as gently massaging and stretching the affected muscle and applying a wrapped hot-water bottle if necessary. Any pain that has no obvious cause or that persists should be discussed with your child's doctor.

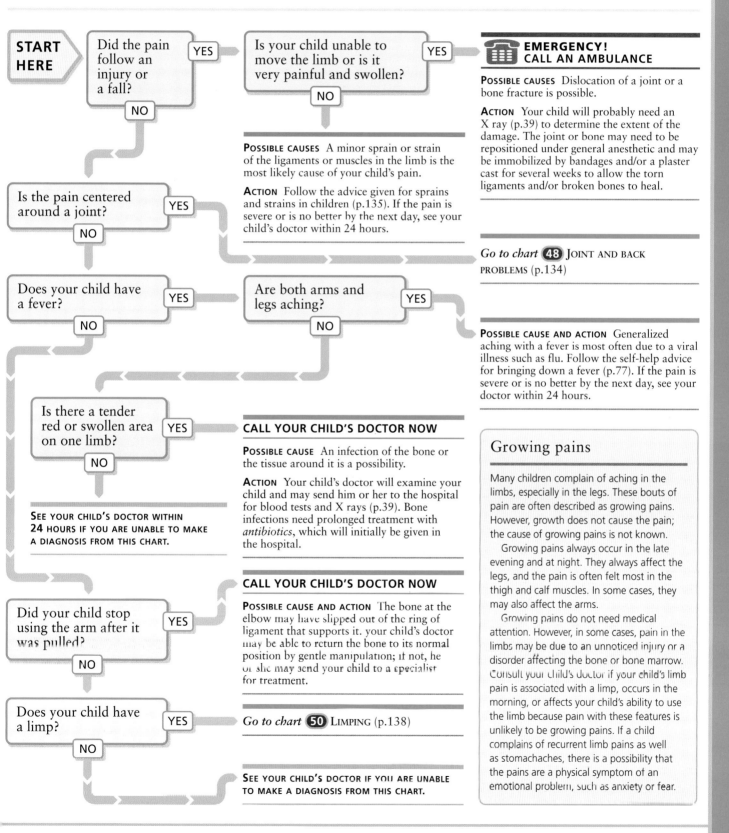

START HERE

Did the pain follow an injury or a fall? — YES → **Is your child unable to move the limb or is it very painful and swollen?** — YES →

EMERGENCY! CALL AN AMBULANCE

POSSIBLE CAUSES Dislocation of a joint or a bone fracture is possible.

ACTION Your child will probably need an X ray (p.39) to determine the extent of the damage. The joint or bone may need to be repositioned under general anesthetic and may be immobilized by bandages and/or a plaster cast for several weeks to allow the torn ligaments and/or broken bones to heal.

(Did the pain follow an injury or a fall?) NO ↓

(Is your child unable to move the limb...?) NO ↓

POSSIBLE CAUSES A minor sprain or strain of the ligaments or muscles in the limb is the most likely cause of your child's pain.

ACTION Follow the advice given for sprains and strains in children (p.135). If the pain is severe or is no better by the next day, see your child's doctor within 24 hours.

Is the pain centered around a joint? — YES → *Go to chart* **48** JOINT AND BACK PROBLEMS (p.134)

(Is the pain centered around a joint?) NO ↓

Does your child have a fever? — YES → **Are both arms and legs aching?** — YES →

POSSIBLE CAUSE AND ACTION Generalized aching with a fever is most often due to a viral illness such as flu. Follow the self-help advice for bringing down a fever (p.77). If the pain is severe or is no better by the next day, see your doctor within 24 hours.

(Does your child have a fever?) NO ↓

(Are both arms and legs aching?) NO ↓

Is there a tender red or swollen area on one limb? — YES →

CALL YOUR CHILD'S DOCTOR NOW

POSSIBLE CAUSE An infection of the bone or the tissue around it is a possibility.

ACTION Your child's doctor will examine your child and may send him or her to the hospital for blood tests and X rays (p.39). Bone infections need prolonged treatment with *antibiotics*, which will initially be given in the hospital.

(Is there a tender red or swollen area on one limb?) NO ↓

SEE YOUR CHILD'S DOCTOR WITHIN 24 HOURS IF YOU ARE UNABLE TO MAKE A DIAGNOSIS FROM THIS CHART.

Did your child stop using the arm after it was pulled? — YES →

CALL YOUR CHILD'S DOCTOR NOW

POSSIBLE CAUSE AND ACTION The bone at the elbow may have slipped out of the ring of ligament that supports it. your child's doctor may be able to return the bone to its normal position by gentle manipulation; if not, he or she may send your child to a specialist for treatment.

(Did your child stop using the arm after it was pulled?) NO ↓

Does your child have a limp? — YES → *Go to chart* **50** LIMPING (p.138)

(Does your child have a limp?) NO ↓

SEE YOUR CHILD'S DOCTOR IF YOU ARE UNABLE TO MAKE A DIAGNOSIS FROM THIS CHART.

Growing pains

Many children complain of aching in the limbs, especially in the legs. These bouts of pain are often described as growing pains. However, growth does not cause the pain; the cause of growing pains is not known.

Growing pains always occur in the late evening and at night. They always affect the legs, and the pain is often felt most in the thigh and calf muscles. In some cases, they may also affect the arms.

Growing pains do not need medical attention. However, in some cases, pain in the limbs may be due to an unnoticed injury or a disorder affecting the bone or bone marrow. Consult your child's doctor if your child's limb pain is associated with a limp, occurs in the morning, or affects your child's ability to use the limb because pain with these features is unlikely to be growing pains. If a child complains of recurrent limb pains as well as stomachaches, there is a possibility that the pains are a physical symptom of an emotional problem, such as anxiety or fear.

48 Joint and back problems

Serious joint and back problems are uncommon in children. A painful or swollen joint is most often the result of a minor strain or sprain of the muscles and ligaments surrounding the joint. However, joint pain or swelling can be caused by arthritis (joint inflammation). Arthritis is less common in children than in adults. However, in childhood the disease can also involve internal organs such as the heart and kidneys. Problems with the spine may be noticed for the first time in adolescence and need medical assessment. Severe back pain in a child of any age needs prompt medical attention.

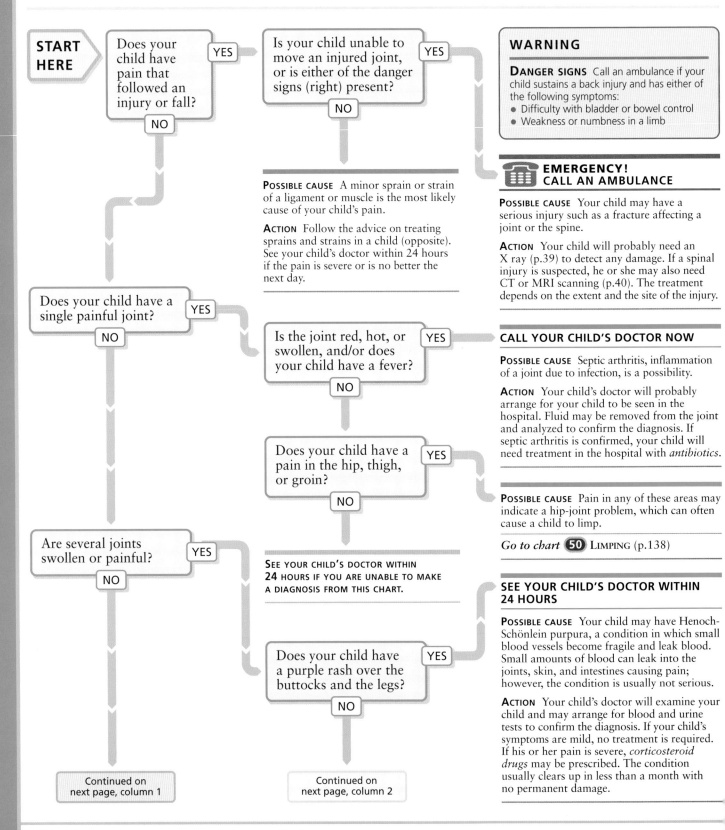

START HERE

Does your child have pain that followed an injury or fall? — YES → **Is your child unable to move an injured joint, or is either of the danger signs (right) present?** — YES →

NO ↓ (from first question)

NO ↓ (from second question)

POSSIBLE CAUSE A minor sprain or strain of a ligament or muscle is the most likely cause of your child's pain.

ACTION Follow the advice on treating sprains and strains in a child (opposite). See your child's doctor within 24 hours if the pain is severe or is no better the next day.

Does your child have a single painful joint? — YES →

NO ↓

Is the joint red, hot, or swollen, and/or does your child have a fever? — YES →

NO ↓

Does your child have a pain in the hip, thigh, or groin? — YES →

NO ↓

Are several joints swollen or painful? — YES →

NO ↓

SEE YOUR CHILD'S DOCTOR WITHIN 24 HOURS IF YOU ARE UNABLE TO MAKE A DIAGNOSIS FROM THIS CHART.

Does your child have a purple rash over the buttocks and the legs? — YES →

NO ↓

Continued on next page, column 1

Continued on next page, column 2

WARNING

DANGER SIGNS Call an ambulance if your child sustains a back injury and has either of the following symptoms:
- Difficulty with bladder or bowel control
- Weakness or numbness in a limb

EMERGENCY! CALL AN AMBULANCE

POSSIBLE CAUSE Your child may have a serious injury such as a fracture affecting a joint or the spine.

ACTION Your child will probably need an X ray (p.39) to detect any damage. If a spinal injury is suspected, he or she may also need CT or MRI scanning (p.40). The treatment depends on the extent and the site of the injury.

CALL YOUR CHILD'S DOCTOR NOW

POSSIBLE CAUSE Septic arthritis, inflammation of a joint due to infection, is a possibility.

ACTION Your child's doctor will probably arrange for your child to be seen in the hospital. Fluid may be removed from the joint and analyzed to confirm the diagnosis. If septic arthritis is confirmed, your child will need treatment in the hospital with *antibiotics*.

POSSIBLE CAUSE Pain in any of these areas may indicate a hip-joint problem, which can often cause a child to limp.

Go to chart **50** LIMPING (p.138)

SEE YOUR CHILD'S DOCTOR WITHIN 24 HOURS

POSSIBLE CAUSE Your child may have Henoch-Schönlein purpura, a condition in which small blood vessels become fragile and leak blood. Small amounts of blood can leak into the joints, skin, and intestines causing pain; however, the condition is usually not serious.

ACTION Your child's doctor will examine your child and may arrange for blood and urine tests to confirm the diagnosis. If your child's symptoms are mild, no treatment is required. If his or her pain is severe, *corticosteroid drugs* may be prescribed. The condition usually clears up in less than a month with no permanent damage.

Continued from
previous page, column 1

Continued from
previous page, column 2

Does your child have a fever, feel generally ill, and/or have a blotchy rash?
YES
NO

Are you concerned that your child may have a problem with his or her back?
YES
NO

SEE YOUR CHILD'S DOCTOR WITHIN 24 HOURS

POSSIBLE CAUSE AND ACTION Your child may have systemic juvenile arthritis, in which the immune system attacks the joints and, in some cases, the internal organs. Your child's doctor will probably refer your child to a specialist for tests. If the diagnosis is confirmed, treatment will include *nonsteroidal anti-inflammatory drugs* and, in some cases, *corticosteroid drugs*.

CONSULT YOUR CHILD'S DOCTOR IF YOU ARE UNABLE TO MAKE A DIAGNOSIS FROM THIS CHART.

Has your child recently had an infection, such as a sore throat or a chest infection?
YES
NO

SEE YOUR CHILD'S DOCTOR WITHIN 24 HOURS

POSSIBLE CAUSE AND ACTION Reactive arthritis, inflammation of the joints in response to a recent infection, is possible. Your child's doctor may arrange for tests to confirm that the infection has cleared up and may prescribe *nonsteroidal anti-inflammatory drugs*. Reactive arthritis usually improves within weeks.

SEE YOUR CHILD'S DOCTOR WITHIN 24 HOURS

POSSIBLE CAUSE Juvenile chronic arthritis, in which the immune system attacks the joints and, in some cases, the eyes, is possible.

ACTION Your child may be referred to a specialist for blood tests and a full eye examination. *Nonsteroidal anti-inflammatory drugs* and *corticosteroids* may be prescribed.

Is your child awakened in the night by back pain, or does he or she have a stiff back on waking?
YES
NO

SEE YOUR CHILD'S DOCTOR WITHIN 24 HOURS

POSSIBLE CAUSES AND ACTION Your child may have a serious problem such as a bone disorder or arthritis of the spine. Your child's doctor will probably arrange for X rays (p.39) of the back and blood tests to make a diagnosis and determine the appropriate treatment.

Does your child's spine appear to be curving sideways?
YES
NO

SEE YOUR CHILD'S DOCTOR WITHIN 24 HOURS

POSSIBLE CAUSE A sideways curvature of the spine is called scoliosis. Some children are born with it and are treated in their first few years. However, some children develop the curvature later in childhood, most often in adolescence.

ACTION Your doctor will assess the curvature of the spine and will probably refer your child to a specialist. In many cases, no treatment is needed, but if the curvature is severe, treatment with exercises and sometimes a brace may be needed to correct the problem and prevent it from progressing.

Did your child's back pain start after strenuous exercise?
YES
NO

POSSIBLE CAUSE A minor sprain or strain of a ligament or muscle in the back is the most likely cause of your child's pain.

ACTION Give your child the recommended dose of a *analgesic*. Your child should avoid sports until he or she is free of pain. See your child's doctor within 24 hours if the pain is severe or has not improved by the next day.

CONSULT YOUR CHILD'S DOCTOR IF YOU ARE UNABLE TO MAKE A DIAGNOSIS FROM THIS CHART.

SELF-HELP Treating sprains and strains in a child

If your child has a sprain or strain or a deep bruise, the appropriate treatment for the injury can be remembered as RICE – Rest, Ice, Compression, and Elevation (*see* TREATING SPRAINS AND STRAINS, p.229). If necessary, give your child the recommended dose of a *analgesic*. If the injury is no better within 24 hours, consult your child's doctor.

Your child should avoid sports or any unnecessary exercise involving the affected part of the body until it is free from pain. If necessary, write your child's school a note explaining the problem.

Cold compress
If your child has a sprain or strain, a cold compress will help reduce the swelling.

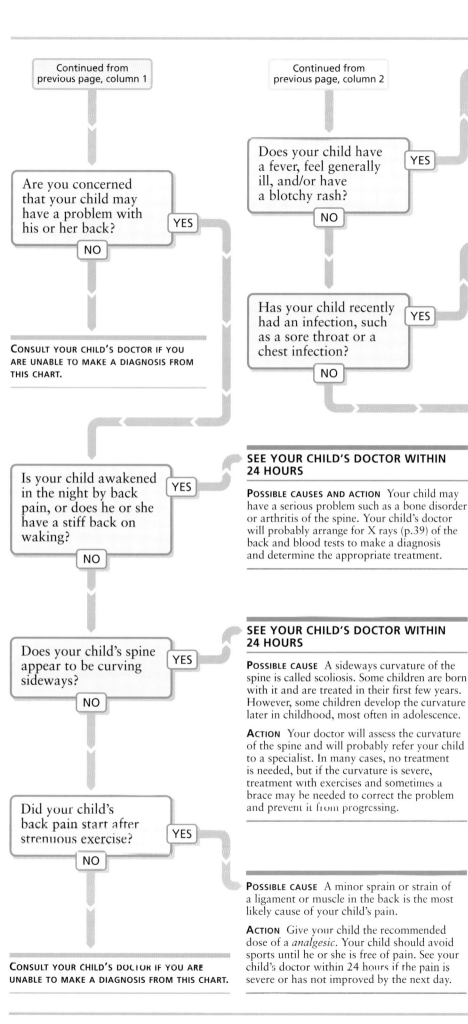

49 Foot problems

The bones in children's feet are soft, unlike bones in other parts of the body, and can be distorted by shoes that do not fit properly. Children's feet grow quickly, and you should check your child's shoes regularly. Feet can also be damaged by wearing high heels or shoes with pointed toes for any length of time. Although wearing ill-fitting shoes may not cause symptoms at the time, it may result in foot problems later in life. Most symptoms affecting children's feet are caused by minor conditions, such as plantar warts, and can be treated at home. However, if your child's foot is very painful or swollen or home treatment has been ineffective, consult your child's doctor.

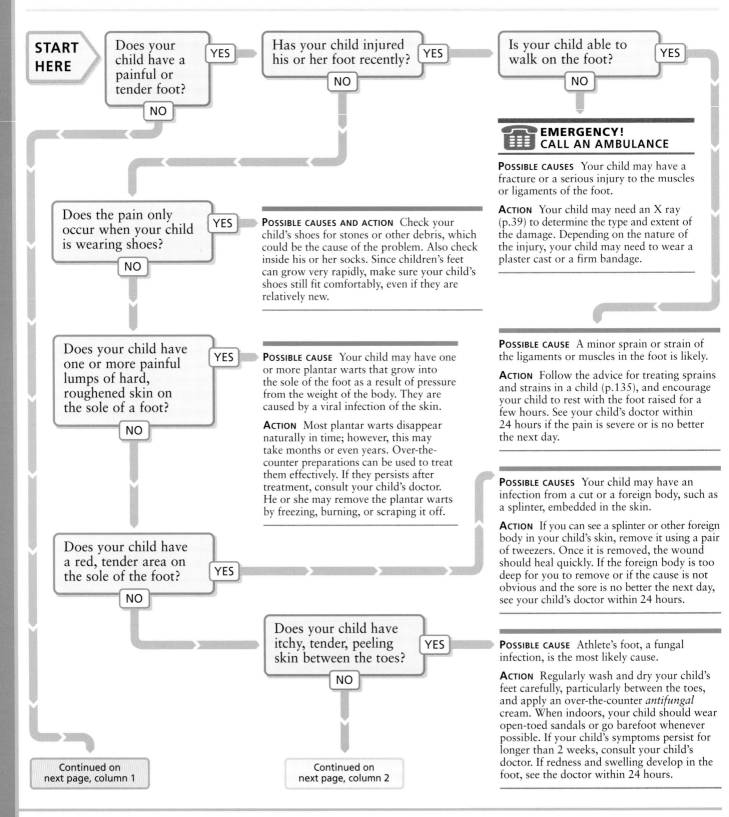

START HERE

Does your child have a painful or tender foot? YES → **Has your child injured his or her foot recently?** YES → **Is your child able to walk on the foot?** YES →

NO / NO / NO

EMERGENCY! CALL AN AMBULANCE

POSSIBLE CAUSES Your child may have a fracture or a serious injury to the muscles or ligaments of the foot.

ACTION Your child may need an X ray (p.39) to determine the type and extent of the damage. Depending on the nature of the injury, your child may need to wear a plaster cast or a firm bandage.

Does the pain only occur when your child is wearing shoes? YES →

NO

POSSIBLE CAUSES AND ACTION Check your child's shoes for stones or other debris, which could be the cause of the problem. Also check inside his or her socks. Since children's feet can grow very rapidly, make sure your child's shoes still fit comfortably, even if they are relatively new.

POSSIBLE CAUSE A minor sprain or strain of the ligaments or muscles in the foot is likely.

ACTION Follow the advice for treating sprains and strains in a child (p.135), and encourage your child to rest with the foot raised for a few hours. See your child's doctor within 24 hours if the pain is severe or is no better the next day.

Does your child have one or more painful lumps of hard, roughened skin on the sole of a foot? YES →

NO

POSSIBLE CAUSE Your child may have one or more plantar warts that grow into the sole of the foot as a result of pressure from the weight of the body. They are caused by a viral infection of the skin.

ACTION Most plantar warts disappear naturally in time; however, this may take months or even years. Over-the-counter preparations can be used to treat them effectively. If they persists after treatment, consult your child's doctor. He or she may remove the plantar warts by freezing, burning, or scraping it off.

POSSIBLE CAUSES Your child may have an infection from a cut or a foreign body, such as a splinter, embedded in the skin.

ACTION If you can see a splinter or other foreign body in your child's skin, remove it using a pair of tweezers. Once it is removed, the wound should heal quickly. If the foreign body is too deep for you to remove or if the cause is not obvious and the sore is no better the next day, see your child's doctor within 24 hours.

Does your child have a red, tender area on the sole of the foot? YES →

NO

Does your child have itchy, tender, peeling skin between the toes? YES →

NO

POSSIBLE CAUSE Athlete's foot, a fungal infection, is the most likely cause.

ACTION Regularly wash and dry your child's feet carefully, particularly between the toes, and apply an over-the-counter *antifungal* cream. When indoors, your child should wear open-toed sandals or go barefoot whenever possible. If your child's symptoms persist for longer than 2 weeks, consult your child's doctor. If redness and swelling develop in the foot, see the doctor within 24 hours.

Continued on next page, column 1

Continued on next page, column 2

Continued from previous page, column 1

Continued from previous page, column 2

Are you concerned about the appearance of your child's feet? **YES**

NO

Does your child have a red, tender swelling around the big toenail? **YES**

NO

POSSIBLE CAUSE An infected, ingrown toenail is a likely cause. This may be the result of cutting the toenails incorrectly or wearing tight shoes. Consult your child's doctor.

ACTION The doctor may prescribe *antibiotics* and drain any pus under a local anesthetic. Surgery is sometimes recommended to remove part or all of the toenail (*see* REMOVAL OF AN INGROWN TOENAIL, p.236). To prevent ingrown toenails, your child should always wear correctly fitting shoes or, if practical, open-toed sandals. Keep the affected area clean and dry, and always cut the toenails straight across rather than in a curve.

CONSULT YOUR CHILD'S DOCTOR IF YOU ARE UNABLE TO MAKE A DIAGNOSIS FROM THIS CHART.

CONSULT YOUR CHILD'S DOCTOR IF YOU ARE UNABLE TO MAKE A DIAGNOSIS FROM THIS CHART.

Does one or both of your child's feet turn inward? **YES**

NO

Does the whole foot including the heel turn inward, and has it been like this since birth? **YES**

NO

POSSIBLE CAUSES The shape of your child's foot may be due to an abnormality in the structure of the bones in the foot or to the position of the baby's foot when it was in the uterus. It is usually noticed by a doctor when the child is born. Consult your child's doctor.

ACTION If the shape of the foot has resulted from its position in the uterus, it should correct itself within a few weeks of birth. If the shape of the foot is due to a structural abnormality, treatment will consist of manipulation and the use of a splint. If this has not corrected the problem by 3 years of age, an operation may be needed.

POSSIBLE CAUSE AND ACTION Your child may have a condition called "intoeing." This is usually noticed when a child begins to walk and is often caused by the inward rotation of the whole leg from the hip or by bow legs, both of which are normal in some children. Consult your child's doctor so that the diagnosis can be confirmed. This condition rarely needs treatment. Bow legs usually correct themselves by the age of 3 years, while hip rotation usually corrects itself by the age of 8 years. In rare cases, an operation is needed to correct the problem.

Are you concerned that your child may have flat feet? **YES**

NO

POSSIBLE CAUSE AND ACTION Children under 3 years of age usually have flat feet because the muscles, ligaments, and bones in their feet are not yet fully developed. The fat pad in the feet of young children also adds to this appearance. There is no cause for concern at this age because a normal arch will probably develop as your child grows.

Is your child under 3 years old? **YES**

NO

Are your child's toes bent or curled under? **YES**

NO

CONSULT YOUR CHILD'S DOCTOR IF YOU ARE UNABLE TO MAKE A DIAGNOSIS FROM THIS CHART.

POSSIBLE CAUSES AND ACTION If your child was born with bent toes, there is probably no cause for concern. If they lead to pain or embarrassment, however, an operation to straighten the toes may be recommended when your child is older. If the condition has developed recently, your child's shoes and/or socks may be too small. Make sure your child always wears well-fitting shoes and socks.

POSSIBLE CAUSE AND ACTION Flat feet are often inherited. In this condition, ligaments in the foot are lax and only form an arch when the child stands on tiptoes. Flat feet are rarely a cause for concern and do not prevent a child from doing well in sports or cause problems in the future. Special exercises and shoe inserts are almost always ineffective and unnecessary. If your child's feet are painful or if you are worried, consult your child's doctor.

50 Limping

For limping due to a painful foot, see chart 49, FOOT PROBLEMS **(p. 136).**
A limp or reluctance to walk may be the first sign of a problem in a child who is too young to explain that something is wrong. A minor injury that causes a limp may get better on its own. However, any child with a limp, even a painless one, should be seen by a doctor within 24 hours. There may be an underlying disorder that requires prompt treatment.

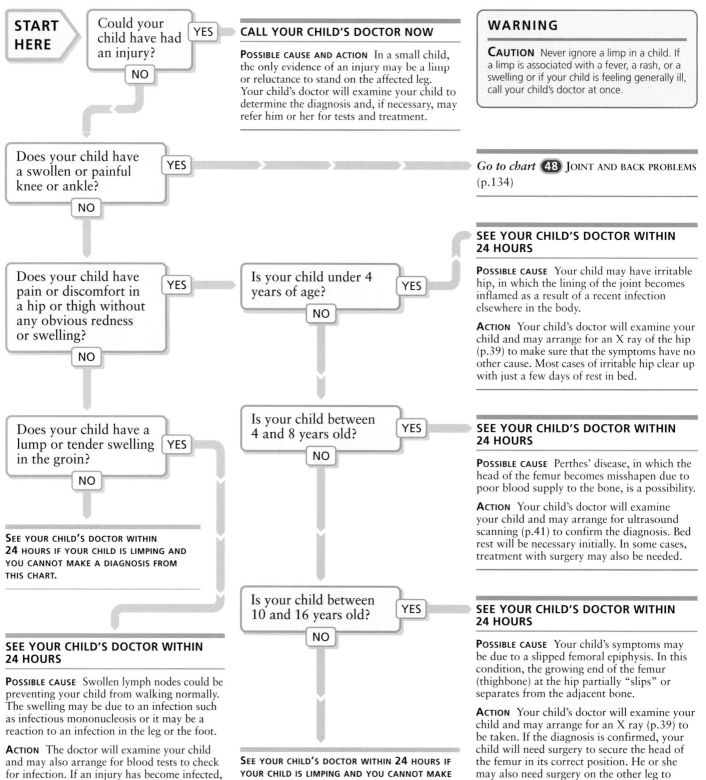

START HERE

Could your child have had an injury?
YES → **CALL YOUR CHILD'S DOCTOR NOW**

POSSIBLE CAUSE AND ACTION In a small child, the only evidence of an injury may be a limp or reluctance to stand on the affected leg. Your child's doctor will examine your child to determine the diagnosis and, if necessary, may refer him or her for tests and treatment.

NO

WARNING

CAUTION Never ignore a limp in a child. If a limp is associated with a fever, a rash, or a swelling or if your child is feeling generally ill, call your child's doctor at once.

Does your child have a swollen or painful knee or ankle?
YES → *Go to chart* **48** JOINT AND BACK PROBLEMS (p.134)

NO

Does your child have pain or discomfort in a hip or thigh without any obvious redness or swelling?
YES → **Is your child under 4 years of age?**
YES → **SEE YOUR CHILD'S DOCTOR WITHIN 24 HOURS**

POSSIBLE CAUSE Your child may have irritable hip, in which the lining of the joint becomes inflamed as a result of a recent infection elsewhere in the body.

ACTION Your child's doctor will examine your child and may arrange for an X ray of the hip (p.39) to make sure that the symptoms have no other cause. Most cases of irritable hip clear up with just a few days of rest in bed.

NO

NO

Is your child between 4 and 8 years old?
YES → **SEE YOUR CHILD'S DOCTOR WITHIN 24 HOURS**

POSSIBLE CAUSE Perthes' disease, in which the head of the femur becomes misshapen due to poor blood supply to the bone, is a possibility.

ACTION Your child's doctor will examine your child and may arrange for ultrasound scanning (p.41) to confirm the diagnosis. Bed rest will be necessary initially. In some cases, treatment with surgery may also be needed.

NO

Does your child have a lump or tender swelling in the groin?
YES

NO

SEE YOUR CHILD'S DOCTOR WITHIN 24 HOURS IF YOUR CHILD IS LIMPING AND YOU CANNOT MAKE A DIAGNOSIS FROM THIS CHART.

Is your child between 10 and 16 years old?
YES → **SEE YOUR CHILD'S DOCTOR WITHIN 24 HOURS**

POSSIBLE CAUSE Your child's symptoms may be due to a slipped femoral epiphysis. In this condition, the growing end of the femur (thighbone) at the hip partially "slips" or separates from the adjacent bone.

NO

SEE YOUR CHILD'S DOCTOR WITHIN 24 HOURS IF YOUR CHILD IS LIMPING AND YOU CANNOT MAKE A DIAGNOSIS FROM THIS CHART.

SEE YOUR CHILD'S DOCTOR WITHIN 24 HOURS

POSSIBLE CAUSE Swollen lymph nodes could be preventing your child from walking normally. The swelling may be due to an infection such as infectious mononucleosis or it may be a reaction to an infection in the leg or the foot.

ACTION The doctor will examine your child and may also arrange for blood tests to check for infection. If an injury has become infected, *antibiotics* may be needed.

ACTION Your child's doctor will examine your child and may arrange for an X ray (p.39) to be taken. If the diagnosis is confirmed, your child will need surgery to secure the head of the femur in its correct position. He or she may also need surgery on the other leg to prevent the same problem from occurring.

51 Adolescent weight problems

An adolescent needs more calories than an adult. The rapid increase in height that occurs in adolescence and the development of adult body proportions sometimes leads a teenager to feel either too thin or too fat. Adolescence is a time when young people are particularly sensitive about their appearance, and as a result, it is a time when eating disorders, such as anorexia nervosa, are most likely to occur. Consult this chart if you are worried about your child's weight or if your child is outside the normal range for his or her height (*see* GROWTH CHARTS, p.26).

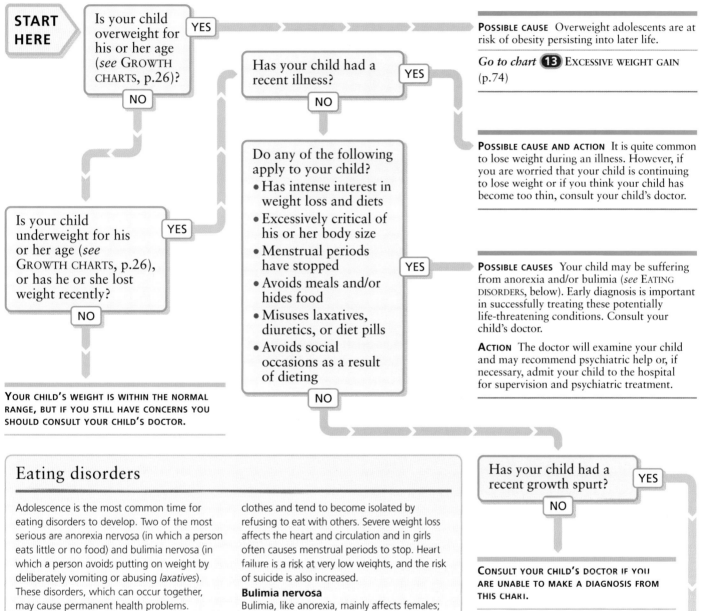

START HERE

Is your child overweight for his or her age (*see* GROWTH CHARTS, p.26)? — **YES** → **POSSIBLE CAUSE** Overweight adolescents are at risk of obesity persisting into later life.

Go to chart **13** EXCESSIVE WEIGHT GAIN (p.74)

NO ↓

Has your child had a recent illness? — **YES** → **POSSIBLE CAUSE AND ACTION** It is quite common to lose weight during an illness. However, if you are worried that your child is continuing to lose weight or if you think your child has become too thin, consult your child's doctor.

NO ↓

Is your child underweight for his or her age (*see* GROWTH CHARTS, p.26), or has he or she lost weight recently? — **YES** →

Do any of the following apply to your child?
- Has intense interest in weight loss and diets
- Excessively critical of his or her body size
- Menstrual periods have stopped
- Avoids meals and/or hides food
- Misuses laxatives, diuretics, or diet pills
- Avoids social occasions as a result of dieting

YES → **POSSIBLE CAUSES** Your child may be suffering from anorexia and/or bulimia (*see* EATING DISORDERS, below). Early diagnosis is important in successfully treating these potentially life-threatening conditions. Consult your child's doctor.

ACTION The doctor will examine your child and may recommend psychiatric help or, if necessary, admit your child to the hospital for supervision and psychiatric treatment.

NO (for underweight question) ↓

YOUR CHILD'S WEIGHT IS WITHIN THE NORMAL RANGE, BUT IF YOU STILL HAVE CONCERNS YOU SHOULD CONSULT YOUR CHILD'S DOCTOR.

NO (for any of the following) →

Has your child had a recent growth spurt? — **YES** →

NO ↓

CONSULT YOUR CHILD'S DOCTOR IF YOU ARE UNABLE TO MAKE A DIAGNOSIS FROM THIS CHART.

POSSIBLE CAUSE AND ACTION A rapid increase in height during a growth spurt may not initially be matched with a similar gain in weight. This is usually no cause for concern, and your child's weight is likely to catch up with his or her height over the next few months. However, if your child seems ill or if his or her weight continues to concern you, consult your child's doctor.

Eating disorders

Adolescence is the most common time for eating disorders to develop. Two of the most serious are anorexia nervosa (in which a person eats little or no food) and bulimia nervosa (in which a person avoids putting on weight by deliberately vomiting or abusing *laxatives*). These disorders, which can occur together, may cause permanent health problems.

Anorexia nervosa
This disorder affects approximately 1 percent of adolescents, mainly girls, although the incidence in boys is rising. It usually occurs in people who are hard workers, overachievers, and conformists, and is often triggered by weight loss after a diet. The person loses weight until he or she is emaciated. Most people with anorexia have an intense desire to be thin and see themselves as fat even when dangerously underweight. They may disguise their weight loss by wearing loose

clothes and tend to become isolated by refusing to eat with others. Severe weight loss affects the heart and circulation and in girls often causes menstrual periods to stop. Heart failure is a risk at very low weights, and the risk of suicide is also increased.

Bulimia nervosa
Bulimia, like anorexia, mainly affects females; 3 percent of women develop it at some time in their lives. People with bulimia often have low self-confidence and use food for comfort. They are usually of normal weight but have episodes (called binges) when they eat excessive amounts, often followed by deliberate vomiting or abuse of *laxatives* or *diuretics*. They may also exercise compulsively. Repeated vomiting causes damage to the teeth. Vomiting and the abuse of *laxatives* can result in chemical imbalances that may affect the internal organs, including the heart.

52 Adolescent behavior problems

Adolescence is the transition between childhood and adulthood. The combined effects of the hormonal changes that begin at puberty and the psychological factors involved in developing independence often lead to behavioral difficulties. An adolescent is much more self-conscious than a child, and the need to fit in with the peer group becomes increasingly important. Concerns about his or her changing body, performance in school, or style of clothing often cause awkwardness. Arguments or misunderstandings at home about dress, language, or general conduct are common. In many cases, offering your support and understanding without making a fuss will be all your child needs at this time. However, if you feel that your child is beyond your control and may be endangering his or her health or risking conflict with the law, consult your child's doctor, who may give advice or recommend relevant support services.

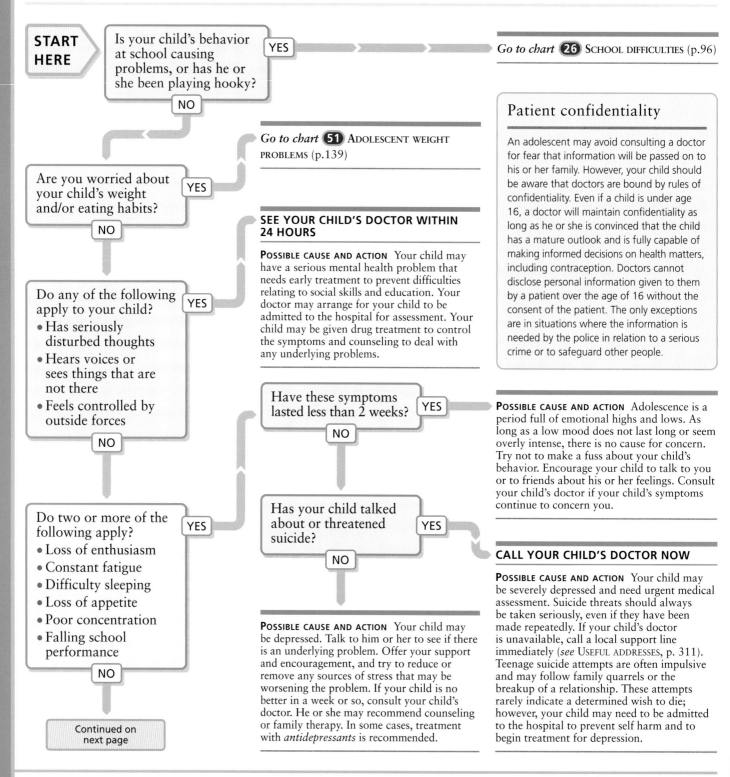

START HERE

Is your child's behavior at school causing problems, or has he or she been playing hooky?

YES → *Go to chart* **26** SCHOOL DIFFICULTIES (p.96)

NO

Are you worried about your child's weight and/or eating habits?

YES → *Go to chart* **51** ADOLESCENT WEIGHT PROBLEMS (p.139)

NO

Do any of the following apply to your child?
- Has seriously disturbed thoughts
- Hears voices or sees things that are not there
- Feels controlled by outside forces

YES →

SEE YOUR CHILD'S DOCTOR WITHIN 24 HOURS

POSSIBLE CAUSE AND ACTION Your child may have a serious mental health problem that needs early treatment to prevent difficulties relating to social skills and education. Your doctor may arrange for your child to be admitted to the hospital for assessment. Your child may be given drug treatment to control the symptoms and counseling to deal with any underlying problems.

NO

Do two or more of the following apply?
- Loss of enthusiasm
- Constant fatigue
- Difficulty sleeping
- Loss of appetite
- Poor concentration
- Falling school performance

YES →

Have these symptoms lasted less than 2 weeks?

YES →

POSSIBLE CAUSE AND ACTION Adolescence is a period full of emotional highs and lows. As long as a low mood does not last long or seem overly intense, there is no cause for concern. Try not to make a fuss about your child's behavior. Encourage your child to talk to you or to friends about his or her feelings. Consult your child's doctor if your child's symptoms continue to concern you.

NO

Has your child talked about or threatened suicide?

YES →

CALL YOUR CHILD'S DOCTOR NOW

POSSIBLE CAUSE AND ACTION Your child may be severely depressed and need urgent medical assessment. Suicide threats should always be taken seriously, even if they have been made repeatedly. If your child's doctor is unavailable, call a local support line immediately (*see* USEFUL ADDRESSES, p. 311). Teenage suicide attempts are often impulsive and may follow family quarrels or the breakup of a relationship. These attempts rarely indicate a determined wish to die; however, your child may need to be admitted to the hospital to prevent self harm and to begin treatment for depression.

NO

POSSIBLE CAUSE AND ACTION Your child may be depressed. Talk to him or her to see if there is an underlying problem. Offer your support and encouragement, and try to reduce or remove any sources of stress that may be worsening the problem. If your child is no better in a week or so, consult your child's doctor. He or she may recommend counseling or family therapy. In some cases, treatment with *antidepressants* is recommended.

NO

Continued on next page

Patient confidentiality

An adolescent may avoid consulting a doctor for fear that information will be passed on to his or her family. However, your child should be aware that doctors are bound by rules of confidentiality. Even if a child is under age 16, a doctor will maintain confidentiality as long as he or she is convinced that the child has a mature outlook and is fully capable of making informed decisions on health matters, including contraception. Doctors cannot disclose personal information given to them by a patient over the age of 16 without the consent of the patient. The only exceptions are in situations where the information is needed by the police in relation to a serious crime or to safeguard other people.

Continued from
previous page

Does your child
seem particularly
apprehensive or tense
much of the time?
— YES →
— NO ↓

Is your child worried
about a problem, such
as exams, difficulties
with friends, or
parental separation?
— YES →
— NO ↓

POSSIBLE CAUSE Most adolescents experience periods of anxiety. This is a cause for concern only if it is severe enough to interfere with day to day functioning.

ACTION Talk to your child, and try to discover any underlying worries that he or she has. Offer your support and understanding. It may help to talk to your child's teachers. If your child's anxiety does not ease with time and extra support, consult your child's doctor, who may recommend counseling or family therapy.

POSSIBLE CAUSE AND ACTION Your child's anxiety may be a symptom of depression. Talk to your child about his or her feelings, and offer your support and understanding. If the symptoms persist for more than 2 weeks, without an obvious cause, consult your child's doctor. He or she may recommend counseling or family therapy.

Do any aspects of your
child's behavior suggest
drug or solvent abuse
or the excess use of
alcohol?
— YES →
— NO ↓

POSSIBLE CAUSE Drug or solvent abuse (below) may be causing your child's behavior problems.

ACTION Talk to your child, to try to find out whether he or she is using drugs or solvents. Explain the dangers of drug abuse, and try to provide your child with support. If your child is unwilling or unable to stop or denies drug usage, consult your child's doctor or a self-help group (see USEFUL ADDRESSES, p.311).

POSSIBLE CAUSE If your child is persistently antisocial or disruptive, he or she may have a conduct disorder. Consult your child's doctor.

ACTION The doctor may refer your child to a specialist for assessment. Counseling or family therapy will probably be recommended. However, long-standing behavior problems may be difficult to change.

Is your child's behavior
aggressive or violent, or
is he or she breaking
the law?
— YES →
— NO ↓

Recognizing drug and solvent abuse

You are unlikely to discover any physical evidence that your child is taking drugs unless he or she wants you to do so. Most adolescent drug users will use the drugs they buy immediately or will be careful to hide any evidence. Behavioral changes are often the only clues. You should bear in mind, however, that most teenagers experience mood swings and other behavioral changes as a normal part of adolescence.

Although different drugs have different effects, the most common signs of regular drug or solvent abuse are:
- Behavioral changes, such as unusual mood swings, irritability, or aggressiveness
- Lying and/or secretiveness about activities
- Lethargy, sleepiness, or drowsiness
- Falling school performance
- Loss of interest in friends or usual activities
- Altered sleep patterns
- Inability to account for money spent
- Disappearance of money or belongings

If you think your child is abusing drugs or solvents, choose a good time to discuss your concerns. If your child denies drug or solvent use or seems unable or unwilling to stop, consult your child's doctor or a self-help group (see USEFUL ADDRESSES, p.311).

Are you concerned
that your child may be
sexually active?
— YES →
— NO ↓

POSSIBLE CAUSE AND ACTION If possible, try to talk to your child about your concerns. Regardless of your opinion about his or her actions, you should make sure that your child is aware of the risk of an unwanted pregnancy and of sexually transmitted infections (see SEX AND HEALTH, p.32). Your child is entitled to confidential medical care from a doctor even if he or she is under 16 (see PATIENT CONFIDENTIALITY, opposite).

Has your child stopped
following his or her
treatment plan for a
long-standing medical
condition?
— YES →
— NO ↓

POSSIBLE CAUSE AND ACTION A reluctance to follow the treatment plan for a long-standing disease, such as diabetes mellitus or asthma, is common in adolescents, even if they have previously been responsible. This is usually due to a child's resentment of being different from others or the need to feel in control of his or her life. Talk to your child, but do not get aggressive or angry. Explain the dangers of not taking a prescribed medication as advised. You should also consult your child's doctor, who may be able to help by talking to your child. He or she may recommend counseling.

CONSULT YOUR CHILD'S DOCTOR IF YOU ARE UNABLE TO FIND AN EXPLANATION FOR YOUR CHILD'S BEHAVIOR ON THIS CHART AND HE OR SHE CONTINUES TO BEHAVE IN A WORRYING WAY.

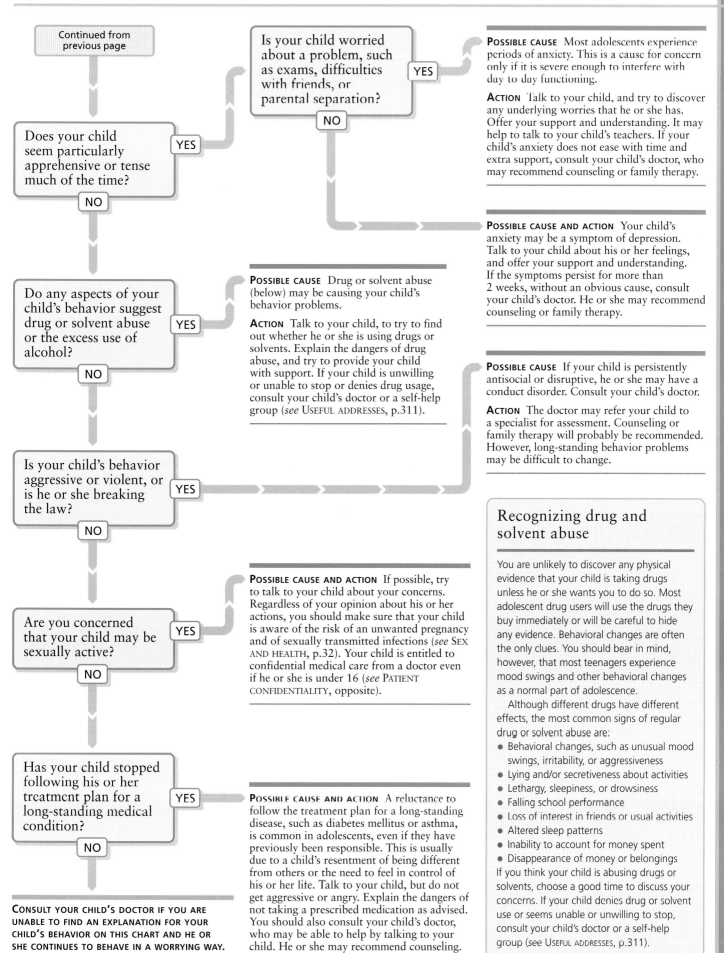

53 Problems with puberty in boys

The time when a child goes through the physical changes involved in becoming an adult is known as puberty. On average, most boys start puberty at 12 years of age; however any age between 9 and 15 years is considered normal. The earliest sign of puberty is usually enlargement of the penis and testes. Other signs of puberty include the ability to ejaculate seminal fluid, the growth of body and facial hair, and deepening of the voice. In boys, the adolescent growth spurt does not tend to occur until puberty is well established. Occasionally, puberty may be associated with a temporary enlargement of breast tissue (*see* BREAST DEVELOPMENT IN MALES, below), which can be embarrassing but is no risk to health.

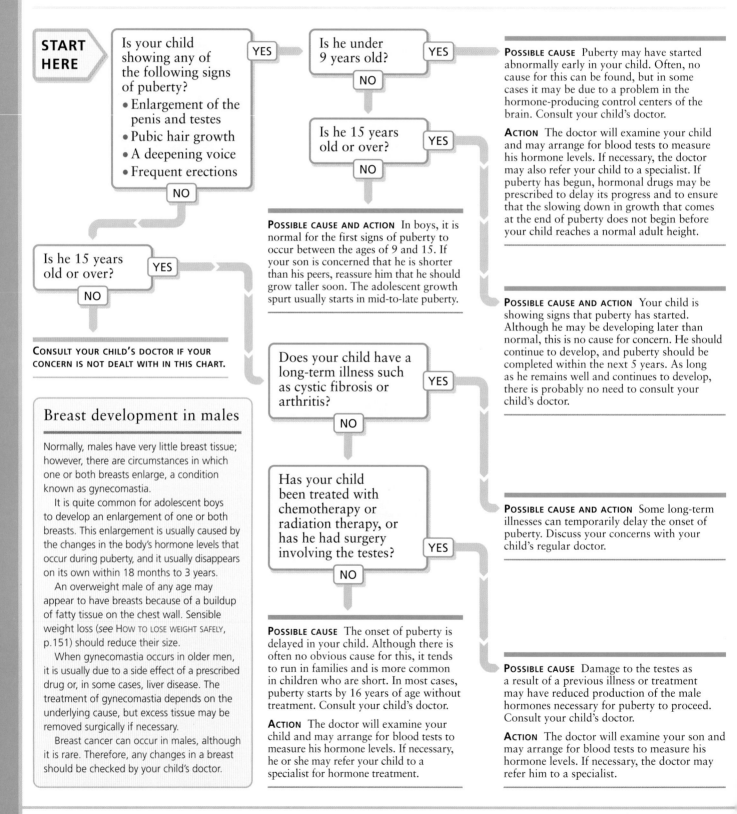

START HERE

Is your child showing any of the following signs of puberty?
- Enlargement of the penis and testes
- Pubic hair growth
- A deepening voice
- Frequent erections

NO → Is he 15 years old or over? → NO

CONSULT YOUR CHILD'S DOCTOR IF YOUR CONCERN IS NOT DEALT WITH IN THIS CHART.

YES → Is he under 9 years old?

YES (under 9) → **POSSIBLE CAUSE** Puberty may have started abnormally early in your child. Often, no cause for this can be found, but in some cases it may be due to a problem in the hormone-producing control centers of the brain. Consult your child's doctor.

ACTION The doctor will examine your child and may arrange for blood tests to measure his hormone levels. If necessary, the doctor may also refer your child to a specialist. If puberty has begun, hormonal drugs may be prescribed to delay its progress and to ensure that the slowing down in growth that comes at the end of puberty does not begin before your child reaches a normal adult height.

NO → Is he 15 years old or over?

YES (15 or over) → **POSSIBLE CAUSE AND ACTION** Your child is showing signs that puberty has started. Although he may be developing later than normal, this is no cause for concern. He should continue to develop, and puberty should be completed within the next 5 years. As long as he remains well and continues to develop, there is probably no need to consult your child's doctor.

NO → **POSSIBLE CAUSE AND ACTION** In boys, it is normal for the first signs of puberty to occur between the ages of 9 and 15. If your son is concerned that he is shorter than his peers, reassure him that he should grow taller soon. The adolescent growth spurt usually starts in mid-to-late puberty.

Does your child have a long-term illness such as cystic fibrosis or arthritis?

YES → **POSSIBLE CAUSE AND ACTION** Some long-term illnesses can temporarily delay the onset of puberty. Discuss your concerns with your child's regular doctor.

NO → Has your child been treated with chemotherapy or radiation therapy, or has he had surgery involving the testes?

YES → **POSSIBLE CAUSE** Damage to the testes as a result of a previous illness or treatment may have reduced production of the male hormones necessary for puberty to proceed. Consult your child's doctor.

ACTION The doctor will examine your son and may arrange for blood tests to measure his hormone levels. If necessary, the doctor may refer him to a specialist.

NO → **POSSIBLE CAUSE** The onset of puberty is delayed in your child. Although there is often no obvious cause for this, it tends to run in families and is more common in children who are short. In most cases, puberty starts by 16 years of age without treatment. Consult your child's doctor.

ACTION The doctor will examine your child and may arrange for blood tests to measure his hormone levels. If necessary, he or she may refer your child to a specialist for hormone treatment.

Breast development in males

Normally, males have very little breast tissue; however, there are circumstances in which one or both breasts enlarge, a condition known as gynecomastia.

It is quite common for adolescent boys to develop an enlargement of one or both breasts. This enlargement is usually caused by the changes in the body's hormone levels that occur during puberty, and it usually disappears on its own within 18 months to 3 years.

An overweight male of any age may appear to have breasts because of a buildup of fatty tissue on the chest wall. Sensible weight loss (*see* HOW TO LOSE WEIGHT SAFELY, p.151) should reduce their size.

When gynecomastia occurs in older men, it is usually due to a side effect of a prescribed drug or, in some cases, liver disease. The treatment of gynecomastia depends on the underlying cause, but excess tissue may be removed surgically if necessary.

Breast cancer can occur in males, although it is rare. Therefore, any changes in a breast should be checked by your child's doctor.

54 Problems with puberty in girls

Puberty is the time when a child goes through the physical changes involved in becoming an adult. The average age for a girl to start puberty is 11½ years, although any age between 8 and 14 years is considered normal. The first signs of puberty are the enlargement of the breasts and the growth of pubic hair, followed by armpit hair. Girls usually have a growth spurt in early puberty, and menstruation usually begins between the ages of 11 and 14. Puberty usually lasts for about 5 years, during which time all of the body features of an adult develop. Consult this chart if you are worried that your child has started puberty too early or that she seems abnormally late in reaching puberty.

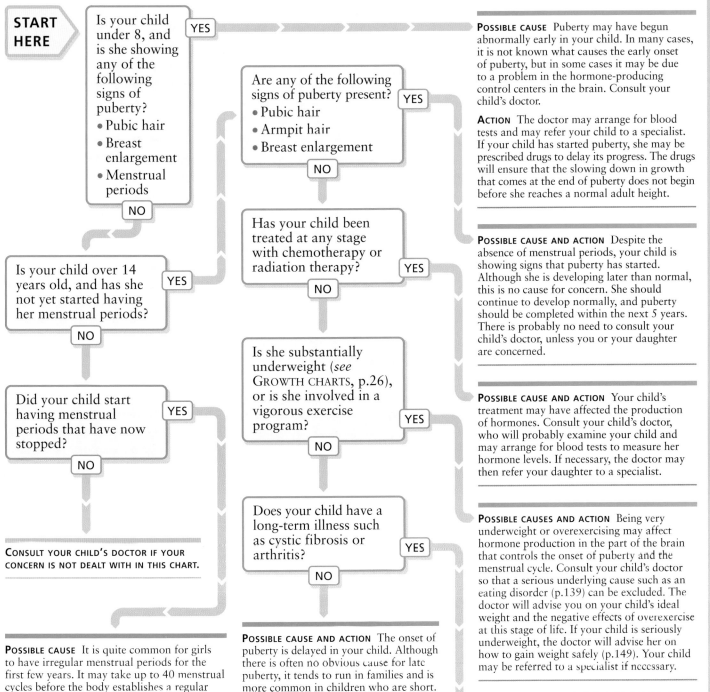

START HERE

Is your child under 8, and is she showing any of the following signs of puberty?
- Pubic hair
- Breast enlargement
- Menstrual periods

YES → **POSSIBLE CAUSE** Puberty may have begun abnormally early in your child. In many cases, it is not known what causes the early onset of puberty, but in some cases it may be due to a problem in the hormone-producing control centers in the brain. Consult your child's doctor.

ACTION The doctor may arrange for blood tests and may refer your child to a specialist. If your child has started puberty, she may be prescribed drugs to delay its progress. The drugs will ensure that the slowing down in growth that comes at the end of puberty does not begin before she reaches a normal adult height.

NO

Are any of the following signs of puberty present?
- Pubic hair
- Armpit hair
- Breast enlargement

YES → (leads to below)

NO

POSSIBLE CAUSE AND ACTION Despite the absence of menstrual periods, your child is showing signs that puberty has started. Although she is developing later than normal, this is no cause for concern. She should continue to develop normally, and puberty should be completed within the next 5 years. There is probably no need to consult your child's doctor, unless you or your daughter are concerned.

Is your child over 14 years old, and has she not yet started having her menstrual periods?

YES

NO

Has your child been treated at any stage with chemotherapy or radiation therapy?

YES → **POSSIBLE CAUSE AND ACTION** Your child's treatment may have affected the production of hormones. Consult your child's doctor, who will probably examine your child and may arrange for blood tests to measure her hormone levels. If necessary, the doctor may then refer your daughter to a specialist.

NO

Did your child start having menstrual periods that have now stopped?

YES

NO

Is she substantially underweight (see GROWTH CHARTS, p.26), or is she involved in a vigorous exercise program?

YES → **POSSIBLE CAUSES AND ACTION** Being very underweight or overexercising may affect hormone production in the part of the brain that controls the onset of puberty and the menstrual cycle. Consult your child's doctor so that a serious underlying cause such as an eating disorder (p.139) can be excluded. The doctor will advise you on your child's ideal weight and the negative effects of overexercise at this stage of life. If your child is seriously underweight, the doctor will advise her on how to gain weight safely (p.149). Your child may be referred to a specialist if necessary.

NO

Does your child have a long-term illness such as cystic fibrosis or arthritis?

YES → **POSSIBLE CAUSE AND ACTION** Some serious long-term illnesses can temporarily delay the onset of puberty. Discuss your concerns with your child's regular doctor.

NO

CONSULT YOUR CHILD'S DOCTOR IF YOUR CONCERN IS NOT DEALT WITH IN THIS CHART.

POSSIBLE CAUSE It is quite common for girls to have irregular menstrual periods for the first few years. It may take up to 40 menstrual cycles before the body establishes a regular pattern. However, the possibility of pregnancy should always be considered.

Go to chart **130** ABSENT MENSTRUAL PERIODS (p.260)

POSSIBLE CAUSE AND ACTION The onset of puberty is delayed in your child. Although there is often no obvious cause for late puberty, it tends to run in families and is more common in children who are short. Consult your child's doctor, who will examine your child and may arrange for blood tests to measure her hormone levels. If necessary, he or she may then refer your child to a specialist.

55 Adolescent skin problems

The onset of adolescence often produces marked changes in the skin. Infantile eczema, which often affects younger children, may clear up altogether before or during adolescence. However, another form of eczema – contact eczema – may occur for the first time during this period. Contact eczema may result from contact with certain metals or cosmetics, causing an itchy, red rash. Other skin problems, such as psoriasis, may also develop for the first time during adolescence. However, the most noticeable skin changes during adolescence are caused by the rising levels of sex hormones. These hormones encourage the sebaceous glands in the skin to produce increasing amounts of sebum – an oily substance that helps lubricate the skin. Not only does the increased sebaceous activity give the skin an oily appearance, but it also encourages the development of acne, which affects almost all adolescents to some extent.

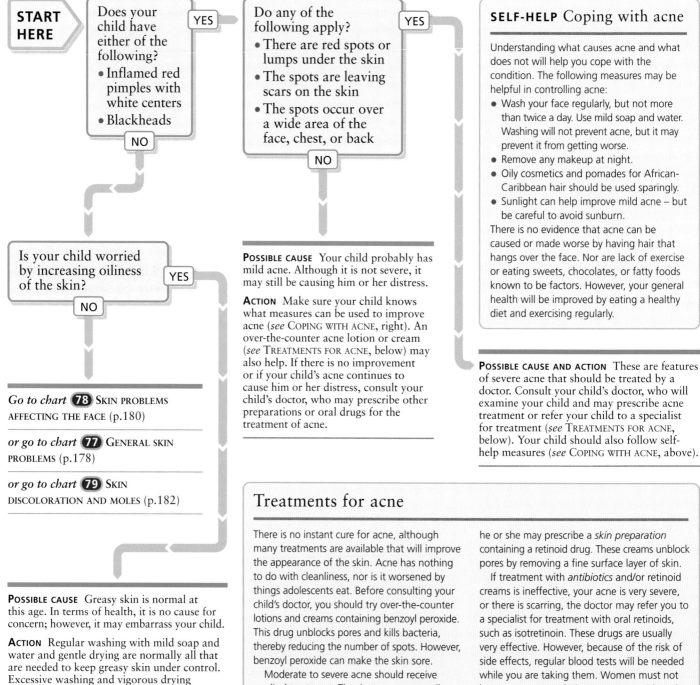

START HERE

Does your child have either of the following?
- Inflamed red pimples with white centers
- Blackheads

YES → Do any of the following apply?
- There are red spots or lumps under the skin
- The spots are leaving scars on the skin
- The spots occur over a wide area of the face, chest, or back

NO

YES

NO

Is your child worried by increasing oiliness of the skin?

YES

NO

POSSIBLE CAUSE Your child probably has mild acne. Although it is not severe, it may still be causing him or her distress.

ACTION Make sure your child knows what measures can be used to improve acne (*see* COPING WITH ACNE, right). An over-the-counter acne lotion or cream (*see* TREATMENTS FOR ACNE, below) may also help. If there is no improvement or if your child's acne continues to cause him or her distress, consult your child's doctor, who may prescribe other preparations or oral drugs for the treatment of acne.

Go to chart **78** SKIN PROBLEMS AFFECTING THE FACE (p.180)

or go to chart **77** GENERAL SKIN PROBLEMS (p.178)

or go to chart **79** SKIN DISCOLORATION AND MOLES (p.182)

POSSIBLE CAUSE Greasy skin is normal at this age. In terms of health, it is no cause for concern; however, it may embarrass your child.

ACTION Regular washing with mild soap and water and gentle drying are normally all that are needed to keep greasy skin under control. Excessive washing and vigorous drying may make oiliness worse. Any makeup that is used should be oil-free and should be removed completely each night.

SELF-HELP Coping with acne

Understanding what causes acne and what does not will help you cope with the condition. The following measures may be helpful in controlling acne:
- Wash your face regularly, but not more than twice a day. Use mild soap and water. Washing will not prevent acne, but it may prevent it from getting worse.
- Remove any makeup at night.
- Oily cosmetics and pomades for African-Caribbean hair should be used sparingly.
- Sunlight can help improve mild acne – but be careful to avoid sunburn.

There is no evidence that acne can be caused or made worse by having hair that hangs over the face. Nor are lack of exercise or eating sweets, chocolates, or fatty foods known to be factors. However, your general health will be improved by eating a healthy diet and exercising regularly.

POSSIBLE CAUSE AND ACTION These are features of severe acne that should be treated by a doctor. Consult your child's doctor, who will examine your child and may prescribe acne treatment or refer your child to a specialist for treatment (*see* TREATMENTS FOR ACNE, below). Your child should also follow self-help measures (*see* COPING WITH ACNE, above).

Treatments for acne

There is no instant cure for acne, although many treatments are available that will improve the appearance of the skin. Acne has nothing to do with cleanliness, nor is it worsened by things adolescents eat. Before consulting your child's doctor, you should try over-the-counter lotions and creams containing benzoyl peroxide. This drug unblocks pores and kills bacteria, thereby reducing the number of spots. However, benzoyl peroxide can make the skin sore.

Moderate to severe acne should receive medical treatment. The doctor may prescribe long-term low-dose *antibiotics*, which need to be taken for at least 6 months. Alternatively, he or she may prescribe a *skin preparation* containing a retinoid drug. These creams unblock pores by removing a fine surface layer of skin.

If treatment with *antibiotics* and/or retinoid creams is ineffective, your acne is very severe, or there is scarring, the doctor may refer you to a specialist for treatment with oral retinoids, such as isotretinoin. These drugs are usually very effective. However, because of the risk of side effects, regular blood tests will be needed while you are taking them. Women must not become pregnant during treatment with oral retinoids because these drugs can cause serious malformations in the fetus.

GENERAL CHARTS FOR ADULTS

56 Not feeling well

Sometimes you may have a vague feeling of being sick without being able to identify a specific symptom such as pain. This feeling is usually the result of a minor infection, psychological pressures, or an unhealthy lifestyle. However, you should always make an appointment to see your doctor if the feeling persists for more than a few days; there is a possibility that it may be a sign of a more serious underlying problem that requires medical treatment.

START HERE

Do you feel continually on edge or worried for no particular reason?
YES →

POSSIBLE CAUSE Feelings of anxiety resulting either from a specific problem or from an accumulation of different stresses and worries can make you feel ill.

Go to chart **73** ANXIETY (p.172)

NO ↓

Have you lost 5 percent of your body weight over 6–12 months without trying?
YES →

POSSIBLE CAUSE Unexplained weight loss combined with a general feeling of being sick may be a sign of an undiagnosed illness.

Go to chart **58** LOSS OF WEIGHT (p.148)

NO ↓

Do you have a temperature of 100.4°F (38°C) or above?
YES →

POSSIBLE CAUSE A viral infection is the most common cause of a general feeling of sickness combined with a fever.

Go to chart **61** FEVER (p.154)

NO ↓

Do you feel tired or do you lack energy most of the time?
YES →

POSSIBLE CAUSE Fatigue is a common symptom of many disorders, some of which require medical treatment.

Go to chart **57** FATIGUE (p.147)

NO ↓

Do you regularly drink more than the recommended safe alcohol limit (p.30)?
YES →

POSSIBLE CAUSE Excessive consumption of alcohol can cause both physical and mental illness (*see* ASSESSING YOUR ALCOHOL CONSUMPTION, right).

ACTION Cut down your alcohol consumption so that you stay within the recommended safe limits. If you are having difficulty reducing your intake, consult your doctor.

NO ↓

Are you taking over-the-counter, prescribed, or recreational drugs?
YES →

NO ↓

POSSIBLE CAUSE AND ACTION Certain drugs can cause a feeling of sickness as a side effect. Consult your doctor. Meanwhile, stop taking any over-the-counter or recreational drugs, but do not stop taking prescribed drugs.

CONSULT YOUR DOCTOR IF YOU ARE UNABLE TO MAKE A DIAGNOSIS FROM THIS CHART.

SELF-HELP Assessing your alcohol consumption

Some people use alcohol to cope with stressful situations or painful emotions. If unchecked, this habit can lead to alcohol dependence. Experiencing severe hangovers or memory loss after drinking alcohol indicates that you are drinking to excess, as do arguments or accidents precipitated by drinking. If you have more than two alcoholic drinks a day on most days, your health may be at risk (*see* SAFE ALCOHOL LIMITS, p.30).

To assess your drinking habits, ask yourself the questions below. The answers may help you judge whether drinking is affecting your life or becoming an uncontrollable habit.

- Have you ever thought that you ought to cut down on your drinking?
- Have other people ever annoyed you by criticizing your drinking?
- Have you ever felt guilty about drinking?
- Have you ever had an "eye-opener" drink first thing in the morning?

If you have answered yes to two or more of these questions, your drinking may be becoming a problem. Consult your doctor.

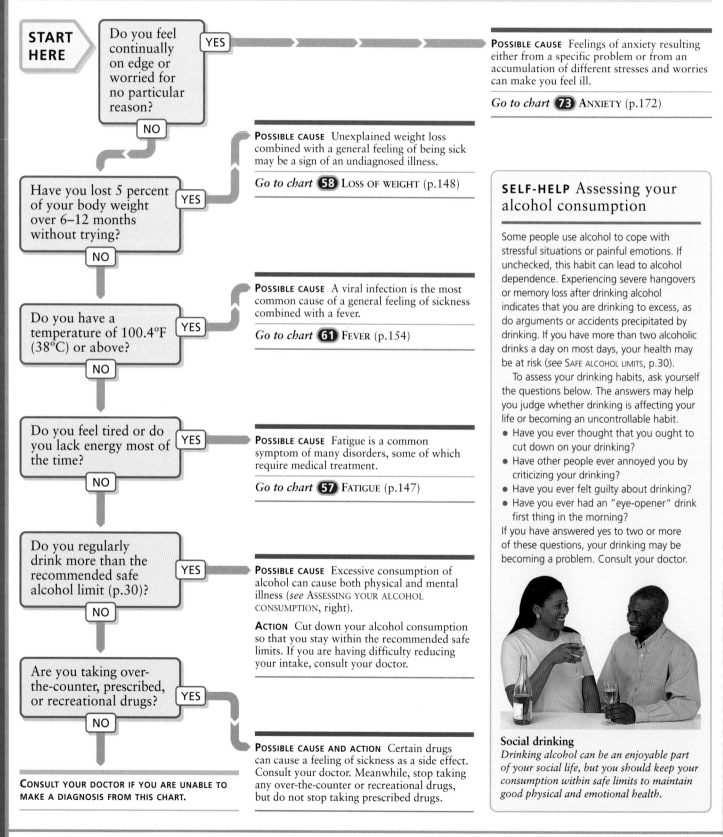

Social drinking
Drinking alcohol can be an enjoyable part of your social life, but you should keep your consumption within safe limits to maintain good physical and emotional health.

57 Fatigue

For problems related to sleeping, see chart 60, DIFFICULTY IN SLEEPING (p.152).
Fatigue is normal after physical exertion or long periods of hard work without a break. It is common after some infectious illnesses, such as flu or other viral infections, but should have cleared up after 2 or 3 weeks. However, if there is no obvious explanation for your fatigue, if it prevents you from carrying out daily activities, or if it is prolonged, you should consult your doctor because in some cases fatigue may indicate a serious health problem.

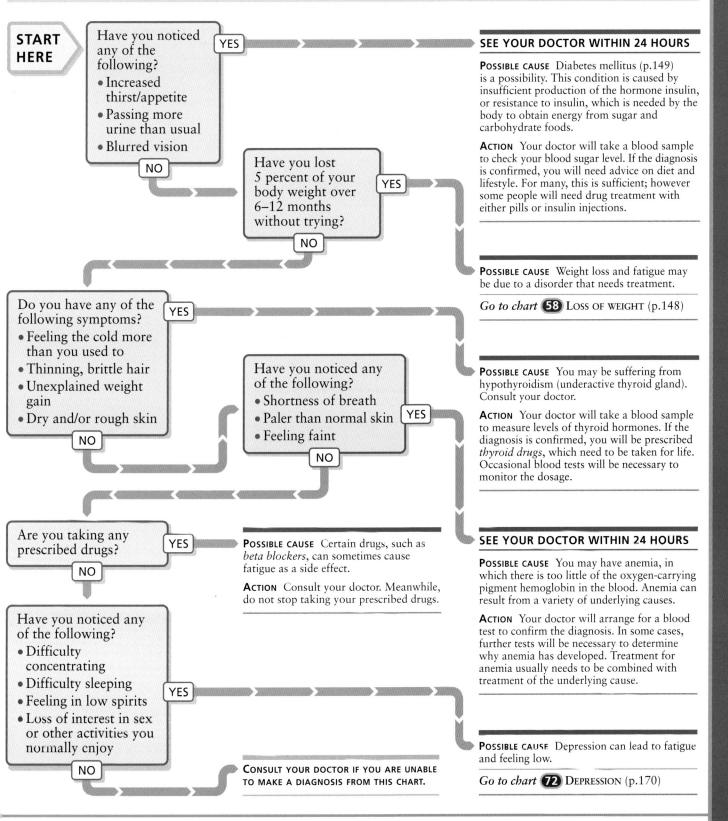

START HERE

Have you noticed any of the following?
- Increased thirst/appetite
- Passing more urine than usual
- Blurred vision

YES →

SEE YOUR DOCTOR WITHIN 24 HOURS

POSSIBLE CAUSE Diabetes mellitus (p.149) is a possibility. This condition is caused by insufficient production of the hormone insulin, or resistance to insulin, which is needed by the body to obtain energy from sugar and carbohydrate foods.

ACTION Your doctor will take a blood sample to check your blood sugar level. If the diagnosis is confirmed, you will need advice on diet and lifestyle. For many, this is sufficient; however some people will need drug treatment with either pills or insulin injections.

NO ↓

Have you lost 5 percent of your body weight over 6–12 months without trying?

YES →

POSSIBLE CAUSE Weight loss and fatigue may be due to a disorder that needs treatment.

Go to chart 58 LOSS OF WEIGHT (p.148)

NO ↓

Do you have any of the following symptoms?
- Feeling the cold more than you used to
- Thinning, brittle hair
- Unexplained weight gain
- Dry and/or rough skin

YES →

POSSIBLE CAUSE You may be suffering from hypothyroidism (underactive thyroid gland). Consult your doctor.

ACTION Your doctor will take a blood sample to measure levels of thyroid hormones. If the diagnosis is confirmed, you will be prescribed *thyroid drugs*, which need to be taken for life. Occasional blood tests will be necessary to monitor the dosage.

NO ↓

Have you noticed any of the following?
- Shortness of breath
- Paler than normal skin
- Feeling faint

YES →

NO ↓

Are you taking any prescribed drugs?

YES →

POSSIBLE CAUSE Certain drugs, such as *beta blockers*, can sometimes cause fatigue as a side effect.

ACTION Consult your doctor. Meanwhile, do not stop taking your prescribed drugs.

NO ↓

SEE YOUR DOCTOR WITHIN 24 HOURS

POSSIBLE CAUSE You may have anemia, in which there is too little of the oxygen-carrying pigment hemoglobin in the blood. Anemia can result from a variety of underlying causes.

ACTION Your doctor will arrange for a blood test to confirm the diagnosis. In some cases, further tests will be necessary to determine why anemia has developed. Treatment for anemia usually needs to be combined with treatment of the underlying cause.

Have you noticed any of the following?
- Difficulty concentrating
- Difficulty sleeping
- Feeling in low spirits
- Loss of interest in sex or other activities you normally enjoy

YES →

POSSIBLE CAUSE Depression can lead to fatigue and feeling low.

Go to chart 72 DEPRESSION (p.170)

NO ↓

CONSULT YOUR DOCTOR IF YOU ARE UNABLE TO MAKE A DIAGNOSIS FROM THIS CHART.

58 Loss of weight

For severe weight loss in adolescents, see chart 51,
ADOLESCENT WEIGHT PROBLEMS (p.139).
Minor fluctuations in weight due to temporary changes in
your diet and/or in the amount of physical exercise you do
are normal. However, severe, unintentional weight loss,

especially if it is combined with loss of appetite or other
symptoms, may be an early warning sign of some cancers or
infections that require urgent medical attention. If you are
worried that you have lost a lot of weight and there is no
obvious cause, you should consult your doctor.

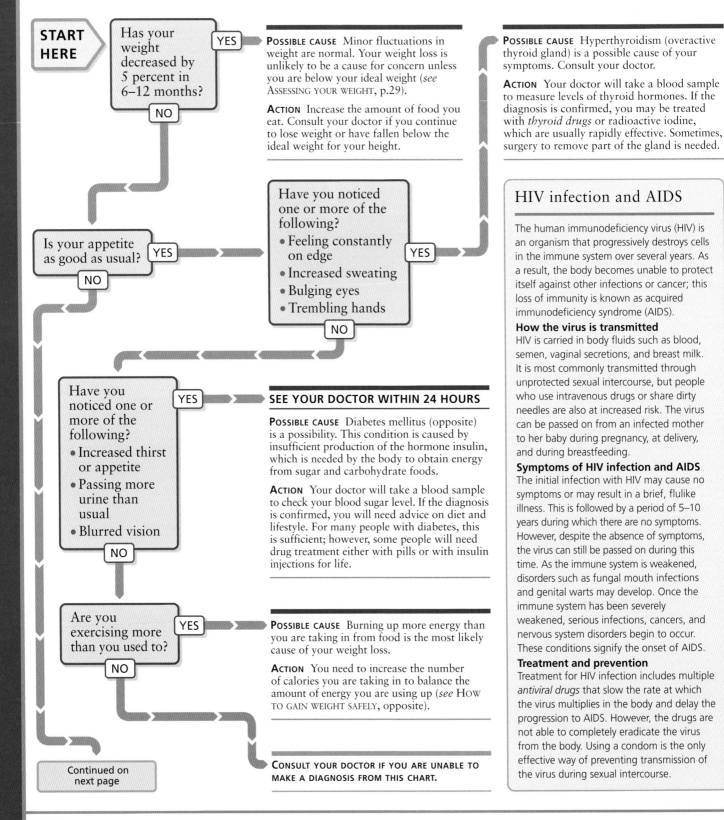

START HERE

Has your weight decreased by 5 percent in 6–12 months? — **YES** → **POSSIBLE CAUSE** Minor fluctuations in weight are normal. Your weight loss is unlikely to be a cause for concern unless you are below your ideal weight (*see* ASSESSING YOUR WEIGHT, p.29).

ACTION Increase the amount of food you eat. Consult your doctor if you continue to lose weight or have fallen below the ideal weight for your height.

NO ↓

Is your appetite as good as usual? — **YES** → **Have you noticed one or more of the following?**
- Feeling constantly on edge
- Increased sweating
- Bulging eyes
- Trembling hands

— **YES** → **POSSIBLE CAUSE** Hyperthyroidism (overactive thyroid gland) is a possible cause of your symptoms. Consult your doctor.

ACTION Your doctor will take a blood sample to measure levels of thyroid hormones. If the diagnosis is confirmed, you may be treated with *thyroid drugs* or radioactive iodine, which are usually rapidly effective. Sometimes, surgery to remove part of the gland is needed.

NO ↓

NO ↓

Have you noticed one or more of the following?
- Increased thirst or appetite
- Passing more urine than usual
- Blurred vision

— **YES** → **SEE YOUR DOCTOR WITHIN 24 HOURS**

POSSIBLE CAUSE Diabetes mellitus (opposite) is a possibility. This condition is caused by insufficient production of the hormone insulin, which is needed by the body to obtain energy from sugar and carbohydrate foods.

ACTION Your doctor will take a blood sample to check your blood sugar level. If the diagnosis is confirmed, you will need advice on diet and lifestyle. For many people with diabetes, this is sufficient; however, some people will need drug treatment either with pills or with insulin injections for life.

NO ↓

Are you exercising more than you used to? — **YES** → **POSSIBLE CAUSE** Burning up more energy than you are taking in from food is the most likely cause of your weight loss.

ACTION You need to increase the number of calories you are taking in to balance the amount of energy you are using up (*see* HOW TO GAIN WEIGHT SAFELY, opposite).

NO ↓

Continued on next page

CONSULT YOUR DOCTOR IF YOU ARE UNABLE TO MAKE A DIAGNOSIS FROM THIS CHART.

HIV infection and AIDS

The human immunodeficiency virus (HIV) is an organism that progressively destroys cells in the immune system over several years. As a result, the body becomes unable to protect itself against other infections or cancer; this loss of immunity is known as acquired immunodeficiency syndrome (AIDS).

How the virus is transmitted
HIV is carried in body fluids such as blood, semen, vaginal secretions, and breast milk. It is most commonly transmitted through unprotected sexual intercourse, but people who use intravenous drugs or share dirty needles are also at increased risk. The virus can be passed on from an infected mother to her baby during pregnancy, at delivery, and during breastfeeding.

Symptoms of HIV infection and AIDS
The initial infection with HIV may cause no symptoms or may result in a brief, flulike illness. This is followed by a period of 5–10 years during which there are no symptoms. However, despite the absence of symptoms, the virus can still be passed on during this time. As the immune system is weakened, disorders such as fungal mouth infections and genital warts may develop. Once the immune system has been severely weakened, serious infections, cancers, and nervous system disorders begin to occur. These conditions signify the onset of AIDS.

Treatment and prevention
Treatment for HIV infection includes multiple *antiviral drugs* that slow the rate at which the virus multiplies in the body and delay the progression to AIDS. However, the drugs are not able to completely eradicate the virus from the body. Using a condom is the only effective way of preventing transmission of the virus during sexual intercourse.

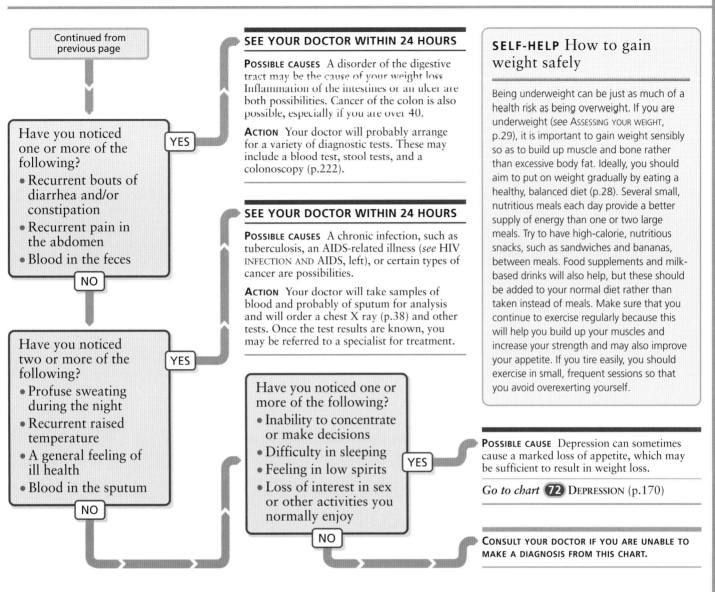

Continued from previous page

Have you noticed one or more of the following?
- Recurrent bouts of diarrhea and/or constipation
- Recurrent pain in the abdomen
- Blood in the feces

YES

NO

Have you noticed two or more of the following?
- Profuse sweating during the night
- Recurrent raised temperature
- A general feeling of ill health
- Blood in the sputum

YES

NO

Have you noticed one or more of the following?
- Inability to concentrate or make decisions
- Difficulty in sleeping
- Feeling in low spirits
- Loss of interest in sex or other activities you normally enjoy

YES

NO

SEE YOUR DOCTOR WITHIN 24 HOURS

POSSIBLE CAUSES A disorder of the digestive tract may be the cause of your weight loss. Inflammation of the intestines or an ulcer are both possibilities. Cancer of the colon is also possible, especially if you are over 40.

ACTION Your doctor will probably arrange for a variety of diagnostic tests. These may include a blood test, stool tests, and a colonoscopy (p.222).

SEE YOUR DOCTOR WITHIN 24 HOURS

POSSIBLE CAUSES A chronic infection, such as tuberculosis, an AIDS-related illness (*see* HIV INFECTION AND AIDS, left), or certain types of cancer are possibilities.

ACTION Your doctor will take samples of blood and probably of sputum for analysis and will order a chest X ray (p.38) and other tests. Once the test results are known, you may be referred to a specialist for treatment.

POSSIBLE CAUSE Depression can sometimes cause a marked loss of appetite, which may be sufficient to result in weight loss.

Go to chart **72** DEPRESSION (p.170)

CONSULT YOUR DOCTOR IF YOU ARE UNABLE TO MAKE A DIAGNOSIS FROM THIS CHART.

SELF-HELP How to gain weight safely

Being underweight can be just as much of a health risk as being overweight. If you are underweight (*see* ASSESSING YOUR WEIGHT, p.29), it is important to gain weight sensibly so as to build up muscle and bone rather than excessive body fat. Ideally, you should aim to put on weight gradually by eating a healthy, balanced diet (p.28). Several small, nutritious meals each day provide a better supply of energy than one or two large meals. Try to have high-calorie, nutritious snacks, such as sandwiches and bananas, between meals. Food supplements and milk-based drinks will also help, but these should be added to your normal diet rather than taken instead of meals. Make sure that you continue to exercise regularly because this will help you build up your muscles and increase your strength and may also improve your appetite. If you tire easily, you should exercise in small, frequent sessions so that you avoid overexerting yourself.

Diabetes mellitus

Diabetes mellitus is a condition in which body cells are not able to utilize enough of the sugar glucose (the body's main energy source) from the blood. This inability is due to a deficiency of, or resistance to, the hormone insulin, normally produced by the pancreas. If there is insufficient insulin, or resistance to insulin, glucose accumulates in the blood and urine. Cells have to use fats as an energy source instead of glucose, which leads to a buildup of toxic by-products. These chemical changes cause the symptoms of diabetes: thirst, excessive passing of urine, and weight loss. Diabetes mellitus affects about 16 million people in the US; once it develops, diabetes is a lifelong condition.

There are two main forms of the disorder: type 1 and type 2. In type 1 diabetes, the pancreas produces too little insulin or none at all; this form usually develops suddenly in childhood or adolescence and causes dramatic weight loss. In type 2 diabetes, the pancreas continues to produce insulin, but body cells are

less responsive to it. This type of diabetes is 10 times more common than type 1. It mainly develops after the age of 40, particularly in those who are overweight. It develops gradually and symptoms may go unrecognized for years.

Complications of diabetes

Uncontrolled diabetes over a prolonged period damages blood vessels throughout the body, which results in problems with the eyes, kidneys, heart, and nervous system. Treatment is aimed at keeping blood sugar levels as normal as possible to delay the onset of complications.

Treating diabetes

Anyone with diabetes will need a special diet. Keeping fit is also an important aspect of treatment. In addition to these measures, people with type 1 diabetes usually need lifelong treatment with insulin injections to replace the missing hormone. The injections are self-administered several times a day, and the doses have to be carefully matched to food intake. Regular monitoring of blood sugar levels is

necessary to ensure that the treatment is effective. People with type 2 diabetes may be able to control their diabetes simply by staying in shape and following the right diet, but most need to take oral drugs and a few need insulin injections.

People with diabetes should visit their doctor every few months so that he or she can assess the control of blood sugar levels and detect and treat any complications of the disease at an early stage.

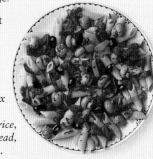

A healthy diet
If you have diabetes, you may need to make sure that your diet is high in complex carbohydrates, such as pasta, rice, cereals, and bread, and low in fats.

59 Overweight

Normally, fat accounts for between 10 and 20 percent of the weight of a man and about 25 percent of a woman; much more than this is unhealthy, increasing the risk of diseases such as diabetes and high blood pressure and of damage to weight-bearing joints, such as the hips or knees. Most people gradually gain a little weight as they grow older, reaching their heaviest at about age 50. Consult this chart if you weigh more than the healthy weight for your height (*see* ASSESSING YOUR WEIGHT, p.29) or if you have excess abdominal fat – a waist measurement of over 35 in (89 cm) for women and over 40 in (102 cm) for men. Excess fat around the abdomen is thought to be a greater risk for heart disease than fat elsewhere. Weight gain is usually due to overeating. Occasionally, there may be a medical reason.

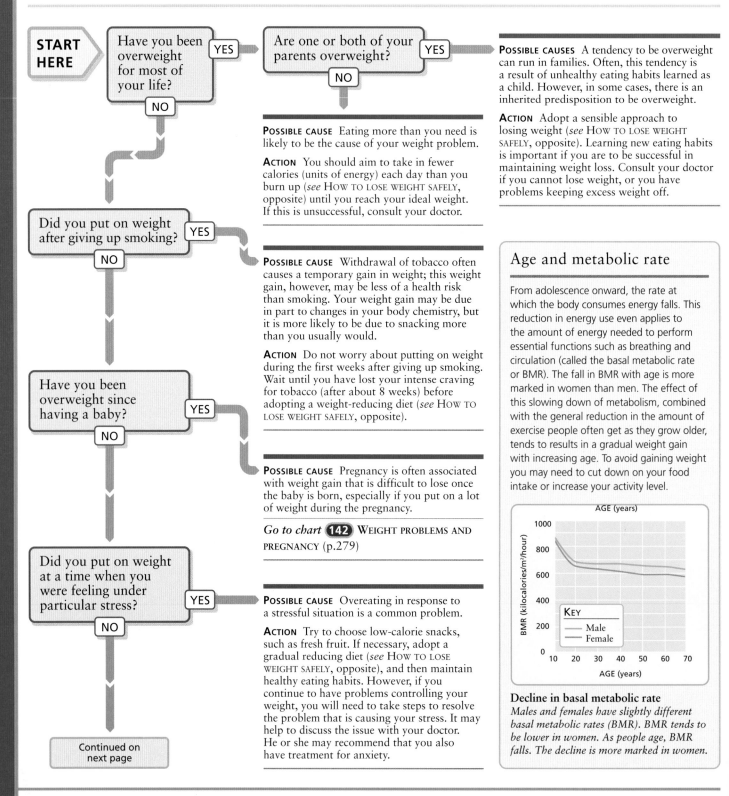

START HERE

Have you been overweight for most of your life? → **YES**
↓ **NO**

Are one or both of your parents overweight? → **YES**
↓ **NO**

POSSIBLE CAUSES A tendency to be overweight can run in families. Often, this tendency is a result of unhealthy eating habits learned as a child. However, in some cases, there is an inherited predisposition to be overweight.

ACTION Adopt a sensible approach to losing weight (*see* HOW TO LOSE WEIGHT SAFELY, opposite). Learning new eating habits is important if you are to be successful in maintaining weight loss. Consult your doctor if you cannot lose weight, or you have problems keeping excess weight off.

POSSIBLE CAUSE Eating more than you need is likely to be the cause of your weight problem.

ACTION You should aim to take in fewer calories (units of energy) each day than you burn up (*see* HOW TO LOSE WEIGHT SAFELY, opposite) until you reach your ideal weight. If this is unsuccessful, consult your doctor.

Did you put on weight after giving up smoking? → **YES**
↓ **NO**

POSSIBLE CAUSE Withdrawal of tobacco often causes a temporary gain in weight; this weight gain, however, may be less of a health risk than smoking. Your weight gain may be due in part to changes in your body chemistry, but it is more likely to be due to snacking more than you usually would.

ACTION Do not worry about putting on weight during the first weeks after giving up smoking. Wait until you have lost your intense craving for tobacco (after about 8 weeks) before adopting a weight-reducing diet (*see* HOW TO LOSE WEIGHT SAFELY, opposite).

Have you been overweight since having a baby? → **YES**
↓ **NO**

POSSIBLE CAUSE Pregnancy is often associated with weight gain that is difficult to lose once the baby is born, especially if you put on a lot of weight during the pregnancy.

Go to chart **142** WEIGHT PROBLEMS AND PREGNANCY (p.279)

Did you put on weight at a time when you were feeling under particular stress? → **YES**
↓ **NO**

POSSIBLE CAUSE Overeating in response to a stressful situation is a common problem.

ACTION Try to choose low-calorie snacks, such as fresh fruit. If necessary, adopt a gradual reducing diet (*see* HOW TO LOSE WEIGHT SAFELY, opposite), and then maintain healthy eating habits. However, if you continue to have problems controlling your weight, you will need to take steps to resolve the problem that is causing your stress. It may help to discuss the issue with your doctor. He or she may recommend that you also have treatment for anxiety.

Continued on next page

Age and metabolic rate

From adolescence onward, the rate at which the body consumes energy falls. This reduction in energy use even applies to the amount of energy needed to perform essential functions such as breathing and circulation (called the basal metabolic rate or BMR). The fall in BMR with age is more marked in women than men. The effect of this slowing down of metabolism, combined with the general reduction in the amount of exercise people often get as they grow older, tends to results in a gradual weight gain with increasing age. To avoid gaining weight you may need to cut down on your food intake or increase your activity level.

AGE (years)

BMR (kilocalories/m²/hour)

KEY
Male
Female

AGE (years)

Decline in basal metabolic rate
Males and females have slightly different basal metabolic rates (BMR). BMR tends to be lower in women. As people age, BMR falls. The decline is more marked in women.

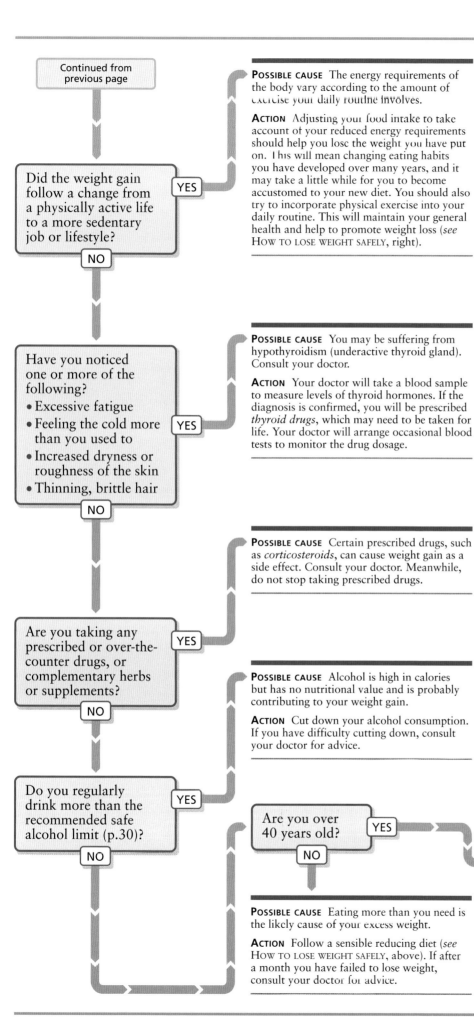

Continued from previous page

Did the weight gain follow a change from a physically active life to a more sedentary job or lifestyle? — YES / NO

POSSIBLE CAUSE The energy requirements of the body vary according to the amount of exercise your daily routine involves.

ACTION Adjusting your food intake to take account of your reduced energy requirements should help you lose the weight you have put on. This will mean changing eating habits you have developed over many years, and it may take a little while for you to become accustomed to your new diet. You should also try to incorporate physical exercise into your daily routine. This will maintain your general health and help to promote weight loss (*see* HOW TO LOSE WEIGHT SAFELY, right).

Have you noticed one or more of the following?
- Excessive fatigue
- Feeling the cold more than you used to
- Increased dryness or roughness of the skin
- Thinning, brittle hair

— YES / NO

POSSIBLE CAUSE You may be suffering from hypothyroidism (underactive thyroid gland). Consult your doctor.

ACTION Your doctor will take a blood sample to measure levels of thyroid hormones. If the diagnosis is confirmed, you will be prescribed *thyroid drugs*, which may need to be taken for life. Your doctor will arrange occasional blood tests to monitor the drug dosage.

Are you taking any prescribed or over-the-counter drugs, or complementary herbs or supplements? — YES / NO

POSSIBLE CAUSE Certain prescribed drugs, such as *corticosteroids*, can cause weight gain as a side effect. Consult your doctor. Meanwhile, do not stop taking prescribed drugs.

Do you regularly drink more than the recommended safe alcohol limit (p.30)? — YES / NO

POSSIBLE CAUSE Alcohol is high in calories but has no nutritional value and is probably contributing to your weight gain.

ACTION Cut down your alcohol consumption. If you have difficulty cutting down, consult your doctor for advice.

Are you over 40 years old? — YES / NO

POSSIBLE CAUSE Eating more than you need is the likely cause of your excess weight.

ACTION Follow a sensible reducing diet (*see* HOW TO LOSE WEIGHT SAFELY, above). If after a month you have failed to lose weight, consult your doctor for advice.

SELF-HELP How to lose weight safely

The most likely cause of being overweight is a combination of overeating and lack of exercise. The best way to lose weight is to combine a reduced calorie intake with regular exercise. Set yourself a realistic, short-term target for weight loss; about ½ to 1 lb per week is sensible. Rapid weight-loss plans and fasting should be avoided.

Calorie reduction
The best type of weight-reducing diet is one that is low in calories but balanced so that you stay well nourished. You should try to reduce your daily calorie intake by 500–1,000 calories. The following suggestions may help:
- Cut down on fatty foods; good alternatives include wholegrain bread, potatoes, and pasta.
- Oven bake or grill rather than fry food.
- Avoid excessive snacking.
- Cut down your alcohol consumption.
- Avoid shopping for food when you are feeling hungry.

Exercise
Regular exercise benefits your general health as well as helping you reduce your weight. Exercise does not have to be strenuous, but you should aim to do 30 minutes, five times a week. Not only are calories burned up during exercise but it also raises basal metabolic rate (BMR), the rate at which your body consumes energy when at rest to maintain basic processes such as breathing and digestion. If your BMR rises, you use up more calories, and, if you have a calorie-controlled diet, you will lose weight.

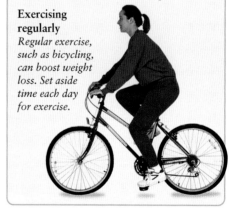

Exercising regularly
Regular exercise, such as bicycling, can boost weight loss. Set aside time each day for exercise.

POSSIBLE CAUSE Growing older is often accompanied by a gain in weight. Your weight gain is probably due to the fact you are doing less exercise at a time when your body needs less food to perform basic functions (*see* AGE AND METABOLIC RATE, opposite).

ACTION Reduce your food intake and/or increase your level of activity to restore the balance of energy intake and expenditure (*see* HOW TO LOSE WEIGHT SAFELY, above).

60 Difficulty sleeping

It is common to have the occasional night when you find it difficult to get to sleep or to stay asleep, and this need not cause concern. Consult this chart if you often find it hard to get to sleep or if you frequently wake during the night. Lifestyle changes can sometimes help with sleeping problems (*see* GETTING A GOOD NIGHT'S SLEEP, opposite).

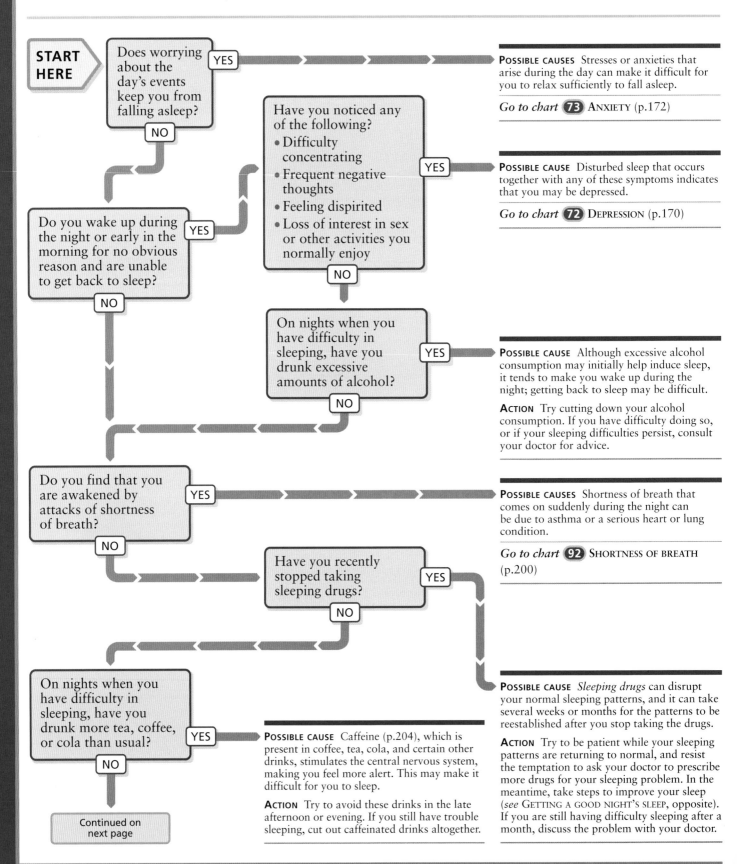

START HERE

Does worrying about the day's events keep you from falling asleep?
- YES →
- NO

POSSIBLE CAUSES Stresses or anxieties that arise during the day can make it difficult for you to relax sufficiently to fall asleep.

Go to chart 73 ANXIETY (p.172)

Have you noticed any of the following?
- Difficulty concentrating
- Frequent negative thoughts
- Feeling dispirited
- Loss of interest in sex or other activities you normally enjoy

- YES →
- NO

POSSIBLE CAUSE Disturbed sleep that occurs together with any of these symptoms indicates that you may be depressed.

Go to chart 72 DEPRESSION (p.170)

Do you wake up during the night or early in the morning for no obvious reason and are unable to get back to sleep?
- YES
- NO

On nights when you have difficulty in sleeping, have you drunk excessive amounts of alcohol?
- YES →
- NO

POSSIBLE CAUSE Although excessive alcohol consumption may initially help induce sleep, it tends to make you wake up during the night; getting back to sleep may be difficult.

ACTION Try cutting down your alcohol consumption. If you have difficulty doing so, or if your sleeping difficulties persist, consult your doctor for advice.

Do you find that you are awakened by attacks of shortness of breath?
- YES →
- NO

POSSIBLE CAUSES Shortness of breath that comes on suddenly during the night can be due to asthma or a serious heart or lung condition.

Go to chart 92 SHORTNESS OF BREATH (p.200)

Have you recently stopped taking sleeping drugs?
- YES →
- NO

POSSIBLE CAUSE *Sleeping drugs* can disrupt your normal sleeping patterns, and it can take several weeks or months for the patterns to be reestablished after you stop taking the drugs.

ACTION Try to be patient while your sleeping patterns are returning to normal, and resist the temptation to ask your doctor to prescribe more drugs for your sleeping problem. In the meantime, take steps to improve your sleep (*see* GETTING A GOOD NIGHT'S SLEEP, opposite). If you are still having difficulty sleeping after a month, discuss the problem with your doctor.

On nights when you have difficulty in sleeping, have you drunk more tea, coffee, or cola than usual?
- YES →
- NO

POSSIBLE CAUSE Caffeine (p.204), which is present in coffee, tea, cola, and certain other drinks, stimulates the central nervous system, making you feel more alert. This may make it difficult for you to sleep.

ACTION Try to avoid these drinks in the late afternoon or evening. If you still have trouble sleeping, cut out caffeinated drinks altogether.

Continued on next page

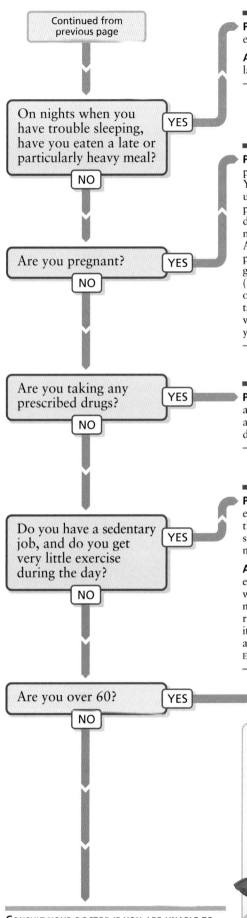

Continued from previous page

On nights when you have trouble sleeping, have you eaten a late or particularly heavy meal? YES

POSSIBLE CAUSE Eating to excess or late in the evening can often make it difficult to sleep.

ACTION Try eating lighter meals or eat your last meal of the day earlier in the evening.

NO

Are you pregnant? YES

POSSIBLE CAUSE AND ACTION Your sleep problems may be related to your pregnancy. You may need to get up during the night to urinate even early in pregnancy. Later in pregnancy, your baby's movements may disturb your sleep and your enlarged abdomen may make it difficult to get comfortable. Anxiety about the birth may also cause sleep problems. Follow the self-help measures for getting a good night's sleep during pregnancy (below). If you still cannot sleep, get up, read, or do odd jobs. Try to catch up on sleep by taking naps during the day. Discuss any worries that you have about the birth with your doctor.

NO

Are you taking any prescribed drugs? YES

POSSIBLE CAUSE AND ACTION Some drugs, such as *beta blockers*, may cause sleep disturbance as a side effect. Consult your doctor. Meanwhile, do not stop taking your prescribed drugs.

NO

Do you have a sedentary job, and do you get very little exercise during the day? YES

POSSIBLE CAUSE A lack of physical exercise during the daytime may mean that you are not sufficiently tired to fall sleep easily, even if you have had a mentally tiring day.

ACTION Try to get some form of regular exercise during the day or evening. This will make you more physically tired and may also help you relax. Not only will regular exercise help you sleep better but it will also improve your general health and feeling of well-being (*see* HOW EXERCISE BENEFITS HEALTH, p.29).

NO

Are you over 60? YES

POSSIBLE CAUSE AND ACTION Most people need less sleep as they grow older; many people over 60 need only 6 hours sleep a night. For this reason, you may find that you wake up earlier in the morning than you used to, or you find it difficult to fall asleep at the same time as when you were younger. Take advantage of your extra time, and try to avoid napping during the day.

NO

CONSULT YOUR DOCTOR IF YOU ARE UNABLE TO MAKE A DIAGNOSIS FROM THIS CHART.

SELF-HELP Getting a good night's sleep

Sleep is an important factor in maintaining good health. If you are having difficulty sleeping, these suggestions may help:

- Exercise during the day to tire yourself physically and help you relax.
- Cut out coffee, tea, cola, and other drinks containing caffeine, particularly during the afternoon and evening.
- Avoid high alcohol consumption: although alcohol may make you sleepy at first, you are more likely to wake up during the night and be unable to get back to sleep.
- Try to establish regular times for going to sleep and waking up; avoid daytime naps.
- Avoid heavy meals in the evening.
- Have a warm drink such as warm milk or camomile tea at bedtime.
- If you need to work in the evening, stop at least 1 hour before bedtime.
- Make sure that your bed is comfortable and your bedroom is well ventilated.

Exercise daily
Regular exercise, such as walking, will make you feel more tired and help you sleep.

SELF-HELP Getting a good night's sleep during pregnancy

Getting a full night's undisturbed sleep may be difficult during pregnancy, especially in later pregnancy when the enlarging abdomen makes it more difficult to find a comfortable position. However, there are several measures you can take to help make sleeping easier. Before going to bed, try to relax. Have a warm bath, listen to the radio, or read until you feel sleepy. Avoid drinks containing caffeine, such as coffee and tea, especially in the evening.

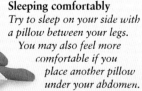

Pillow between legs

Sleeping comfortably
Try to sleep on your side with a pillow between your legs. You may also feel more comfortable if you place another pillow under your abdomen.

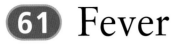

61 Fever

A fever is a body temperature higher than 100.4°F (38°C). It can be a symptom of many diseases, but it usually indicates that your body is fighting an infection. Heat exposure and certain drugs can also raise your body temperature. You may suspect that you have a fever if you feel shivery, alternately hot and cold, and generally sick. To check if you do have a fever, use a thermometer to measure your temperature accurately (*see* MANAGING A FEVER, below).

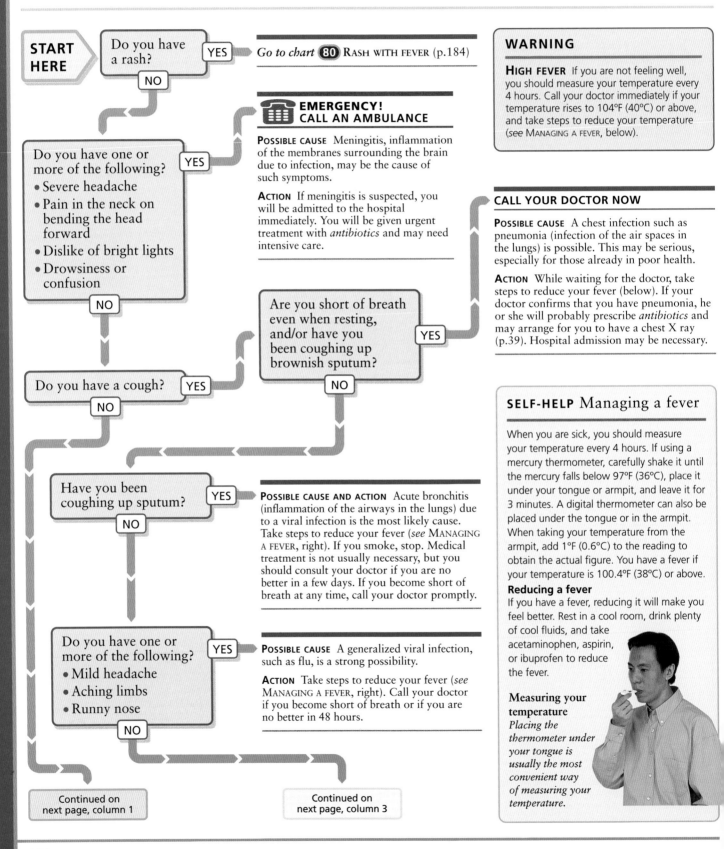

START HERE

Do you have a rash? → **YES** → *Go to chart* **80** RASH WITH FEVER (p.184)

↓ NO

Do you have one or more of the following?
- Severe headache
- Pain in the neck on bending the head forward
- Dislike of bright lights
- Drowsiness or confusion

→ **YES** →

☎ **EMERGENCY! CALL AN AMBULANCE**

POSSIBLE CAUSE Meningitis, inflammation of the membranes surrounding the brain due to infection, may be the cause of such symptoms.

ACTION If meningitis is suspected, you will be admitted to the hospital immediately. You will be given urgent treatment with *antibiotics* and may need intensive care.

↓ NO

Do you have a cough? → **YES** →

Are you short of breath even when resting, and/or have you been coughing up brownish sputum? → **YES** →

CALL YOUR DOCTOR NOW

POSSIBLE CAUSE A chest infection such as pneumonia (infection of the air spaces in the lungs) is possible. This may be serious, especially for those already in poor health.

ACTION While waiting for the doctor, take steps to reduce your fever (below). If your doctor confirms that you have pneumonia, he or she will probably prescribe *antibiotics* and may arrange for you to have a chest X ray (p.39). Hospital admission may be necessary.

↓ NO (cough)   ↓ NO (short of breath)

Have you been coughing up sputum? → **YES** →

POSSIBLE CAUSE AND ACTION Acute bronchitis (inflammation of the airways in the lungs) due to a viral infection is the most likely cause. Take steps to reduce your fever (*see* MANAGING A FEVER, right). If you smoke, stop. Medical treatment is not usually necessary, but you should consult your doctor if you are no better in a few days. If you become short of breath at any time, call your doctor promptly.

↓ NO

Do you have one or more of the following?
- Mild headache
- Aching limbs
- Runny nose

→ **YES** →

POSSIBLE CAUSE A generalized viral infection, such as flu, is a strong possibility.

ACTION Take steps to reduce your fever (*see* MANAGING A FEVER, right). Call your doctor if you become short of breath or if you are no better in 48 hours.

↓ NO

WARNING

HIGH FEVER If you are not feeling well, you should measure your temperature every 4 hours. Call your doctor immediately if your temperature rises to 104°F (40°C) or above, and take steps to reduce your temperature (*see* MANAGING A FEVER, below).

SELF-HELP Managing a fever

When you are sick, you should measure your temperature every 4 hours. If using a mercury thermometer, carefully shake it until the mercury falls below 97°F (36°C), place it under your tongue or armpit, and leave it for 3 minutes. A digital thermometer can also be placed under the tongue or in the armpit. When taking your temperature from the armpit, add 1°F (0.6°C) to the reading to obtain the actual figure. You have a fever if your temperature is 100.4°F (38°C) or above.

Reducing a fever
If you have a fever, reducing it will make you feel better. Rest in a cool room, drink plenty of cool fluids, and take acetaminophen, aspirin, or ibuprofen to reduce the fever.

Measuring your temperature
Placing the thermometer under your tongue is usually the most convenient way of measuring your temperature.

Continued on next page, column 1

Continued on next page, column 3

Continued from previous page, column 1

Go to chart **88** SORE THROAT (p.195)

Continued from previous page, column 2

Do you have a sore throat? — **YES**

NO

Do you have one or more of the following?
- Pain in the flank on one or both sides
- Abnormally frequent urination
- Pain when urinating
- Discolored or cloudy urine

YES

NO

Have you recently returned from a trip abroad? — **YES**

NO

Are you female, and do you have an abnormal vaginal discharge with or without lower abdominal pain? — **YES**

NO

Have you spent several hours either in strong sunlight or in very hot conditions? — **YES**

NO

Over the last few weeks, have you had a recurrent fever, possibly with unintentional weight loss? — **YES**

NO

Are you coughing up more than 3 teaspoons of blood in a day? — **YES**

NO

SEE YOUR DOCTOR WITHIN 24 HOURS

POSSIBLE CAUSES Inflammation of the kidney (pyelonephritis) or inflammation of the bladder (cystitis) as a result of an infection may be the cause of your symptoms.

ACTION Your doctor will examine you and test your urine for signs of infection. You will probably be prescribed *antibiotics*. Women who have repeated infections or men who have had one previous infection may need further tests, such as ultrasound scanning (p.41), to exclude an underlying cause.

SEE YOUR DOCTOR WITHIN 24 HOURS

POSSIBLE CAUSE A tropical disease that is rare in the US, such as malaria or typhoid, is a possibility.

ACTION Tell your doctor about your trip and about any medications that you have taken, such as antimalarial drugs. If your doctor suspects a tropical disease after examining you, he or she may send you for tests, including blood tests and tests on feces. Any treatment will depend on the test results.

POSSIBLE CAUSE AND ACTION Exposure to heat may have caused your temperature to rise. To bring it down, rest in a cool room and drink plenty of cold drinks. If your temperature has not started to fall within an hour, call your doctor.

SEE A DOCTOR WITHIN 24 HOURS IF YOU ARE STILL FEVERISH AFTER 2 DAYS AND CANNOT MAKE A DIAGNOSIS FROM THIS CHART.

SEE YOUR DOCTOR WITHIN 24 HOURS

POSSIBLE CAUSE You may have a serious lung disorder, such as tuberculosis or lung cancer.

ACTION Your doctor will probably arrange for initial blood and sputum tests and a chest X ray (p.39). You may then be referred to a specialist for tests, such as bronchoscopy (p.199), which will help determine what treatment is necessary.

SEE YOUR DOCTOR WITHIN 24 HOURS

POSSIBLE CAUSE Pelvic inflammatory disease, inflammation of the reproductive organs, often due to a sexually transmitted infection, may be the cause.

ACTION Your doctor will examine you and may arrange for tests to confirm the diagnosis. You will probably be given *analgesics* and prescribed *antibiotics*.

SEE YOUR DOCTOR WITHIN 24 HOURS

POSSIBLE CAUSE A serious disorder such as tuberculosis, cancer of the lymph nodes, or an AIDS-related illness (*see* HIV INFECTION AND AIDS, p.148) is possible.

ACTION Your doctor will examine you and will probably arrange blood and/or sputum tests. He or she may also order a chest X ray (p.39) and other tests. You may need to be referred to a specialist for further investigations and for treatment.

SEE A DOCTOR WITHIN 24 HOURS IF YOU ARE STILL FEVERISH AFTER 2 DAYS AND ARE UNABLE TO MAKE A DIAGNOSIS FROM THIS CHART.

62 Excessive sweating

Sweating is one of the natural mechanisms for regulating body temperature and is the normal response to hot conditions or strenuous exercise. Some people naturally sweat more than others, and if you have always sweated profusely, there is unlikely to be anything wrong. However, sweating that is not brought on by heat or exercise or that is more profuse than you are used to may be a sign of one of a number of medical conditions.

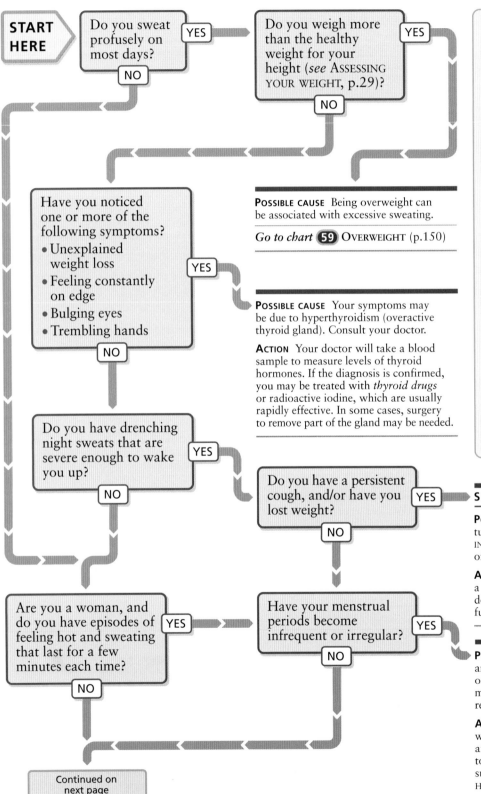

START HERE

Do you sweat profusely on most days? YES → **Do you weigh more than the healthy weight for your height (see ASSESSING YOUR WEIGHT, p.29)?** YES →

NO

NO

POSSIBLE CAUSE Being overweight can be associated with excessive sweating.

Go to chart 59 OVERWEIGHT (p.150)

Have you noticed one or more of the following symptoms?
• Unexplained weight loss
• Feeling constantly on edge
• Bulging eyes
• Trembling hands

YES →

NO

POSSIBLE CAUSE Your symptoms may be due to hyperthyroidism (overactive thyroid gland). Consult your doctor.

ACTION Your doctor will take a blood sample to measure levels of thyroid hormones. If the diagnosis is confirmed, you may be treated with *thyroid drugs* or radioactive iodine, which are usually rapidly effective. In some cases, surgery to remove part of the gland may be needed.

Do you have drenching night sweats that are severe enough to wake you up? YES →

NO

Do you have a persistent cough, and/or have you lost weight? YES →

NO

Are you a woman, and do you have episodes of feeling hot and sweating that last for a few minutes each time? YES →

NO

Have your menstrual periods become infrequent or irregular? YES →

NO

Continued on next page

Controlling excessive sweating

Excessive sweating can be very embarrassing, especially if it results in a noticeable body odor or causes the hands to be particularly wet and slippery. Washing regularly and wearing comfortable, loose clothing made from natural fibers that absorb sweat should help prevent body odor. An underarm deodorant containing an antiperspirant should help reduce the amount of sweat produced from the armpits. Such deodorants may be bought in the form of a spray, a roll-on applicator, or a cream. All of these forms of deodorant are equally effective.

If these measures do not help combat excessive sweating, consult your pharmacist or doctor. Stronger treatments are available over the counter. Alternatively, your doctor may prescribe a cream or gel containing aluminum chloride that is applied to the skin to reduce the activity of the sweat glands. If you still sweat heavily, particularly on your hands, your doctor may suggest that you have an operation to destroy nerves near the back of the neck that supply the sweat glands under the arms and on the palms of the hands. This operation dramatically reduces sweating in these areas.

SEE YOUR DOCTOR WITHIN 24 HOURS

POSSIBLE CAUSES A chronic infection such as tuberculosis, an AIDS-related illness (*see* HIV INFECTION AND AIDS, p.148), or certain types of cancer are possibilities.

ACTION After initial investigations, such as a chest X ray (p.39) and blood tests, your doctor may refer you to a specialist for any further tests or appropriate treatment.

POSSIBLE CAUSE Sudden episodes of feeling hot and sweating, known as hot flashes, are one of the most common symptoms of the onset of menopause or any abnormality of the ovaries resulting in decreased levels of estrogen (p.21).

ACTION Many women are prepared to put up with hot flashes, knowing that they will stop after a year or so. However, you may wish to consult your doctor to discuss treatments such as hormone replacement therapy (*see* A HEALTHY MENOPAUSE, p.261).

Continued from previous page

POSSIBLE CAUSE Sweating is the body's response to fever and is part of the normal temperature control mechanism.

Go to chart **61** FEVER (p.154)

Do you have a temperature of 100.4°F (38°C) or above?
YES →

NO ↓

POSSIBLE CAUSE AND ACTION In some women, changes in the levels of sex hormones can cause increased sweating during menstruation. This is no cause for concern, but consult your doctor if you are worried.

Are you female, and does the excessive sweating occur only during your menstrual periods?
YES →

NO ↓

Do you regularly drink more than the recommended safe alcohol limit (p.30)?
YES →

NO ↓

POSSIBLE CAUSE Excessive alcohol consumption can be a cause of increased sweating.

ACTION Cut down your alcohol intake so that you stay within the recommended safe limit. If you are having difficulty reducing your alcohol consumption, consult your doctor for advice.

Are you taking any prescribed or over-the-counter drugs?
YES →

NO ↓

POSSIBLE CAUSE AND ACTION Certain drugs, such as some *antidepressants* and aspirin, can cause excessive sweating as a side effect. Stop taking over-the-counter drugs, and consult your doctor. Meanwhile, do not stop taking your prescribed drugs.

Is the excessive sweating confined to your hands or feet?
YES →

NO ↓

POSSIBLE CAUSE The hands and feet have a high concentration of sweat glands (left). For this reason, these parts of the body react most noticeably to a rise in temperature. However, this is not a cause for concern.

ACTION If the sweating becomes worse when you are worried or feeling anxious, learn relaxation exercises (p.32) to use in stressful situations. Wash your hands and feet regularly. If these measures do not help, consult your doctor. For severe cases of sweating of the hands, surgery to destroy the nerves that control sweating in the palms may be considered.

Do you notice the sweating only when you are anxious or excited?
YES →

NO ↓

POSSIBLE CAUSE AND ACTION Emotional stress can easily cause an increase in sweating. This in itself is not a cause for concern, but if it happens regularly or causes embarrassment, try doing some relaxation exercises (p.32). Consult your doctor if these exercises do not help.

Are you in your teens?
YES →

NO ↓

CONSULT YOUR DOCTOR IF YOU ARE UNABLE TO MAKE A DIAGNOSIS FROM THIS CHART AND YOUR EXCESSIVE SWEATING CONTINUES TO WORRY YOU. THERE IS, HOWEVER, UNLIKELY TO BE A SERIOUS CAUSE FOR THIS SYMPTOM.

POSSIBLE CAUSE In adolescence, the apocrine sweat glands (*see* SWEAT GLANDS, left) become active. This is usually associated with an increase in sweating that is particularly noticeable under the arms. It is perfectly normal.

ACTION Make sure you wash regularly. You may also want to use an antiperspirant deodorant to reduce wetness and prevent body odor (*see* CONTROLLING EXCESSIVE SWEATING, opposite).

Sweat glands

Sweat glands are found in the layer of the skin called the dermis and release moisture (sweat) through pores in the surface of the skin. There are two types of sweat glands – eccrine glands and apocrine glands – and these produce different kinds of sweat.

Eccrine glands
These glands are found all over the body and are active from birth onward. The sweat from them is a clear, salty fluid containing various waste chemicals. This sweat evaporates on the surface of the skin to reduce body temperature as necessary. The eccrine glands may also produce sweat in response to anxiety or fear. Eccrine glands are most concentrated on the forehead, palms, and soles of the feet, and profuse sweating is likely to become apparent first in these areas.

Apocrine glands
During adolescence, apocrine glands become active. They are concentrated mainly in the armpit, in the groin, and around the nipples. These glands produce a fluid that contains fats and proteins. The scent from this type of gland is thought to play a role in attracting the opposite sex. However, if it is allowed to remain on the skin for long, it may interact with bacteria to produce body odor.

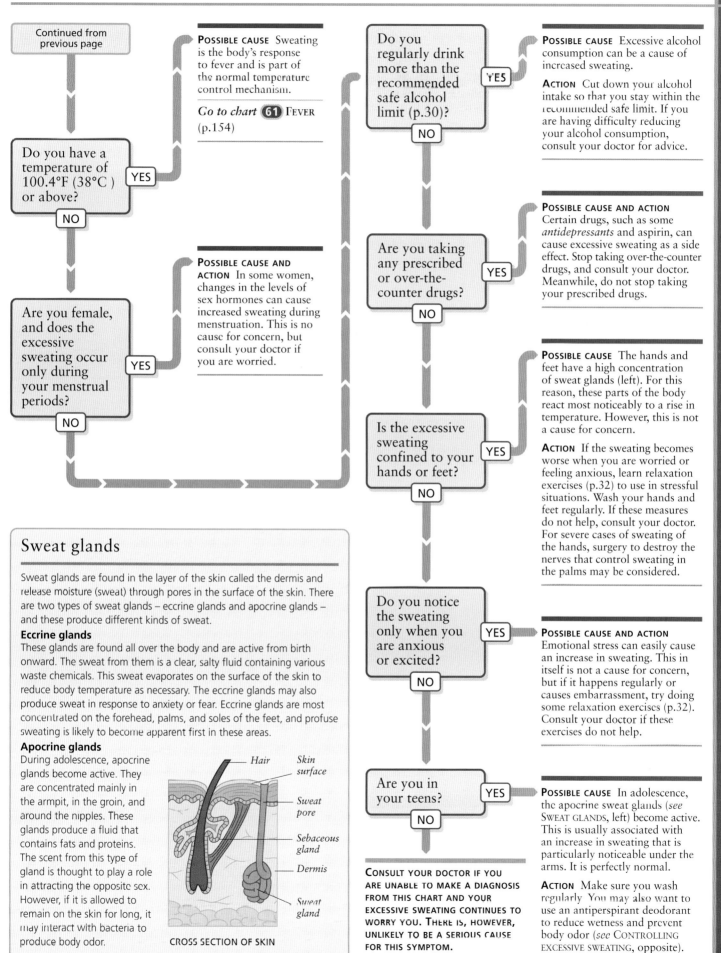

Labels: Hair — Skin surface — Sweat pore — Sebaceous gland — Dermis — Sweat gland

CROSS SECTION OF SKIN

63 Headache

From time to time nearly everyone suffers from mild-to-moderate headaches that develop gradually and clear up after a few hours, leaving no after-effects. Headaches like this are extremely unlikely to be a sign of a serious underlying disorder and are usually the result of factors such as tension, fatigue, or an excessive consumption of alcohol. However, if you have a headache that is severe, lasts for more than 24 hours, is not improved by taking over-the-counter *analgesic*, or recurs several times during one week, you should see your doctor promptly.

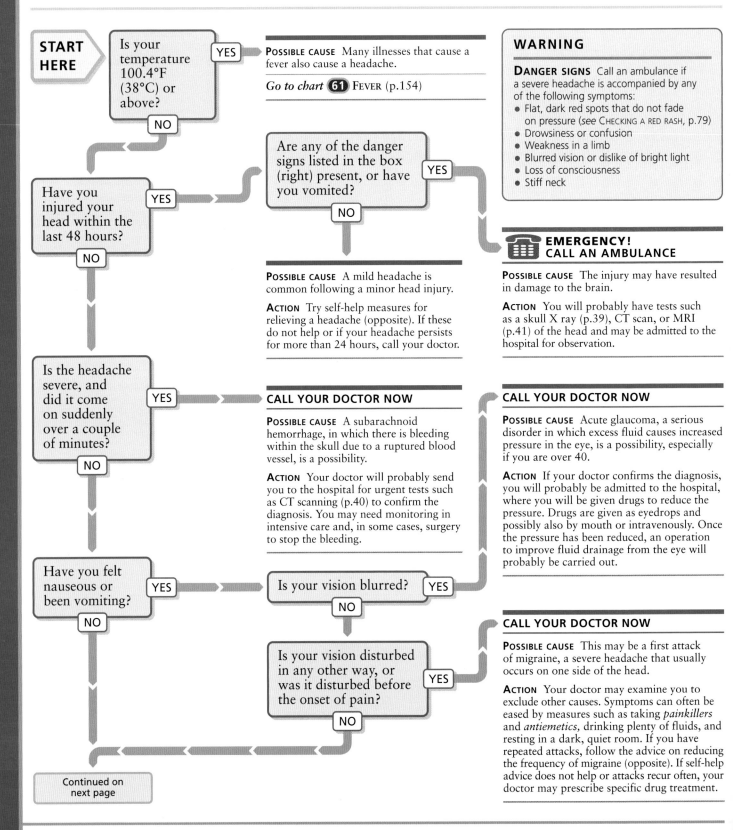

START HERE

Is your temperature 100.4°F (38°C) or above? — **YES** → **POSSIBLE CAUSE** Many illnesses that cause a fever also cause a headache.

Go to chart **61** FEVER (p.154)

NO

Have you injured your head within the last 48 hours? — **YES** → Are any of the danger signs listed in the box (right) present, or have you vomited? — **YES** →

NO

POSSIBLE CAUSE A mild headache is common following a minor head injury.

ACTION Try self-help measures for relieving a headache (opposite). If these do not help or if your headache persists for more than 24 hours, call your doctor.

WARNING

DANGER SIGNS Call an ambulance if a severe headache is accompanied by any of the following symptoms:
- Flat, dark red spots that do not fade on pressure (*see* CHECKING A RED RASH, p.79)
- Drowsiness or confusion
- Weakness in a limb
- Blurred vision or dislike of bright light
- Loss of consciousness
- Stiff neck

EMERGENCY! CALL AN AMBULANCE

POSSIBLE CAUSE The injury may have resulted in damage to the brain.

ACTION You will probably have tests such as a skull X ray (p.39), CT scan, or MRI (p.41) of the head and may be admitted to the hospital for observation.

NO

Is the headache severe, and did it come on suddenly over a couple of minutes? — **YES** →

NO

CALL YOUR DOCTOR NOW

POSSIBLE CAUSE A subarachnoid hemorrhage, in which there is bleeding within the skull due to a ruptured blood vessel, is a possibility.

ACTION Your doctor will probably send you to the hospital for urgent tests such as CT scanning (p.40) to confirm the diagnosis. You may need monitoring in intensive care and, in some cases, surgery to stop the bleeding.

CALL YOUR DOCTOR NOW

POSSIBLE CAUSE Acute glaucoma, a serious disorder in which excess fluid causes increased pressure in the eye, is a possibility, especially if you are over 40.

ACTION If your doctor confirms the diagnosis, you will probably be admitted to the hospital, where you will be given drugs to reduce the pressure. Drugs are given as eyedrops and possibly also by mouth or intravenously. Once the pressure has been reduced, an operation to improve fluid drainage from the eye will probably be carried out.

Have you felt nauseous or been vomiting? — **YES** → Is your vision blurred? — **YES** →

NO / **NO**

Is your vision disturbed in any other way, or was it disturbed before the onset of pain? — **YES** →

NO

CALL YOUR DOCTOR NOW

POSSIBLE CAUSE This may be a first attack of migraine, a severe headache that usually occurs on one side of the head.

ACTION Your doctor may examine you to exclude other causes. Symptoms can often be eased by measures such as taking *painkillers* and *antiemetics*, drinking plenty of fluids, and resting in a dark, quiet room. If you have repeated attacks, follow the advice on reducing the frequency of migraine (opposite). If self-help advice does not help or attacks recur often, your doctor may prescribe specific drug treatment.

Continued on next page

Continued from previous page

Is the pain felt mainly in the face, and is the pain worse when you bend down?

YES

NO

POSSIBLE CAUSE Sinusitis (inflammation of the membranes lining the air spaces in the skull) may be the cause of this problem, especially if you have recently had a cold or a runny or stuffy nose.

ACTION Try steam inhalation (*see* TREATING A COLD, p.194). *Pain medication* may also help. Consult your doctor if your symptoms are no better in 48 hours; you may need *antibiotics*.

Are you over 55 and is the pain felt mainly in the temples, and/or are these areas tender to touch?

YES

NO

CALL YOUR DOCTOR NOW

POSSIBLE CAUSE Temporal arteritis (inflammation of the arteries in the scalp and elsewhere in the body) is a possibility. Urgent treatment may be needed to prevent the condition from affecting the arteries supplying the eyes.

ACTION Your doctor will probably prescribe *corticosteroid drugs* to reduce the inflammation. It may be necessary for you to have regular blood tests to confirm that the dose you are taking is sufficient to control the inflammation.

Did the headache occur after you had been reading or doing close work?

YES

NO

SELF-HELP Reducing the frequency of migraine

Many factors are known to trigger a migraine. You need to identify the particular ones that affect you. Keeping a migraine diary for a few weeks may help pinpoint any triggering factors, which should then be avoided if possible. The following self-help measures may also help in reducing the frequency of your migraine attacks:

- Avoid foods such as cheese or chocolate, which are common triggering factors.
- Eat regularly, because missing a meal may trigger an attack.
- Follow a regular sleep pattern if possible, because changing it may trigger an attack.
- If stress is a trigger, try doing relaxation exercises (p.32).

POSSIBLE CAUSE Muscle strain in your neck, as a result of poor posture or tension from concentration, is the most likely cause of your headache.

ACTION Try self-help measures for relieving a headache (below). In order to prevent the problem from recurring, make sure that when you read, you are not sitting in an awkward position. Periodic rest from whatever you are doing will also help. If headaches do recur, either arrange for a vision test (p.189) with an ophthalmologist or consult your doctor.

Are you sleeping poorly, and/or are you feeling tense or under stress?

YES

NO

POSSIBLE CAUSE AND ACTION Headaches can be caused by lack of sleep. Psychological stress often causes tension headaches. Try self-help measures for relieving a headache (left).

Go to chart **73** ANXIETY (p.172)

Are you taking any prescription drugs?

YES

NO

POSSIBLE CAUSE AND ACTION Certain drugs, including oral contraceptives, can cause headaches as a side effect. Consult your doctor, who may offer you an alternative drug if your medication is a possible cause. Meanwhile, do not stop taking any prescription drugs.

SELF-HELP Relieving a headache

Most headaches are not serious and are simply due to the pressures of everyday life. To ease the pain of a headache, take a break and get some fresh air. Try massaging your neck and shoulder muscles. If these measures do not help, rest in a quiet, cool, darkened room and take the recommended dose of a standard *analgesic*.

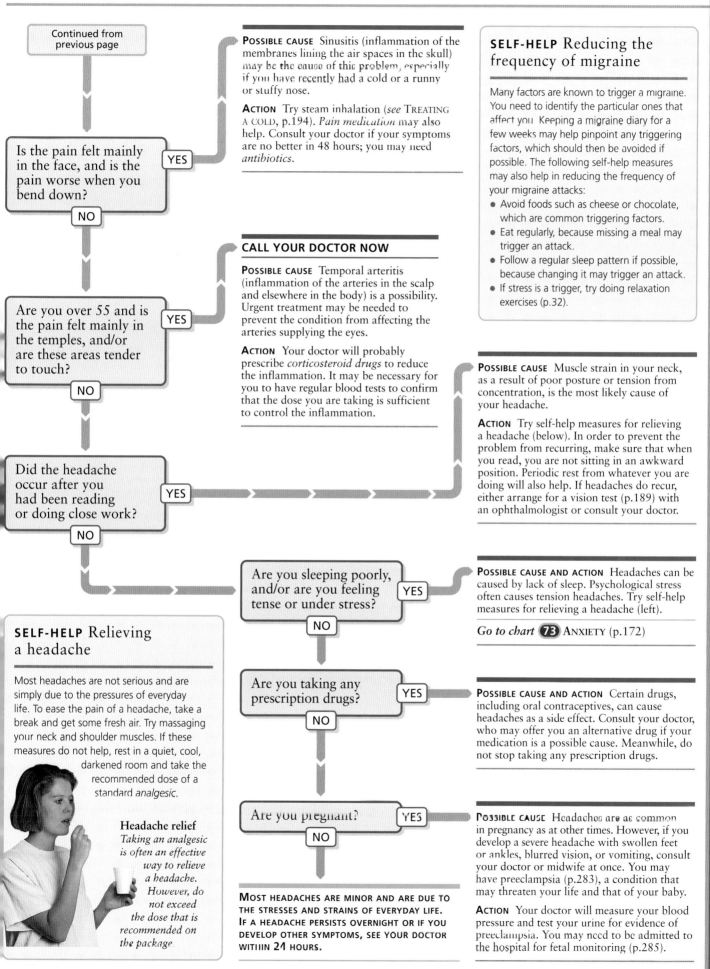

Headache relief
Taking an analgesic is often an effective way to relieve a headache. However, do not exceed the dose that is recommended on the package.

Are you pregnant?

YES

NO

MOST HEADACHES ARE MINOR AND ARE DUE TO THE STRESSES AND STRAINS OF EVERYDAY LIFE. IF A HEADACHE PERSISTS OVERNIGHT OR IF YOU DEVELOP OTHER SYMPTOMS, SEE YOUR DOCTOR WITHIN 24 HOURS.

POSSIBLE CAUSE Headaches are as common in pregnancy as at other times. However, if you develop a severe headache with swollen feet or ankles, blurred vision, or vomiting, consult your doctor or midwife at once. You may have preeclampsia (p.283), a condition that may threaten your life and that of your baby.

ACTION Your doctor will measure your blood pressure and test your urine for evidence of preeclampsia. You may need to be admitted to the hospital for fetal monitoring (p.285).

64 Feeling faint and passing out

People who feel faint usually experience a sensation of lightheadedness or dizziness and possibly nausea. Such feelings of faintness may sometimes progress to passing out – a brief loss of consciousness known as fainting. Feeling faint and passing out are usually caused by a sudden drop in blood pressure – as a result, for example, of emotional shock – or they may be due to an abnormally low level of sugar in the blood. Isolated episodes of feeling faint are hardly ever a cause for concern, but if you suffer repeated episodes, or if you pass out for no obvious reason, you should seek medical advice. Loss of consciousness may sometimes be due to a serious underlying medical condition.

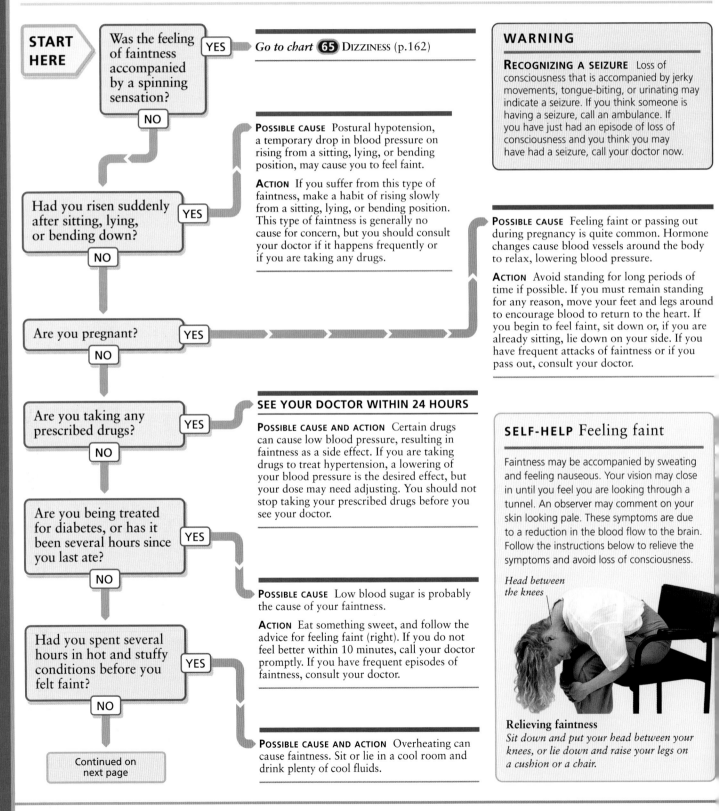

START HERE

Was the feeling of faintness accompanied by a spinning sensation?
YES → *Go to chart* **65** DIZZINESS (p.162)
NO ↓

Had you risen suddenly after sitting, lying, or bending down?
YES →
NO ↓

POSSIBLE CAUSE Postural hypotension, a temporary drop in blood pressure on rising from a sitting, lying, or bending position, may cause you to feel faint.

ACTION If you suffer from this type of faintness, make a habit of rising slowly from a sitting, lying, or bending position. This type of faintness is generally no cause for concern, but you should consult your doctor if it happens frequently or if you are taking any drugs.

Are you pregnant?
YES →
NO ↓

Are you taking any prescribed drugs?
YES →
NO ↓

Are you being treated for diabetes, or has it been several hours since you last ate?
YES →
NO ↓

Had you spent several hours in hot and stuffy conditions before you felt faint?
YES →
NO ↓

Continued on next page

POSSIBLE CAUSE Feeling faint or passing out during pregnancy is quite common. Hormone changes cause blood vessels around the body to relax, lowering blood pressure.

ACTION Avoid standing for long periods of time if possible. If you must remain standing for any reason, move your feet and legs around to encourage blood to return to the heart. If you begin to feel faint, sit down or, if you are already sitting, lie down on your side. If you have frequent attacks of faintness or if you pass out, consult your doctor.

SEE YOUR DOCTOR WITHIN 24 HOURS

POSSIBLE CAUSE AND ACTION Certain drugs can cause low blood pressure, resulting in faintness as a side effect. If you are taking drugs to treat hypertension, a lowering of your blood pressure is the desired effect, but your dose may need adjusting. You should not stop taking your prescribed drugs before you see your doctor.

POSSIBLE CAUSE Low blood sugar is probably the cause of your faintness.

ACTION Eat something sweet, and follow the advice for feeling faint (right). If you do not feel better within 10 minutes, call your doctor promptly. If you have frequent episodes of faintness, consult your doctor.

POSSIBLE CAUSE AND ACTION Overheating can cause faintness. Sit or lie in a cool room and drink plenty of cool fluids.

WARNING

RECOGNIZING A SEIZURE Loss of consciousness that is accompanied by jerky movements, tongue-biting, or urinating may indicate a seizure. If you think someone is having a seizure, call an ambulance. If you have just had an episode of loss of consciousness and you think you may have had a seizure, call your doctor now.

SELF-HELP Feeling faint

Faintness may be accompanied by sweating and feeling nauseous. Your vision may close in until you feel you are looking through a tunnel. An observer may comment on your skin looking pale. These symptoms are due to a reduction in the blood flow to the brain. Follow the instructions below to relieve the symptoms and avoid loss of consciousness.

Head between the knees

Relieving faintness
Sit down and put your head between your knees, or lie down and raise your legs on a cushion or a chair.

Continued from previous page

Do you have one or more of the following symptoms?
• Difficulty speaking
• Disturbed vision
• Numbness, tingling, or weakness in any part of the body
• Confusion

YES →

Have these symptoms now disappeared?

YES →

NO ↓

☎ EMERGENCY! CALL AN AMBULANCE

POSSIBLE CAUSES If you are over 40, the most likely cause of your symptoms is a stroke, in which there is permanent damage to part of the brain due to a disruption in its blood supply. In younger people, a disorder of the nervous system is a possibility.

ACTION Regardless of your age, your symptoms need urgent assessment in a hospital. You may need tests such as MRI (p.41) to help determine the cause and appropriate treatment.

CALL YOUR DOCTOR NOW

POSSIBLE CAUSES If you are over 40, the most likely cause of your symptoms is a transient ischemic attack (TIA), in which a blood clot temporarily blocks a blood vessel supplying the brain. In younger people, a disorder of the nervous system is a possibility.

ACTION Regardless of your age, your symptoms require urgent assessment. You may need to be hospitalized and have tests such as MRI (p.41) to help determine the cause and appropriate treatment.

NO ↓

Do you have any form of heart disease, and/or did you notice your heart rate speed up or slow down before the onset of faintness?

YES →

CALL YOUR DOCTOR NOW

POSSIBLE CAUSES There are a number of potentially serious conditions, such as an irregular heartbeat and heart valve problems, that reduce the output of blood from the heart, resulting in faintness and passing out.

ACTION Your doctor may arrange for you to be admitted urgently to a hospital, where your condition can be monitored. You will need tests such as ECG (p.203) or a chest X ray (p.39) to look for the cause of your faintness.

NO ↓

Did the faintness follow an emotional shock?

YES →

POSSIBLE CAUSE AND ACTION A sudden emotional shock can cause a fall in blood pressure, resulting in feelings of faintness. This is a normal response and does not need medical treatment.

SEE YOUR DOCTOR WITHIN 24 HOURS

POSSIBLE CAUSE Your symptoms may be due to anemia. In this condition, there is too little of the oxygen-carrying pigment hemoglobin in the blood. Anemia can be the result of a variety of underlying causes.

ACTION Your doctor will arrange for a blood test to confirm the diagnosis. In some cases, further tests will be necessary to determine why anemia has developed. Treatment for the anemia will usually need to be combined with treatment of the underlying cause.

NO ↓

Have you noticed one or more of the following symptoms?
• Excessive fatigue
• Shortness of breath
• Paler than normal skin

YES →

NO ↓

Have you vomited blood or coffeeground-like material, or have your stools become black or bloody?

YES →

☎ EMERGENCY! CALL AN AMBULANCE

POSSIBLE CAUSE Bleeding in the digestive tract, for example from a peptic ulcer, is a likely cause of these symptoms.

ACTION You will probably be admitted to the hospital. If the bleeding was severe, you may be given a blood transfusion. You may also have tests such as endoscopy (p.213) to determine the cause of the bleeding.

NO ↓

Does turning your head or looking upward bring on a feeling of faintness?

YES →

POSSIBLE CAUSE Cervical spondylosis, arthritis in the bones in the neck, may be the cause, especially if you are over 50. This can cause compression of blood vessels in the neck when you turn your head, leading to faintness. Consult your doctor.

ACTION If your doctor thinks your faintness is due to cervical spondylosis, an X ray or MRI of the neck might be ordered to confirm the diagnosis and guide treatment.

NO ↓

CONSULT YOUR DOCTOR IF YOU ARE UNABLE TO MAKE A DIAGNOSIS FROM THIS CHART.

65 Dizziness

Feeling unsteady on your feet for a moment is a common experience and need not be a matter for concern. However, true dizziness (also known as vertigo), in which there is a sensation that everything is moving or spinning around, is not normal unless you have drunk too much alcohol or have been spinning around, as on an amusement park ride. Dizziness may be a symptom of an underlying disorder and should be brought to your doctor's attention.

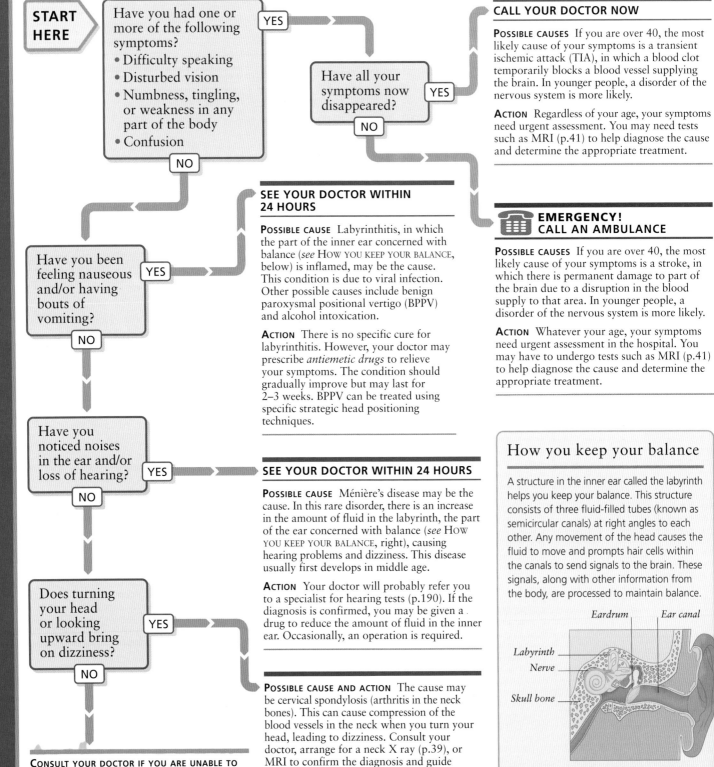

START HERE

Have you had one or more of the following symptoms?
- **Difficulty speaking**
- **Disturbed vision**
- **Numbness, tingling, or weakness in any part of the body**
- **Confusion**

YES → **Have all your symptoms now disappeared?**

NO

Have all your symptoms now disappeared? YES →

NO ↓

Have you been feeling nauseous and/or having bouts of vomiting?

YES →

NO ↓

Have you noticed noises in the ear and/or loss of hearing?

YES →

NO ↓

Does turning your head or looking upward bring on dizziness?

YES →

NO ↓

CONSULT YOUR DOCTOR IF YOU ARE UNABLE TO MAKE A DIAGNOSIS FROM THIS CHART.

CALL YOUR DOCTOR NOW

POSSIBLE CAUSES If you are over 40, the most likely cause of your symptoms is a transient ischemic attack (TIA), in which a blood clot temporarily blocks a blood vessel supplying the brain. In younger people, a disorder of the nervous system is more likely.

ACTION Regardless of your age, your symptoms need urgent assessment. You may need tests such as MRI (p.41) to help diagnose the cause and determine the appropriate treatment.

SEE YOUR DOCTOR WITHIN 24 HOURS

POSSIBLE CAUSE Labyrinthitis, in which the part of the inner ear concerned with balance (*see* HOW YOU KEEP YOUR BALANCE, below) is inflamed, may be the cause. This condition is due to viral infection. Other possible causes include benign paroxysmal positional vertigo (BPPV) and alcohol intoxication.

ACTION There is no specific cure for labyrinthitis. However, your doctor may prescribe *antiemetic drugs* to relieve your symptoms. The condition should gradually improve but may last for 2–3 weeks. BPPV can be treated using specific strategic head positioning techniques.

EMERGENCY! CALL AN AMBULANCE

POSSIBLE CAUSES If you are over 40, the most likely cause of your symptoms is a stroke, in which there is permanent damage to part of the brain due to a disruption in the blood supply to that area. In younger people, a disorder of the nervous system is more likely.

ACTION Whatever your age, your symptoms need urgent assessment in the hospital. You may have to undergo tests such as MRI (p.41) to help diagnose the cause and determine the appropriate treatment.

SEE YOUR DOCTOR WITHIN 24 HOURS

POSSIBLE CAUSE Ménière's disease may be the cause. In this rare disorder, there is an increase in the amount of fluid in the labyrinth, the part of the ear concerned with balance (*see* HOW YOU KEEP YOUR BALANCE, right), causing hearing problems and dizziness. This disease usually first develops in middle age.

ACTION Your doctor will probably refer you to a specialist for hearing tests (p.190). If the diagnosis is confirmed, you may be given a drug to reduce the amount of fluid in the inner ear. Occasionally, an operation is required.

POSSIBLE CAUSE AND ACTION The cause may be cervical spondylosis (arthritis in the neck bones). This can cause compression of the blood vessels in the neck when you turn your head, leading to dizziness. Consult your doctor, arrange for a neck X ray (p.39), or MRI to confirm the diagnosis and guide further treatment.

How you keep your balance

A structure in the inner ear called the labyrinth helps you keep your balance. This structure consists of three fluid-filled tubes (known as semicircular canals) at right angles to each other. Any movement of the head causes the fluid to move and prompts hair cells within the canals to send signals to the brain. These signals, along with other information from the body, are processed to maintain balance.

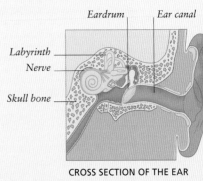

Eardrum
Ear canal
Labyrinth
Nerve
Skull bone

CROSS SECTION OF THE EAR

66 Numbness and/or tingling

It is normal to experience numbness and/or tingling if you have been sitting in an awkward position. This is commonly called "pins and needles" and can occur in any part of the body. The feeling disappears as soon as you move around. Numbness or tingling that occurs without apparent cause may be due to a disorder that needs medical treatment.

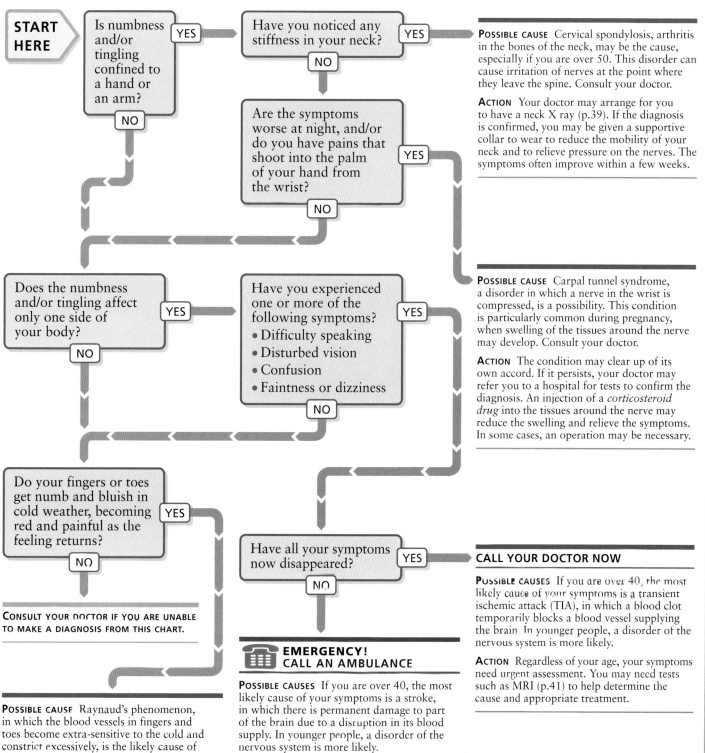

START HERE

Is numbness and/or tingling confined to a hand or an arm?
- **YES** → Have you noticed any stiffness in your neck?
  - **YES** → **POSSIBLE CAUSE** Cervical spondylosis, arthritis in the bones of the neck, may be the cause, especially if you are over 50. This disorder can cause irritation of nerves at the point where they leave the spine. Consult your doctor.

    ACTION Your doctor may arrange for you to have a neck X ray (p.39). If the diagnosis is confirmed, you may be given a supportive collar to wear to reduce the mobility of your neck and to relieve pressure on the nerves. The symptoms often improve within a few weeks.
  - **NO** → Are the symptoms worse at night, and/or do you have pains that shoot into the palm of your hand from the wrist?
    - **YES** → **POSSIBLE CAUSE** Carpal tunnel syndrome, a disorder in which a nerve in the wrist is compressed, is a possibility. This condition is particularly common during pregnancy, when swelling of the tissues around the nerve may develop. Consult your doctor.

      ACTION The condition may clear up of its own accord. If it persists, your doctor may refer you to a hospital for tests to confirm the diagnosis. An injection of a *corticosteroid drug* into the tissues around the nerve may reduce the swelling and relieve the symptoms. In some cases, an operation may be necessary.
    - **NO** ↓
- **NO** ↓

Does the numbness and/or tingling affect only one side of your body?
- **YES** → Have you experienced one or more of the following symptoms?
  - Difficulty speaking
  - Disturbed vision
  - Confusion
  - Faintness or dizziness
    - **YES** → Have all your symptoms now disappeared?
      - **YES** → **CALL YOUR DOCTOR NOW**

        POSSIBLE CAUSES If you are over 40, the most likely cause of your symptoms is a transient ischemic attack (TIA), in which a blood clot temporarily blocks a blood vessel supplying the brain. In younger people, a disorder of the nervous system is more likely.

        ACTION Regardless of your age, your symptoms need urgent assessment. You may need tests such as MRI (p.41) to help determine the cause and appropriate treatment.
      - **NO** → ☎ **EMERGENCY! CALL AN AMBULANCE**

        POSSIBLE CAUSES If you are over 40, the most likely cause of your symptoms is a stroke, in which there is permanent damage to part of the brain due to a disruption in its blood supply. In younger people, a disorder of the nervous system is more likely.

        ACTION Regardless of your age, your symptoms need urgent assessment in a hospital. You may need tests such as MRI (p.41) to help determine the cause and appropriate treatment.
    - **NO** ↓
- **NO** ↓

Do your fingers or toes get numb and bluish in cold weather, becoming red and painful as the feeling returns?
- **YES** → **POSSIBLE CAUSE** Raynaud's phenomenon, in which the blood vessels in fingers and toes become extra-sensitive to the cold and constrict excessively, is the likely cause of these symptoms. Consult your doctor.

  ACTION Keep your hands and feet warm and dry. Do not smoke. In some cases, drug treatment or, rarely, surgery may be needed.
- **NO** → **CONSULT YOUR DOCTOR IF YOU ARE UNABLE TO MAKE A DIAGNOSIS FROM THIS CHART.**

67 Forgetfulness and/or confusion

We all suffer from mild forgetfulness from time to time, especially in later life when such "absent-mindedness" is a natural part of aging. People often forget details when they have been preoccupied with other things, which is no cause for concern. However, confusion, especially if it comes on suddenly, or forgetfulness and confusion severe enough to disrupt everyday life, may be due to an underlying medical problem. This chart deals with sudden or severe confusion or forgetfulness that you are aware of in yourself or in someone else who may not realize he or she has a problem.

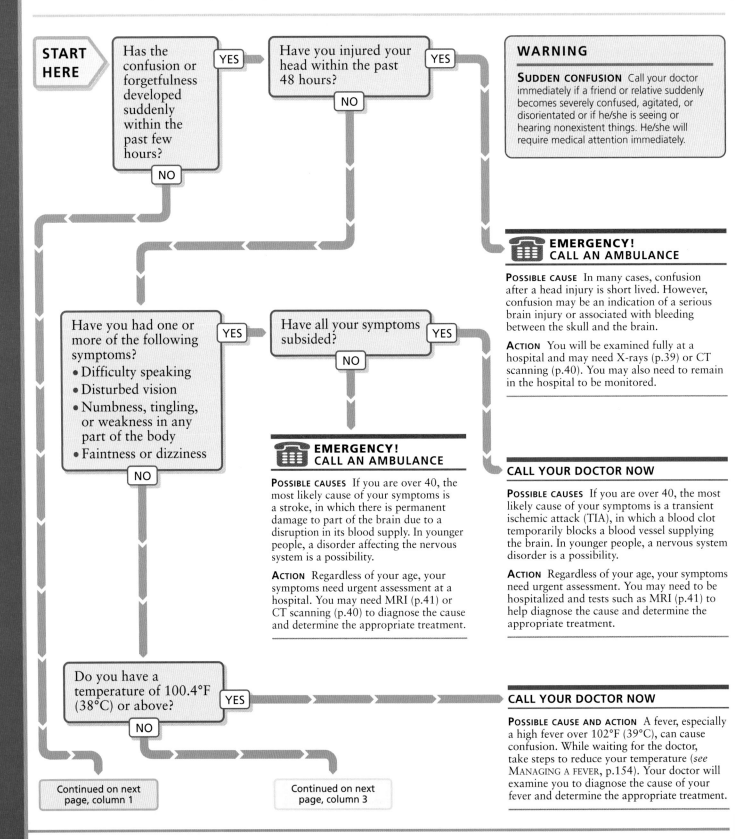

START HERE

Has the confusion or forgetfulness developed suddenly within the past few hours? — **YES** → Have you injured your head within the past 48 hours? — **YES** →

NO

NO

WARNING

SUDDEN CONFUSION Call your doctor immediately if a friend or relative suddenly becomes severely confused, agitated, or disorientated or if he/she is seeing or hearing nonexistent things. He/she will require medical attention immediately.

Have you had one or more of the following symptoms? — **YES** → Have all your symptoms subsided? — **YES** →
• Difficulty speaking
• Disturbed vision
• Numbness, tingling, or weakness in any part of the body
• Faintness or dizziness

NO

NO

☎ EMERGENCY! CALL AN AMBULANCE

POSSIBLE CAUSE In many cases, confusion after a head injury is short lived. However, confusion may be an indication of a serious brain injury or associated with bleeding between the skull and the brain.

ACTION You will be examined fully at a hospital and may need X-rays (p.39) or CT scanning (p.40). You may also need to remain in the hospital to be monitored.

☎ EMERGENCY! CALL AN AMBULANCE

POSSIBLE CAUSES If you are over 40, the most likely cause of your symptoms is a stroke, in which there is permanent damage to part of the brain due to a disruption in its blood supply. In younger people, a disorder affecting the nervous system is a possibility.

ACTION Regardless of your age, your symptoms need urgent assessment at a hospital. You may need MRI (p.41) or CT scanning (p.40) to diagnose the cause and determine the appropriate treatment.

CALL YOUR DOCTOR NOW

POSSIBLE CAUSES If you are over 40, the most likely cause of your symptoms is a transient ischemic attack (TIA), in which a blood clot temporarily blocks a blood vessel supplying the brain. In younger people, a nervous system disorder is a possibility.

ACTION Regardless of your age, your symptoms need urgent assessment. You may need to be hospitalized and tests such as MRI (p.41) to help diagnose the cause and determine the appropriate treatment.

Do you have a temperature of 100.4°F (38°C) or above? — **YES** →

NO

CALL YOUR DOCTOR NOW

POSSIBLE CAUSE AND ACTION A fever, especially a high fever over 102°F (39°C), can cause confusion. While waiting for the doctor, take steps to reduce your temperature (*see* MANAGING A FEVER, p.154). Your doctor will examine you to diagnose the cause of your fever and determine the appropriate treatment.

Continued on next page, column 1

Continued on next page, column 3

Continued from previous page, column 1

Have you noticed any of the following symptoms?
- Inability to concentrate or make decisions
- Difficulty sleeping
- Feeling in low spirits
- Loss of interest in sex or activities you normally enjoy

YES → **POSSIBLE CAUSE** Depression can cause forgetfulness and confusion, particularly in elderly people. Consult your doctor.

ACTION If your doctor confirms that you are depressed, he/she may prescribe *antidepressant drugs*. These drugs often improve mental functioning as well as treating depression, but they may take a few weeks to take effect.

NO ↓

Have you noticed that you have difficulty coping with everyday matters or in following complex instructions?

YES → **POSSIBLE CAUSE** Progressive loss of mental function (dementia) due to a disorder such as Alzheimer's disease or recurrent small strokes is a possibility. Dementia is most likely to occur in people over the age of 65, although in rare cases the condition can affect younger people. Consult your doctor.

ACTION Your doctor will examine you and he/she may refer you to a specialist. You may need blood tests or an MRI (p.41) to exclude other underlying causes. In most cases, treatments cannot reverse dementia, but drug treatments may slow deterioration. Support groups (*see* USEFUL ADDRESSES, p.311) can provide self-help information, and social services may provide practical help.

NO ↓

Are you taking any prescribed drugs?

YES →

NO ↓

Do you regularly drink more than the recommended safe alcohol limit (p.30)?

YES → **POSSIBLE CAUSE** Excessive alcohol consumption commonly causes memory loss and confusion.

ACTION If you regularly drink an amount of alcohol that leaves you confused, you should cut down your consumption. If you have difficulty doing so, consult your doctor for advice.

NO ↓

Do you use recreational drugs or inhale solvents?

YES →

NO ↓

Continued from previous page, column 2

Are you suffering from a serious heart or lung condition?

YES → ### CALL YOUR DOCTOR NOW

POSSIBLE CAUSE A sudden worsening of disorders affecting the heart or lungs may reduce the supply of oxygen to the brain, leading to confusion.

ACTION You may need to be admitted to a hospital where you will be given oxygen and drugs to stabilize your condition.

NO ↓

Are you being treated for diabetes?

YES → **POSSIBLE CAUSES** Your blood sugar level may be too low, particularly if the symptoms started suddenly. Less commonly, these symptoms may be due to an abnormally high blood sugar level.

ACTION Eat or drink something very sweet. This should balance your blood sugar level. If you are not better within 10 minutes, call your doctor immediately.

NO ↓

SEE YOUR DOCTOR WITHIN 24 HOURS

POSSIBLE CAUSE AND ACTION Certain drugs may be the cause of forgetfulness or confusion as a side effect. Do not stop taking your prescribed drugs unless otherwise advised by your doctor.

POSSIBLE CAUSE AND ACTION Recreational drugs may cause confusion and prolonged use can lead to irreversible brain damage. Stop using recreational drugs or inhaling solvents. If you have trouble stopping, consult your doctor, who may be able to help or may put you in contact with a counselor or a self-help group (*see* USEFUL ADDRESSES, p.311).

CONSULT YOUR DOCTOR IF YOU ARE UNABLE TO MAKE A DIAGNOSIS FROM THIS CHART.

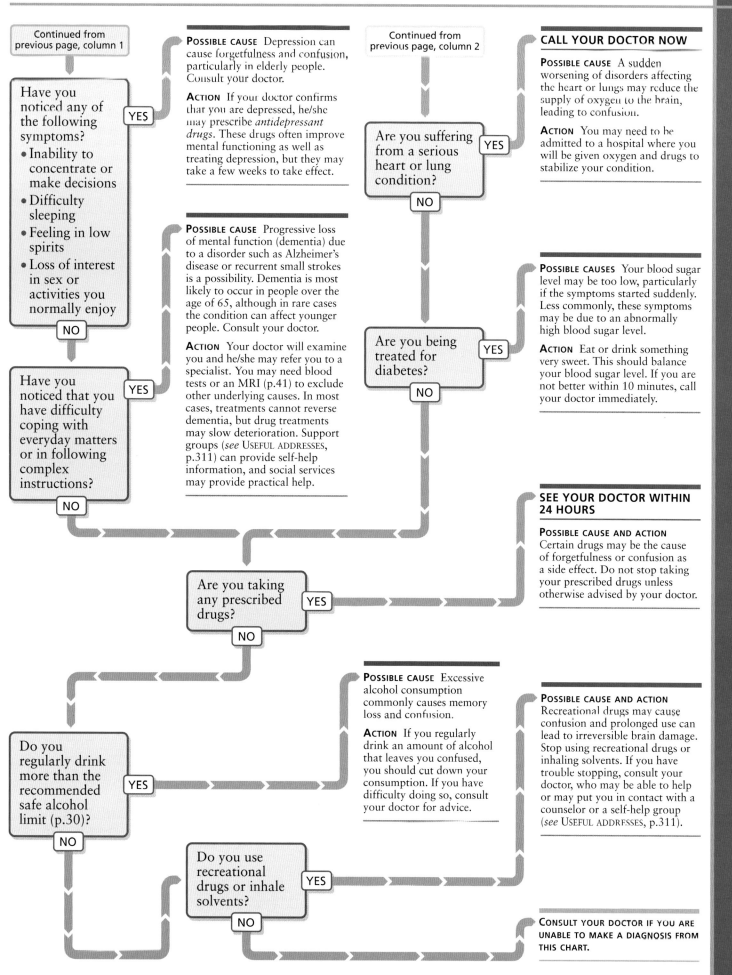

68 Twitching and/or trembling

Consult this chart if you experience any involuntary or uncontrolled movements. Such movements may range from slight twitching to prolonged, repeated trembling or shaking of the arms, legs, or head. Brief episodes are often simply the result of fatigue or stress and are rarely a cause for concern.

Jerking movements that happen while you are falling asleep are also common and harmless. Occasionally, however, involuntary movements may be caused by problems that require medical treatment, such as excessive alcohol consumption or a neurological disorder.

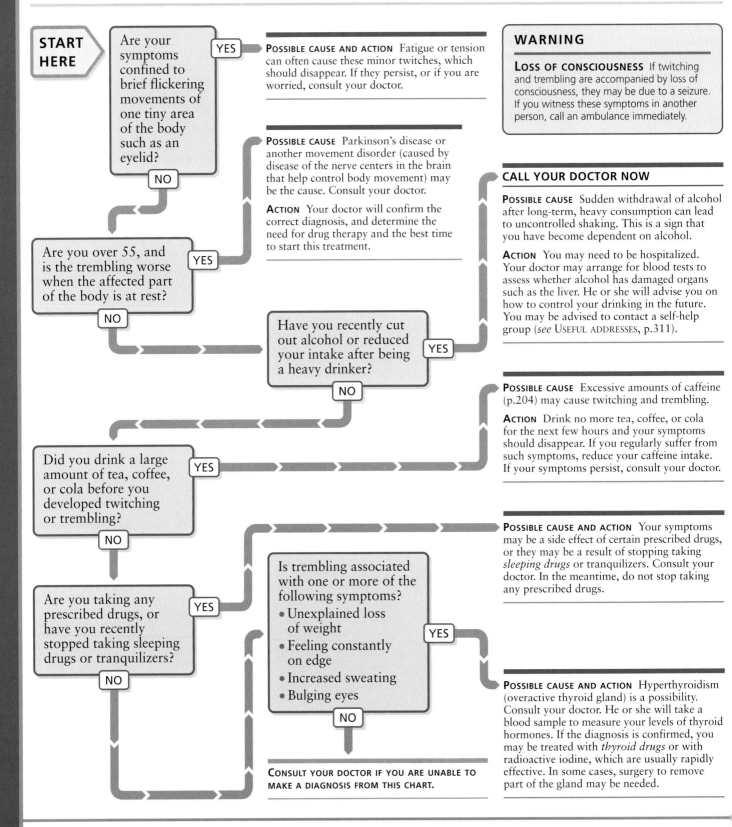

START HERE

Are your symptoms confined to brief flickering movements of one tiny area of the body such as an eyelid?
YES → **POSSIBLE CAUSE AND ACTION** Fatigue or tension can often cause these minor twitches, which should disappear. If they persist, or if you are worried, consult your doctor.

NO

Are you over 55, and is the trembling worse when the affected part of the body is at rest?
YES → **POSSIBLE CAUSE** Parkinson's disease or another movement disorder (caused by disease of the nerve centers in the brain that help control body movement) may be the cause. Consult your doctor.

ACTION Your doctor will confirm the correct diagnosis, and determine the need for drug therapy and the best time to start this treatment.

NO

Have you recently cut out alcohol or reduced your intake after being a heavy drinker?
YES → (see CALL YOUR DOCTOR NOW)

NO

Did you drink a large amount of tea, coffee, or cola before you developed twitching or trembling?
YES → (see caffeine POSSIBLE CAUSE)

NO

Are you taking any prescribed drugs, or have you recently stopped taking sleeping drugs or tranquilizers?
YES → **POSSIBLE CAUSE AND ACTION** Your symptoms may be a side effect of certain prescribed drugs, or they may be a result of stopping taking *sleeping drugs* or tranquilizers. Consult your doctor. In the meantime, do not stop taking any prescribed drugs.

NO

Is trembling associated with one or more of the following symptoms?
- Unexplained loss of weight
- Feeling constantly on edge
- Increased sweating
- Bulging eyes

YES → **POSSIBLE CAUSE AND ACTION** Hyperthyroidism (overactive thyroid gland) is a possibility. Consult your doctor. He or she will take a blood sample to measure your levels of thyroid hormones. If the diagnosis is confirmed, you may be treated with *thyroid drugs* or with radioactive iodine, which are usually rapidly effective. In some cases, surgery to remove part of the gland may be needed.

NO

CONSULT YOUR DOCTOR IF YOU ARE UNABLE TO MAKE A DIAGNOSIS FROM THIS CHART.

WARNING

LOSS OF CONSCIOUSNESS If twitching and trembling are accompanied by loss of consciousness, they may be due to a seizure. If you witness these symptoms in another person, call an ambulance immediately.

CALL YOUR DOCTOR NOW

POSSIBLE CAUSE Sudden withdrawal of alcohol after long-term, heavy consumption can lead to uncontrolled shaking. This is a sign that you have become dependent on alcohol.

ACTION You may need to be hospitalized. Your doctor may arrange for blood tests to assess whether alcohol has damaged organs such as the liver. He or she will advise you on how to control your drinking in the future. You may be advised to contact a self-help group (*see* USEFUL ADDRESSES, p.311).

POSSIBLE CAUSE Excessive amounts of caffeine (p.204) may cause twitching and trembling.

ACTION Drink no more tea, coffee, or cola for the next few hours and your symptoms should disappear. If you regularly suffer from such symptoms, reduce your caffeine intake. If your symptoms persist, consult your doctor.

69 Facial pain

For toothache, see chart 95 TEETH PROBLEMS (p.206). For pain in or around the mouth, see chart 96, MOUTH PROBLEMS (p.208). For a headache, see chart 63, HEADACHE (p.158). Consult this chart if you develop pain or discomfort that is limited to the area of the face and/or the forehead. Facial pain may be a dull, throbbing ache or a sharp, stabbing sensation. It is often caused by infection or inflammation of the underlying tissues or irritation of a nerve. Although pain in the face can be distressing and may require medical treatment, it is rarely a sign of a serious disorder.

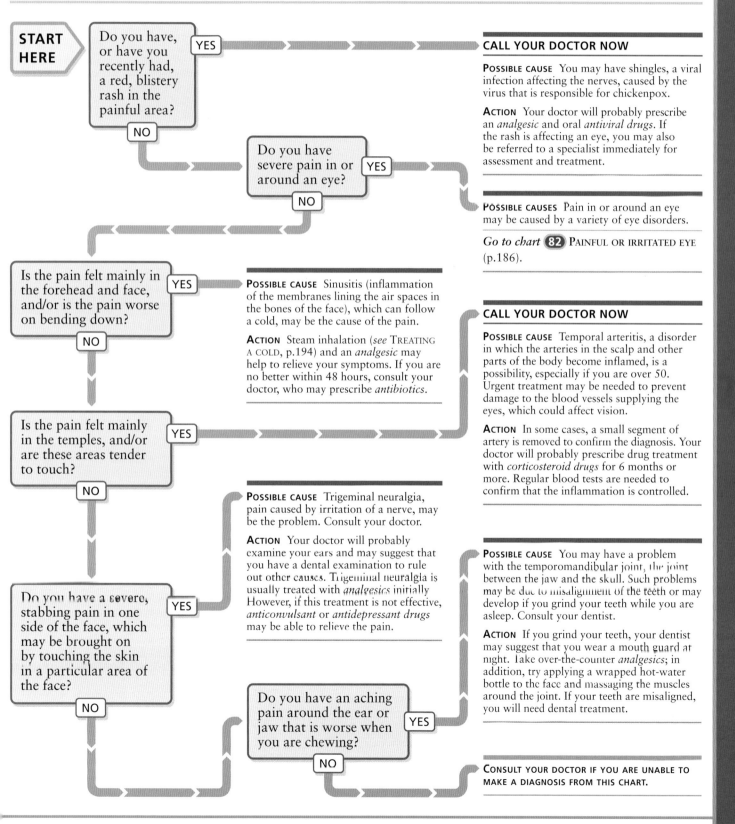

START HERE

Do you have, or have you recently had, a red, blistery rash in the painful area?
YES →

NO

Do you have severe pain in or around an eye?
YES →

NO

Is the pain felt mainly in the forehead and face, and/or is the pain worse on bending down?
YES →

NO

Is the pain felt mainly in the temples, and/or are these areas tender to touch?
YES →

NO

Do you have a severe, stabbing pain in one side of the face, which may be brought on by touching the skin in a particular area of the face?
YES →

NO

Do you have an aching pain around the ear or jaw that is worse when you are chewing?
YES →

NO

CALL YOUR DOCTOR NOW

POSSIBLE CAUSE You may have shingles, a viral infection affecting the nerves, caused by the virus that is responsible for chickenpox.

ACTION Your doctor will probably prescribe an *analgesic* and oral *antiviral drugs*. If the rash is affecting an eye, you may also be referred to a specialist immediately for assessment and treatment.

POSSIBLE CAUSES Pain in or around an eye may be caused by a variety of eye disorders.

Go to chart **82** PAINFUL OR IRRITATED EYE (p.186).

POSSIBLE CAUSE Sinusitis (inflammation of the membranes lining the air spaces in the bones of the face), which can follow a cold, may be the cause of the pain.

ACTION Steam inhalation (*see* TREATING A COLD, p.194) and an *analgesic* may help to relieve your symptoms. If you are no better within 48 hours, consult your doctor, who may prescribe *antibiotics*.

CALL YOUR DOCTOR NOW

POSSIBLE CAUSE Temporal arteritis, a disorder in which the arteries in the scalp and other parts of the body become inflamed, is a possibility, especially if you are over 50. Urgent treatment may be needed to prevent damage to the blood vessels supplying the eyes, which could affect vision.

ACTION In some cases, a small segment of artery is removed to confirm the diagnosis. Your doctor will probably prescribe drug treatment with *corticosteroid drugs* for 6 months or more. Regular blood tests are needed to confirm that the inflammation is controlled.

POSSIBLE CAUSE Trigeminal neuralgia, pain caused by irritation of a nerve, may be the problem. Consult your doctor.

ACTION Your doctor will probably examine your ears and may suggest that you have a dental examination to rule out other causes. Trigeminal neuralgia is usually treated with *analgesics* initially. However, if this treatment is not effective, *anticonvulsant* or *antidepressant drugs* may be able to relieve the pain.

POSSIBLE CAUSE You may have a problem with the temporomandibular joint, the joint between the jaw and the skull. Such problems may be due to misalignment of the teeth or may develop if you grind your teeth while you are asleep. Consult your dentist.

ACTION If you grind your teeth, your dentist may suggest that you wear a mouth guard at night. Take over-the-counter *analgesics*; in addition, try applying a wrapped hot-water bottle to the face and massaging the muscles around the joint. If your teeth are misaligned, you will need dental treatment.

CONSULT YOUR DOCTOR IF YOU ARE UNABLE TO MAKE A DIAGNOSIS FROM THIS CHART.

70 Difficulty speaking

Consult this chart if you have, or recently have had, difficulty finding or using words or if your speech has become unclear. Such speech difficulties may be related to disorders affecting the brain, the mouth, or the facial nerves. In some cases, speech may be affected permanently, although speech therapy (below) is often beneficial.

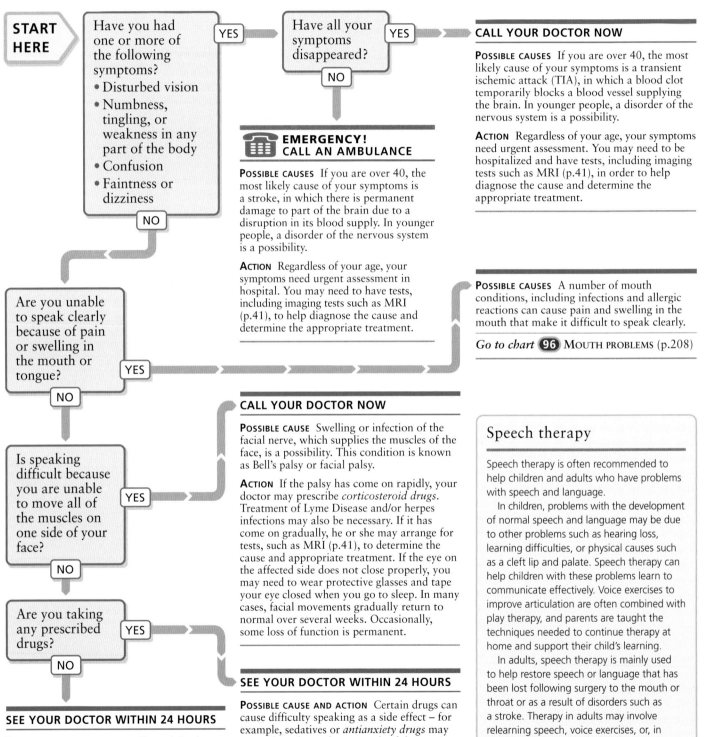

START HERE

Have you had one or more of the following symptoms?
- Disturbed vision
- Numbness, tingling, or weakness in any part of the body
- Confusion
- Faintness or dizziness

YES → **Have all your symptoms disappeared?**

YES →

CALL YOUR DOCTOR NOW

POSSIBLE CAUSES If you are over 40, the most likely cause of your symptoms is a transient ischemic attack (TIA), in which a blood clot temporarily blocks a blood vessel supplying the brain. In younger people, a disorder of the nervous system is a possibility.

ACTION Regardless of your age, your symptoms need urgent assessment. You may need to be hospitalized and have tests, including imaging tests such as MRI (p.41), in order to help diagnose the cause and determine the appropriate treatment.

NO →

☎ EMERGENCY! CALL AN AMBULANCE

POSSIBLE CAUSES If you are over 40, the most likely cause of your symptoms is a stroke, in which there is permanent damage to part of the brain due to a disruption in its blood supply. In younger people, a disorder of the nervous system is a possibility.

ACTION Regardless of your age, your symptoms need urgent assessment in hospital. You may need to have tests, including imaging tests such as MRI (p.41), to help diagnose the cause and determine the appropriate treatment.

NO (from first question)

Are you unable to speak clearly because of pain or swelling in the mouth or tongue?

YES →

POSSIBLE CAUSES A number of mouth conditions, including infections and allergic reactions can cause pain and swelling in the mouth that make it difficult to speak clearly.

Go to chart **96** MOUTH PROBLEMS (p.208)

NO →

Is speaking difficult because you are unable to move all of the muscles on one side of your face?

YES →

CALL YOUR DOCTOR NOW

POSSIBLE CAUSE Swelling or infection of the facial nerve, which supplies the muscles of the face, is a possibility. This condition is known as Bell's palsy or facial palsy.

ACTION If the palsy has come on rapidly, your doctor may prescribe *corticosteroid drugs*. Treatment of Lyme Disease and/or herpes infections may also be necessary. If it has come on gradually, he or she may arrange for tests, such as MRI (p.41), to determine the cause and appropriate treatment. If the eye on the affected side does not close properly, you may need to wear protective glasses and tape your eye closed when you go to sleep. In many cases, facial movements gradually return to normal over several weeks. Occasionally, some loss of function is permanent.

NO →

Are you taking any prescribed drugs?

YES →

SEE YOUR DOCTOR WITHIN 24 HOURS

POSSIBLE CAUSE AND ACTION Certain drugs can cause difficulty speaking as a side effect – for example, sedatives or *antianxiety drugs* may cause slurred speech as a result of their action on the brain, and *antidepressants* may make speech difficult by causing a dry mouth. However, you should not stop taking your prescribed drugs unless you are advised to do so by your doctor.

NO →

SEE YOUR DOCTOR WITHIN 24 HOURS

POSSIBLE CAUSE AND ACTION Unexplained difficulty speaking may be an early sign of an underlying disorder of the brain or nervous system and needs prompt medical assessment. Your doctor may arrange for tests to diagnose the cause and determine the treatment.

Speech therapy

Speech therapy is often recommended to help children and adults who have problems with speech and language.

In children, problems with the development of normal speech and language may be due to other problems such as hearing loss, learning difficulties, or physical causes such as a cleft lip and palate. Speech therapy can help children with these problems learn to communicate effectively. Voice exercises to improve articulation are often combined with play therapy, and parents are taught the techniques needed to continue therapy at home and support their child's learning.

In adults, speech therapy is mainly used to help restore speech or language that has been lost following surgery to the mouth or throat or as a result of disorders such as a stroke. Therapy in adults may involve relearning speech, voice exercises, or, in some cases, using electronic devices to aid speech production. If speech cannot be restored, help with communication – for example, with the use of pictures or specialized computers – may be offered.

71 Disturbing thoughts and feelings

Consult this chart if you begin to have thoughts and feelings that worry you or that seem to you or to other people to be abnormal or unhealthy. You may be having upsetting or intrusive thoughts or you may be experiencing unfamiliar or uncontrolled emotions. If your thoughts and feelings continue to worry you, whatever your particular problem, talk to your doctor about them. He or she may be able to help you put your feelings into context by discussing them with you. If your concerns are justified, he or she may suggest treatment or refer you to a specialized therapist.

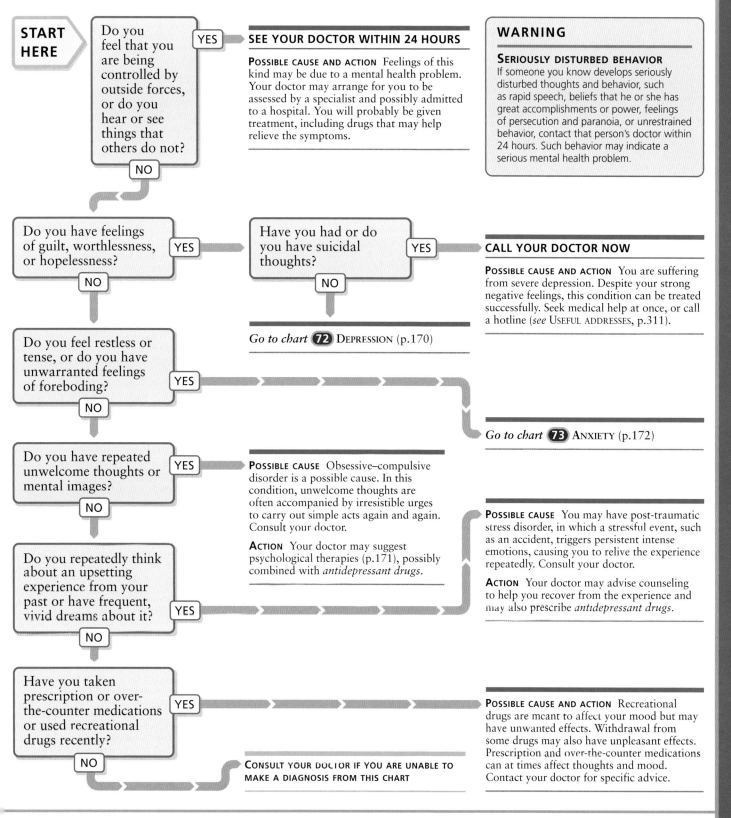

START HERE

Do you feel that you are being controlled by outside forces, or do you hear or see things that others do not? — YES →

SEE YOUR DOCTOR WITHIN 24 HOURS

POSSIBLE CAUSE AND ACTION Feelings of this kind may be due to a mental health problem. Your doctor may arrange for you to be assessed by a specialist and possibly admitted to a hospital. You will probably be given treatment, including drugs that may help relieve the symptoms.

WARNING

SERIOUSLY DISTURBED BEHAVIOR
If someone you know develops seriously disturbed thoughts and behavior, such as rapid speech, beliefs that he or she has great accomplishments or power, feelings of persecution and paranoia, or unrestrained behavior, contact that person's doctor within 24 hours. Such behavior may indicate a serious mental health problem.

NO ↓

Do you have feelings of guilt, worthlessness, or hopelessness? — YES → **Have you had or do you have suicidal thoughts?** — YES →

CALL YOUR DOCTOR NOW

POSSIBLE CAUSE AND ACTION You are suffering from severe depression. Despite your strong negative feelings, this condition can be treated successfully. Seek medical help at once, or call a hotline (*see* USEFUL ADDRESSES, p.311).

NO ↓

Go to chart **72** DEPRESSION (p.170)

NO ↓

Do you feel restless or tense, or do you have unwarranted feelings of foreboding? — YES →

Go to chart **73** ANXIETY (p.172)

NO ↓

Do you have repeated unwelcome thoughts or mental images? — YES →

POSSIBLE CAUSE Obsessive–compulsive disorder is a possible cause. In this condition, unwelcome thoughts are often accompanied by irresistible urges to carry out simple acts again and again. Consult your doctor.

ACTION Your doctor may suggest psychological therapies (p.171), possibly combined with *antidepressant drugs*.

NO ↓

Do you repeatedly think about an upsetting experience from your past or have frequent, vivid dreams about it? — YES →

POSSIBLE CAUSE You may have post-traumatic stress disorder, in which a stressful event, such as an accident, triggers persistent intense emotions, causing you to relive the experience repeatedly. Consult your doctor.

ACTION Your doctor may advise counseling to help you recover from the experience and may also prescribe *antidepressant drugs*.

NO ↓

Have you taken prescription or over-the-counter medications or used recreational drugs recently? — YES →

POSSIBLE CAUSE AND ACTION Recreational drugs are meant to affect your mood but may have unwanted effects. Withdrawal from some drugs may also have unpleasant effects. Prescription and over-the-counter medications can at times affect thoughts and mood. Contact your doctor for specific advice.

NO ↓

CONSULT YOUR DOCTOR IF YOU ARE UNABLE TO MAKE A DIAGNOSIS FROM THIS CHART

72 Depression

Most people have minor ups and downs in mood, feeling good one day but low the next. These changes often have an identifiable cause and usually pass quickly. True depression is associated with physical symptoms including excessive fatigue, changes in weight, and sleep disturbances, such as early waking (*see* RECOGNIZING DEPRESSION, below). In some cases, a depressive illness follows a traumatic event, such as divorce, bereavement, or loss of a job. In other cases, it follows a major life change, such as retirement. It may also be precipitated by hormonal changes at menopause or after childbirth. In many cases, however, depression has no apparent cause. Some people have repeated episodes. Depression is a treatable disorder, and you should always see your doctor if you think you might be depressed.

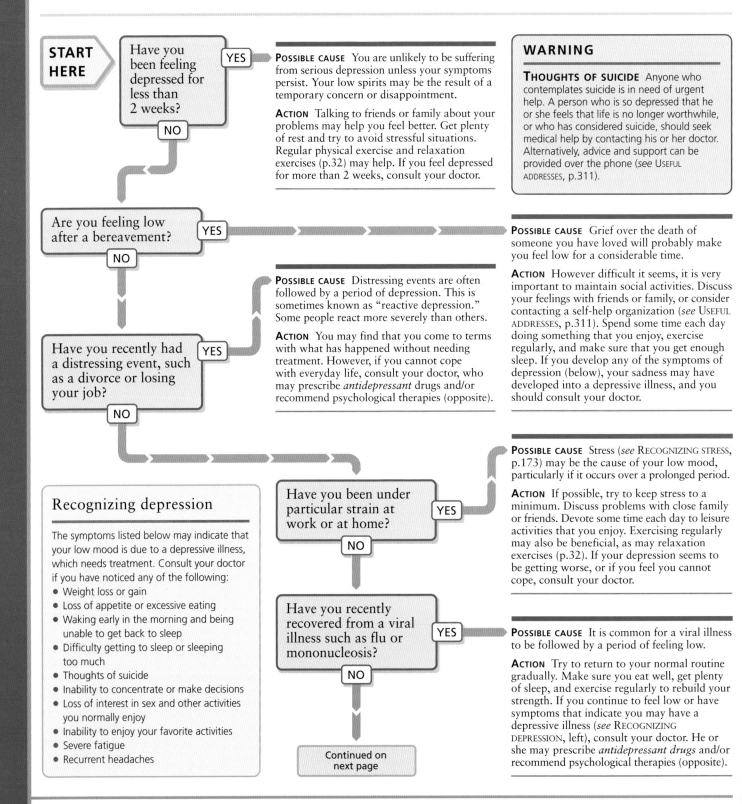

START HERE

Have you been feeling depressed for less than 2 weeks? — YES

POSSIBLE CAUSE You are unlikely to be suffering from serious depression unless your symptoms persist. Your low spirits may be the result of a temporary concern or disappointment.

ACTION Talking to friends or family about your problems may help you feel better. Get plenty of rest and try to avoid stressful situations. Regular physical exercise and relaxation exercises (p.32) may help. If you feel depressed for more than 2 weeks, consult your doctor.

NO

Are you feeling low after a bereavement? — YES

NO

Have you recently had a distressing event, such as a divorce or losing your job? — YES

POSSIBLE CAUSE Distressing events are often followed by a period of depression. This is sometimes known as "reactive depression." Some people react more severely than others.

ACTION You may find that you come to terms with what has happened without needing treatment. However, if you cannot cope with everyday life, consult your doctor, who may prescribe *antidepressant* drugs and/or recommend psychological therapies (opposite).

NO

WARNING

THOUGHTS OF SUICIDE Anyone who contemplates suicide is in need of urgent help. A person who is so depressed that he or she feels that life is no longer worthwhile, or who has considered suicide, should seek medical help by contacting his or her doctor. Alternatively, advice and support can be provided over the phone (*see* USEFUL ADDRESSES, p.311).

POSSIBLE CAUSE Grief over the death of someone you have loved will probably make you feel low for a considerable time.

ACTION However difficult it seems, it is very important to maintain social activities. Discuss your feelings with friends or family, or consider contacting a self-help organization (*see* USEFUL ADDRESSES, p.311). Spend some time each day doing something that you enjoy, exercise regularly, and make sure that you get enough sleep. If you develop any of the symptoms of depression (below), your sadness may have developed into a depressive illness, and you should consult your doctor.

Recognizing depression

The symptoms listed below may indicate that your low mood is due to a depressive illness, which needs treatment. Consult your doctor if you have noticed any of the following:

- Weight loss or gain
- Loss of appetite or excessive eating
- Waking early in the morning and being unable to get back to sleep
- Difficulty getting to sleep or sleeping too much
- Thoughts of suicide
- Inability to concentrate or make decisions
- Loss of interest in sex and other activities you normally enjoy
- Inability to enjoy your favorite activities
- Severe fatigue
- Recurrent headaches

Have you been under particular strain at work or at home? — YES

NO

Have you recently recovered from a viral illness such as flu or mononucleosis? — YES

NO

POSSIBLE CAUSE Stress (*see* RECOGNIZING STRESS, p.173) may be the cause of your low mood, particularly if it occurs over a prolonged period.

ACTION If possible, try to keep stress to a minimum. Discuss problems with close family or friends. Devote some time each day to leisure activities that you enjoy. Exercising regularly may also be beneficial, as may relaxation exercises (p.32). If your depression seems to be getting worse, or if you feel you cannot cope, consult your doctor.

POSSIBLE CAUSE It is common for a viral illness to be followed by a period of feeling low.

ACTION Try to return to your normal routine gradually. Make sure you eat well, get plenty of sleep, and exercise regularly to rebuild your strength. If you continue to feel low or have symptoms that indicate you may have a depressive illness (*see* RECOGNIZING DEPRESSION, left), consult your doctor. He or she may prescribe *antidepressant drugs* and/or recommend psychological therapies (opposite).

Continued on next page

Continued from previous page

Have you recently had a serious illness or accident?
YES → NO

POSSIBLE CAUSES A serious physical illness, such as a heart attack, or a major accident may often be followed by depression. This may slow down your physical recovery. Consult your doctor.

ACTION Your doctor will talk to you about your current health and will explain that this is a common reaction. *Antidepressant drugs* may be prescribed, and/or your doctor may recommend psychological therapies (below).

POSSIBLE CAUSE Regularly drinking too much alcohol may lead to depression. You should also be aware of why you drink. Some people may use alcohol to help them cope with stress or unrecognized depression. Drinking too much may be compounding the problem.

ACTION Cut down the amount of alcohol you drink. If you find this difficult, or you continue to feel depressed, consult your doctor for advice.

Do you regularly drink more than the recommended safe alcohol limit (p.30)?
YES → NO

Are you using, or have you ever used, recreational drugs?
YES → NO

POSSIBLE CAUSE Many recreational drugs can cause profound psychological disturbances, both during use and after withdrawal. Some drugs can cause problems even years later.

ACTION If you still take recreational drugs, stop now. If you find you cannot stop or are still having problems after you have stopped, consult your doctor, who may be able to help or may put you in contact with a counselor or self-help group (*see* USEFUL ADDRESSES, p.311).

Are you taking any prescribed drugs?
YES → NO

POSSIBLE CAUSE AND ACTION Certain drugs, such as *antihypertensives* (drugs used to treat hypertension) and oral contraceptives, can cause depression as a side effect. Consult your doctor. Meanwhile, do not stop taking your prescribed drugs.

Psychological therapies

There are a variety of psychological therapies available, some of which explore a person's past, while others focus on current behavior or thought processes. All involve a therapist who usually encourages you to talk about your feelings and fears, while he or she provides help and advice.

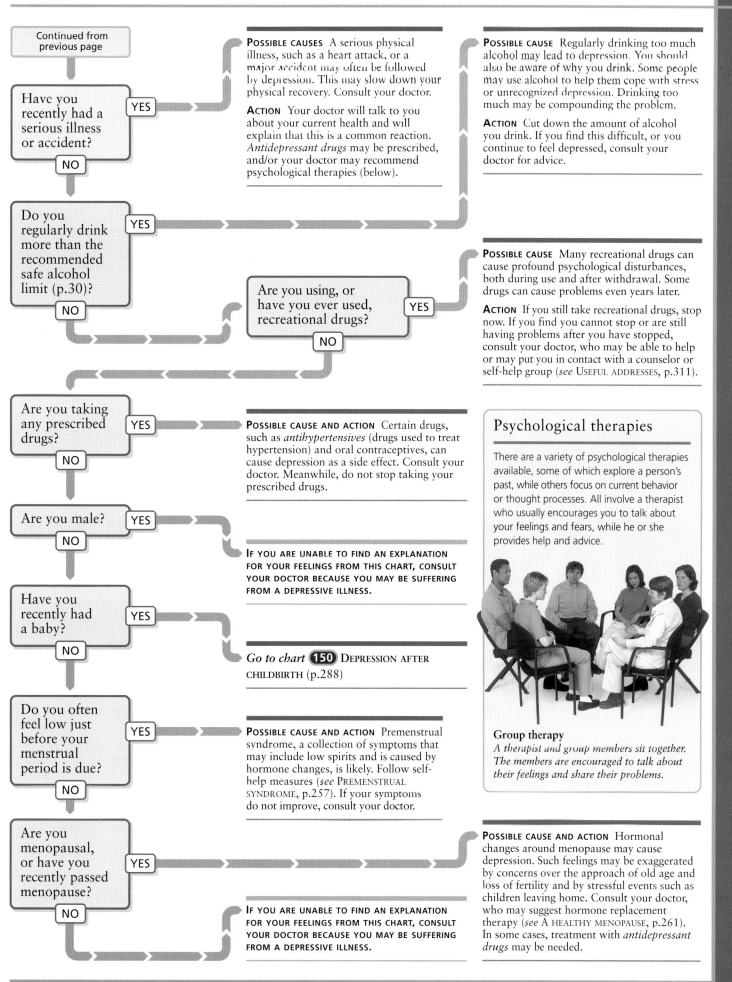

Are you male?
YES → NO

IF YOU ARE UNABLE TO FIND AN EXPLANATION FOR YOUR FEELINGS FROM THIS CHART, CONSULT YOUR DOCTOR BECAUSE YOU MAY BE SUFFERING FROM A DEPRESSIVE ILLNESS.

Have you recently had a baby?
YES → NO

Go to chart **150** DEPRESSION AFTER CHILDBIRTH (p.288)

Group therapy
A therapist and group members sit together. The members are encouraged to talk about their feelings and share their problems.

Do you often feel low just before your menstrual period is due?
YES → NO

POSSIBLE CAUSE AND ACTION Premenstrual syndrome, a collection of symptoms that may include low spirits and is caused by hormone changes, is likely. Follow self-help measures (*see* PREMENSTRUAL SYNDROME, p.257). If your symptoms do not improve, consult your doctor.

Are you menopausal, or have you recently passed menopause?
YES → NO

IF YOU ARE UNABLE TO FIND AN EXPLANATION FOR YOUR FEELINGS FROM THIS CHART, CONSULT YOUR DOCTOR BECAUSE YOU MAY BE SUFFERING FROM A DEPRESSIVE ILLNESS.

POSSIBLE CAUSE AND ACTION Hormonal changes around menopause may cause depression. Such feelings may be exaggerated by concerns over the approach of old age and loss of fertility and by stressful events such as children leaving home. Consult your doctor, who may suggest hormone replacement therapy (*see* A HEALTHY MENOPAUSE, p.261). In some cases, treatment with *antidepressant drugs* may be needed.

73 Anxiety

If you are suffering from anxiety, you will probably feel apprehensive and tense and be unable to concentrate, think clearly, or sleep well. You may have a sense of foreboding for no obvious reason or have repetitive worrying thoughts. Some people also have physical symptoms such as headaches, excessive sweating, chest pains, palpitations, abdominal cramps, and a general feeling of fatigue. Anxiety is a natural reaction to stress, and it is normal to feel anxious if, for example, you are worried about money or family matters or if you have exams coming up. Such anxiety may help you deal with stressful events and can help improve your performance in certain situations. However, anxiety is not normal if it comes on without an apparent cause or if it is so severe that you can no longer cope with everyday life.

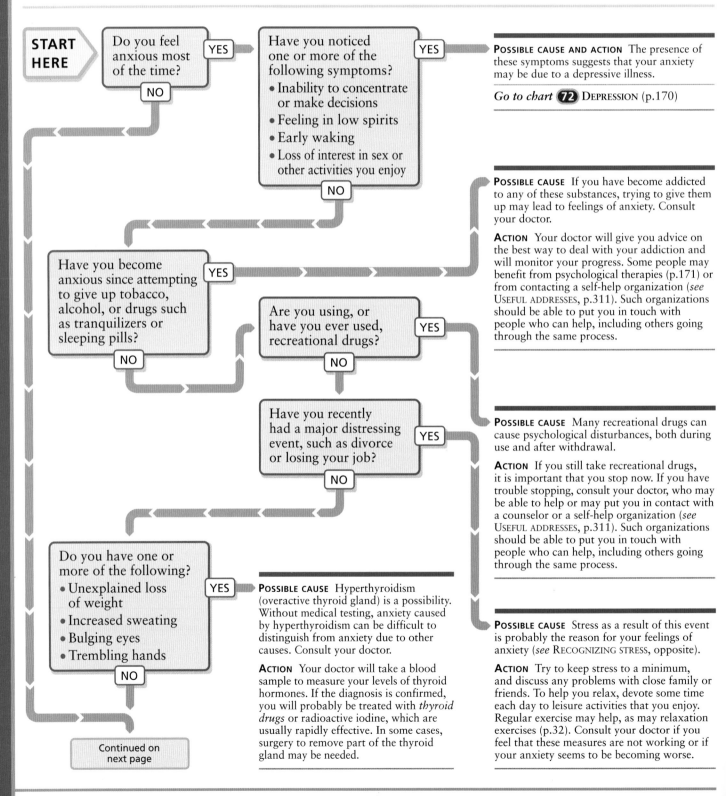

START HERE

Do you feel anxious most of the time? **YES** →

Have you noticed one or more of the following symptoms?
- Inability to concentrate or make decisions
- Feeling in low spirits
- Early waking
- Loss of interest in sex or other activities you enjoy

YES →

POSSIBLE CAUSE AND ACTION The presence of these symptoms suggests that your anxiety may be due to a depressive illness.

Go to chart **72** DEPRESSION (p.170)

NO ↓ (from "Do you feel anxious most of the time?")

NO ↓ (from symptoms box)

Have you become anxious since attempting to give up tobacco, alcohol, or drugs such as tranquilizers or sleeping pills? **YES** →

POSSIBLE CAUSE If you have become addicted to any of these substances, trying to give them up may lead to feelings of anxiety. Consult your doctor.

ACTION Your doctor will give you advice on the best way to deal with your addiction and will monitor your progress. Some people may benefit from psychological therapies (p.171) or from contacting a self-help organization (*see* USEFUL ADDRESSES, p.311). Such organizations should be able to put you in touch with people who can help, including others going through the same process.

NO ↓

Are you using, or have you ever used, recreational drugs? **YES** →

NO ↓

POSSIBLE CAUSE Many recreational drugs can cause psychological disturbances, both during use and after withdrawal.

ACTION If you still take recreational drugs, it is important that you stop now. If you have trouble stopping, consult your doctor, who may be able to help or may put you in contact with a counselor or a self-help organization (*see* USEFUL ADDRESSES, p.311). Such organizations should be able to put you in touch with people who can help, including others going through the same process.

Have you recently had a major distressing event, such as divorce or losing your job? **YES** →

NO ↓

POSSIBLE CAUSE Stress as a result of this event is probably the reason for your feelings of anxiety (*see* RECOGNIZING STRESS, opposite).

ACTION Try to keep stress to a minimum, and discuss any problems with close family or friends. To help you relax, devote some time each day to leisure activities that you enjoy. Regular exercise may help, as may relaxation exercises (p.32). Consult your doctor if you feel that these measures are not working or if your anxiety seems to be becoming worse.

Do you have one or more of the following?
- Unexplained loss of weight
- Increased sweating
- Bulging eyes
- Trembling hands

YES →

POSSIBLE CAUSE Hyperthyroidism (overactive thyroid gland) is a possibility. Without medical testing, anxiety caused by hyperthyroidism can be difficult to distinguish from anxiety due to other causes. Consult your doctor.

ACTION Your doctor will take a blood sample to measure your levels of thyroid hormones. If the diagnosis is confirmed, you will probably be treated with *thyroid drugs* or radioactive iodine, which are usually rapidly effective. In some cases, surgery to remove part of the thyroid gland may be needed.

NO ↓

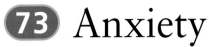

Continued on next page

Continued from previous page

Recognizing stress

Stress is a normal part of life for many people and has a beneficial effect under certain circumstances, readying the body for action. The normal stress response causes the release of the hormone epinephrine (adrenaline), which increases heart rate and maximizes blood flow to the muscles in preparation for action. These responses are beneficial if stress is relieved. However, prolonged or excessive stress can result in a range of symptoms, including chest pain, stomach upsets, headaches, fatigue, insomnia, and anxiety. Having a series of infections, such as colds, or getting recurrent mouth ulcers may be a sign of stress because stress may depress the immune system. Stress can also result in flare-ups of existing disorders such as eczema. In the long term, stress may seriously damage health. It is important that you learn to recognize signs of stress and take action to deal with it (*see* STRESS, p.32).

Do you have any worries related to sex? YES

NO

Do you feel anxious only in certain social situations – for instance, meeting people or going to parties? YES

NO

POSSIBLE CAUSE In some situations, a degree of anxiety is natural, and the problem usually improves with experience. If your anxiety is so severe that you avoid certain types of social interaction, consult your doctor.

ACTION Your doctor may be able to teach you coping strategies for dealing with social situations, or he or she may refer you to a counselor for help. If your anxiety is severe, drug treatment with *beta blockers* or some types of *antidepressant* may be helpful.

Do you feel anxious only when confronted with specific objects or situations or if you are prevented from doing things in your usual way? YES

NO

POSSIBLE CAUSES Your anxiety may be caused by a phobia, which is an irrational fear of a specific object or situation. You may, for example, be afraid of spiders. Otherwise, you may have obsessive–compulsive disorder, in which you feel an irresistible need to behave in a certain fashion, even though you may know that it is not necessary. You may, for example, feel the need to repeatedly wash your hands and become excessively anxious if you are unable to do so. Consult your doctor.

ACTION Your doctor will ask you about your feelings. He or she may advise psychological therapies (p.171) or drug treatment for your anxiety. Most people can learn to manage their fears and anxiety so that they do not affect their lives on a day-to day basis.

Do you have episodes of intense anxiety coupled with sweating, trembling, nausea, and/or dizziness? YES

NO

SEE YOUR DOCTOR WITHIN 24 HOURS

POSSIBLE CAUSE You may be having panic attacks, in which feelings of intense anxiety are coupled with alarming physical symptoms. Panic attacks are unpredictable and usually have no obvious cause.

ACTION It is important to see your doctor as soon as possible so that he or she can confirm the diagnosis and rule out a physical cause for your symptoms. If you are having panic attacks, you will need treatment with psychological therapies (p.171) and/or drug treatment. Follow self-help measures for coping with panic attacks (right).

CONSULT YOUR DOCTOR IF YOU ARE UNABLE TO FIND A CAUSE FOR YOUR ANXIETY FROM THIS CHART AND/OR UNEXPLAINED ANXIETY PERSISTS FOR MORE THAN A FEW DAYS.

POSSIBLE CAUSES Anxiety about sex is common, particularly during early adult life. A specific difficulty affecting you or your partner, such as premature ejaculation or a fear of pregnancy or contracting a sexually transmitted disease, can be a source of anxiety. Worries about sexual orientation (p.251) may also cause anxiety. In later life, anxiety may be related to decreasing sexual activity or worries about attractiveness (*see* SEX IN LATER LIFE, p.270).

ACTION If you have a regular partner, you should discuss your feelings with him or her. Talking about sex openly (*see* COMMUNICATING YOUR SEXUAL NEEDS, p.273) is often the best way to deal with anxiety. If you are unable to communicate satisfactorily or if you do not have a regular partner with whom you can talk, consult your doctor. He or she may be able to advise you or may suggest that you receive counseling (*see* SEX COUNSELING, p.251).

SELF-HELP Coping with a panic attack

Rapid breathing during a panic attack reduces carbon dioxide levels in the blood and may lead to frightening physical symptoms, such as palpitations and muscle spasms. You can control the symptoms by breathing into and out of a paper bag. When you do this, you rebreathe carbon dioxide, restoring your blood levels. Place the bag over your mouth, and breathe in and out 10 times. Then, remove the bag and breathe normally for 15 seconds. Repeat this process until your breathing rate is back to normal.

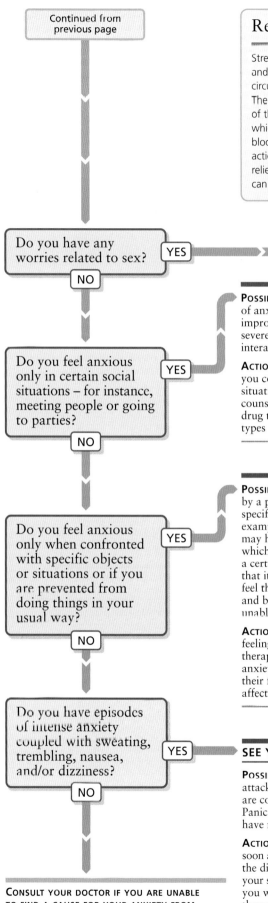

Rebreathing from a bag
Hold a paper bag tightly over the mouth, and breathe in and out slowly.

74 Lumps and swellings

For breast lumps, see chart 128, BREAST PROBLEMS (p.256).
For lumps and swellings in the scrotum, see chart 123,
TESTES AND SCROTUM PROBLEMS (p.248).
Consult this chart if you develop one or more swellings
or lumps beneath the surface of the skin. In some cases,

a swelling is due to enlargement of a lymph gland in
response to an infection. However, multiple swellings that
last longer than a month may be the result of an underlying
disorder. Always consult your doctor if you have one or
more painless or persistent lumps or swellings.

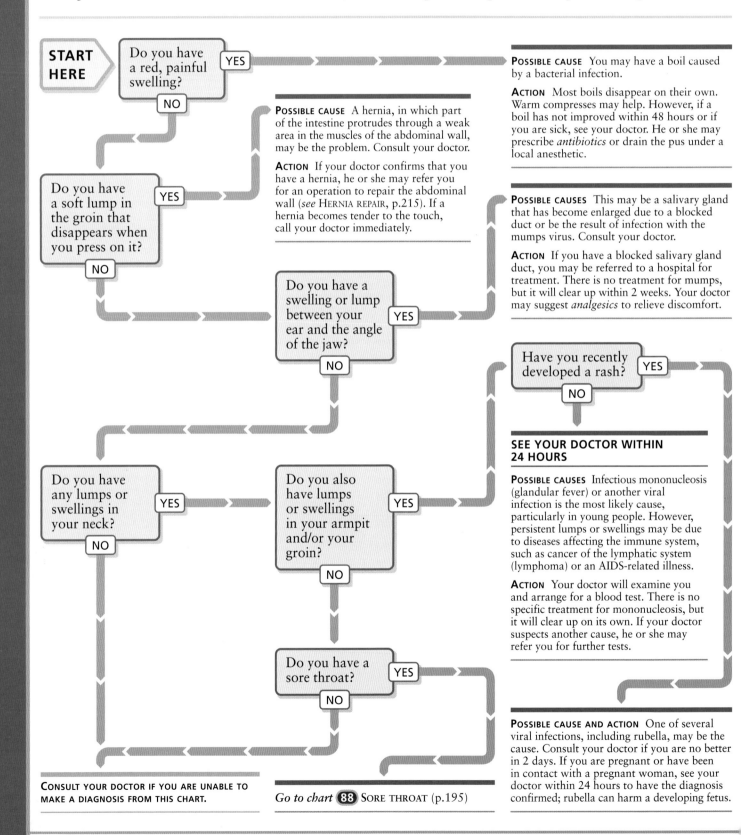

START HERE

Do you have a red, painful swelling?
YES → **POSSIBLE CAUSE** You may have a boil caused by a bacterial infection.

ACTION Most boils disappear on their own. Warm compresses may help. However, if a boil has not improved within 48 hours or if you are sick, see your doctor. He or she may prescribe *antibiotics* or drain the pus under a local anesthetic.

NO

Do you have a soft lump in the groin that disappears when you press on it?
YES → **POSSIBLE CAUSE** A hernia, in which part of the intestine protrudes through a weak area in the muscles of the abdominal wall, may be the problem. Consult your doctor.

ACTION If your doctor confirms that you have a hernia, he or she may refer you for an operation to repair the abdominal wall (*see* HERNIA REPAIR, p.215). If a hernia becomes tender to the touch, call your doctor immediately.

NO

Do you have a swelling or lump between your ear and the angle of the jaw?
YES → **POSSIBLE CAUSES** This may be a salivary gland that has become enlarged due to a blocked duct or be the result of infection with the mumps virus. Consult your doctor.

ACTION If you have a blocked salivary gland duct, you may be referred to a hospital for treatment. There is no treatment for mumps, but it will clear up within 2 weeks. Your doctor may suggest *analgesics* to relieve discomfort.

NO

Do you have any lumps or swellings in your neck?
YES → **Do you also have lumps or swellings in your armpit and/or your groin?**
YES → **Have you recently developed a rash?**
YES →

NO

SEE YOUR DOCTOR WITHIN 24 HOURS

POSSIBLE CAUSES Infectious mononucleosis (glandular fever) or another viral infection is the most likely cause, particularly in young people. However, persistent lumps or swellings may be due to diseases affecting the immune system, such as cancer of the lymphatic system (lymphoma) or an AIDS-related illness.

ACTION Your doctor will examine you and arrange for a blood test. There is no specific treatment for mononucleosis, but it will clear up on its own. If your doctor suspects another cause, he or she may refer you for further tests.

NO

Do you have a sore throat?
YES →

NO

CONSULT YOUR DOCTOR IF YOU ARE UNABLE TO MAKE A DIAGNOSIS FROM THIS CHART.

Go to chart **88** SORE THROAT (p.195)

POSSIBLE CAUSE AND ACTION One of several viral infections, including rubella, may be the cause. Consult your doctor if you are no better in 2 days. If you are pregnant or have been in contact with a pregnant woman, see your doctor within 24 hours to have the diagnosis confirmed; rubella can harm a developing fetus.

75 Itching

For itching confined to the scalp, see chart 76, HAIR AND SCALP PROBLEMS (p.176). For itching confined to the anus, see chart 107, ANAL PROBLEMS (p.223).
Itching (irritation of the skin that leads to an intense desire to scratch) may be caused by an infection or by an allergic reaction to a particular substance. In other cases, itching can be a feature of a skin disorder or may even indicate an underlying disease or psychological stress. Loss of natural oils in the skin as a result of aging or from excessive washing may cause dryness and itching of the skin.

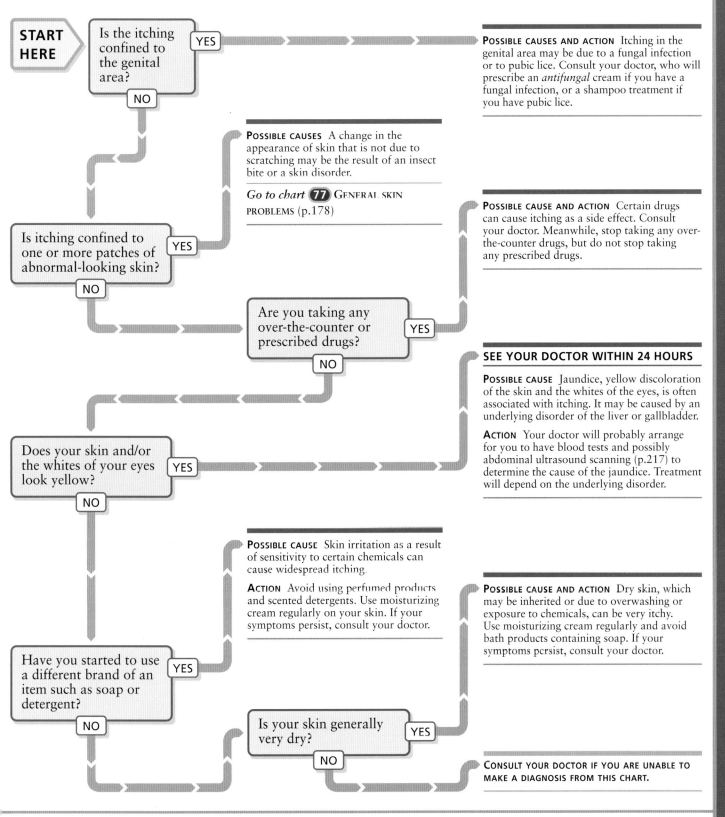

START HERE

Is the itching confined to the genital area?
YES →
POSSIBLE CAUSES AND ACTION Itching in the genital area may be due to a fungal infection or to pubic lice. Consult your doctor, who will prescribe an *antifungal* cream if you have a fungal infection, or a shampoo treatment if you have pubic lice.

NO ↓

Is itching confined to one or more patches of abnormal-looking skin?
YES →
POSSIBLE CAUSES A change in the appearance of skin that is not due to scratching may be the result of an insect bite or a skin disorder.

Go to chart 77 GENERAL SKIN PROBLEMS (p.178)

NO ↓

Are you taking any over-the-counter or prescribed drugs?
YES →
POSSIBLE CAUSE AND ACTION Certain drugs can cause itching as a side effect. Consult your doctor. Meanwhile, stop taking any over-the-counter drugs, but do not stop taking any prescribed drugs.

NO ↓

Does your skin and/or the whites of your eyes look yellow?
YES →
SEE YOUR DOCTOR WITHIN 24 HOURS

POSSIBLE CAUSE Jaundice, yellow discoloration of the skin and the whites of the eyes, is often associated with itching. It may be caused by an underlying disorder of the liver or gallbladder.

ACTION Your doctor will probably arrange for you to have blood tests and possibly abdominal ultrasound scanning (p.217) to determine the cause of the jaundice. Treatment will depend on the underlying disorder.

NO ↓

Have you started to use a different brand of an item such as soap or detergent?
YES →
POSSIBLE CAUSE Skin irritation as a result of sensitivity to certain chemicals can cause widespread itching.

ACTION Avoid using perfumed products and scented detergents. Use moisturizing cream regularly on your skin. If your symptoms persist, consult your doctor.

NO ↓

Is your skin generally very dry?
YES →
POSSIBLE CAUSE AND ACTION Dry skin, which may be inherited or due to overwashing or exposure to chemicals, can be very itchy. Use moisturizing cream regularly and avoid bath products containing soap. If your symptoms persist, consult your doctor.

NO ↓

CONSULT YOUR DOCTOR IF YOU ARE UNABLE TO MAKE A DIAGNOSIS FROM THIS CHART.

76 Hair and scalp problems

Fine hairs grow on most areas of the body. The hair on the head is usually much thicker, and problems affecting its growth are therefore very noticeable. Your hair color and type (straight, wavy, or curly) are inherited, but the condition of your hair may be affected by your overall state of health and factors such as your diet and age. This chart deals with some of the more common problems affecting the hair on the head and the condition of the scalp.

START HERE

Has your hair become generally thin?
- NO
- YES →

Has thinning occurred within 4 months of one of the following events?
- A prolonged or serious illness
- Childbirth
- Stopping oral contraceptives
- NO
- YES →

POSSIBLE CAUSE A long illness or hormonal changes can disrupt the normal hair growth cycle (*see* HAIR STRUCTURE AND FUNCTION, below), resulting in a large number of hairs being lost at the same time.

ACTION The hair growth cycle should resume, and hair should return to normal within 6 months. However, if you are concerned, consult your doctor.

Are you taking any prescribed drugs?
- NO
- YES →

POSSIBLE CAUSE AND ACTION Certain drugs, particularly those used to treat cancer, can cause hair loss as a side effect. Consult your doctor. Meanwhile, do not stop taking your prescribed drugs. Hair often returns to normal at the end of treatment or if alternative drugs can be prescribed.

Have you noticed one or more of the following symptoms?
- Excessive fatigue
- Unexplained weight gain
- Feeling the cold more than you used to
- Increased dryness or roughness of the skin
- NO
- YES →

POSSIBLE CAUSE You may be suffering from hypothyroidism (underactive thyroid gland). Consult your doctor.

ACTION Your doctor will take a blood sample to measure your levels of thyroid hormones. If the diagnosis is confirmed, you will be prescribed *thyroid drugs*, which may need to be taken for life. Your doctor will arrange for periodic blood tests to monitor the dosage.

POSSIBLE CAUSE AND ACTION Hairdressing methods such as these may damage your hair if used inexpertly or excessively. If you adopt a more natural hairstyle, your hair will probably regain its thickness. You may need to have your hair cut short if it has been severely damaged.

Do you use any of the following hairdressing techniques?
- Bleaching
- Dyeing
- Perming
- Tight braiding
- NO
- YES →

Hair structure and function

Hair helps provide the body with insulation and protection from the environment. Hairs are made of dead cells that grow from a living base. Each hair grows in a hair follicle, which has a rest phase followed by a growth phase. During the rest phase, cell activity slows and then stops, and the hair dies. During the growth phase, cells in the follicle divide rapidly to form a new hair. The new, growing hair pushes the dead hair out of the follicle. Every day some hairs grow while others are shed. A single hair grows between ¼ in (6mm) and ⅓ in (8mm) a month.

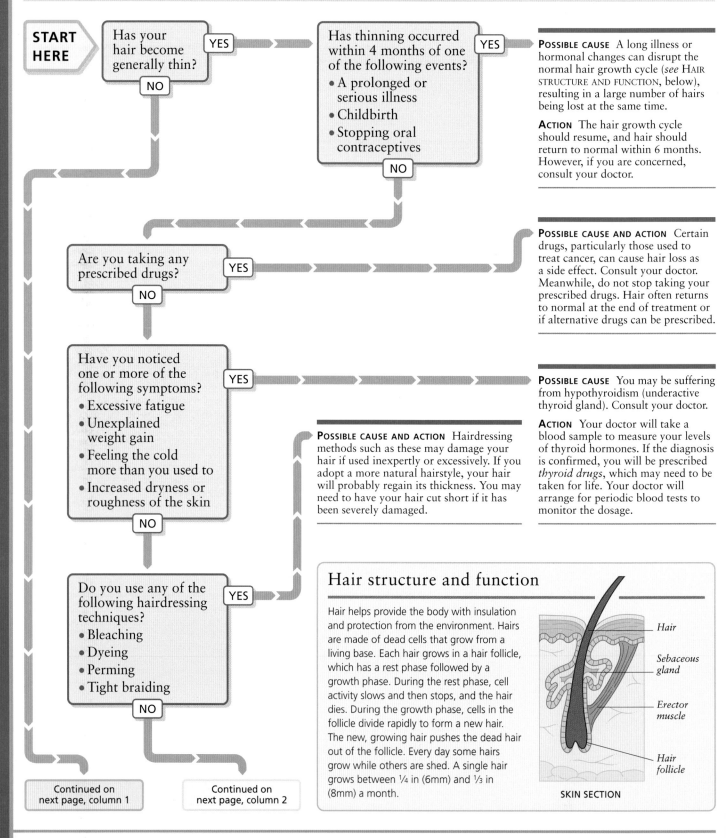

- Hair
- Sebaceous gland
- Erector muscle
- Hair follicle

SKIN SECTION

Continued on next page, column 1

Continued on next page, column 2

Hair transplant

Baldness can be treated surgically by several different methods of hair transplantation. In the method shown, skin and hair are taken from a donor site, often at the back of the scalp or behind the ears. The removed hairs and their attached follicles are then inserted in the bald area (the recipient site). A mild sedative is usually given, and both sites are anesthetized. The transplanted hairs will fall out shortly after the transplant, but new hair starts to grow from the transplanted follicles 3 weeks to 3 months later.

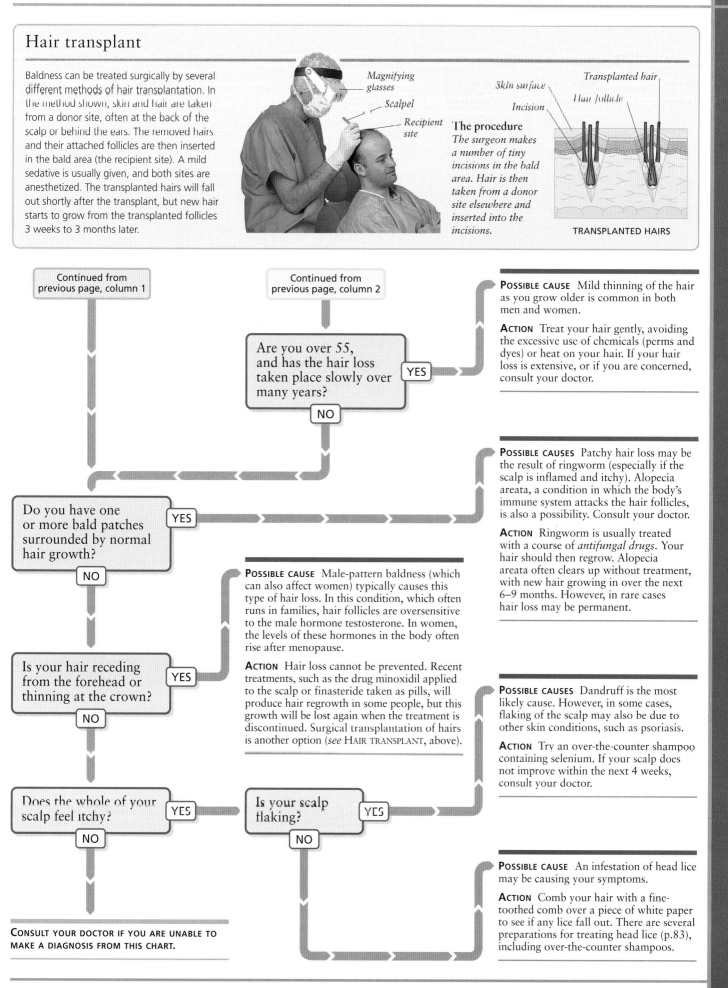

Magnifying glasses

Scalpel

Recipient site

Skin surface

Incision

Transplanted hair

Hair follicle

The procedure
The surgeon makes a number of tiny incisions in the bald area. Hair is then taken from a donor site elsewhere and inserted into the incisions.

TRANSPLANTED HAIRS

Continued from previous page, column 1

Continued from previous page, column 2

Are you over 55, and has the hair loss taken place slowly over many years? YES / NO

POSSIBLE CAUSE Mild thinning of the hair as you grow older is common in both men and women.

ACTION Treat your hair gently, avoiding the excessive use of chemicals (perms and dyes) or heat on your hair. If your hair loss is extensive, or if you are concerned, consult your doctor.

Do you have one or more bald patches surrounded by normal hair growth? YES / NO

POSSIBLE CAUSES Patchy hair loss may be the result of ringworm (especially if the scalp is inflamed and itchy). Alopecia areata, a condition in which the body's immune system attacks the hair follicles, is also a possibility. Consult your doctor.

ACTION Ringworm is usually treated with a course of *antifungal drugs*. Your hair should then regrow. Alopecia areata often clears up without treatment, with new hair growing in over the next 6–9 months. However, in rare cases hair loss may be permanent.

Is your hair receding from the forehead or thinning at the crown? YES / NO

POSSIBLE CAUSE Male-pattern baldness (which can also affect women) typically causes this type of hair loss. In this condition, which often runs in families, hair follicles are oversensitive to the male hormone testosterone. In women, the levels of these hormones in the body often rise after menopause.

ACTION Hair loss cannot be prevented. Recent treatments, such as the drug minoxidil applied to the scalp or finasteride taken as pills, will produce hair regrowth in some people, but this growth will be lost again when the treatment is discontinued. Surgical transplantation of hairs is another option (*see* HAIR TRANSPLANT, above).

Does the whole of your scalp feel itchy? YES / NO

Is your scalp flaking? YES / NO

POSSIBLE CAUSES Dandruff is the most likely cause. However, in some cases, flaking of the scalp may also be due to other skin conditions, such as psoriasis.

ACTION Try an over-the-counter shampoo containing selenium. If your scalp does not improve within the next 4 weeks, consult your doctor.

POSSIBLE CAUSE An infestation of head lice may be causing your symptoms.

ACTION Comb your hair with a fine-toothed comb over a piece of white paper to see if any lice fall out. There are several preparations for treating head lice (p.83), including over-the-counter shampoos.

CONSULT YOUR DOCTOR IF YOU ARE UNABLE TO MAKE A DIAGNOSIS FROM THIS CHART.

77 General skin problems

For itching in skin that appears normal, see chart 75,
ITCHING *(p.175).*
Short-term skin problems are often the result of a minor injury
or a superficial infection and are easily treated. Many skin
conditions can be distressing if they persist or affect visible
areas of skin, but most do not pose a serious risk to health.
It is important, however, that potentially serious conditions,
such as skin cancer, be recognized and treated early.

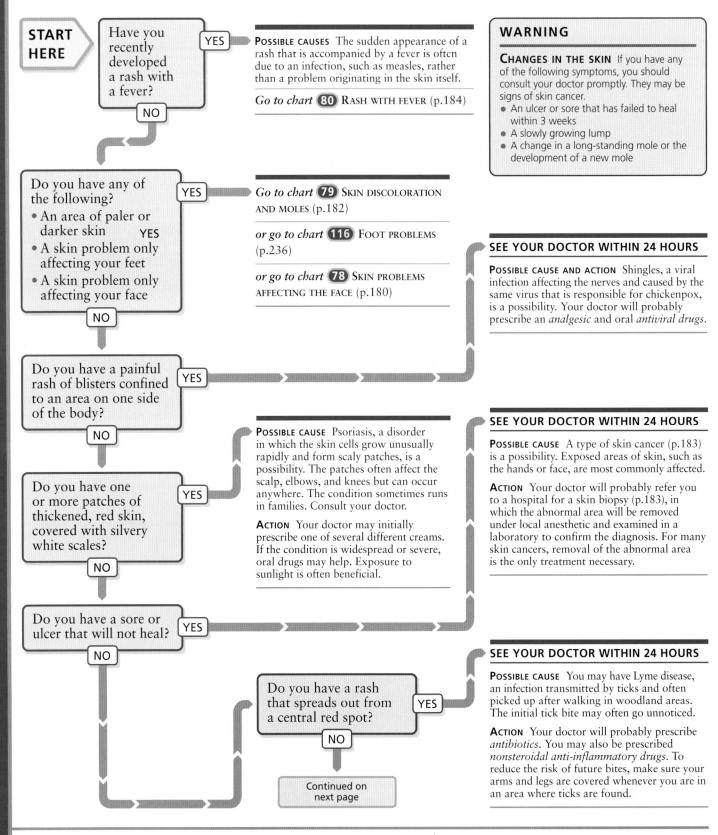

START HERE

Have you recently developed a rash with a fever?
YES →

POSSIBLE CAUSES The sudden appearance of a rash that is accompanied by a fever is often due to an infection, such as measles, rather than a problem originating in the skin itself.

Go to chart 80 RASH WITH FEVER *(p.184)*

NO ↓

Do you have any of the following?
- An area of paler or darker skin
- A skin problem only affecting your feet
- A skin problem only affecting your face
YES →

Go to chart 79 SKIN DISCOLORATION AND MOLES *(p.182)*

or go to chart 116 FOOT PROBLEMS *(p.236)*

or go to chart 78 SKIN PROBLEMS AFFECTING THE FACE *(p.180)*

NO ↓

Do you have a painful rash of blisters confined to an area on one side of the body?
YES →

NO ↓

Do you have one or more patches of thickened, red skin, covered with silvery white scales?
YES →

POSSIBLE CAUSE Psoriasis, a disorder in which the skin cells grow unusually rapidly and form scaly patches, is a possibility. The patches often affect the scalp, elbows, and knees but can occur anywhere. The condition sometimes runs in families. Consult your doctor.

ACTION Your doctor may initially prescribe one of several different creams. If the condition is widespread or severe, oral drugs may help. Exposure to sunlight is often beneficial.

NO ↓

Do you have a sore or ulcer that will not heal?
YES →

NO ↓

Do you have a rash that spreads out from a central red spot?
YES →

NO ↓

Continued on next page

WARNING

CHANGES IN THE SKIN If you have any of the following symptoms, you should consult your doctor promptly. They may be signs of skin cancer.
- An ulcer or sore that has failed to heal within 3 weeks
- A slowly growing lump
- A change in a long-standing mole or the development of a new mole

---

SEE YOUR DOCTOR WITHIN 24 HOURS

POSSIBLE CAUSE AND ACTION Shingles, a viral infection affecting the nerves and caused by the same virus that is responsible for chickenpox, is a possibility. Your doctor will probably prescribe an *analgesic* and oral *antiviral drugs.*

SEE YOUR DOCTOR WITHIN 24 HOURS

POSSIBLE CAUSE A type of skin cancer (p.183) is a possibility. Exposed areas of skin, such as the hands or face, are most commonly affected.

ACTION Your doctor will probably refer you to a hospital for a skin biopsy (p.183), in which the abnormal area will be removed under local anesthetic and examined in a laboratory to confirm the diagnosis. For many skin cancers, removal of the abnormal area is the only treatment necessary.

SEE YOUR DOCTOR WITHIN 24 HOURS

POSSIBLE CAUSE You may have Lyme disease, an infection transmitted by ticks and often picked up after walking in woodland areas. The initial tick bite may often go unnoticed.

ACTION Your doctor will probably prescribe *antibiotics.* You may also be prescribed *nonsteroidal anti-inflammatory drugs.* To reduce the risk of future bites, make sure your arms and legs are covered whenever you are in an area where ticks are found.

Continued from previous page

Do you have one or more areas of itchy, abnormal-looking skin? — **NO** / **YES**

Are you taking any over-the-counter or prescribed drugs? — **NO** / **YES**

CONSULT YOUR DOCTOR IF YOU ARE UNABLE TO MAKE A DIAGNOSIS FROM THIS CHART.

POSSIBLE CAUSE AND ACTION Some drugs commonly cause a rash, and others, such as penicillin, may cause a rash only in people who are allergic to them. If the rash has developed suddenly, call your doctor before the next dose of any prescribed drugs is due. Otherwise, make an appointment with your doctor. Meanwhile, stop taking any over-the-counter drugs.

Do the abnormal areas of skin have clearly defined, scaly edges? — **NO** / **YES**

POSSIBLE CAUSES You may have a fungal infection such as ringworm. Warm, moist areas, such as the groin or the armpit, are most likely to be affected. Alternatively, a type of eczema, known as discoid eczema, is a possibility, particularly if the affected areas are on the limbs. Consult your doctor.

ACTION Your doctor may want to take skin scrapings to see if fungi are present. If they are, treatment is with *antifungal* cream or pills. If eczema is the cause, you will be prescribed *corticosteroid* cream.

Do you have intense itching, with or without gray lines between your fingers and/or on your wrists? — **NO** / **YES**

POSSIBLE CAUSE You may have atopic eczema. This condition often appears first during childhood and can flare up during adulthood.

ACTION An over-the-counter *corticosteroid* cream will probably relieve the irritation. Use an emollient, such as moisturizing cream, to keep the skin from becoming dry. If these measures do not help, consult your doctor.

Are these areas raised, red lumps? — **YES** / **NO**

Does the rash mainly affect your hands, and do you spend a lot of time with your hands in water or do you handle chemicals? — **YES** / **NO**

Does the area of itching clear up and then recur, and is it always in the same place? — **YES** / **NO**

POSSIBLE CAUSES You may have urticaria, also known as hives. This condition may occur as an allergic reaction to a particular type of food, such as shellfish, but, in many cases, no cause can be found. Insect bites, such as flea or mosquito bites, are another possibility.

ACTION If the itching is severe, over-the-counter *antihistamine* creams or tablets should provide relief. In most cases, urticaria clears up within hours, and insect bites clear up within a few days. If urticaria recurs, you should consult your doctor. Tests may be needed to look for an underlying cause.

POSSIBLE CAUSE You probably have dyshydrotic eczema. This is a common problem for people who work in occupations such as hairdressing and cleaning, where hands are frequently in water or exposed to chemicals.

ACTION Try to keep your hands out of water. If this is not possible or if you are using chemicals, wear cotton-lined rubber gloves. Apply a barrier cream or an emollient, such as moisturizing cream, frequently throughout the day, and wash your hands with a mild soap. If these measures do not help, consult your doctor, who may prescribe a *corticosteroid* cream to relieve the itching and irritation.

POSSIBLE CAUSE Allergic contact dermatitis, in which inflammation of the skin occurs in response to contact with a particular substance, is possible. Nickel, found in earrings and in the studs in jeans, is a common cause, although a wide variety of substances can cause allergic contact dermatitis.

ACTION If you can identify the cause and avoid it, the condition will probably clear up without any treatment. If you are unsure why the condition is occurring, consult your doctor, who may refer you to a hospital for tests to identify the cause.

SEE YOUR DOCTOR WITHIN 24 HOURS

POSSIBLE CAUSE Scabies, a parasitic infection, may be causing your symptoms. Scabies mites burrow under the skin between the fingers and can cause a widespread rash. Scabies is very contagious and often affects a whole family.

ACTION Your doctor will probably prescribe a treatment lotion, which you will need to apply to your entire body from the neck down. Everyone else in the household will need to be treated at the same time, and clothing and bedding also need to be washed. The mites should die within 3 days of treatment, but the itching may continue for up to 2 weeks.

78 Skin problems affecting the face

Consult this chart if you have a skin problem confined to the face. The skin of the face can be affected by conditions that rarely appear on other parts of the body, such as cold sores. Facial skin may also be at risk of damage from external factors that are not as likely to affect other areas of the body. For example, the face is exposed to weather conditions such as sunlight, cold, and wind, and cosmetics are a common cause of skin irritation and allergy in women. Abnormal areas of skin on the face are more noticeable than on other parts of the body and may therefore be more distressing.

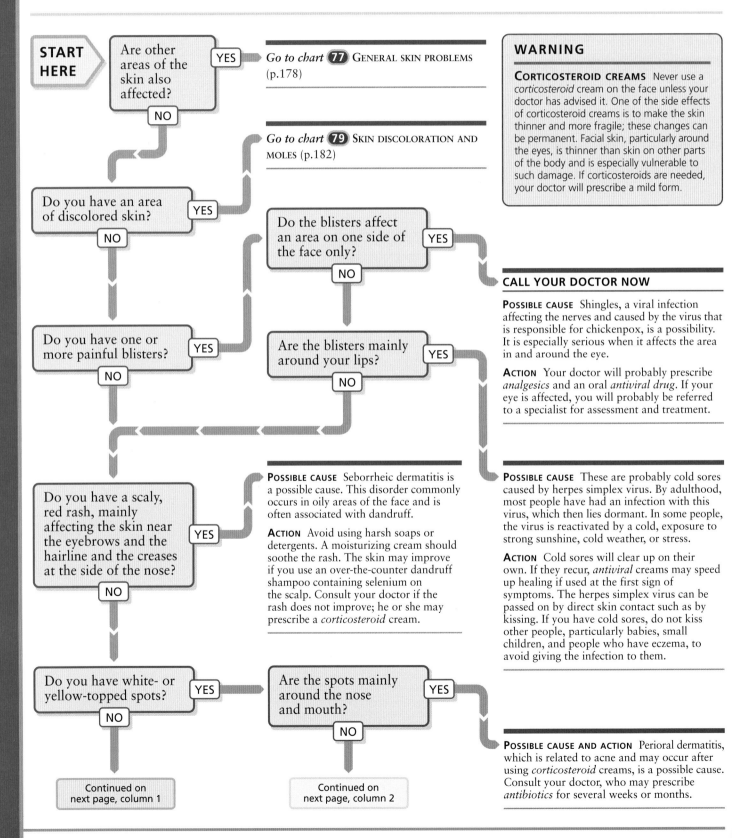

START HERE

Are other areas of the skin also affected?
YES → *Go to chart* **77** GENERAL SKIN PROBLEMS (p.178)
NO

Do you have an area of discolored skin?
YES → *Go to chart* **79** SKIN DISCOLORATION AND MOLES (p.182)
NO

Do you have one or more painful blisters?
YES →
NO

Do the blisters affect an area on one side of the face only?
YES →
NO

Are the blisters mainly around your lips?
YES →
NO

Do you have a scaly, red rash, mainly affecting the skin near the eyebrows and the hairline and the creases at the side of the nose?
YES →
NO

Do you have white- or yellow-topped spots?
YES →
NO

Are the spots mainly around the nose and mouth?
YES →
NO

| Continued on next page, column 1 |

| Continued on next page, column 2 |

WARNING

CORTICOSTEROID CREAMS Never use a *corticosteroid* cream on the face unless your doctor has advised it. One of the side effects of corticosteroid creams is to make the skin thinner and more fragile; these changes can be permanent. Facial skin, particularly around the eyes, is thinner than skin on other parts of the body and is especially vulnerable to such damage. If corticosteroids are needed, your doctor will prescribe a mild form.

CALL YOUR DOCTOR NOW

POSSIBLE CAUSE Shingles, a viral infection affecting the nerves and caused by the virus that is responsible for chickenpox, is a possibility. It is especially serious when it affects the area in and around the eye.

ACTION Your doctor will probably prescribe *analgesics* and an oral *antiviral drug*. If your eye is affected, you will probably be referred to a specialist for assessment and treatment.

POSSIBLE CAUSE Seborrheic dermatitis is a possible cause. This disorder commonly occurs in oily areas of the face and is often associated with dandruff.

ACTION Avoid using harsh soaps or detergents. A moisturizing cream should soothe the rash. The skin may improve if you use an over-the-counter dandruff shampoo containing selenium on the scalp. Consult your doctor if the rash does not improve; he or she may prescribe a *corticosteroid* cream.

POSSIBLE CAUSE These are probably cold sores caused by herpes simplex virus. By adulthood, most people have had an infection with this virus, which then lies dormant. In some people, the virus is reactivated by a cold, exposure to strong sunshine, cold weather, or stress.

ACTION Cold sores will clear up on their own. If they recur, *antiviral* creams may speed up healing if used at the first sign of symptoms. The herpes simplex virus can be passed on by direct skin contact such as by kissing. If you have cold sores, do not kiss other people, particularly babies, small children, and people who have eczema, to avoid giving the infection to them.

POSSIBLE CAUSE AND ACTION Perioral dermatitis, which is related to acne and may occur after using *corticosteroid* creams, is a possible cause. Consult your doctor, who may prescribe *antibiotics* for several weeks or months.

Continued from previous page, column 1

Continued from previous page, column 2

POSSIBLE CAUSE AND ACTION Acne, which is associated with certain skin bacteria and occurs when hair follicles are blocked by sebum (an oily substance secreted by skin glands), is likely. It usually starts during adolescence but often persists into adulthood. Try self-help measures (see COPING WITH ACNE, p.144) and over-the-counter treatments for acne (p.144). If these steps do not help, consult your doctor.

Do you also have blackheads and/or tender, red spots? **YES**

NO

Do you have a growth with a raised pearly edge, with or without a central depression or ulcer? **YES**

NO

Does your face become easily flushed – for example when you have been drinking alcohol or when you enter a warm room? **YES**

NO

POSSIBLE CAUSE Basal cell carcinoma, a type of skin cancer (p.183), is a possible cause. Consult your doctor.

ACTION Your doctor will probably refer you to a dermatologist for a skin biopsy (p.183), in which the abnormal area is removed under a local anesthetic and examined in a laboratory to confirm the diagnosis. More extensive surgery is often needed but, once the abnormal area has been removed, further treatment is usually not necessary.

Do you have an ulcer that will not heal? **YES**

NO

CONSULT YOUR DOCTOR IF YOU ARE UNABLE TO MAKE A DIAGNOSIS FROM THIS CHART.

POSSIBLE CAUSE Squamous cell carcinoma, a type of skin cancer (p.183), is a possibility. Consult your doctor.

ACTION Your doctor will probably refer you to a dermatologist for a skin biopsy (p.183), in which the abnormal area is removed under a local anesthetic and examined in a laboratory to confirm the diagnosis. You may not need any further treatment if all of the abnormal area has been removed. In some cases, further surgery may be necessary.

POSSIBLE CAUSE Rosacea, a condition similar to acne, is possible. It usually develops between the ages of 40 and 60 and is often worst on the cheeks and nose. Consult your doctor.

ACTION Your doctor may prescribe *antibiotic* pills or cream to be used for several weeks or months. You should avoid excessive exposure to the sun and cut down your alcohol intake, because they may make the condition worse.

Is the affected skin red and swollen, and do you have a high temperature? **YES**

NO

CALL YOUR DOCTOR NOW

POSSIBLE CAUSE Erysipelas, a bacterial infection of the facial skin and the underlying tissues, is a possible cause. If not treated, this condition can spread, resulting in a serious blood infection known as septicemia.

ACTION If the diagnosis is confirmed, your doctor will probably prescribe oral *antibiotics*. If the infection is severe, you may need to be admitted to a hospital so that you can be given intravenous *antibiotics*.

Does the problem seem related to cosmetics or perfumed products? **YES**

NO

POSSIBLE CAUSE AND ACTION You may be allergic to a new product, or you may have recently become allergic to a product you have been using for some time. Stop using all the products that could be responsible; the skin should return to normal in a few days. You can then reintroduce one item every few days so that the cause of the problem can be identified.

Have you been taking any over-the-counter or prescribed drugs? **YES**

NO

POSSIBLE CAUSE AND ACTION Certain drugs increase the sensitivity of skin to sunlight and can cause a reaction confined to the face. Stop taking any over-the-counter drugs, and consult your doctor. Meanwhile, continue taking any prescribed drugs and consult your doctor.

CONSULT YOUR DOCTOR IF YOU ARE UNABLE TO MAKE A DIAGNOSIS FROM THIS CHART.

79 Skin discoloration and moles

For birthmarks, see chart 8, SKIN PROBLEMS IN BABIES (p.64). Consult this chart if areas of your skin have become darker or paler than the surrounding skin or if you are worried about a new mole or changes in a mole. Although changes in skin color are most often due to exposure to the sun, you may have a skin condition that needs medical attention. Too much exposure to the sun can cause the skin to burn and increases the risk of developing skin cancer in later life.

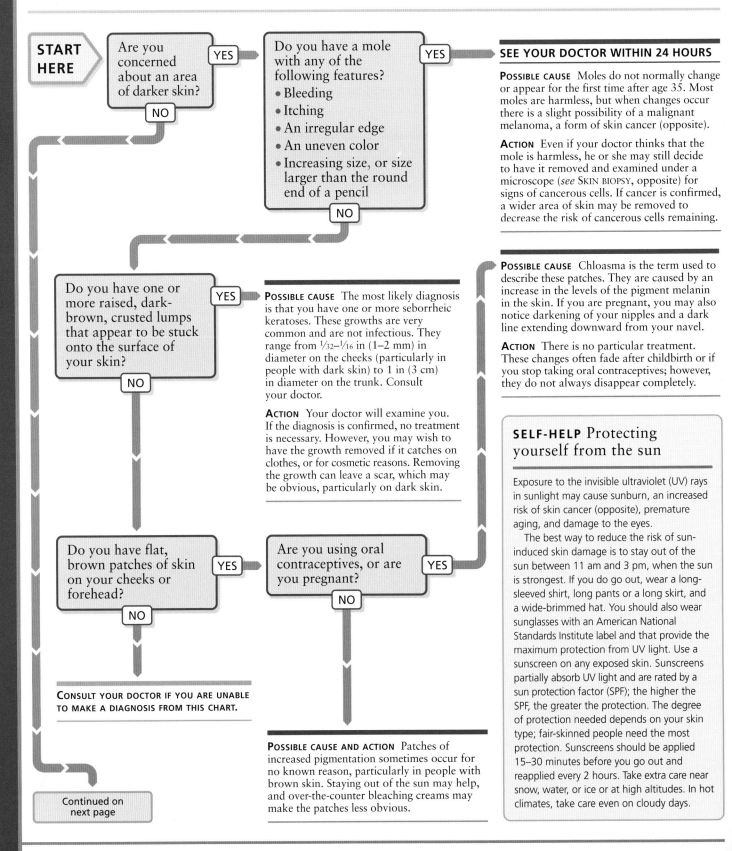

START HERE

Are you concerned about an area of darker skin? — NO / YES

Do you have a mole with any of the following features?
- Bleeding
- Itching
- An irregular edge
- An uneven color
- Increasing size, or size larger than the round end of a pencil

YES / NO

Do you have one or more raised, dark-brown, crusted lumps that appear to be stuck onto the surface of your skin? — YES / NO

Do you have flat, brown patches of skin on your cheeks or forehead? — YES / NO

Are you using oral contraceptives, or are you pregnant? — YES / NO

SEE YOUR DOCTOR WITHIN 24 HOURS

POSSIBLE CAUSE Moles do not normally change or appear for the first time after age 35. Most moles are harmless, but when changes occur there is a slight possibility of a malignant melanoma, a form of skin cancer (opposite).

ACTION Even if your doctor thinks that the mole is harmless, he or she may still decide to have it removed and examined under a microscope (*see* SKIN BIOPSY, opposite) for signs of cancerous cells. If cancer is confirmed, a wider area of skin may be removed to decrease the risk of cancerous cells remaining.

POSSIBLE CAUSE Chloasma is the term used to describe these patches. They are caused by an increase in the levels of the pigment melanin in the skin. If you are pregnant, you may also notice darkening of your nipples and a dark line extending downward from your navel.

ACTION There is no particular treatment. These changes often fade after childbirth or if you stop taking oral contraceptives; however, they do not always disappear completely.

POSSIBLE CAUSE The most likely diagnosis is that you have one or more seborrheic keratoses. These growths are very common and are not infectious. They range from 1/32–1/16 in (1–2 mm) in diameter on the cheeks (particularly in people with dark skin) to 1 in (3 cm) in diameter on the trunk. Consult your doctor.

ACTION Your doctor will examine you. If the diagnosis is confirmed, no treatment is necessary. However, you may wish to have the growth removed if it catches on clothes, or for cosmetic reasons. Removing the growth can leave a scar, which may be obvious, particularly on dark skin.

POSSIBLE CAUSE AND ACTION Patches of increased pigmentation sometimes occur for no known reason, particularly in people with brown skin. Staying out of the sun may help, and over-the-counter bleaching creams may make the patches less obvious.

CONSULT YOUR DOCTOR IF YOU ARE UNABLE TO MAKE A DIAGNOSIS FROM THIS CHART.

Continued on next page

SELF-HELP Protecting yourself from the sun

Exposure to the invisible ultraviolet (UV) rays in sunlight may cause sunburn, an increased risk of skin cancer (opposite), premature aging, and damage to the eyes.

The best way to reduce the risk of sun-induced skin damage is to stay out of the sun between 11 am and 3 pm, when the sun is strongest. If you do go out, wear a long-sleeved shirt, long pants or a long skirt, and a wide-brimmed hat. You should also wear sunglasses with an American National Standards Institute label and that provide the maximum protection from UV light. Use a sunscreen on any exposed skin. Sunscreens partially absorb UV light and are rated by a sun protection factor (SPF); the higher the SPF, the greater the protection. The degree of protection needed depends on your skin type; fair-skinned people need the most protection. Sunscreens should be applied 15–30 minutes before you go out and reapplied every 2 hours. Take extra care near snow, water, or ice or at high altitudes. In hot climates, take care even on cloudy days.

Continued from previous page

Do you have patches of paler skin? NO / YES

CONSULT YOUR DOCTOR IF YOU ARE UNABLE TO MAKE A DIAGNOSIS FROM THIS CHART.

Skin biopsy

A skin biopsy is a procedure used to make or confirm a diagnosis of a variety of skin diseases such as cancers. The biopsy site is anesthetized with local anesthetic. In one form of the procedure (excision biopsy), the entire abnormal area is removed. Another form of the procedure is used if a skin condition is widespread. In this case, a small representative area of skin, about ⅜–¾ in (1–2 cm) in diameter, which includes both normal and abnormal skin, is removed. It is usually removed in an ellipse shape to ease stitching of the biopsy site. The removed tissue is then examined under a microscope in a laboratory.

Normal skin · Abnormal area of skin · Epidermis · Dermis · Line of incision

Excision biopsy
After the biopsy site is anesthetized, an incision is made to remove the abnormality and the whole thickness of skin.

Do the patches have clearly defined edges, and do they affect the same area on both sides of the body? NO / YES

POSSIBLE CAUSE Vitiligo, an autoimmune disorder in which the body attacks its own tissue, causing patches of skin to lose pigment, is a likely cause. Consult your doctor.

ACTION Your doctor may test for other autoimmune conditions. Although there is no treatment, in some cases, strong *corticosteroid* creams or other medication can sometimes help. Cosmetics may help disguise the discolored areas. Because these paler patches cannot tan and will burn, you should avoid exposing them to the sun (*see* PROTECTING YOURSELF FROM THE SUN, opposite).

Do you have several small patches of paler skin affecting only your back and/or chest? NO / YES

POSSIBLE CAUSE AND ACTION This is probably a halo nevus, which occurs when pigment disappears from a mole. Eventually the mole may disappear completely, and skin color will return to normal. No treatment is necessary, but consult your doctor if you are concerned.

POSSIBLE CAUSE This may be due to pityriasis versicolor, a minor fungal skin infection.

ACTION This condition is harmless and does not need treatment. However, if you are concerned about its appearance, consult your doctor, who may advise you to use an over-the-counter *antifungal* shampoo on the body as a lotion. Your skin color may take several weeks to return to normal after treatment.

Skin cancer

Skin cancer is the most common form of cancer worldwide. It is usually caused by exposure to ultraviolet rays in sunlight. Fair-skinned people are particularly at risk. There are three main types of skin cancer: basal cell carcinoma, squamous cell carcinoma, and malignant melanoma. All three can usually be cured by surgical removal if they are diagnosed at an early stage.

Basal cell carcinoma
This is the most common type of skin cancer but the least dangerous because it very rarely spreads to other parts of the body. A typical lesion develops as a small, painless lump of a pink to brownish-gray color with a waxy or pearl-like border. It may form a shallow ulcer.

Squamous cell carcinoma
Another common skin cancer is squamous cell carcinoma. It often affects the face, taking the form of a hard, painless, slowly enlarging lump with an irregular edge. It is red or reddish brown and may form a nonhealing ulcer.

Malignant melanoma
This serious form of cancer can spread and may be fatal if not treated early. A new mole or a fast-growing, irregularly shaped, unevenly colored, itchy, or bleeding mole may be malignant and needs urgent attention.

Malignant melanoma
The uneven color and irregular edges of this growth are characteristic of a malignant melanoma.

Do you have a pale area of skin surrounding a mole? NO / YES

CONSULT YOUR DOCTOR IF YOU ARE UNABLE TO MAKE A DIAGNOSIS FROM THIS CHART.

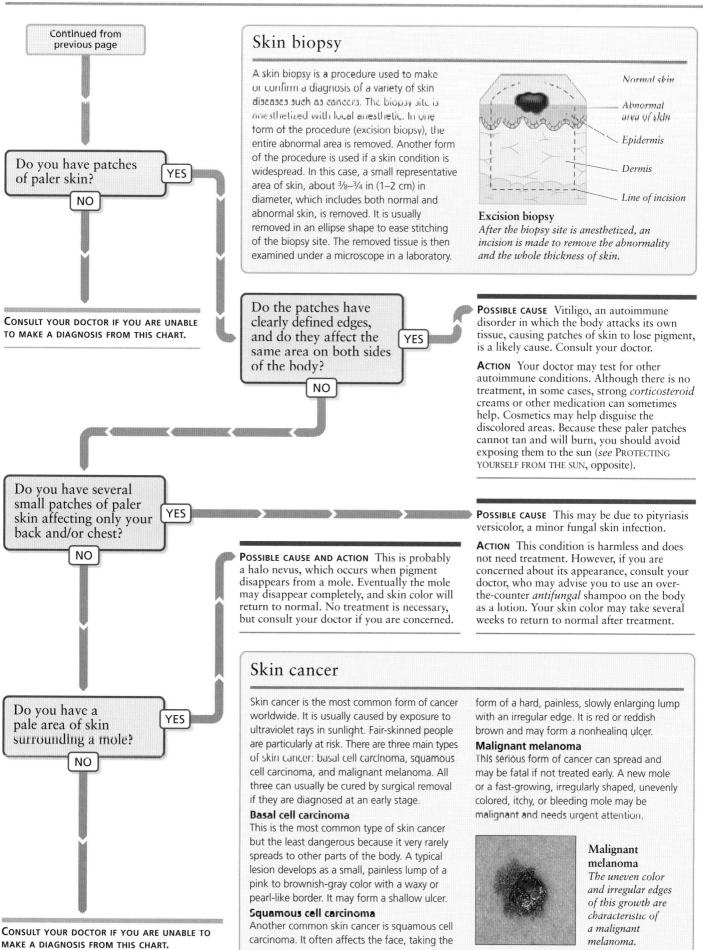

80 Rash with fever

Consult this chart if you have a widespread rash or discolored areas of skin and a temperature of 100.4°F (38°C) or above, since you may have an infectious disease. These diseases are more likely to cause complications in adults than children. To find out if you have a fever, measure your temperature with a thermometer (*see* MANAGING A FEVER, p.154).

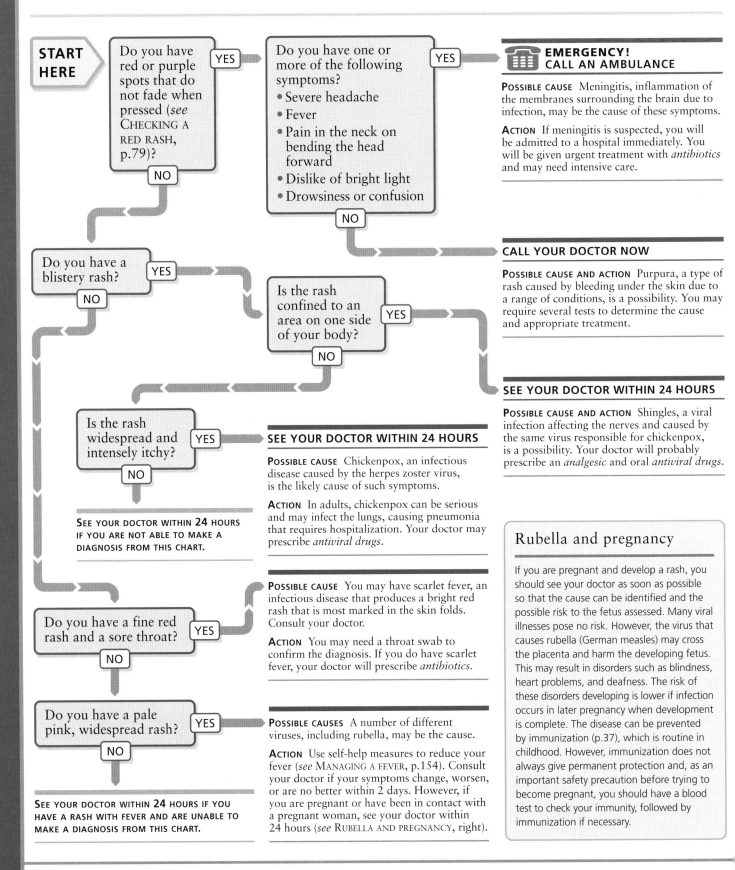

START HERE

Do you have red or purple spots that do not fade when pressed (*see* CHECKING A RED RASH, p.79)? — YES → **Do you have one or more of the following symptoms?**
- Severe headache
- Fever
- Pain in the neck on bending the head forward
- Dislike of bright light
- Drowsiness or confusion

YES →

📞 EMERGENCY! CALL AN AMBULANCE

POSSIBLE CAUSE Meningitis, inflammation of the membranes surrounding the brain due to infection, may be the cause of these symptoms.

ACTION If meningitis is suspected, you will be admitted to a hospital immediately. You will be given urgent treatment with *antibiotics* and may need intensive care.

NO ↓ (from symptoms box)

CALL YOUR DOCTOR NOW

POSSIBLE CAUSE AND ACTION Purpura, a type of rash caused by bleeding under the skin due to a range of conditions, is a possibility. You may require several tests to determine the cause and appropriate treatment.

Do you have a blistery rash? — YES → **Is the rash confined to an area on one side of your body?** — YES →

SEE YOUR DOCTOR WITHIN 24 HOURS

POSSIBLE CAUSE AND ACTION Shingles, a viral infection affecting the nerves and caused by the same virus responsible for chickenpox, is a possibility. Your doctor will probably prescribe an *analgesic* and oral *antiviral drugs*.

NO (blistery rash) ↓

NO (rash confined) ↓

Is the rash widespread and intensely itchy? — YES →

SEE YOUR DOCTOR WITHIN 24 HOURS

POSSIBLE CAUSE Chickenpox, an infectious disease caused by the herpes zoster virus, is the likely cause of such symptoms.

ACTION In adults, chickenpox can be serious and may infect the lungs, causing pneumonia that requires hospitalization. Your doctor may prescribe *antiviral drugs*.

NO ↓

SEE YOUR DOCTOR WITHIN 24 HOURS IF YOU ARE NOT ABLE TO MAKE A DIAGNOSIS FROM THIS CHART.

Do you have a fine red rash and a sore throat? — YES →

POSSIBLE CAUSE You may have scarlet fever, an infectious disease that produces a bright red rash that is most marked in the skin folds. Consult your doctor.

ACTION You may need a throat swab to confirm the diagnosis. If you do have scarlet fever, your doctor will prescribe *antibiotics*.

NO ↓

Do you have a pale pink, widespread rash? — YES →

POSSIBLE CAUSES A number of different viruses, including rubella, may be the cause.

ACTION Use self-help measures to reduce your fever (*see* MANAGING A FEVER, p.154). Consult your doctor if your symptoms change, worsen, or are no better within 2 days. However, if you are pregnant or have been in contact with a pregnant woman, see your doctor within 24 hours (*see* RUBELLA AND PREGNANCY, right).

NO ↓

SEE YOUR DOCTOR WITHIN 24 HOURS IF YOU HAVE A RASH WITH FEVER AND ARE UNABLE TO MAKE A DIAGNOSIS FROM THIS CHART.

Rubella and pregnancy

If you are pregnant and develop a rash, you should see your doctor as soon as possible so that the cause can be identified and the possible risk to the fetus assessed. Many viral illnesses pose no risk. However, the virus that causes rubella (German measles) may cross the placenta and harm the developing fetus. This may result in disorders such as blindness, heart problems, and deafness. The risk of these disorders developing is lower if infection occurs in later pregnancy when development is complete. The disease can be prevented by immunization (p.37), which is routine in childhood. However, immunization does not always give permanent protection and, as an important safety precaution before trying to become pregnant, you should have a blood test to check your immunity, followed by immunization if necessary.

81 Nail problems

Nails are made of hard, dead tissue called keratin, which protects the sensitive tips of the fingers and toes from damage. Common problems affecting the nails include distortion of the nail and painful or inflamed skin around the nail. The most common causes of misshapen nails are injury and fungal infections. However, most widespread skin conditions, including psoriasis and eczema, can also affect the growth and appearance of the nails. Since it takes between 6 months and 1 year for a nail to replace itself, treatment for nail problems often needs to be continued for some time.

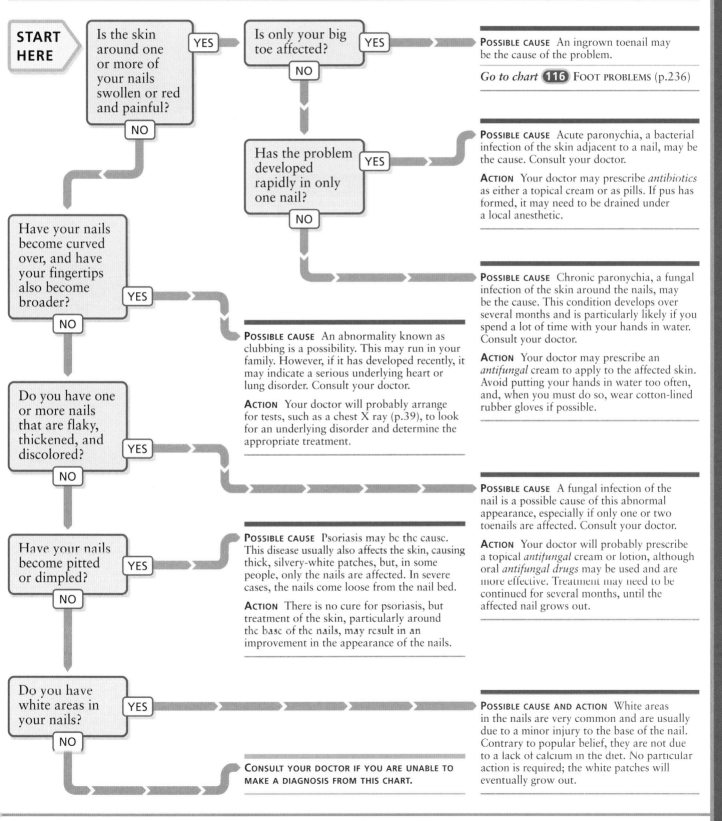

START HERE

Is the skin around one or more of your nails swollen or red and painful?
YES → **Is only your big toe affected?**
YES →

POSSIBLE CAUSE An ingrown toenail may be the cause of the problem.

Go to chart **116** FOOT PROBLEMS (p.236)

Is only your big toe affected? NO →
Has the problem developed rapidly in only one nail? YES →

POSSIBLE CAUSE Acute paronychia, a bacterial infection of the skin adjacent to a nail, may be the cause. Consult your doctor.

ACTION Your doctor may prescribe *antibiotics* as either a topical cream or as pills. If pus has formed, it may need to be drained under a local anesthetic.

Has the problem developed rapidly in only one nail? NO →

POSSIBLE CAUSE Chronic paronychia, a fungal infection of the skin around the nails, may be the cause. This condition develops over several months and is particularly likely if you spend a lot of time with your hands in water. Consult your doctor.

ACTION Your doctor may prescribe an *antifungal* cream to apply to the affected skin. Avoid putting your hands in water too often, and, when you must do so, wear cotton-lined rubber gloves if possible.

Is the skin around one or more of your nails swollen or red and painful? NO →
Have your nails become curved over, and have your fingertips also become broader? YES →

POSSIBLE CAUSE An abnormality known as clubbing is a possibility. This may run in your family. However, if it has developed recently, it may indicate a serious underlying heart or lung disorder. Consult your doctor.

ACTION Your doctor will probably arrange for tests, such as a chest X ray (p.39), to look for an underlying disorder and determine the appropriate treatment.

Have your nails become curved over...? NO →
Do you have one or more nails that are flaky, thickened, and discolored? YES →

POSSIBLE CAUSE A fungal infection of the nail is a possible cause of this abnormal appearance, especially if only one or two toenails are affected. Consult your doctor.

ACTION Your doctor will probably prescribe a topical *antifungal* cream or lotion, although oral *antifungal drugs* may be used and are more effective. Treatment may need to be continued for several months, until the affected nail grows out.

Do you have one or more nails that are flaky...? NO →
Have your nails become pitted or dimpled? YES →

POSSIBLE CAUSE Psoriasis may be the cause. This disease usually also affects the skin, causing thick, silvery-white patches, but, in some people, only the nails are affected. In severe cases, the nails come loose from the nail bed.

ACTION There is no cure for psoriasis, but treatment of the skin, particularly around the base of the nails, may result in an improvement in the appearance of the nails.

Have your nails become pitted or dimpled? NO →
Do you have white areas in your nails? YES →

POSSIBLE CAUSE AND ACTION White areas in the nails are very common and are usually due to a minor injury to the base of the nail. Contrary to popular belief, they are not due to a lack of calcium in the diet. No particular action is required; the white patches will eventually grow out.

Do you have white areas in your nails? NO →

CONSULT YOUR DOCTOR IF YOU ARE UNABLE TO MAKE A DIAGNOSIS FROM THIS CHART.

82 Painful or irritated eye

For blurred vision, see chart 83, DISTURBED OR IMPAIRED VISION (p.188).

In most cases, a painful or irritated eye is due to a relatively minor problem and, unless you wear contact lenses, may not need professional attention. However, an eye problem that persists or impairs vision should always be seen by a doctor. A red, painless area in the white of the eye is probably a burst blood vessel and should clear up on its own.

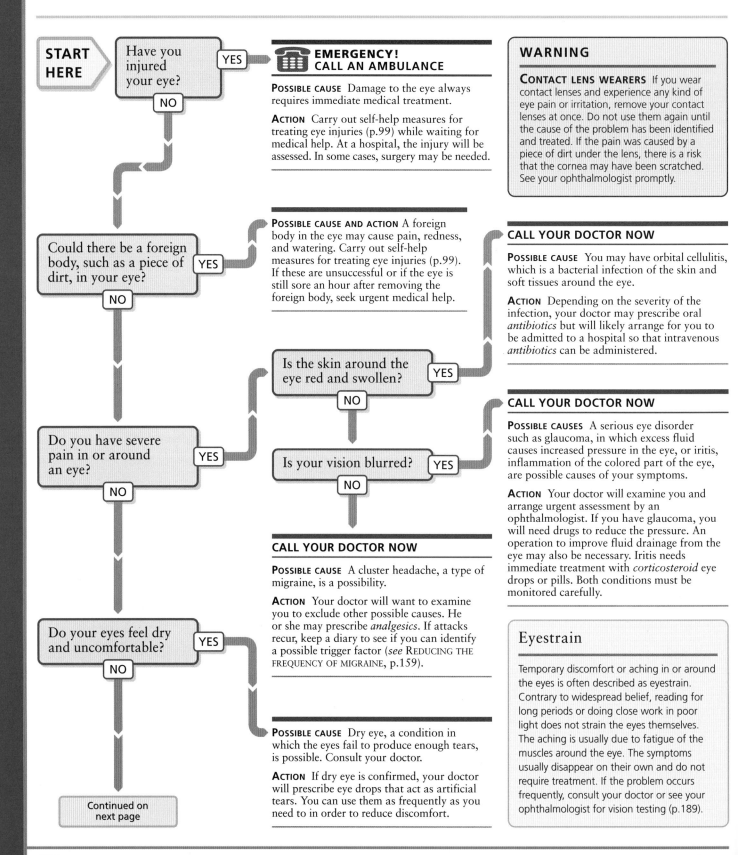

START HERE

Have you injured your eye? — YES →

📞 EMERGENCY! CALL AN AMBULANCE

POSSIBLE CAUSE Damage to the eye always requires immediate medical treatment.

ACTION Carry out self-help measures for treating eye injuries (p.99) while waiting for medical help. At a hospital, the injury will be assessed. In some cases, surgery may be needed.

NO ↓

Could there be a foreign body, such as a piece of dirt, in your eye? — YES →

POSSIBLE CAUSE AND ACTION A foreign body in the eye may cause pain, redness, and watering. Carry out self-help measures for treating eye injuries (p.99). If these are unsuccessful or if the eye is still sore an hour after removing the foreign body, seek urgent medical help.

NO ↓

Do you have severe pain in or around an eye? — YES →

Is the skin around the eye red and swollen? — YES →

CALL YOUR DOCTOR NOW

POSSIBLE CAUSE You may have orbital cellulitis, which is a bacterial infection of the skin and soft tissues around the eye.

ACTION Depending on the severity of the infection, your doctor may prescribe oral *antibiotics* but will likely arrange for you to be admitted to a hospital so that intravenous *antibiotics* can be administered.

NO ↓

Is your vision blurred? — YES →

CALL YOUR DOCTOR NOW

POSSIBLE CAUSES A serious eye disorder such as glaucoma, in which excess fluid causes increased pressure in the eye, or iritis, inflammation of the colored part of the eye, are possible causes of your symptoms.

ACTION Your doctor will examine you and arrange urgent assessment by an ophthalmologist. If you have glaucoma, you will need drugs to reduce the pressure. An operation to improve fluid drainage from the eye may also be necessary. Iritis needs immediate treatment with *corticosteroid* eye drops or pills. Both conditions must be monitored carefully.

NO ↓

CALL YOUR DOCTOR NOW

POSSIBLE CAUSE A cluster headache, a type of migraine, is a possibility.

ACTION Your doctor will want to examine you to exclude other possible causes. He or she may prescribe *analgesics*. If attacks recur, keep a diary to see if you can identify a possible trigger factor (*see* REDUCING THE FREQUENCY OF MIGRAINE, p.159).

NO ↓

Do your eyes feel dry and uncomfortable? — YES →

POSSIBLE CAUSE Dry eye, a condition in which the eyes fail to produce enough tears, is possible. Consult your doctor.

ACTION If dry eye is confirmed, your doctor will prescribe eye drops that act as artificial tears. You can use them as frequently as you need to in order to reduce discomfort.

NO ↓

Continued on next page

WARNING

CONTACT LENS WEARERS If you wear contact lenses and experience any kind of eye pain or irritation, remove your contact lenses at once. Do not use them again until the cause of the problem has been identified and treated. If the pain was caused by a piece of dirt under the lens, there is a risk that the cornea may have been scratched. See your ophthalmologist promptly.

Eyestrain

Temporary discomfort or aching in or around the eyes is often described as eyestrain. Contrary to widespread belief, reading for long periods or doing close work in poor light does not strain the eyes themselves. The aching is usually due to fatigue of the muscles around the eye. The symptoms usually disappear on their own and do not require treatment. If the problem occurs frequently, consult your doctor or see your ophthalmologist for vision testing (p.189).

Continued from previous page

Do you have bloodshot eyes with or without a sticky discharge? — YES / NO

Do you have a problem with one or more of your eyelids? — YES / NO

CONSULT YOUR DOCTOR IF YOU ARE UNABLE TO MAKE A DIAGNOSIS FROM THIS CHART.

Is an eyelid turned inward or outward? — YES / NO

CONSULT YOUR DOCTOR IF YOU ARE UNABLE TO MAKE A DIAGNOSIS FROM THIS CHART.

SELF-HELP Avoiding contact lens problems

Most people who wear contact lenses to correct their vision and have few problems with them. If your eyes become irritated during or after wearing contact lenses, you may have an allergy to the cleaning or soaking solutions. To prevent potentially serious eye infections, use strict hygiene when cleaning nondisposable lenses and never moisten contact lenses with saliva. If not treated promptly, an infection may result in permanent damage to your vision. If you wear contact lenses, always consult your pharmacist before using any over-the-counter eyedrops because some may be incompatible with contact lenses.

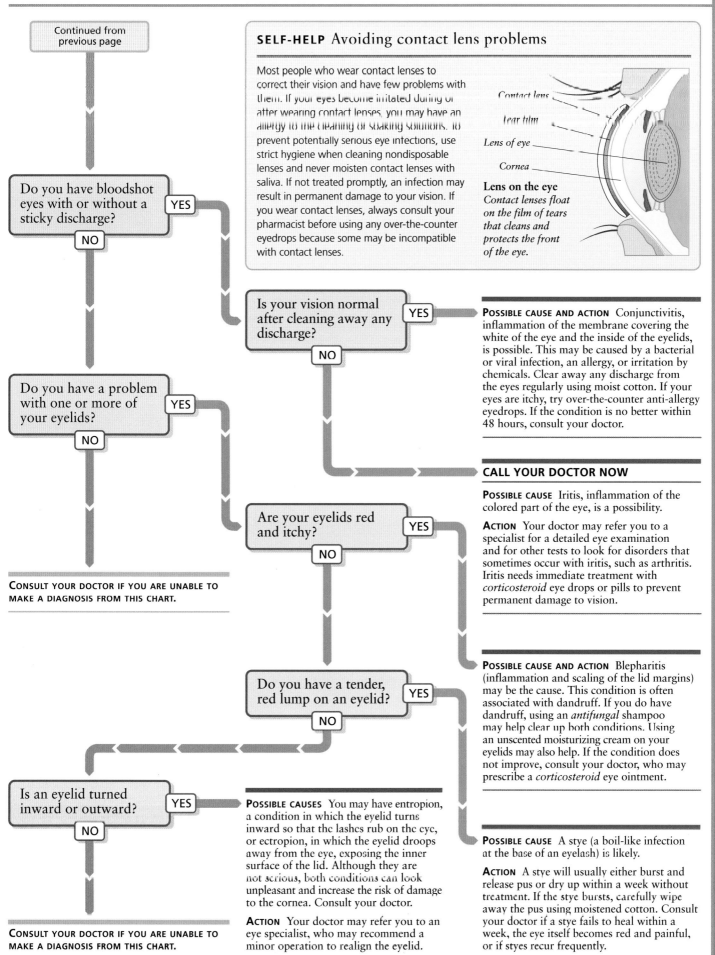

Contact lens
Tear film
Lens of eye
Cornea

Lens on the eye
Contact lenses float on the film of tears that cleans and protects the front of the eye.

Is your vision normal after cleaning away any discharge? — YES / NO

POSSIBLE CAUSE AND ACTION Conjunctivitis, inflammation of the membrane covering the white of the eye and the inside of the eyelids, is possible. This may be caused by a bacterial or viral infection, an allergy, or irritation by chemicals. Clear away any discharge from the eyes regularly using moist cotton. If your eyes are itchy, try over-the-counter anti-allergy eyedrops. If the condition is no better within 48 hours, consult your doctor.

CALL YOUR DOCTOR NOW

POSSIBLE CAUSE Iritis, inflammation of the colored part of the eye, is a possibility.

ACTION Your doctor may refer you to a specialist for a detailed eye examination and for other tests to look for disorders that sometimes occur with iritis, such as arthritis. Iritis needs immediate treatment with *corticosteroid* eye drops or pills to prevent permanent damage to vision.

Are your eyelids red and itchy? — YES / NO

POSSIBLE CAUSE AND ACTION Blepharitis (inflammation and scaling of the lid margins) may be the cause. This condition is often associated with dandruff. If you do have dandruff, using an *antifungal* shampoo may help clear up both conditions. Using an unscented moisturizing cream on your eyelids may also help. If the condition does not improve, consult your doctor, who may prescribe a *corticosteroid* eye ointment.

Do you have a tender, red lump on an eyelid? — YES / NO

POSSIBLE CAUSES You may have entropion, a condition in which the eyelid turns inward so that the lashes rub on the eye, or ectropion, in which the eyelid droops away from the eye, exposing the inner surface of the lid. Although they are not serious, both conditions can look unpleasant and increase the risk of damage to the cornea. Consult your doctor.

ACTION Your doctor may refer you to an eye specialist, who may recommend a minor operation to realign the eyelid.

POSSIBLE CAUSE A stye (a boil-like infection at the base of an eyelash) is likely.

ACTION A stye will usually either burst and release pus or dry up within a week without treatment. If the stye bursts, carefully wipe away the pus using moistened cotton. Consult your doctor if a stye fails to heal within a week, the eye itself becomes red and painful, or if styes recur frequently.

83 Disturbed or impaired vision

This chart deals with any change in your vision, including blurring, double vision, seeing flashing lights or floating spots, and loss of part or all of your field of vision. Any such change in vision should be brought to your doctor's attention to rule out the possibility of a serious nervous system or eye disorder, some of which could damage your sight. Successful treatment of many of these disorders may depend on detecting the disease in its early stages.

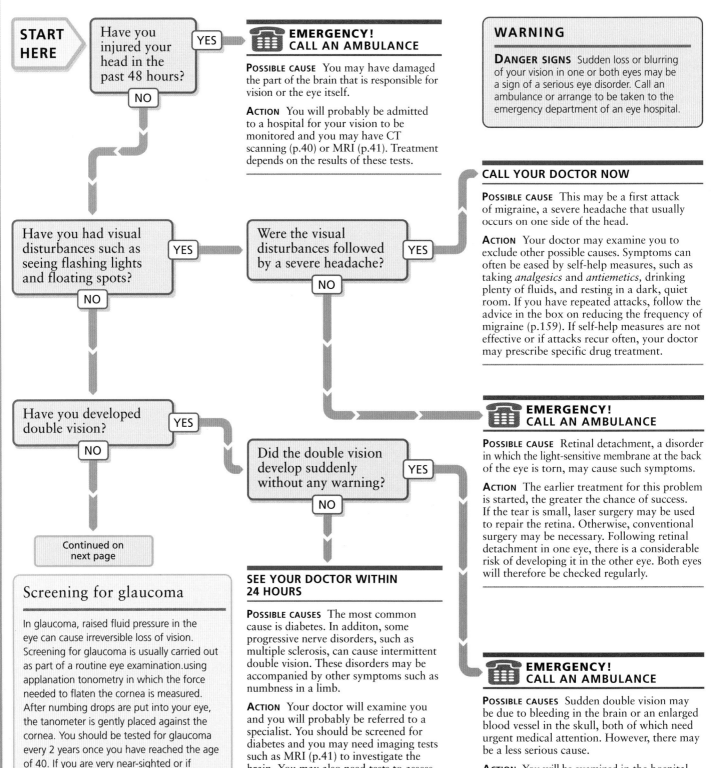

START HERE

Have you injured your head in the past 48 hours? — YES

NO

☎ EMERGENCY! CALL AN AMBULANCE

POSSIBLE CAUSE You may have damaged the part of the brain that is responsible for vision or the eye itself.

ACTION You will probably be admitted to a hospital for your vision to be monitored and you may have CT scanning (p.40) or MRI (p.41). Treatment depends on the results of these tests.

Have you had visual disturbances such as seeing flashing lights and floating spots? — YES

NO

Were the visual disturbances followed by a severe headache? — YES

NO

CALL YOUR DOCTOR NOW

POSSIBLE CAUSE This may be a first attack of migraine, a severe headache that usually occurs on one side of the head.

ACTION Your doctor may examine you to exclude other possible causes. Symptoms can often be eased by self-help measures, such as taking *analgesics* and *antiemetics,* drinking plenty of fluids, and resting in a dark, quiet room. If you have repeated attacks, follow the advice in the box on reducing the frequency of migraine (p.159). If self-help measures are not effective or if attacks recur often, your doctor may prescribe specific drug treatment.

Have you developed double vision? — YES

NO

Did the double vision develop suddenly without any warning? — YES

NO

☎ EMERGENCY! CALL AN AMBULANCE

POSSIBLE CAUSE Retinal detachment, a disorder in which the light-sensitive membrane at the back of the eye is torn, may cause such symptoms.

ACTION The earlier treatment for this problem is started, the greater the chance of success. If the tear is small, laser surgery may be used to repair the retina. Otherwise, conventional surgery may be necessary. Following retinal detachment in one eye, there is a considerable risk of developing it in the other eye. Both eyes will therefore be checked regularly.

Continued on next page

SEE YOUR DOCTOR WITHIN 24 HOURS

POSSIBLE CAUSES The most common cause is diabetes. In additon, some progressive nerve disorders, such as multiple sclerosis, can cause intermittent double vision. These disorders may be accompanied by other symptoms such as numbness in a limb.

ACTION Your doctor will examine you and you will probably be referred to a specialist. You should be screened for diabetes and you may need imaging tests such as MRI (p.41) to investigate the brain. You may also need tests to assess the optic nerves supplying the eyes. Treatment depends on the results.

☎ EMERGENCY! CALL AN AMBULANCE

POSSIBLE CAUSES Sudden double vision may be due to bleeding in the brain or an enlarged blood vessel in the skull, both of which need urgent medical attention. However, there may be a less serious cause.

ACTION You will be examined in the hospital and may have CT scanning (p.40) to look for the cause and determine the appropriate treatment.

WARNING

DANGER SIGNS Sudden loss or blurring of your vision in one or both eyes may be a sign of a serious eye disorder. Call an ambulance or arrange to be taken to the emergency department of an eye hospital.

Screening for glaucoma

In glaucoma, raised fluid pressure in the eye can cause irreversible loss of vision. Screening for glaucoma is usually carried out as part of a routine eye examination.using applanation tonometry in which the force needed to flaten the cornea is measured. After numbing drops are put into your eye, the tanometer is gently placed against the cornea. You should be tested for glaucoma every 2 years once you have reached the age of 40. If you are very near-sighted or if glaucoma runs in your family, testing should start at an earlier age.

Continued from previous page

Vision testing

You should have your vision tested every 2 years, especially once you are over 40. The most common test gauges the sharpness of your distance vision by assessing how well you can read letters lined up in decreasing size on a Snellen chart. Your ability to focus on near objects may also be measured by asking you to read very small print on a chart held at normal reading distance. These tests show if you need corrective lenses, and which ones. In addition, your ophthalmologist will examine your eyes to look for disorders such as diabetes and high blood pressure, which can cause changes in the back of the eye, sometimes before general symptoms develop. You may also be tested for glaucoma (*see* SCREENING FOR GLAUCOMA, opposite).

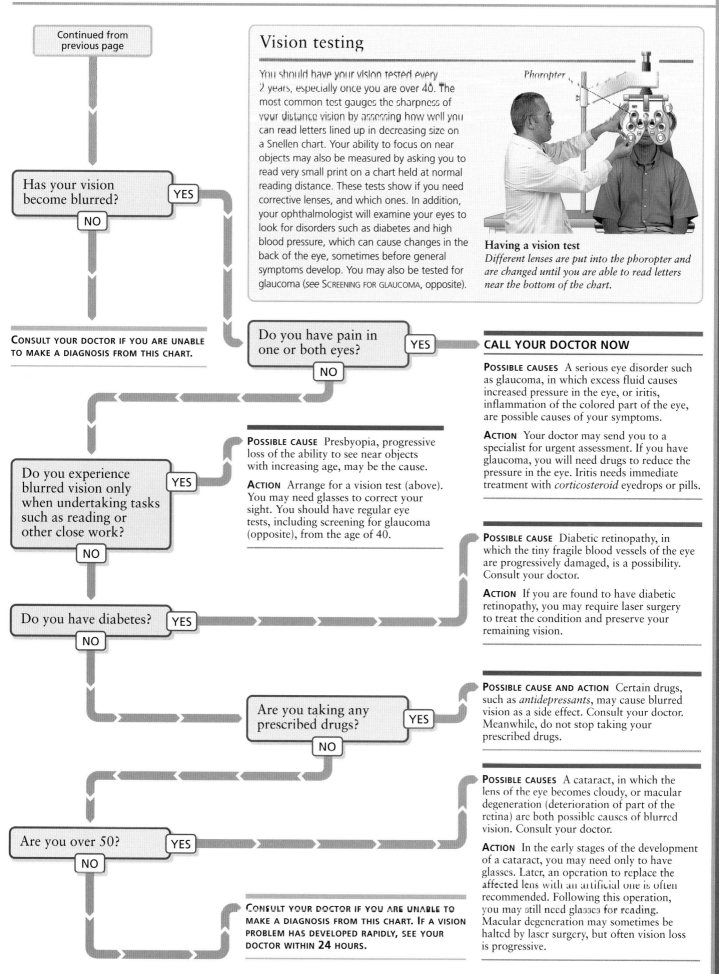

Phoropter

Having a vision test
Different lenses are put into the phoropter and are changed until you are able to read letters near the bottom of the chart.

Has your vision become blurred? — YES / NO

CONSULT YOUR DOCTOR IF YOU ARE UNABLE TO MAKE A DIAGNOSIS FROM THIS CHART.

Do you have pain in one or both eyes? — YES / NO

CALL YOUR DOCTOR NOW

POSSIBLE CAUSES A serious eye disorder such as glaucoma, in which excess fluid causes increased pressure in the eye, or iritis, inflammation of the colored part of the eye, are possible causes of your symptoms.

ACTION Your doctor may send you to a specialist for urgent assessment. If you have glaucoma, you will need drugs to reduce the pressure in the eye. Iritis needs immediate treatment with *corticosteroid* eyedrops or pills.

Do you experience blurred vision only when undertaking tasks such as reading or other close work? — YES / NO

POSSIBLE CAUSE Presbyopia, progressive loss of the ability to see near objects with increasing age, may be the cause.

ACTION Arrange for a vision test (above). You may need glasses to correct your sight. You should have regular eye tests, including screening for glaucoma (opposite), from the age of 40.

POSSIBLE CAUSE Diabetic retinopathy, in which the tiny fragile blood vessels of the eye are progressively damaged, is a possibility. Consult your doctor.

ACTION If you are found to have diabetic retinopathy, you may require laser surgery to treat the condition and preserve your remaining vision.

Do you have diabetes? — YES / NO

Are you taking any prescribed drugs? — YES / NO

POSSIBLE CAUSE AND ACTION Certain drugs, such as *antidepressants*, may cause blurred vision as a side effect. Consult your doctor. Meanwhile, do not stop taking your prescribed drugs.

POSSIBLE CAUSES A cataract, in which the lens of the eye becomes cloudy, or macular degeneration (deterioration of part of the retina) are both possible causes of blurred vision. Consult your doctor.

ACTION In the early stages of the development of a cataract, you may need only to have glasses. Later, an operation to replace the affected lens with an artificial one is often recommended. Following this operation, you may still need glasses for reading. Macular degeneration may sometimes be halted by laser surgery, but often vision loss is progressive.

Are you over 50? — YES / NO

CONSULT YOUR DOCTOR IF YOU ARE UNABLE TO MAKE A DIAGNOSIS FROM THIS CHART. IF A VISION PROBLEM HAS DEVELOPED RAPIDLY, SEE YOUR DOCTOR WITHIN **24** HOURS.

84 Hearing problems

Deterioration in the ability to hear some or all sounds may come on gradually over a period of several months or years or may occur suddenly over a matter of hours or days. In many cases, hearing loss is the result of an ear infection or a wax blockage and can be treated easily. Hearing loss is also a common feature of aging. However, if you suddenly develop severe hearing loss in one or both ears for no obvious reason, always consult your doctor.

START HERE

Do you have an earache?

YES → *Go to chart* **86** EARACHE (p.193)

NO ↓

Did the hearing loss start during or immediately after an airplane flight?

YES →

POSSIBLE CAUSE Barotrauma, damage to the eardrum resulting from a pressure difference between the middle and outer ear is possible, especially if you already had a stuffy nose.

ACTION Try blowing through your nose while pinching the nostrils closed. If the hearing loss persists for more than 24 hours, consult your doctor. Follow the advice on preventing ear problems caused by flying (p.193) in the future.

NO ↓

Is there a discharge from the ear?

YES →

POSSIBLE CAUSE An infection of the outer ear canal, resulting in discharge blocking the canal, may be the cause, particularly if you experience pain when pulling on the earlobe. Consult your doctor.

ACTION Your doctor may prescribe *antibiotic* eardrops for an outer ear infection. If the infection is severe, you may be given oral antibiotics. Your doctor may also clean the ear canal to remove debris.

NO ↓

Have you had a runny or stuffy nose, or a sore throat in the past week?

YES →

POSSIBLE CAUSE A cold or allergic rhinitis may result in blockage of the eustachian tube, which connects the middle ear to the throat. This may account for your hearing problem.

ACTION This is usually no cause for concern and should clear up without treatment within a week. Try steam inhalation (p.194). Consult your doctor if your symptoms do not improve.

NO ↓

Have you experienced attacks of dizziness, during which everything around you seems to spin, and do you also have noises in your ear?

YES →

POSSIBLE CAUSE Ménière's disease may be the problem. This is a relatively uncommon disorder in which there is an increase in the amount of fluid in the inner ear (*see* HOW YOU KEEP YOUR BALANCE, p.162). The problem is most common in middle age. Consult your doctor.

ACTION Your doctor may arrange for tests, including hearing tests (p.190). If you are diagnosed with Ménière's disease, you may be given drug treatment to reduce the amount of fluid in the inner ear.

NO ↓

Continued on next page

Hearing tests

Preliminary hearing tests assess the type of hearing loss you might have.

Audiometry measures the degree of hearing loss. Sounds of increasing volume and at different frequencies are transmitted to one ear at a time through headphones.

Tympanometry shows whether the eardrum moves normally when sounds hit it. A probe with a sound generator, microphone, and air pump is placed in the ear canal. Sounds are played while the air pressure is varied and the pattern of the sound waves reflected by the eardrum is recorded.

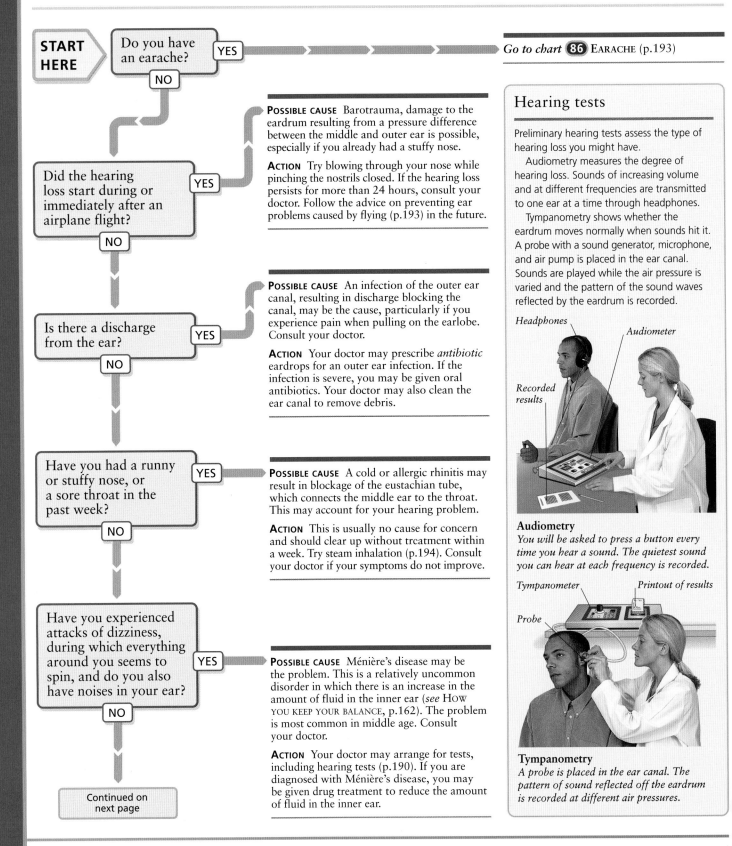

Headphones

Audiometer

Recorded results

Audiometry
You will be asked to press a button every time you hear a sound. The quietest sound you can hear at each frequency is recorded.

Tympanometer *Printout of results*

Probe

Tympanometry
A probe is placed in the ear canal. The pattern of sound reflected off the eardrum is recorded at different air pressures.

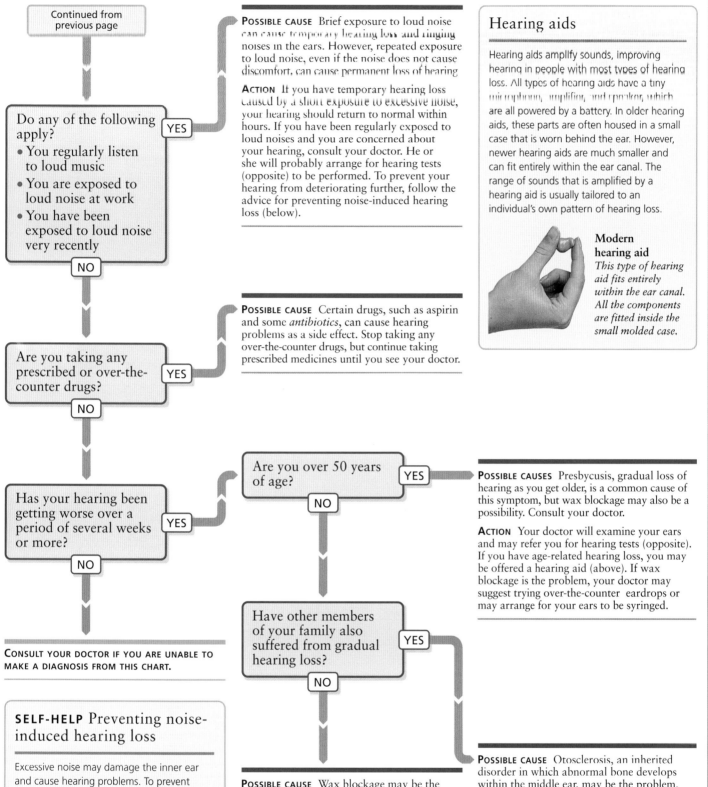

Continued from previous page

Do any of the following apply?
- You regularly listen to loud music
- You are exposed to loud noise at work
- You have been exposed to loud noise very recently

YES →

POSSIBLE CAUSE Brief exposure to loud noise can cause temporary hearing loss and ringing noises in the ears. However, repeated exposure to loud noise, even if the noise does not cause discomfort, can cause permanent loss of hearing.

ACTION If you have temporary hearing loss caused by a short exposure to excessive noise, your hearing should return to normal within hours. If you have been regularly exposed to loud noises and you are concerned about your hearing, consult your doctor. He or she will probably arrange for hearing tests (opposite) to be performed. To prevent your hearing from deteriorating further, follow the advice for preventing noise-induced hearing loss (below).

NO ↓

Are you taking any prescribed or over-the-counter drugs?

YES →

POSSIBLE CAUSE Certain drugs, such as aspirin and some *antibiotics*, can cause hearing problems as a side effect. Stop taking any over-the-counter drugs, but continue taking prescribed medicines until you see your doctor.

NO ↓

Has your hearing been getting worse over a period of several weeks or more?

YES →

Are you over 50 years of age?

YES →

POSSIBLE CAUSES Presbycusis, gradual loss of hearing as you get older, is a common cause of this symptom, but wax blockage may also be a possibility. Consult your doctor.

ACTION Your doctor will examine your ears and may refer you for hearing tests (opposite). If you have age-related hearing loss, you may be offered a hearing aid (above). If wax blockage is the problem, your doctor may suggest trying over-the-counter eardrops or may arrange for your ears to be syringed.

NO ↓

Have other members of your family also suffered from gradual hearing loss?

YES →

NO ↓

NO ↓

CONSULT YOUR DOCTOR IF YOU ARE UNABLE TO MAKE A DIAGNOSIS FROM THIS CHART.

Hearing aids

Hearing aids amplify sounds, improving hearing in people with most types of hearing loss. All types of hearing aids have a tiny microphone, amplifier, and speaker, which are all powered by a battery. In older hearing aids, these parts are often housed in a small case that is worn behind the ear. However, newer hearing aids are much smaller and can fit entirely within the ear canal. The range of sounds that is amplified by a hearing aid is usually tailored to an individual's own pattern of hearing loss.

Modern hearing aid
This type of hearing aid fits entirely within the ear canal. All the components are fitted inside the small molded case.

SELF-HELP Preventing noise-induced hearing loss

Excessive noise may damage the inner ear and cause hearing problems. To prevent such problems, avoid exposure to loud noise whenever possible. For example, do not listen to very loud music, especially through headphones. If you do listen to music through headphones, make sure that the volume is low enough for you to hear conversation above the music. If you are exposed to loud noise at work, always wear ear protectors or ear plugs. These should be provided by your employer to protect you.

POSSIBLE CAUSE Wax blockage may be the cause of your hearing problem.

ACTION To remove ear wax yourself, soften it with over-the-counter eardrops or olive oil for several days. Then try to wash the wax out while in a warm shower. Do not insert anything, such as cotton swabs, into the ear because this may make the blockage worse and may damage the eardrum. If you cannot remove the wax, consult your doctor, who will probably arrange for your ear to be washed out with water in a syringe.

POSSIBLE CAUSE Otosclerosis, an inherited disorder in which abnormal bone develops within the middle ear, may be the problem. This type of deafness can affect young adults and is more common in women. It may get worse during pregnancy. Consult your doctor.

ACTION If your doctor suspects otosclerosis, he or she will probably arrange for you to undergo hearing tests (opposite). Treatment is often initially with a hearing aid. In some cases, an operation known as a stapedectomy is performed. In this procedure, the abnormal bone in the middle ear is removed and then replaced with a prosthesis.

85 Noises in the ear

Hearing noises inside your ear, such as buzzing, ringing, or hissing, is known as tinnitus. Some people have brief episodes of tinnitus that are not due to a serious ear disorder and that clear up without needing medical treatment. Others have persistent tinnitus that is not only distressing but may also indicate an ear problem that should be investigated.

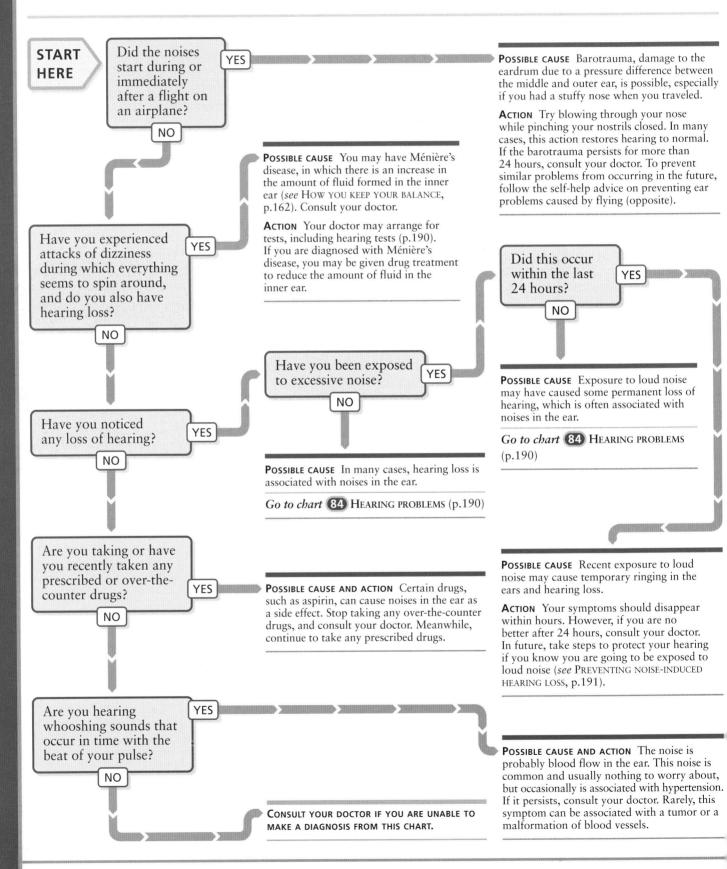

START HERE

Did the noises start during or immediately after a flight on an airplane?

YES →

POSSIBLE CAUSE Barotrauma, damage to the eardrum due to a pressure difference between the middle and outer ear, is possible, especially if you had a stuffy nose when you traveled.

ACTION Try blowing through your nose while pinching your nostrils closed. In many cases, this action restores hearing to normal. If the barotrauma persists for more than 24 hours, consult your doctor. To prevent similar problems from occurring in the future, follow the self-help advice on preventing ear problems caused by flying (opposite).

NO ↓

Have you experienced attacks of dizziness during which everything seems to spin around, and do you also have hearing loss?

YES →

POSSIBLE CAUSE You may have Ménière's disease, in which there is an increase in the amount of fluid formed in the inner ear (*see* HOW YOU KEEP YOUR BALANCE, p.162). Consult your doctor.

ACTION Your doctor may arrange for tests, including hearing tests (p.190). If you are diagnosed with Ménière's disease, you may be given drug treatment to reduce the amount of fluid in the inner ear.

NO ↓

Have you noticed any loss of hearing?

YES →

Have you been exposed to excessive noise?

YES →

Did this occur within the last 24 hours?

YES →

NO ↓

POSSIBLE CAUSE Exposure to loud noise may have caused some permanent loss of hearing, which is often associated with noises in the ear.

Go to chart **84** HEARING PROBLEMS (p.190)

NO ↓

POSSIBLE CAUSE In many cases, hearing loss is associated with noises in the ear.

Go to chart **84** HEARING PROBLEMS (p.190)

POSSIBLE CAUSE Recent exposure to loud noise may cause temporary ringing in the ears and hearing loss.

ACTION Your symptoms should disappear within hours. However, if you are no better after 24 hours, consult your doctor. In future, take steps to protect your hearing if you know you are going to be exposed to loud noise (*see* PREVENTING NOISE-INDUCED HEARING LOSS, p.191).

NO ↓

Are you taking or have you recently taken any prescribed or over-the-counter drugs?

YES →

POSSIBLE CAUSE AND ACTION Certain drugs, such as aspirin, can cause noises in the ear as a side effect. Stop taking any over-the-counter drugs, and consult your doctor. Meanwhile, continue to take any prescribed drugs.

NO ↓

Are you hearing whooshing sounds that occur in time with the beat of your pulse?

YES →

POSSIBLE CAUSE AND ACTION The noise is probably blood flow in the ear. This noise is common and usually nothing to worry about, but occasionally is associated with hypertension. If it persists, consult your doctor. Rarely, this symptom can be associated with a tumor or a malformation of blood vessels.

NO ↓

CONSULT YOUR DOCTOR IF YOU ARE UNABLE TO MAKE A DIAGNOSIS FROM THIS CHART.

86 Earache

Earache may vary from a dull, throbbing sensation to a sharp, severe, stabbing pain. Although it is very common in childhood, it occurs much less frequently in adults. The pain is often due to infection of the ear canal or of the middle ear behind the eardrum. If severe, the pain will require medical attention and, in some cases, **treatment with antibiotics**.

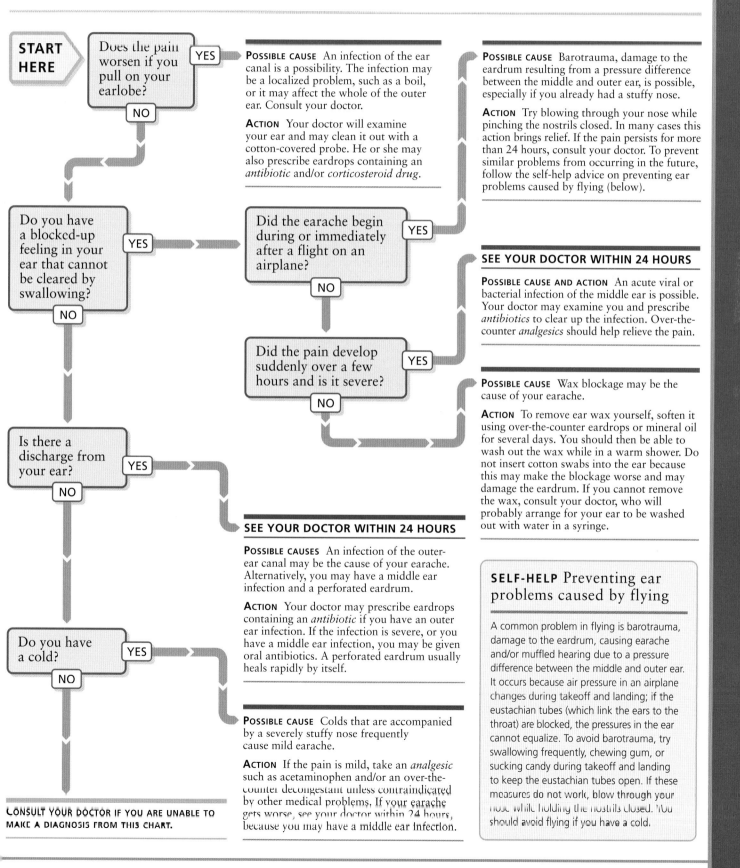

START HERE

Does the pain worsen if you pull on your earlobe? — **YES** →

POSSIBLE CAUSE An infection of the ear canal is a possibility. The infection may be a localized problem, such as a boil, or it may affect the whole of the outer ear. Consult your doctor.

ACTION Your doctor will examine your ear and may clean it out with a cotton-covered probe. He or she may also prescribe eardrops containing an *antibiotic* and/or *corticosteroid drug*.

NO ↓

Do you have a blocked-up feeling in your ear that cannot be cleared by swallowing? — **YES** →

Did the earache begin during or immediately after a flight on an airplane? — **YES** →

POSSIBLE CAUSE Barotrauma, damage to the eardrum resulting from a pressure difference between the middle and outer ear, is possible, especially if you already had a stuffy nose.

ACTION Try blowing through your nose while pinching the nostrils closed. In many cases this action brings relief. If the pain persists for more than 24 hours, consult your doctor. To prevent similar problems from occurring in the future, follow the self-help advice on preventing ear problems caused by flying (below).

NO ↓

Did the pain develop suddenly over a few hours and is it severe? — **YES** →

SEE YOUR DOCTOR WITHIN 24 HOURS

POSSIBLE CAUSE AND ACTION An acute viral or bacterial infection of the middle ear is possible. Your doctor may examine you and prescribe *antibiotics* to clear up the infection. Over-the-counter *analgesics* should help relieve the pain.

NO ↓

POSSIBLE CAUSE Wax blockage may be the cause of your earache.

ACTION To remove ear wax yourself, soften it using over-the-counter eardrops or mineral oil for several days. You should then be able to wash out the wax while in a warm shower. Do not insert cotton swabs into the ear because this may make the blockage worse and may damage the eardrum. If you cannot remove the wax, consult your doctor, who will probably arrange for your ear to be washed out with water in a syringe.

NO ↓

Is there a discharge from your ear? — **YES** →

SEE YOUR DOCTOR WITHIN 24 HOURS

POSSIBLE CAUSES An infection of the outer-ear canal may be the cause of your earache. Alternatively, you may have a middle ear infection and a perforated eardrum.

ACTION Your doctor may prescribe eardrops containing an *antibiotic* if you have an outer ear infection. If the infection is severe, or you have a middle ear infection, you may be given oral antibiotics. A perforated eardrum usually heals rapidly by itself.

NO ↓

Do you have a cold? — **YES** →

POSSIBLE CAUSE Colds that are accompanied by a severely stuffy nose frequently cause mild earache.

ACTION If the pain is mild, take an *analgesic* such as acetaminophen and/or an over-the-counter decongestant unless contraindicated by other medical problems. If your earache gets worse, see your doctor within 24 hours, because you may have a middle ear infection.

NO ↓

CONSULT YOUR DOCTOR IF YOU ARE UNABLE TO MAKE A DIAGNOSIS FROM THIS CHART.

SELF-HELP Preventing ear problems caused by flying

A common problem in flying is barotrauma, damage to the eardrum, causing earache and/or muffled hearing due to a pressure difference between the middle and outer ear. It occurs because air pressure in an airplane changes during takeoff and landing; if the eustachian tubes (which link the ears to the throat) are blocked, the pressures in the ear cannot equalize. To avoid barotrauma, try swallowing frequently, chewing gum, or sucking candy during takeoff and landing to keep the eustachian tubes open. If these measures do not work, blow through your nose while holding the nostrils closed. You should avoid flying if you have a cold.

87 Runny or stuffy nose

Most people have a stuffy or runny nose at least once a year. The usual cause of these symptoms is irritation of the lining of the nose. This irritation can be caused by a viral infection, such as a cold, or it can result from an allergic reaction, such as seasonal allergic rhinitis (hay fever). Nosebleeds (below) may have a specific cause, such as injury or forceful nose blowing, but they may occur spontaneously. They can be serious in people over the age of 50.

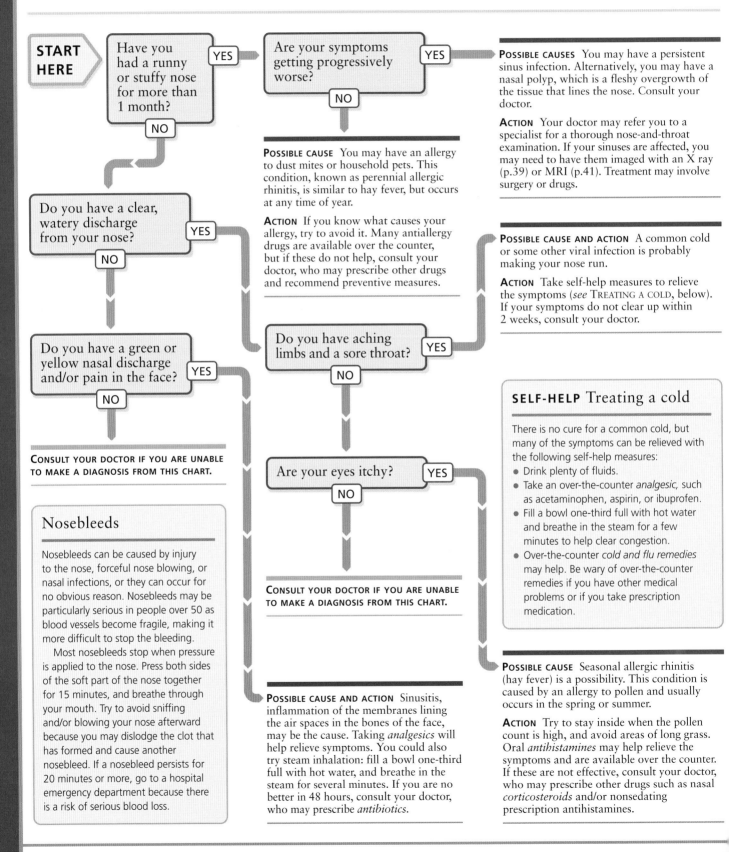

START HERE

Have you had a runny or stuffy nose for more than 1 month?
YES → / NO ↓

Are your symptoms getting progressively worse?
YES → / NO ↓

POSSIBLE CAUSES You may have a persistent sinus infection. Alternatively, you may have a nasal polyp, which is a fleshy overgrowth of the tissue that lines the nose. Consult your doctor.

ACTION Your doctor may refer you to a specialist for a thorough nose-and-throat examination. If your sinuses are affected, you may need to have them imaged with an X ray (p.39) or MRI (p.41). Treatment may involve surgery or drugs.

POSSIBLE CAUSE You may have an allergy to dust mites or household pets. This condition, known as perennial allergic rhinitis, is similar to hay fever, but occurs at any time of year.

ACTION If you know what causes your allergy, try to avoid it. Many antiallergy drugs are available over the counter, but if these do not help, consult your doctor, who may prescribe other drugs and recommend preventive measures.

Do you have a clear, watery discharge from your nose?
YES → / NO ↓

Do you have a green or yellow nasal discharge and/or pain in the face?
YES → / NO ↓

Do you have aching limbs and a sore throat?
YES → / NO ↓

POSSIBLE CAUSE AND ACTION A common cold or some other viral infection is probably making your nose run.

ACTION Take self-help measures to relieve the symptoms (*see* TREATING A COLD, below). If your symptoms do not clear up within 2 weeks, consult your doctor.

CONSULT YOUR DOCTOR IF YOU ARE UNABLE TO MAKE A DIAGNOSIS FROM THIS CHART.

Are your eyes itchy?
YES → / NO ↓

CONSULT YOUR DOCTOR IF YOU ARE UNABLE TO MAKE A DIAGNOSIS FROM THIS CHART.

Nosebleeds

Nosebleeds can be caused by injury to the nose, forceful nose blowing, or nasal infections, or they can occur for no obvious reason. Nosebleeds may be particularly serious in people over 50 as blood vessels become fragile, making it more difficult to stop the bleeding.

Most nosebleeds stop when pressure is applied to the nose. Press both sides of the soft part of the nose together for 15 minutes, and breathe through your mouth. Try to avoid sniffing and/or blowing your nose afterward because you may dislodge the clot that has formed and cause another nosebleed. If a nosebleed persists for 20 minutes or more, go to a hospital emergency department because there is a risk of serious blood loss.

POSSIBLE CAUSE AND ACTION Sinusitis, inflammation of the membranes lining the air spaces in the bones of the face, may be the cause. Taking *analgesics* will help relieve symptoms. You could also try steam inhalation: fill a bowl one-third full with hot water, and breathe in the steam for several minutes. If you are no better in 48 hours, consult your doctor, who may prescribe *antibiotics*.

SELF-HELP Treating a cold

There is no cure for a common cold, but many of the symptoms can be relieved with the following self-help measures:
- Drink plenty of fluids.
- Take an over-the-counter *analgesic*, such as acetaminophen, aspirin, or ibuprofen.
- Fill a bowl one-third full with hot water and breathe in the steam for a few minutes to help clear congestion.
- Over-the-counter *cold and flu remedies* may help. Be wary of over-the-counter remedies if you have other medical problems or if you take prescription medication.

POSSIBLE CAUSE Seasonal allergic rhinitis (hay fever) is a possibility. This condition is caused by an allergy to pollen and usually occurs in the spring or summer.

ACTION Try to stay inside when the pollen count is high, and avoid areas of long grass. Oral *antihistamines* may help relieve the symptoms and are available over the counter. If these are not effective, consult your doctor, who may prescribe other drugs such as nasal *corticosteroids* and/or nonsedating prescription antihistamines.

88 Sore throat

Most people suffer from a painful, rough, or raw feeling in the throat from time to time. A sore throat usually clears up within a few days and is most commonly due to a minor infection, such as a cold, or irritation from smoke. Swallowing something sharp, such as a fishbone, can scratch the throat. The cause of the soreness in this case is usually obvious.

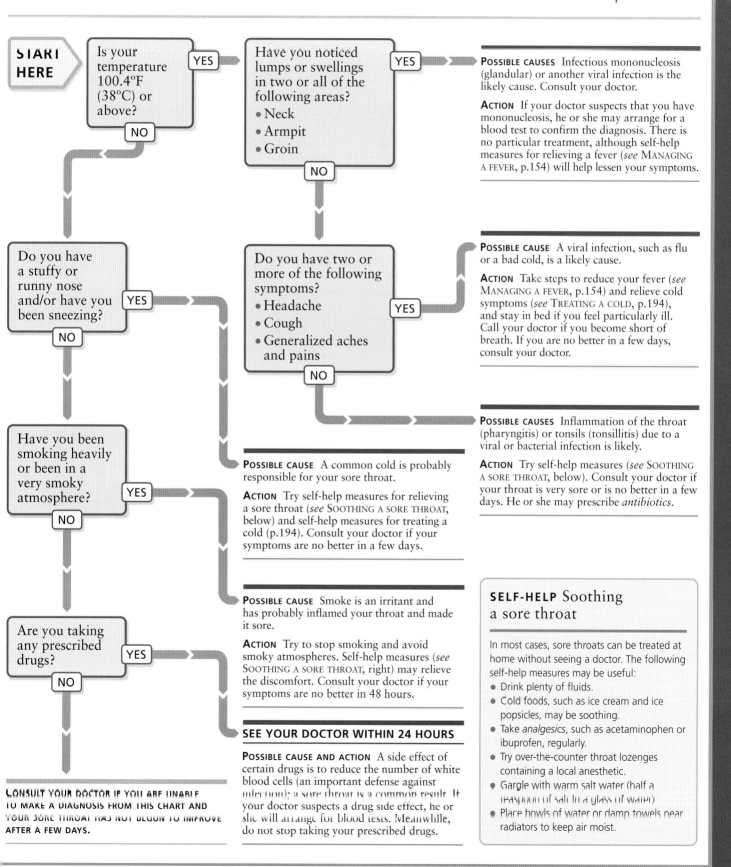

START HERE

Is your temperature 100.4°F (38°C) or above?
YES / NO

Have you noticed lumps or swellings in two or all of the following areas?
- Neck
- Armpit
- Groin

YES / NO

POSSIBLE CAUSES Infectious mononucleosis (glandular) or another viral infection is the likely cause. Consult your doctor.

ACTION If your doctor suspects that you have mononucleosis, he or she may arrange for a blood test to confirm the diagnosis. There is no particular treatment, although self-help measures for relieving a fever (see MANAGING A FEVER, p.154) will help lessen your symptoms.

Do you have a stuffy or runny nose and/or have you been sneezing?
YES / NO

Do you have two or more of the following symptoms?
- Headache
- Cough
- Generalized aches and pains

YES / NO

POSSIBLE CAUSE A viral infection, such as flu or a bad cold, is a likely cause.

ACTION Take steps to reduce your fever (see MANAGING A FEVER, p.154) and relieve cold symptoms (see TREATING A COLD, p.194), and stay in bed if you feel particularly ill. Call your doctor if you become short of breath. If you are no better in a few days, consult your doctor.

Have you been smoking heavily or been in a very smoky atmosphere?
YES / NO

POSSIBLE CAUSE A common cold is probably responsible for your sore throat.

ACTION Try self-help measures for relieving a sore throat (see SOOTHING A SORE THROAT, below) and self-help measures for treating a cold (p.194). Consult your doctor if your symptoms are no better in a few days.

POSSIBLE CAUSES Inflammation of the throat (pharyngitis) or tonsils (tonsillitis) due to a viral or bacterial infection is likely.

ACTION Try self-help measures (see SOOTHING A SORE THROAT, below). Consult your doctor if your throat is very sore or is no better in a few days. He or she may prescribe antibiotics.

POSSIBLE CAUSE Smoke is an irritant and has probably inflamed your throat and made it sore.

ACTION Try to stop smoking and avoid smoky atmospheres. Self-help measures (see SOOTHING A SORE THROAT, right) may relieve the discomfort. Consult your doctor if your symptoms are no better in 48 hours.

Are you taking any prescribed drugs?
YES / NO

SEE YOUR DOCTOR WITHIN 24 HOURS

POSSIBLE CAUSE AND ACTION A side effect of certain drugs is to reduce the number of white blood cells (an important defense against infection); a sore throat is a common result. If your doctor suspects a drug side effect, he or she will arrange for blood tests. Meanwhile, do not stop taking your prescribed drugs.

> **SELF-HELP** Soothing a sore throat
>
> In most cases, sore throats can be treated at home without seeing a doctor. The following self-help measures may be useful:
> - Drink plenty of fluids.
> - Cold foods, such as ice cream and ice popsicles, may be soothing.
> - Take analgesics, such as acetaminophen or ibuprofen, regularly.
> - Try over-the-counter throat lozenges containing a local anesthetic.
> - Gargle with warm salt water (half a teaspoon of salt in a glass of water).
> - Place bowls of water or damp towels near radiators to keep air moist.

CONSULT YOUR DOCTOR IF YOU ARE UNABLE TO MAKE A DIAGNOSIS FROM THIS CHART AND YOUR SORE THROAT HAS NOT BEGUN TO IMPROVE AFTER A FEW DAYS.

89 Hoarseness or loss of voice

Hoarseness, huskiness, or loss of voice is almost always due to laryngitis – inflammation and swelling of the vocal cords. In most cases, the cause of the inflammation is a viral infection or overuse of the voice. Symptoms can be relieved by using self-help measures, and there is no need to consult your doctor. However, persistent or recurrent hoarseness or loss or change of voice may have a serious cause, and, in these cases, you should always consult your doctor.

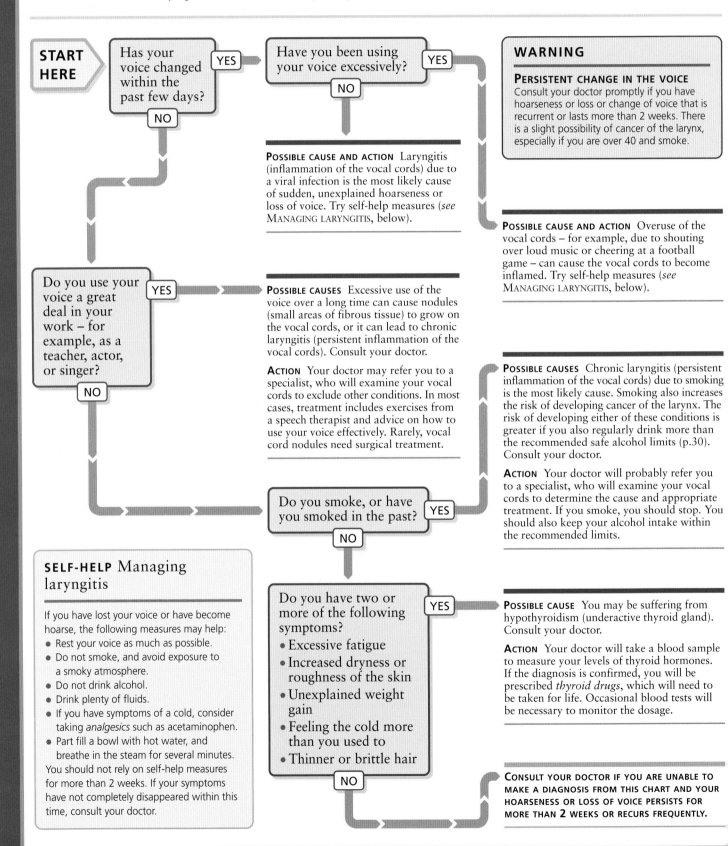

START HERE

Has your voice changed within the past few days? — YES →

Have you been using your voice excessively? — YES →

NO ↓

POSSIBLE CAUSE AND ACTION Laryngitis (inflammation of the vocal cords) due to a viral infection is the most likely cause of sudden, unexplained hoarseness or loss of voice. Try self-help measures (*see* MANAGING LARYNGITIS, below).

NO ↓

Do you use your voice a great deal in your work – for example, as a teacher, actor, or singer? — YES →

POSSIBLE CAUSES Excessive use of the voice over a long time can cause nodules (small areas of fibrous tissue) to grow on the vocal cords, or it can lead to chronic laryngitis (persistent inflammation of the vocal cords). Consult your doctor.

ACTION Your doctor may refer you to a specialist, who will examine your vocal cords to exclude other conditions. In most cases, treatment includes exercises from a speech therapist and advice on how to use your voice effectively. Rarely, vocal cord nodules need surgical treatment.

NO ↓

Do you smoke, or have you smoked in the past? — YES →

NO ↓

Do you have two or more of the following symptoms?
- Excessive fatigue
- Increased dryness or roughness of the skin
- Unexplained weight gain
- Feeling the cold more than you used to
- Thinner or brittle hair

— YES →

NO ↓

WARNING

PERSISTENT CHANGE IN THE VOICE
Consult your doctor promptly if you have hoarseness or loss or change of voice that is recurrent or lasts more than 2 weeks. There is a slight possibility of cancer of the larynx, especially if you are over 40 and smoke.

POSSIBLE CAUSE AND ACTION Overuse of the vocal cords – for example, due to shouting over loud music or cheering at a football game – can cause the vocal cords to become inflamed. Try self-help measures (*see* MANAGING LARYNGITIS, below).

POSSIBLE CAUSES Chronic laryngitis (persistent inflammation of the vocal cords) due to smoking is the most likely cause. Smoking also increases the risk of developing cancer of the larynx. The risk of developing either of these conditions is greater if you also regularly drink more than the recommended safe alcohol limits (p.30). Consult your doctor.

ACTION Your doctor will probably refer you to a specialist, who will examine your vocal cords to determine the cause and appropriate treatment. If you smoke, you should stop. You should also keep your alcohol intake within the recommended limits.

POSSIBLE CAUSE You may be suffering from hypothyroidism (underactive thyroid gland). Consult your doctor.

ACTION Your doctor will take a blood sample to measure your levels of thyroid hormones. If the diagnosis is confirmed, you will be prescribed *thyroid drugs*, which will need to be taken for life. Occasional blood tests will be necessary to monitor the dosage.

SELF-HELP Managing laryngitis

If you have lost your voice or have become hoarse, the following measures may help:
- Rest your voice as much as possible.
- Do not smoke, and avoid exposure to a smoky atmosphere.
- Do not drink alcohol.
- Drink plenty of fluids.
- If you have symptoms of a cold, consider taking *analgesics* such as acetaminophen.
- Part fill a bowl with hot water, and breathe in the steam for several minutes.

You should not rely on self-help measures for more than 2 weeks. If your symptoms have not completely disappeared within this time, consult your doctor.

CONSULT YOUR DOCTOR IF YOU ARE UNABLE TO MAKE A DIAGNOSIS FROM THIS CHART AND YOUR HOARSENESS OR LOSS OF VOICE PERSISTS FOR MORE THAN 2 WEEKS OR RECURS FREQUENTLY.

90 Wheezing

Wheezing is a whistling or rasping sound made when you exhale. It is usually due to narrowing of the airways as a result of inflammation caused by infection, asthma, or smoking. Rarely, wheezing is due to a small foreign body or a tumor partially blocking an airway. If you suddenly start to wheeze or are short of breath, get medical help at once.

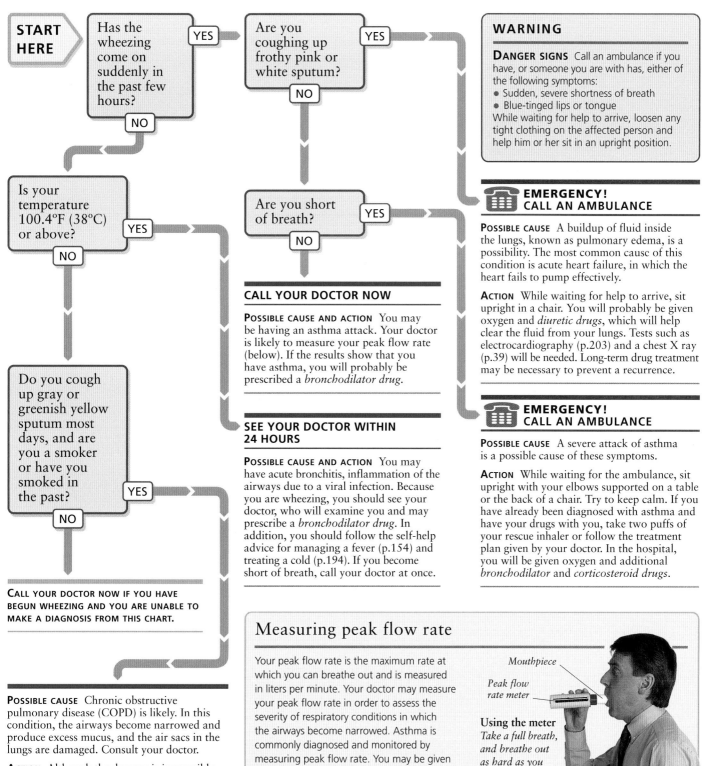

START HERE

Has the wheezing come on suddenly in the past few hours? — YES → **Are you coughing up frothy pink or white sputum?** — YES →

Are you coughing up frothy pink or white sputum? — NO → **Are you short of breath?**

Has the wheezing come on suddenly in the past few hours? — NO → **Is your temperature 100.4°F (38°C) or above?**

Is your temperature 100.4°F (38°C) or above? — YES →

Is your temperature 100.4°F (38°C) or above? — NO → **Do you cough up gray or greenish yellow sputum most days, and are you a smoker or have you smoked in the past?**

Are you short of breath? — YES →

Are you short of breath? — NO → **CALL YOUR DOCTOR NOW**

Do you cough up gray or greenish yellow sputum most days, and are you a smoker or have you smoked in the past? — YES →

Do you cough up gray or greenish yellow sputum most days, and are you a smoker or have you smoked in the past? — NO →

WARNING

DANGER SIGNS Call an ambulance if you have, or someone you are with has, either of the following symptoms:
- Sudden, severe shortness of breath
- Blue-tinged lips or tongue

While waiting for help to arrive, loosen any tight clothing on the affected person and help him or her sit in an upright position.

📞 EMERGENCY! CALL AN AMBULANCE

POSSIBLE CAUSE A buildup of fluid inside the lungs, known as pulmonary edema, is a possibility. The most common cause of this condition is acute heart failure, in which the heart fails to pump effectively.

ACTION While waiting for help to arrive, sit upright in a chair. You will probably be given oxygen and *diuretic drugs*, which will help clear the fluid from your lungs. Tests such as electrocardiography (p.203) and a chest X ray (p.39) will be needed. Long-term drug treatment may be necessary to prevent a recurrence.

📞 EMERGENCY! CALL AN AMBULANCE

POSSIBLE CAUSE A severe attack of asthma is a possible cause of these symptoms.

ACTION While waiting for the ambulance, sit upright with your elbows supported on a table or the back of a chair. Try to keep calm. If you have already been diagnosed with asthma and have your drugs with you, take two puffs of your rescue inhaler or follow the treatment plan given by your doctor. In the hospital, you will be given oxygen and additional *bronchodilator* and *corticosteroid drugs*.

CALL YOUR DOCTOR NOW

POSSIBLE CAUSE AND ACTION You may be having an asthma attack. Your doctor is likely to measure your peak flow rate (below). If the results show that you have asthma, you will probably be prescribed a *bronchodilator drug.*

SEE YOUR DOCTOR WITHIN 24 HOURS

POSSIBLE CAUSE AND ACTION You may have acute bronchitis, inflammation of the airways due to a viral infection. Because you are wheezing, you should see your doctor, who will examine you and may prescribe a *bronchodilator drug.* In addition, you should follow the self-help advice for managing a fever (p.154) and treating a cold (p.194). If you become short of breath, call your doctor at once.

CALL YOUR DOCTOR NOW IF YOU HAVE BEGUN WHEEZING AND YOU ARE UNABLE TO MAKE A DIAGNOSIS FROM THIS CHART.

POSSIBLE CAUSE Chronic obstructive pulmonary disease (COPD) is likely. In this condition, the airways become narrowed and produce excess mucus, and the air sacs in the lungs are damaged. Consult your doctor.

ACTION Although the damage is irreversible, your doctor may prescribe a *bronchodilator drug* to help relieve symptoms. Stop smoking to prevent the condition from worsening.

Measuring peak flow rate

Your peak flow rate is the maximum rate at which you can breathe out and is measured in liters per minute. Your doctor may measure your peak flow rate in order to assess the severity of respiratory conditions in which the airways become narrowed. Asthma is commonly diagnosed and monitored by measuring peak flow rate. You may be given a peak flow rate meter to use at home so that you can check your condition regularly and adjust your treatment as necessary.

Mouthpiece

Peak flow rate meter

Using the meter
Take a full breath, and breathe out as hard as you can. The pointer on the meter shows the result.

91 Coughing

Coughing is the body's response to irritation or inflammation in the lungs or the throat and may either produce sputum or be "dry." The most common causes of coughing are colds, smoking, asthma, or inhaling a foreign body. Sometimes, however, a persistent cough may signal a more serious respiratory disorder or a tumor.

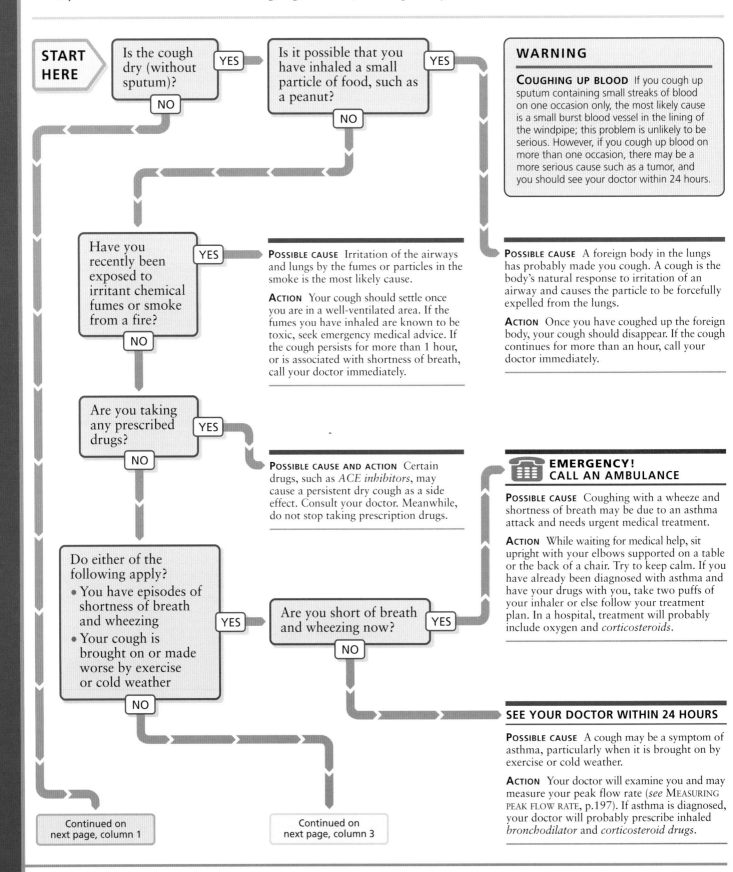

START HERE

Is the cough dry (without sputum)? — YES → **Is it possible that you have inhaled a small particle of food, such as a peanut?** — YES →

Have you recently been exposed to irritant chemical fumes or smoke from a fire? — YES →

POSSIBLE CAUSE Irritation of the airways and lungs by the fumes or particles in the smoke is the most likely cause.

ACTION Your cough should settle once you are in a well-ventilated area. If the fumes you have inhaled are known to be toxic, seek emergency medical advice. If the cough persists for more than 1 hour, or is associated with shortness of breath, call your doctor immediately.

Are you taking any prescribed drugs? — YES →

POSSIBLE CAUSE AND ACTION Certain drugs, such as *ACE inhibitors*, may cause a persistent dry cough as a side effect. Consult your doctor. Meanwhile, do not stop taking prescription drugs.

Do either of the following apply?
- You have episodes of shortness of breath and wheezing
- Your cough is brought on or made worse by exercise or cold weather

— YES → **Are you short of breath and wheezing now?** — YES →

WARNING

COUGHING UP BLOOD If you cough up sputum containing small streaks of blood on one occasion only, the most likely cause is a small burst blood vessel in the lining of the windpipe; this problem is unlikely to be serious. However, if you cough up blood on more than one occasion, there may be a more serious cause such as a tumor, and you should see your doctor within 24 hours.

POSSIBLE CAUSE A foreign body in the lungs has probably made you cough. A cough is the body's natural response to irritation of an airway and causes the particle to be forcefully expelled from the lungs.

ACTION Once you have coughed up the foreign body, your cough should disappear. If the cough continues for more than an hour, call your doctor immediately.

EMERGENCY! CALL AN AMBULANCE

POSSIBLE CAUSE Coughing with a wheeze and shortness of breath may be due to an asthma attack and needs urgent medical treatment.

ACTION While waiting for medical help, sit upright with your elbows supported on a table or the back of a chair. Try to keep calm. If you have already been diagnosed with asthma and have your drugs with you, take two puffs of your inhaler or else follow your treatment plan. In a hospital, treatment will probably include oxygen and *corticosteroids*.

SEE YOUR DOCTOR WITHIN 24 HOURS

POSSIBLE CAUSE A cough may be a symptom of asthma, particularly when it is brought on by exercise or cold weather.

ACTION Your doctor will examine you and may measure your peak flow rate (*see* MEASURING PEAK FLOW RATE, p.197). If asthma is diagnosed, your doctor will probably prescribe inhaled *bronchodilator* and *corticosteroid drugs*.

Continued on next page, column 1

Continued on next page, column 3

Continued from previous page, column 1

Has the cough started within the past week? **NO** / **YES**

Do you have shortness of breath, with or without a fever? **NO** / **YES**

Continued from previous page, column 2

Do you have burning discomfort in the center of your chest that may get worse when you bend over or lie down? **NO** / **YES**

POSSIBLE CAUSE AND ACTION You may have acute bronchitis or another viral infection such as a common cold. Take *analgesics* and try steam inhalation (p.194). If you smoke, you should stop. Call your doctor if you become short of breath. Otherwise, consult your doctor if you are no better in a few days.

Is your cough associated with any of the following?
- Weight loss
- Coughing up blood
- Persistent hoarse voice
- Night sweats

NO / **YES**

CALL YOUR DOCTOR NOW

POSSIBLE CAUSE A chest infection such as pneumonia (infection of the air sacs in the lungs) is possible.

ACTION If you have a fever, take steps to reduce it (*see* MANAGING A FEVER, p.154). If your doctor confirms that you have pneumonia, he or she will probably prescribe *antibiotics* and may arrange for you to have a chest X ray (p.39). Hospital admission is sometimes necessary.

CONSULT YOUR DOCTOR IF YOU ARE UNABLE TO MAKE A DIAGNOSIS FROM THIS CHART.

POSSIBLE CAUSE Gastroesophageal reflux, in which the acid stomach contents regurgitate back up the esophagus, may be the cause of your cough, since some regurgitated matter can enter the lungs. Consult your doctor.

ACTION Your doctor will advise you on how to reduce episodes of gastroesophageal reflux (*see* COPING WITH GASTROESOPHAGEAL REFLUX, p.209). If the symptoms do not improve with these measures, your doctor may prescribe an *ulcer-healing drug* in order to reduce the production of stomach acid.

SEE YOUR DOCTOR WITHIN 24 HOURS

POSSIBLE CAUSE You may have a serious lung disorder such as tuberculosis or lung cancer.

ACTION Your doctor will probably arrange for blood and sputum tests and a chest X ray (p.39). Depending on the results, you may then be referred to a specialist for tests such as bronchoscopy (below).

Do you cough up thick, grayish sputum most days, and do you smoke, or have you smoked in the past? **NO** / **YES**

CONSULT YOUR DOCTOR IF YOU ARE UNABLE TO MAKE A DIAGNOSIS FROM THIS CHART.

POSSIBLE CAUSE Chronic obstructive pulmonary disease (COPD) is likely. In this condition the airways become narrowed and produce excess mucus and the air sacs in the lungs are damaged. Consult your doctor.

ACTION The damage is irreversible, but your doctor may prescribe *bronchodilators* to help relieve your symptoms. Stop smoking to prevent the condition form worsening.

Bronchoscopy

Bronchoscopy can be used to diagnose lung disorders, such as lung cancer. In most cases, a flexible bronchoscope is passed through the nose or mouth down into the lungs to view the bronchi (airways). Before the procedure, you will be given a local anesthetic spray to numb the back of your throat or nose and/or offered mild sedation. Sometimes, surgical instruments can also be passed down through the bronchoscope to remove tissue samples or carry out treatments during the procedure.

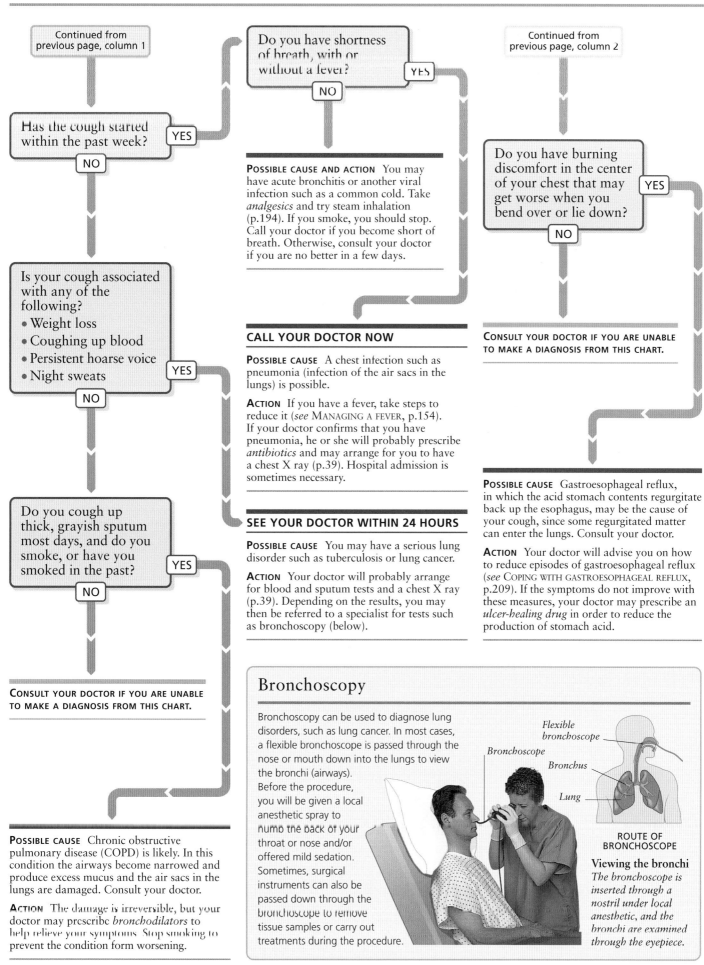

Flexible bronchoscope

Bronchoscope

Bronchus

Lung

ROUTE OF BRONCHOSCOPE

Viewing the bronchi
The bronchoscope is inserted through a nostril under local anesthetic, and the bronchi are examined through the eyepiece.

92 Shortness of breath

It is normal to become short of breath after strenuous exercise. Pregnant women and people who are overweight become short of breath most easily. If, however, you are breathing rapidly or you are "puffing" at rest or after very gentle exercise, you may have a problem affecting the heart or respiratory system. Because such problems may be serious and threaten the oxygen supply to the tissues, it is very important to seek medical advice without delay if you become short of breath for no apparent reason. Sudden shortness of breath and an inability to make any sound that comes on while eating is probably due to choking and needs urgent first-aid treatment (see CHOKING, p.294).

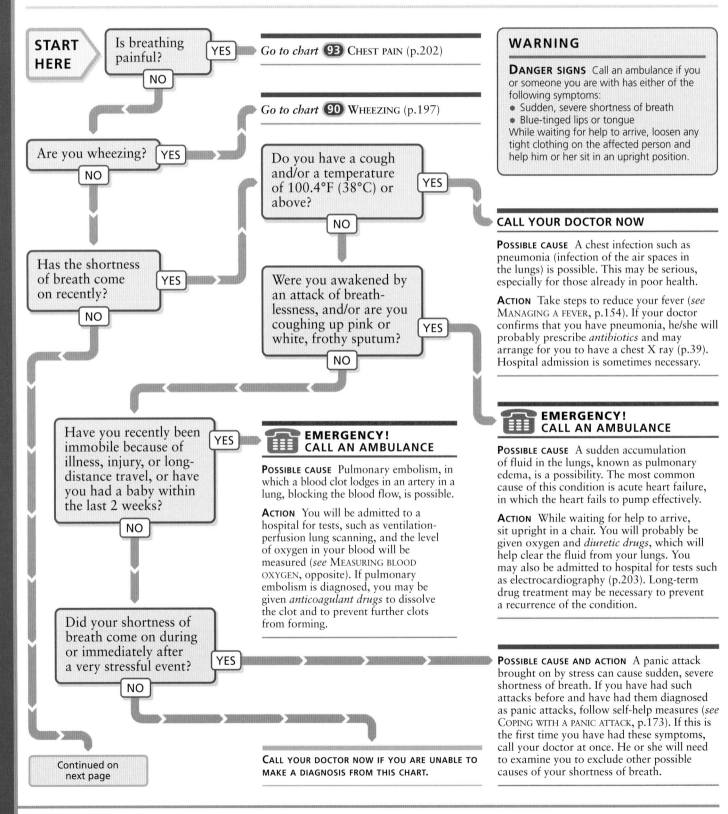

START HERE → **Is breathing painful?** — YES → *Go to chart* **93** CHEST PAIN (p.202)
NO

Are you wheezing? — YES → *Go to chart* **90** WHEEZING (p.197)
NO

Do you have a cough and/or a temperature of 100.4°F (38°C) or above? — YES →
NO

Has the shortness of breath come on recently? — YES →
NO

Were you awakened by an attack of breathlessness, and/or are you coughing up pink or white, frothy sputum? — YES →
NO

Have you recently been immobile because of illness, injury, or long-distance travel, or have you had a baby within the last 2 weeks? — YES →
NO

Did your shortness of breath come on during or immediately after a very stressful event? — YES →
NO

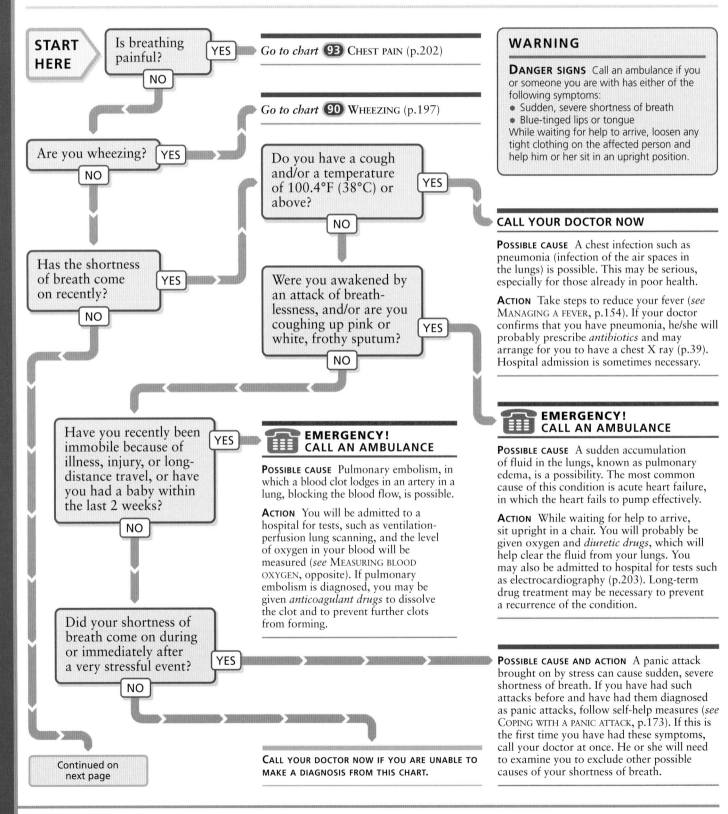
Continued on next page

WARNING

DANGER SIGNS Call an ambulance if you or someone you are with has either of the following symptoms:
- Sudden, severe shortness of breath
- Blue-tinged lips or tongue

While waiting for help to arrive, loosen any tight clothing on the affected person and help him or her sit in an upright position.

CALL YOUR DOCTOR NOW

POSSIBLE CAUSE A chest infection such as pneumonia (infection of the air spaces in the lungs) is possible. This may be serious, especially for those already in poor health.

ACTION Take steps to reduce your fever (see MANAGING A FEVER, p.154). If your doctor confirms that you have pneumonia, he/she will probably prescribe *antibiotics* and may arrange for you to have a chest X ray (p.39). Hospital admission is sometimes necessary.

EMERGENCY! CALL AN AMBULANCE

POSSIBLE CAUSE A sudden accumulation of fluid in the lungs, known as pulmonary edema, is a possibility. The most common cause of this condition is acute heart failure, in which the heart fails to pump effectively.

ACTION While waiting for help to arrive, sit upright in a chair. You will probably be given oxygen and *diuretic drugs*, which will help clear the fluid from your lungs. You may also be admitted to hospital for tests such as electrocardiography (p.203). Long-term drug treatment may be necessary to prevent a recurrence of the condition.

POSSIBLE CAUSE AND ACTION A panic attack brought on by stress can cause sudden, severe shortness of breath. If you have had such attacks before and have had them diagnosed as panic attacks, follow self-help measures (see COPING WITH A PANIC ATTACK, p.173). If this is the first time you have had these symptoms, call your doctor at once. He or she will need to examine you to exclude other possible causes of your shortness of breath.

EMERGENCY! CALL AN AMBULANCE

POSSIBLE CAUSE Pulmonary embolism, in which a blood clot lodges in an artery in a lung, blocking the blood flow, is possible.

ACTION You will be admitted to a hospital for tests, such as ventilation-perfusion lung scanning, and the level of oxygen in your blood will be measured (see MEASURING BLOOD OXYGEN, opposite). If pulmonary embolism is diagnosed, you may be given *anticoagulant drugs* to dissolve the clot and to prevent further clots from forming.

CALL YOUR DOCTOR NOW IF YOU ARE UNABLE TO MAKE A DIAGNOSIS FROM THIS CHART.

Continued from previous page

Do you cough up thick, grayish sputum on most days? — **YES** →

Do you work or have you worked in a dusty atmosphere such as in a mine or quarry? — **YES** →

NO

POSSIBLE CAUSE An occupational lung disease, such as a pneumoconiosis, in which the lungs are progressively damaged by inhaled particles, may be the cause. Consult your doctor.

ACTION Your doctor will ask you about your current and past occupations. He or she will also arrange for a chest X ray (p.39) and lung function tests to assess how well your lungs are working. If you smoke, you should stop. In severe cases, you may have to consider a change of employment.

POSSIBLE CAUSE Chronic obstructive pulmonary disease (COPD) is likely, especially if you smoke or have smoked in the past. In this condition, the airways become narrowed and produce excess mucus, and the air sacs in the lungs are damaged. Consult your doctor.

ACTION Although the damage is irreversible, your doctor may prescribe *bronchodilator drugs* to help relieve your symptoms. If you smoke, you must stop to prevent the condition from worsening.

NO

Are your ankles swollen? — **YES** →

NO

SEE YOUR DOCTOR WITHIN 24 HOURS

POSSIBLE CAUSE A gradual accumulation of fluid in the lungs and in other tissues is probably the cause of your symptoms. This problem is most commonly due to heart failure (in which the heart fails to pump effectively), especially in people over 60 years of age. It can also result from a kidney or liver disorder.

ACTION Your doctor will examine you. Regardless of the underlying cause, he/she may prescribe drugs, including *diuretics*, which will help clear excess fluid. You will need other tests, including blood tests and electrocardiography (p.203), to establish the underlying cause and appropriate treatment.

Does your work or hobby involve regular contact with grain or other crops and/or caged birds or animals? — **YES** →

NO

POSSIBLE CAUSE A lung disorder known as extrinsic allergic alveolitis or hypersensitivity pneumonitis, in which the air sacs in the lungs become inflamed in response to certain inhaled substances, is a possibility. The disorder can sometimes cause a fever. Consult your doctor.

ACTION Your doctor will probably arrange for diagnostic tests, including a chest X ray (p.39) and skin tests to look for sensitivity to different substances. If the diagnosis is confirmed, you will probably be advised to avoid further exposure to the substance causing the reaction. If this is not possible, you may have to consider changing your job or hobby. You may be given *corticosteroid drugs* to reduce the inflammation.

Have you noticed any of the following symptoms with the shortness of breath?
• Excessive fatigue
• Feeling faint or passing out
• Paler than normal skin — **YES** →

NO

SEE YOUR DOCTOR WITHIN 24 HOURS

POSSIBLE CAUSE You may have anemia, in which there is too little of the oxygen-carrying pigment hemoglobin in the blood. Anemia can result from a variety of underlying causes. Consult your doctor.

ACTION Your doctor will arrange for a blood test to confirm the diagnosis. In some cases, further tests will be necessary to determine why anemia has developed. Treatment for anemia will usually need to be combined with treatment of the underlying cause.

SEE YOUR DOCTOR WITHIN 24 HOURS IF YOU ARE UNABLE TO MAKE A DIAGNOSIS FROM THIS CHART.

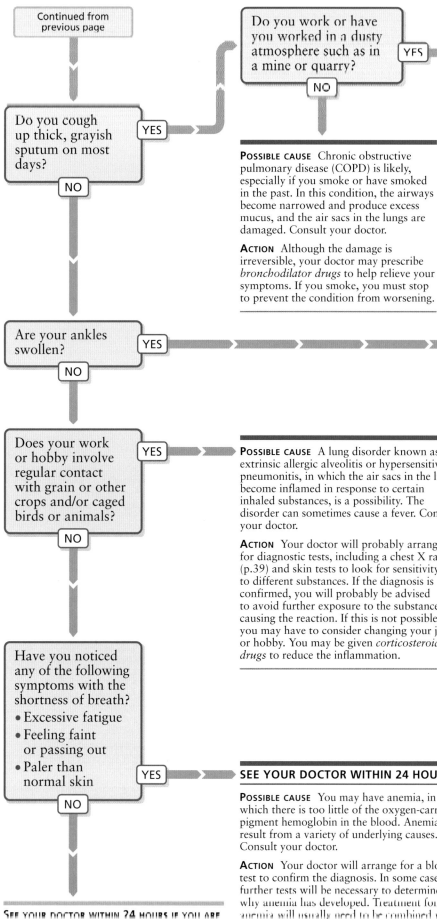

Measuring blood oxygen

Tests that measure the amount of oxygen in the blood show how efficiently the lungs are working and are used to help diagnose and monitor lung disorders such as pneumonia and pulmonary embolism. Blood oxygen levels can be measured by taking a blood sample from an artery, usually in the wrist. However, an easier and painless method is pulse oximetry, which indirectly measures the concentration of oxygen in blood in the tissues. The pulse oximeter is clipped over the fingertip and shines a light through the tissues. Changes in the amount of light absorbed by the tissues are detected and displayed on a monitor. Tissues containing oxygen-rich blood absorb more light than those in which the blood is low in oxygen.

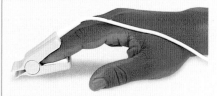

Pulse oximetry
The pulse oximeter is clipped over a fingertip. It shines light through the tissues of the finger and measures how much light is absorbed, which indicates the blood oxygen level.

93 Chest pain

Pain in the chest (anywhere between the neck and the bottom of the ribcage) may be alarming and may or may not have a serious cause. Most chest pain is due to minor disorders such as muscle strain or indigestion. Severe,

crushing, central chest pain, or pain that is associated with shortness of breath, an irregular heartbeat, nausea, sweating, or faintness, may be a sign of a serious disorder of the heart or lungs and may need emergency treatment.

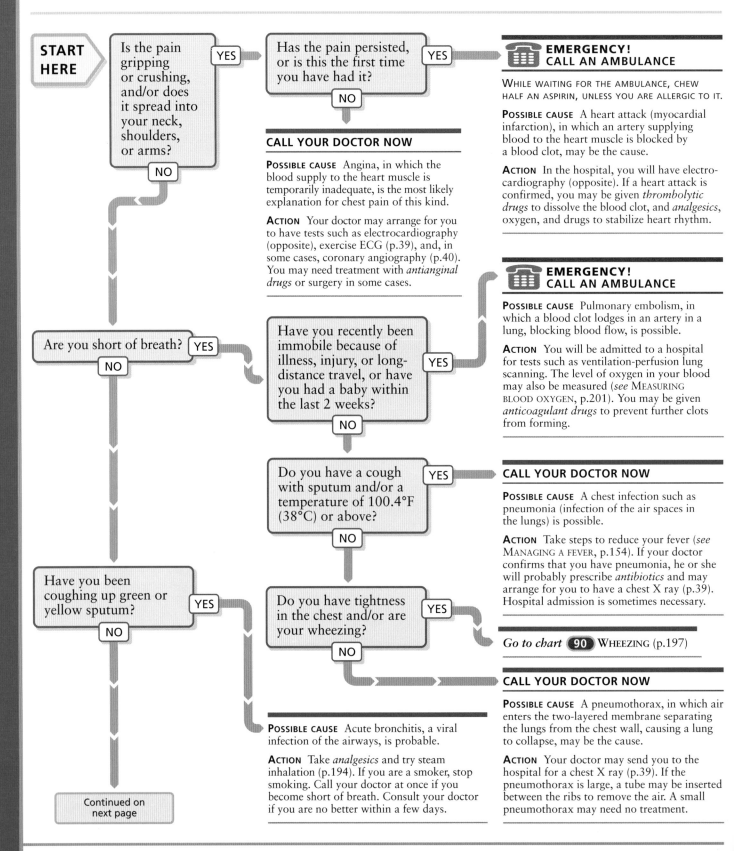

START HERE

Is the pain gripping or crushing, and/or does it spread into your neck, shoulders, or arms?
YES →
NO ↓

Has the pain persisted, or is this the first time you have had it?
YES →
NO ↓

EMERGENCY! CALL AN AMBULANCE

WHILE WAITING FOR THE AMBULANCE, CHEW HALF AN ASPIRIN, UNLESS YOU ARE ALLERGIC TO IT.

POSSIBLE CAUSE A heart attack (myocardial infarction), in which an artery supplying blood to the heart muscle is blocked by a blood clot, may be the cause.

ACTION In the hospital, you will have electro-cardiography (opposite). If a heart attack is confirmed, you may be given *thrombolytic drugs* to dissolve the blood clot, and *analgesics*, oxygen, and drugs to stabilize heart rhythm.

CALL YOUR DOCTOR NOW

POSSIBLE CAUSE Angina, in which the blood supply to the heart muscle is temporarily inadequate, is the most likely explanation for chest pain of this kind.

ACTION Your doctor may arrange for you to have tests such as electrocardiography (opposite), exercise ECG (p.39), and, in some cases, coronary angiography (p.40). You may need treatment with *antianginal drugs* or surgery in some cases.

Are you short of breath?
YES →
NO ↓

Have you recently been immobile because of illness, injury, or long-distance travel, or have you had a baby within the last 2 weeks?
YES →
NO ↓

EMERGENCY! CALL AN AMBULANCE

POSSIBLE CAUSE Pulmonary embolism, in which a blood clot lodges in an artery in a lung, blocking blood flow, is possible.

ACTION You will be admitted to a hospital for tests such as ventilation-perfusion lung scanning. The level of oxygen in your blood may also be measured (*see* MEASURING BLOOD OXYGEN, p.201). You may be given *anticoagulant drugs* to prevent further clots from forming.

Do you have a cough with sputum and/or a temperature of 100.4°F (38°C) or above?
YES →
NO ↓

CALL YOUR DOCTOR NOW

POSSIBLE CAUSE A chest infection such as pneumonia (infection of the air spaces in the lungs) is possible.

ACTION Take steps to reduce your fever (*see* MANAGING A FEVER, p.154). If your doctor confirms that you have pneumonia, he or she will probably prescribe *antibiotics* and may arrange for you to have a chest X ray (p.39). Hospital admission is sometimes necessary.

Have you been coughing up green or yellow sputum?
YES →
NO ↓

Do you have tightness in the chest and/or are your wheezing?
YES →
NO ↓

Go to chart **90** WHEEZING (p.197)

CALL YOUR DOCTOR NOW

POSSIBLE CAUSE A pneumothorax, in which air enters the two-layered membrane separating the lungs from the chest wall, causing a lung to collapse, may be the cause.

ACTION Your doctor may send you to the hospital for a chest X ray (p.39). If the pneumothorax is large, a tube may be inserted between the ribs to remove the air. A small pneumothorax may need no treatment.

POSSIBLE CAUSE Acute bronchitis, a viral infection of the airways, is probable.

ACTION Take *analgesics* and try steam inhalation (p.194). If you are a smoker, stop smoking. Call your doctor at once if you become short of breath. Consult your doctor if you are no better within a few days.

Continued on next page

Continued from previous page

Is the pain in the center of the chest, and does it get worse when you bend over or lie down? **YES**

POSSIBLE CAUSE Gastroesophageal reflux, in which the acidic stomach contents leak back up the esophagus, may be the cause. Consult your doctor.

ACTION Your doctor will give you advice on how to cope with gastroesophageal reflux (*see* COPING WITH GASTROESOPHAGEAL REFLUX, p.209). If your symptoms do not improve, you may be prescribed *ulcer-healing drugs* to reduce the production of stomach acid.

NO

Have you had this type of pain before, and does it come on after eating? **YES**

POSSIBLE CAUSE Indigestion is the most likely explanation.

ACTION Take an over the counter *antacid* to relieve the symptoms. To avoid further attacks try self-help measures for preventing indigestion (p.217). Consult your doctor if you often have indigestion.

NO

Is the pain on only one side of the chest? **YES**

NO

SEE YOUR DOCTOR WITHIN 24 HOURS IF YOU ARE NOT ABLE TO MAKE A DIAGNOSIS FROM THIS CHART.

Is the pain worse if you take a deep breath? **YES**

NO

Do you have a burning pain in your skin that is unaffected by breathing? **YES**

NO

SEE YOUR DOCTOR WITHIN 24 HOURS IF YOU ARE NOT ABLE TO MAKE A DIAGNOSIS FROM THIS CHART.

SEE YOUR DOCTOR WITHIN 24 HOURS

POSSIBLE CAUSE AND ACTION Shingles, a viral infection affecting the nerves, is possible. This causes pain before a blistery rash develops. Your doctor will probably prescribe an *analgesic* and oral *antiviral drugs*.

Is your chest tender to touch? **YES**

NO

SEE YOUR DOCTOR WITHIN 24 HOURS

POSSIBLE CAUSE Pleurisy, inflammation of the two-layered membrane separating the lungs from the chest wall, is possible. This condition is often the result of a viral infection.

ACTION Your doctor will examine you and may arrange tests such as a chest X ray (p.39). Over-the-counter *nonsteroidal anti-inflammatory drugs* will help relieve the pain.

POSSIBLE CAUSES Inflammation or injury affecting a muscle, a ligament, or cartilage of the ribcage are the probable causes.

ACTION Stay as active as feels comfortable. For pain relief, take an over-the-counter *nonsteroidal anti-inflammatory drug*. Consult your doctor if the pain is no better after 48 hours.

Electrocardiography

Electrocardiography (ECG) is used to record the electrical activity produced by the heart as it beats. The procedure is frequently used to investigate the cause of chest pain and to diagnose abnormal heart rhythms. Electrodes are attached to the skin of the chest, wrists, and ankles and transmit the electrical activity of the heart to an ECG machine. This records the transmitted information as a tracing on a moving graph paper or a screen. Each of the tracings shows electrical activity in a different area of the heart. The test usually takes several minutes to complete, is safe, and causes no discomfort.

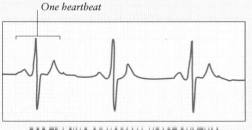

One heartbeat

ECG TRACING OF NORMAL HEART RHYTHM

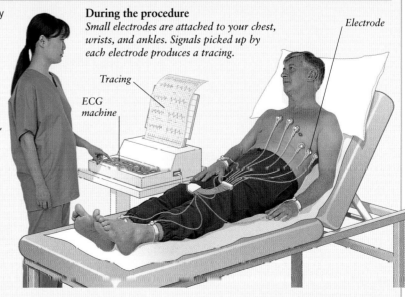

During the procedure
Small electrodes are attached to your chest, wrists, and ankles. Signals picked up by each electrode produces a tracing.

Electrode

Tracing

ECG machine

94 Palpitations

Palpitation is the sensation of unusually rapid, strong, or irregular beating of the heart. It is normal for the heart rate to speed up during strenuous exercise, and you may feel your heart "thumping" for some minutes afterward. This is usually no cause for concern. In most cases, palpitations that occur at rest are caused by the effect of drugs such as caffeine or nicotine or may simply be due to anxiety. In a small proportion of people, however, palpitations that occur at rest are a symptom of an underlying illness. If you experience recurrent palpitations that have no obvious cause or that are associated with chest pain or shortness of breath, you should always seek medical advice.

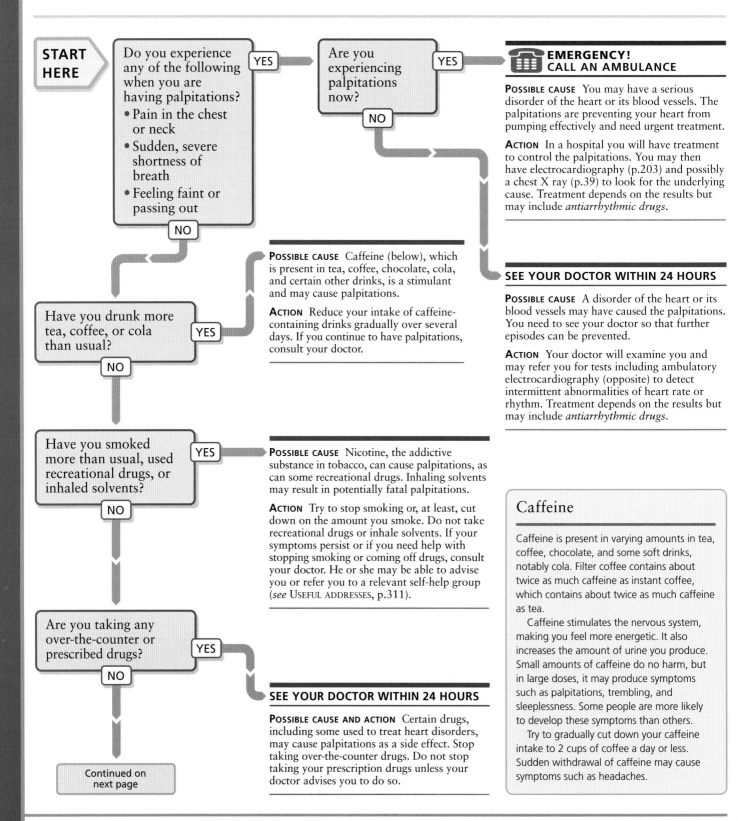

START HERE

Do you experience any of the following when you are having palpitations?
• Pain in the chest or neck
• Sudden, severe shortness of breath
• Feeling faint or passing out

YES → Are you experiencing palpitations now? **YES** →

EMERGENCY! CALL AN AMBULANCE

POSSIBLE CAUSE You may have a serious disorder of the heart or its blood vessels. The palpitations are preventing your heart from pumping effectively and need urgent treatment.

ACTION In a hospital you will have treatment to control the palpitations. You may then have electrocardiography (p.203) and possibly a chest X ray (p.39) to look for the underlying cause. Treatment depends on the results but may include *antiarrhythmic drugs*.

NO ↓

SEE YOUR DOCTOR WITHIN 24 HOURS

POSSIBLE CAUSE A disorder of the heart or its blood vessels may have caused the palpitations. You need to see your doctor so that further episodes can be prevented.

ACTION Your doctor will examine you and may refer you for tests including ambulatory electrocardiography (opposite) to detect intermittent abnormalities of heart rate or rhythm. Treatment depends on the results but may include *antiarrhythmic drugs*.

NO ↓

Have you drunk more tea, coffee, or cola than usual? **YES** →

POSSIBLE CAUSE Caffeine (below), which is present in tea, coffee, chocolate, cola, and certain other drinks, is a stimulant and may cause palpitations.

ACTION Reduce your intake of caffeine-containing drinks gradually over several days. If you continue to have palpitations, consult your doctor.

NO ↓

Have you smoked more than usual, used recreational drugs, or inhaled solvents? **YES** →

POSSIBLE CAUSE Nicotine, the addictive substance in tobacco, can cause palpitations, as can some recreational drugs. Inhaling solvents may result in potentially fatal palpitations.

ACTION Try to stop smoking or, at least, cut down on the amount you smoke. Do not take recreational drugs or inhale solvents. If your symptoms persist or if you need help with stopping smoking or coming off drugs, consult your doctor. He or she may be able to advise you or refer you to a relevant self-help group (*see* USEFUL ADDRESSES, p.311).

NO ↓

Are you taking any over-the-counter or prescribed drugs? **YES** →

SEE YOUR DOCTOR WITHIN 24 HOURS

POSSIBLE CAUSE AND ACTION Certain drugs, including some used to treat heart disorders, may cause palpitations as a side effect. Stop taking over-the-counter drugs. Do not stop taking your prescription drugs unless your doctor advises you to do so.

NO ↓

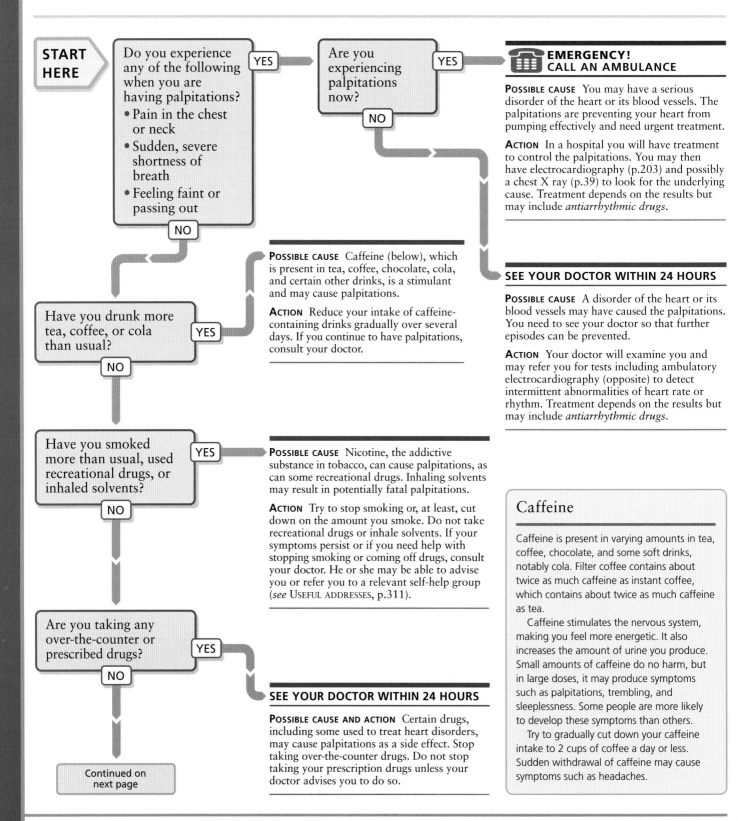

Continued on next page

Caffeine

Caffeine is present in varying amounts in tea, coffee, chocolate, and some soft drinks, notably cola. Filter coffee contains about twice as much caffeine as instant coffee, which contains about twice as much caffeine as tea.

Caffeine stimulates the nervous system, making you feel more energetic. It also increases the amount of urine you produce. Small amounts of caffeine do no harm, but in large doses, it may produce symptoms such as palpitations, trembling, and sleeplessness. Some people are more likely to develop these symptoms than others.

Try to gradually cut down your caffeine intake to 2 cups of coffee a day or less. Sudden withdrawal of caffeine may cause symptoms such as headaches.

Continued from previous page

Ambulatory electrocardiography

In one type of ambulatory electrocardiography (ECG), a wearable device called a Holter monitor records the electrical activity of the heart by means of electrodes attached to the chest. The device is usually worn for 24 hours or longer and detects intermittent arrhythmias (abnormal heart rates and rhythms). Whenever symptoms occur, you press a button, which adds a mark to the recording. The recording is analyzed to check for any periods of arrhythmia and if they coincide with the marks denoting symptoms.

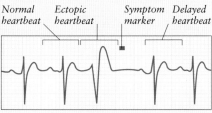

Normal heartbeat   Ectopic heartbeat   Symptom marker   Delayed heartbeat

AMBULATORY ECG TRACING

Using a Holter monitor
The device is worn under clothing. This trace (left) produced by the device shows an early abnormal beat (ectopic beat), which coincides with a symptom marker.

Shoulder strap
Electrode
Symptom marker button
Monitor

Do you have any of the following symptoms?
- Weight loss with increased appetite
- Feeling constantly on edge
- Bulging eyes
- Increased sweating

YES →

POSSIBLE CAUSE Hyperthyroidism (overactive thyroid gland) is a possible cause of these symptoms. Consult your doctor.

ACTION Your doctor will take a blood sample to measure levels of thyroid hormones. If the diagnosis is confirmed, you may be treated with *thyroid drugs* or radioactive iodine, which are usually rapidly effective. In some cases, surgery to remove part of the gland may be needed.

NO ↓

Have you been feeling generally tired, been short of breath after mild exercise, and do you have pale skin?

YES →

SEE YOUR DOCTOR WITHIN 24 HOURS

POSSIBLE CAUSE You may have anemia, in which there is too little of the oxygen-carrying pigment hemoglobin in the blood. Anemia can result from a variety of underlying causes.

ACTION Your doctor will take a sample of blood to measure your hemoglobin levels. If anemia is confirmed, you will probably need further tests to determine why the condition has developed. You will need treatment for anemia and for the underlying cause.

NO ↓

Do you have a pre-existing heart condition?

YES →

CALL YOUR DOCTOR NOW

POSSIBLE CAUSE The palpitations may indicate that your condition has worsened. Whatever the cause, the palpitations will put additional strain on your heart and require investigation.

ACTION Your doctor will arrange for you to have tests such as electrocardiography (p.203) and a chest X ray (p.39). Treatment will depend on the results, but you may be prescribed *antiarrhythmic drugs*.

NO ↓

Do either of the following describe your palpitations?
- Missed beats
- Particularly strong or early beats

YES →

POSSIBLE CAUSE AND ACTION Ectopic beats, in which a heartbeat is slightly delayed or early compared with the regular pattern, is a likely cause. Ectopic beats are more common when resting quietly and disappear during exercise. Occasional ectopic beats are common and are very unlikely to be a sign of heart disease. Caffeine (opposite) and stress make ectopic beats more likely and should be avoided.

NO ↓

Are you tense and under stress?

YES →

POSSIBLE CAUSE AND ACTION Anxiety can increase your awareness of your heartbeat, as well as increase the heart rate itself. Try to keep stress to a minimum and use relaxation techniques (p.32). If these measures do not help, consult your doctor.

NO ↓

CONSULT YOUR DOCTOR IF YOU ARE UNABLE TO MAKE A DIAGNOSIS FROM THIS CHART.

95 Teeth problems

For pain affecting other parts of the mouth, see chart 96,
MOUTH PROBLEMS (p.208).
Teeth are at constant risk of decay because bacteria act on
sugars in our diet to create acids that erode the surface of the
teeth. If untreated, decay can spread to the center of the teeth.
The same conditions that cause decay can also cause gum

disorders and are often associated with poor dental hygiene
(*see* CARING FOR YOUR TEETH AND GUMS, opposite). You
should see your dentist every 6–12 months. If you have a
heart valve disorder, tell your dentist; you may need to have
antibiotics before dental treatment. Let your dentist know if
you are pregnant so that any X rays can be postponed.

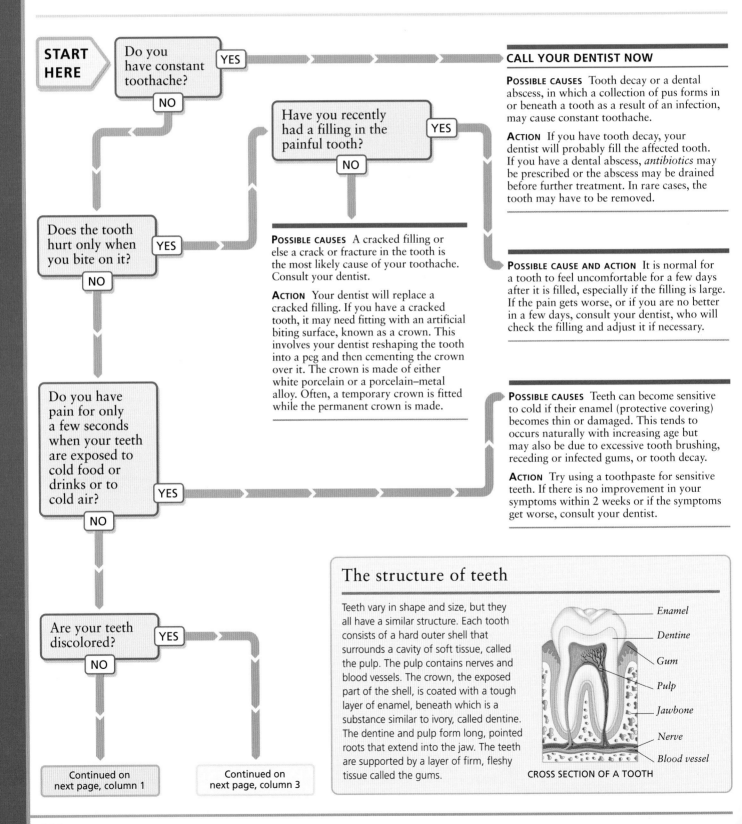

START HERE

Do you have constant toothache? — YES →

NO

Have you recently had a filling in the painful tooth? — YES →

NO

Does the tooth hurt only when you bite on it? — YES →

NO

Do you have pain for only a few seconds when your teeth are exposed to cold food or drinks or to cold air? — YES →

NO

Are your teeth discolored? — YES →

NO

CALL YOUR DENTIST NOW

POSSIBLE CAUSES Tooth decay or a dental
abscess, in which a collection of pus forms in
or beneath a tooth as a result of an infection,
may cause constant toothache.

ACTION If you have tooth decay, your
dentist will probably fill the affected tooth.
If you have a dental abscess, *antibiotics* may
be prescribed or the abscess may be drained
before further treatment. In rare cases, the
tooth may have to be removed.

POSSIBLE CAUSE AND ACTION It is normal for
a tooth to feel uncomfortable for a few days
after it is filled, especially if the filling is large.
If the pain gets worse, or if you are no better
in a few days, consult your dentist, who will
check the filling and adjust it if necessary.

POSSIBLE CAUSES A cracked filling or
else a crack or fracture in the tooth is
the most likely cause of your toothache.
Consult your dentist.

ACTION Your dentist will replace a
cracked filling. If you have a cracked
tooth, it may need fitting with an artificial
biting surface, known as a crown. This
involves your dentist reshaping the tooth
into a peg and then cementing the crown
over it. The crown is made of either
white porcelain or a porcelain–metal
alloy. Often, a temporary crown is fitted
while the permanent crown is made.

POSSIBLE CAUSES Teeth can become sensitive
to cold if their enamel (protective covering)
becomes thin or damaged. This tends to
occurs naturally with increasing age but
may also be due to excessive tooth brushing,
receding or infected gums, or tooth decay.

ACTION Try using a toothpaste for sensitive
teeth. If there is no improvement in your
symptoms within 2 weeks or if the symptoms
get worse, consult your dentist.

The structure of teeth

Teeth vary in shape and size, but they
all have a similar structure. Each tooth
consists of a hard outer shell that
surrounds a cavity of soft tissue, called
the pulp. The pulp contains nerves and
blood vessels. The crown, the exposed
part of the shell, is coated with a tough
layer of enamel, beneath which is a
substance similar to ivory, called dentine.
The dentine and pulp form long, pointed
roots that extend into the jaw. The teeth
are supported by a layer of firm, fleshy
tissue called the gums.

Enamel
Dentine
Gum
Pulp
Jawbone
Nerve
Blood vessel

CROSS SECTION OF A TOOTH

Continued on next page, column 1

Continued on next page, column 3

SELF-HELP Caring for your teeth and gums

Daily care is vital to maintain dental health. You need to limit your intake of foods and drinks containing sugar because these contribute to tooth decay. You should also brush and floss your teeth regularly to prevent food particles from building up on your teeth and reduce the risk of tooth decay and gum disease.

Brush your teeth at least twice a day, or, if possible, after every meal. Use a soft electric or manual toothbrush with a small head and a fluoride toothpaste. Brush for at least 2 minutes, cleaning all the surfaces of your teeth, especially where they meet the gum. Next, use dental floss or tape to clean between the teeth, removing food particles that a brush cannot reach.

Toothbrush held at angle to teeth

Dental floss

Floss curved around tooth

Brushing your teeth
Brush your teeth in small circular motions, using a small-headed toothbrush held at an angle to the teeth. Make sure you clean each tooth.

Using dental floss
Keeping the floss taut, guide it between the teeth. Gently scrape the side of the tooth, working away from the gum.

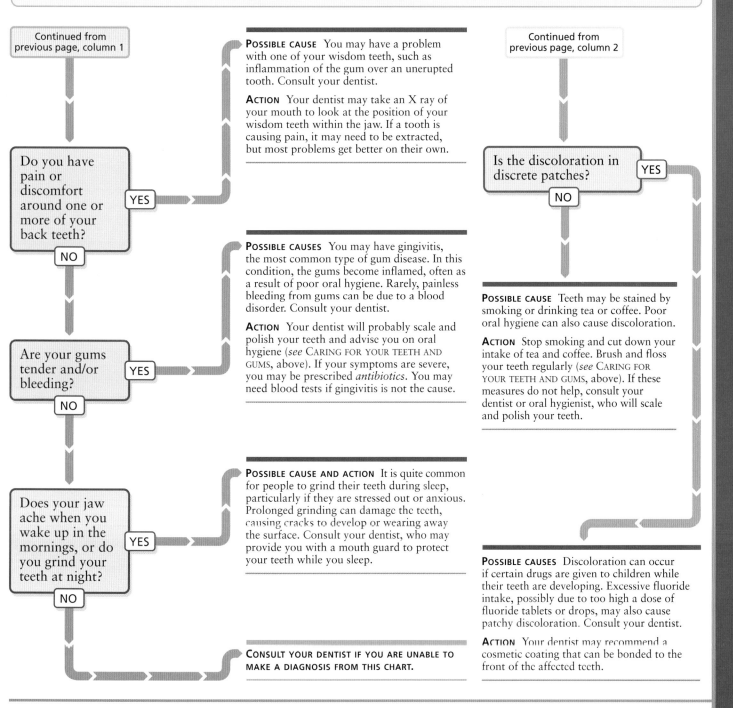

Continued from previous page, column 1

Do you have pain or discomfort around one or more of your back teeth?

YES →

POSSIBLE CAUSE You may have a problem with one of your wisdom teeth, such as inflammation of the gum over an unerupted tooth. Consult your dentist.

ACTION Your dentist may take an X ray of your mouth to look at the position of your wisdom teeth within the jaw. If a tooth is causing pain, it may need to be extracted, but most problems get better on their own.

NO ↓

Are your gums tender and/or bleeding?

YES →

POSSIBLE CAUSES You may have gingivitis, the most common type of gum disease. In this condition, the gums become inflamed, often as a result of poor oral hygiene. Rarely, painless bleeding from gums can be due to a blood disorder. Consult your dentist.

ACTION Your dentist will probably scale and polish your teeth and advise you on oral hygiene (*see* CARING FOR YOUR TEETH AND GUMS, above). If your symptoms are severe, you may be prescribed *antibiotics*. You may need blood tests if gingivitis is not the cause.

NO ↓

Does your jaw ache when you wake up in the mornings, or do you grind your teeth at night?

YES →

POSSIBLE CAUSE AND ACTION It is quite common for people to grind their teeth during sleep, particularly if they are stressed out or anxious. Prolonged grinding can damage the teeth, causing cracks to develop or wearing away the surface. Consult your dentist, who may provide you with a mouth guard to protect your teeth while you sleep.

NO ↓

CONSULT YOUR DENTIST IF YOU ARE UNABLE TO MAKE A DIAGNOSIS FROM THIS CHART.

Continued from previous page, column 2

Is the discoloration in discrete patches?

YES →
NO ↓

POSSIBLE CAUSE Teeth may be stained by smoking or drinking tea or coffee. Poor oral hygiene can also cause discoloration.

ACTION Stop smoking and cut down your intake of tea and coffee. Brush and floss your teeth regularly (*see* CARING FOR YOUR TEETH AND GUMS, above). If these measures do not help, consult your dentist or oral hygienist, who will scale and polish your teeth.

POSSIBLE CAUSES Discoloration can occur if certain drugs are given to children while their teeth are developing. Excessive fluoride intake, possibly due to too high a dose of fluoride tablets or drops, may also cause patchy discoloration. Consult your dentist.

ACTION Your dentist may recommend a cosmetic coating that can be bonded to the front of the affected teeth.

96 Mouth problems

For problems with the skin around the mouth, see chart 78,
SKIN PROBLEMS AFFECTING THE FACE (**p.180**).
A sore mouth or tongue is most commonly due to a minor
injury. For example, biting your tongue or cheek may cause
a painful area. Such injuries should heal within a week.
Minor infections are another relatively common cause of

soreness in the mouth. Occasionally, a widespread skin
condition or an intestinal disorder such as Crohn's disease
may also affect the mouth, causing sore areas to develop. It
is important that you keep your mouth and gums healthy by
maintaining good oral hygiene (*see* CARING FOR YOUR TEETH
AND GUMS, **p.207**) and having regular dental checkups.

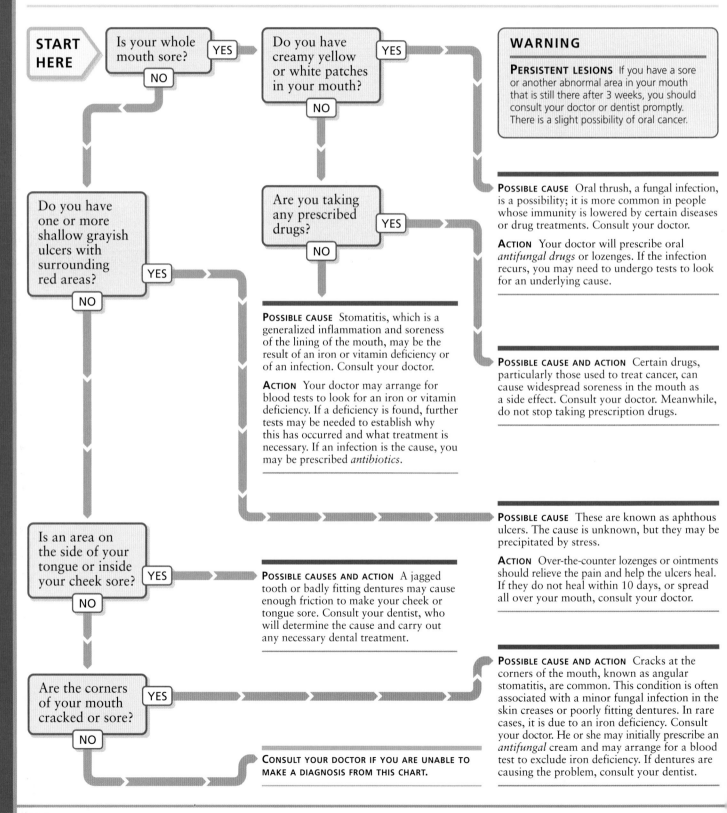

START HERE

Is your whole mouth sore? — NO / YES

Do you have creamy yellow or white patches in your mouth? — NO / YES

WARNING

PERSISTENT LESIONS If you have a sore or another abnormal area in your mouth that is still there after 3 weeks, you should consult your doctor or dentist promptly. There is a slight possibility of oral cancer.

Do you have one or more shallow grayish ulcers with surrounding red areas? — NO / YES

Are you taking any prescribed drugs? — NO / YES

POSSIBLE CAUSE Oral thrush, a fungal infection, is a possibility; it is more common in people whose immunity is lowered by certain diseases or drug treatments. Consult your doctor.

ACTION Your doctor will prescribe oral *antifungal drugs* or lozenges. If the infection recurs, you may need to undergo tests to look for an underlying cause.

POSSIBLE CAUSE Stomatitis, which is a generalized inflammation and soreness of the lining of the mouth, may be the result of an iron or vitamin deficiency or of an infection. Consult your doctor.

ACTION Your doctor may arrange for blood tests to look for an iron or vitamin deficiency. If a deficiency is found, further tests may be needed to establish why this has occurred and what treatment is necessary. If an infection is the cause, you may be prescribed *antibiotics*.

POSSIBLE CAUSE AND ACTION Certain drugs, particularly those used to treat cancer, can cause widespread soreness in the mouth as a side effect. Consult your doctor. Meanwhile, do not stop taking prescription drugs.

POSSIBLE CAUSE These are known as aphthous ulcers. The cause is unknown, but they may be precipitated by stress.

ACTION Over-the-counter lozenges or ointments should relieve the pain and help the ulcers heal. If they do not heal within 10 days, or spread all over your mouth, consult your doctor.

Is an area on the side of your tongue or inside your cheek sore? — NO / YES

POSSIBLE CAUSES AND ACTION A jagged tooth or badly fitting dentures may cause enough friction to make your cheek or tongue sore. Consult your dentist, who will determine the cause and carry out any necessary dental treatment.

Are the corners of your mouth cracked or sore? — NO / YES

POSSIBLE CAUSE AND ACTION Cracks at the corners of the mouth, known as angular stomatitis, are common. This condition is often associated with a minor fungal infection in the skin creases or poorly fitting dentures. In rare cases, it is due to an iron deficiency. Consult your doctor. He or she may initially prescribe an *antifungal* cream and may arrange for a blood test to exclude iron deficiency. If dentures are causing the problem, consult your dentist.

CONSULT YOUR DOCTOR IF YOU ARE UNABLE TO MAKE A DIAGNOSIS FROM THIS CHART.

97 Difficulty swallowing

Difficulty swallowing is most often due to a sore throat caused by an infection and usually clears up within a few days. However, difficulty swallowing or pain that is not related to a sore throat may be due to a disorder of the esophagus, the tube that leads from the throat to the stomach. In this case, you should seek medical advice.

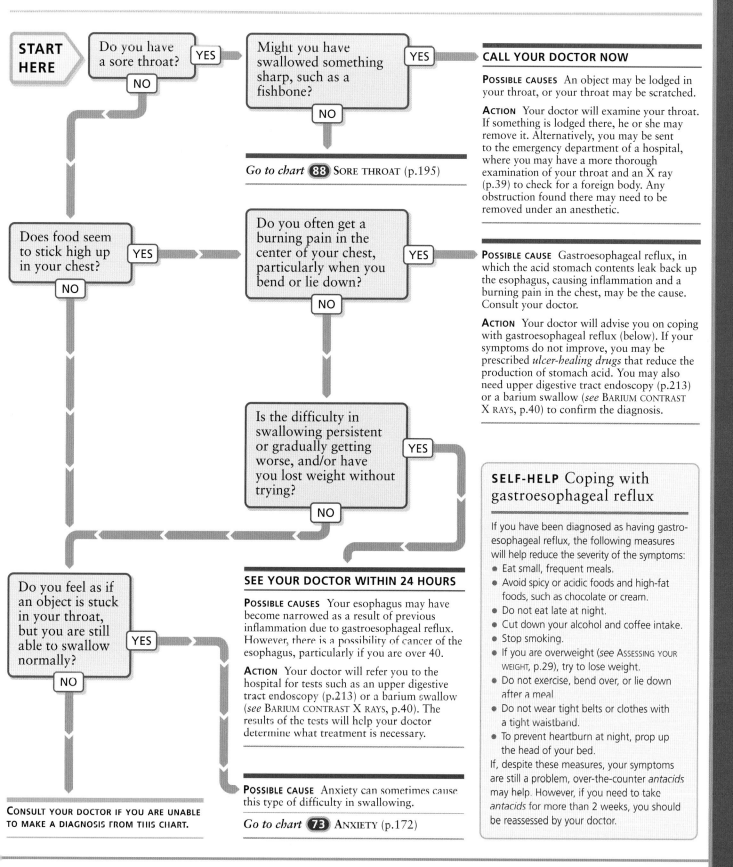

START HERE → **Do you have a sore throat?** — YES → **Might you have swallowed something sharp, such as a fishbone?** — YES → **CALL YOUR DOCTOR NOW**

Do you have a sore throat? — NO

Might you have swallowed something sharp, such as a fishbone? — NO → Go to chart **88** SORE THROAT (p.195)

Does food seem to stick high up in your chest? — YES → **Do you often get a burning pain in the center of your chest, particularly when you bend or lie down?** — YES

Does food seem to stick high up in your chest? — NO

Do you often get a burning pain in the center of your chest, particularly when you bend or lie down? — NO → **Is the difficulty in swallowing persistent or gradually getting worse, and/or have you lost weight without trying?** — YES

Is the difficulty in swallowing persistent or gradually getting worse, and/or have you lost weight without trying? — NO

Do you feel as if an object is stuck in your throat, but you are still able to swallow normally? — YES

Do you feel as if an object is stuck in your throat, but you are still able to swallow normally? — NO

CALL YOUR DOCTOR NOW

POSSIBLE CAUSES An object may be lodged in your throat, or your throat may be scratched.

ACTION Your doctor will examine your throat. If something is lodged there, he or she may remove it. Alternatively, you may be sent to the emergency department of a hospital, where you may have a more thorough examination of your throat and an X ray (p.39) to check for a foreign body. Any obstruction found there may need to be removed under an anesthetic.

POSSIBLE CAUSE Gastroesophageal reflux, in which the acid stomach contents leak back up the esophagus, causing inflammation and a burning pain in the chest, may be the cause. Consult your doctor.

ACTION Your doctor will advise you on coping with gastroesophageal reflux (below). If your symptoms do not improve, you may be prescribed *ulcer-healing drugs* that reduce the production of stomach acid. You may also need upper digestive tract endoscopy (p.213) or a barium swallow (*see* BARIUM CONTRAST X RAYS, p.40) to confirm the diagnosis.

SELF-HELP Coping with gastroesophageal reflux

If you have been diagnosed as having gastro-esophageal reflux, the following measures will help reduce the severity of the symptoms:

- Eat small, frequent meals.
- Avoid spicy or acidic foods and high-fat foods, such as chocolate or cream.
- Do not eat late at night.
- Cut down your alcohol and coffee intake.
- Stop smoking.
- If you are overweight (*see* ASSESSING YOUR WEIGHT, p.29), try to lose weight.
- Do not exercise, bend over, or lie down after a meal
- Do not wear tight belts or clothes with a tight waistband.
- To prevent heartburn at night, prop up the head of your bed.

If, despite these measures, your symptoms are still a problem, over-the-counter *antacids* may help. However, if you need to take *antacids* for more than 2 weeks, you should be reassessed by your doctor.

SEE YOUR DOCTOR WITHIN 24 HOURS

POSSIBLE CAUSES Your esophagus may have become narrowed as a result of previous inflammation due to gastroesophageal reflux. However, there is a possibility of cancer of the esophagus, particularly if you are over 40.

ACTION Your doctor will refer you to the hospital for tests such as an upper digestive tract endoscopy (p.213) or a barium swallow (*see* BARIUM CONTRAST X RAYS, p.40). The results of the tests will help your doctor determine what treatment is necessary.

POSSIBLE CAUSE Anxiety can sometimes cause this type of difficulty in swallowing.

Go to chart **73** ANXIETY (p.172)

CONSULT YOUR DOCTOR IF YOU ARE UNABLE TO MAKE A DIAGNOSIS FROM THIS CHART.

98 Vomiting

For recurrent vomiting, see chart 99, RECURRENT NAUSEA AND VOMITING (p.212).

Vomiting is often the result of irritation of the stomach from infection or overindulgence in rich food or alcohol, but it may also follow a disturbance elsewhere in the digestive tract. Occasionally, a disorder affecting the nerve signals from the

brain or from the balance mechanism in the inner ear can produce vomiting. People who have recurrent migraine attacks recognize the familiar symptoms of headache with nausea or vomiting. In other cases of vomiting accompanied by severe headache, or when vomiting occurs with acute abdominal pain, urgent medical attention is needed.

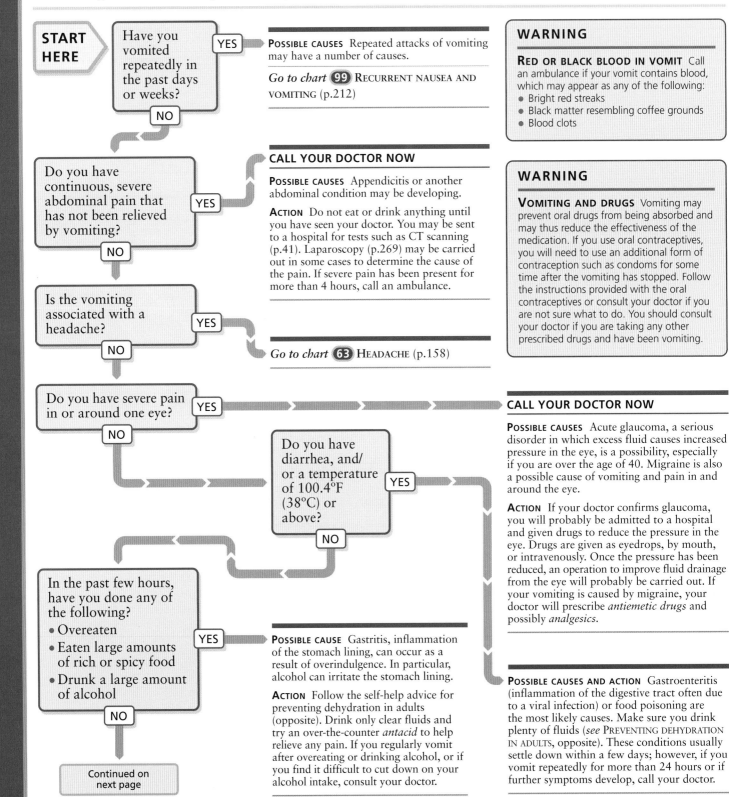

START HERE

Have you vomited repeatedly in the past days or weeks? — YES →

POSSIBLE CAUSES Repeated attacks of vomiting may have a number of causes.

Go to chart **99** RECURRENT NAUSEA AND VOMITING (p.212)

NO ↓

Do you have continuous, severe abdominal pain that has not been relieved by vomiting? — YES →

CALL YOUR DOCTOR NOW

POSSIBLE CAUSES Appendicitis or another abdominal condition may be developing.

ACTION Do not eat or drink anything until you have seen your doctor. You may be sent to a hospital for tests such as CT scanning (p.41). Laparoscopy (p.269) may be carried out in some cases to determine the cause of the pain. If severe pain has been present for more than 4 hours, call an ambulance.

NO ↓

Is the vomiting associated with a headache? — YES →

Go to chart **63** HEADACHE (p.158)

NO ↓

Do you have severe pain in or around one eye? — YES →

NO ↓

Do you have diarrhea, and/or a temperature of 100.4°F (38°C) or above? — YES →

NO ↓

In the past few hours, have you done any of the following?
- Overeaten
- Eaten large amounts of rich or spicy food
- Drunk a large amount of alcohol

— YES →

POSSIBLE CAUSE Gastritis, inflammation of the stomach lining, can occur as a result of overindulgence. In particular, alcohol can irritate the stomach lining.

ACTION Follow the self-help advice for preventing dehydration in adults (opposite). Drink only clear fluids and try an over-the-counter *antacid* to help relieve any pain. If you regularly vomit after overeating or drinking alcohol, or if you find it difficult to cut down on your alcohol intake, consult your doctor.

NO ↓

Continued on next page

WARNING

RED OR BLACK BLOOD IN VOMIT Call an ambulance if your vomit contains blood, which may appear as any of the following:
- Bright red streaks
- Black matter resembling coffee grounds
- Blood clots

WARNING

VOMITING AND DRUGS Vomiting may prevent oral drugs from being absorbed and may thus reduce the effectiveness of the medication. If you use oral contraceptives, you will need to use an additional form of contraception such as condoms for some time after the vomiting has stopped. Follow the instructions provided with the oral contraceptives or consult your doctor if you are not sure what to do. You should consult your doctor if you are taking any other prescribed drugs and have been vomiting.

CALL YOUR DOCTOR NOW

POSSIBLE CAUSES Acute glaucoma, a serious disorder in which excess fluid causes increased pressure in the eye, is a possibility, especially if you are over the age of 40. Migraine is also a possible cause of vomiting and pain in and around the eye.

ACTION If your doctor confirms glaucoma, you will probably be admitted to a hospital and given drugs to reduce the pressure in the eye. Drugs are given as eyedrops, by mouth, or intravenously. Once the pressure has been reduced, an operation to improve fluid drainage from the eye will probably be carried out. If your vomiting is caused by migraine, your doctor will prescribe *antiemetic drugs* and possibly *analgesics*.

POSSIBLE CAUSES AND ACTION Gastroenteritis (inflammation of the digestive tract often due to a viral infection) or food poisoning are the most likely causes. Make sure you drink plenty of fluids (*see* PREVENTING DEHYDRATION IN ADULTS, opposite). These conditions usually settle down within a few days; however, if you vomit repeatedly for more than 24 hours or if further symptoms develop, call your doctor.

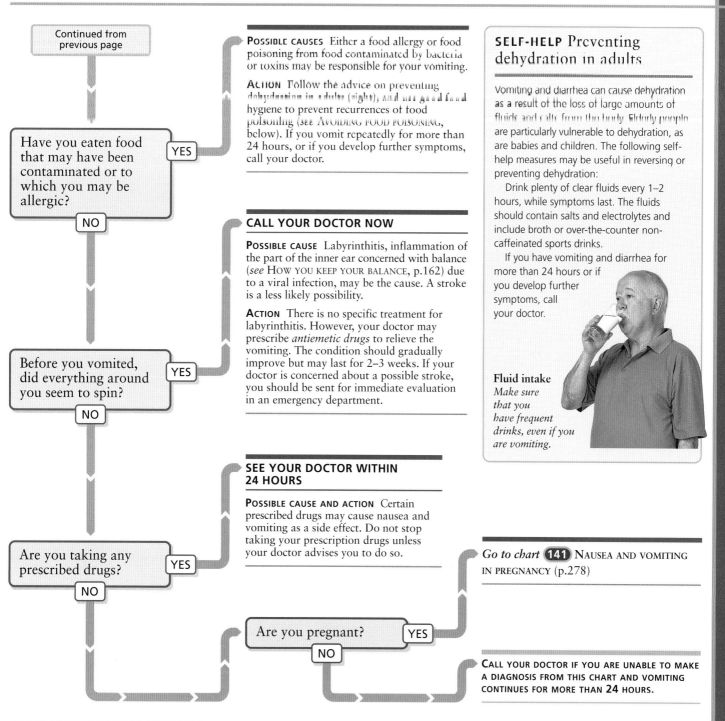

Continued from previous page

Have you eaten food that may have been contaminated or to which you may be allergic?

YES

POSSIBLE CAUSES Either a food allergy or food poisoning from food contaminated by bacteria or toxins may be responsible for your vomiting.

ACTION Follow the advice on preventing dehydration in adults (right), and use good food hygiene to prevent recurrences of food poisoning (see AVOIDING FOOD POISONING, below). If you vomit repeatedly for more than 24 hours, or if you develop further symptoms, call your doctor.

NO

Before you vomited, did everything around you seem to spin?

YES

CALL YOUR DOCTOR NOW

POSSIBLE CAUSE Labyrinthitis, inflammation of the part of the inner ear concerned with balance (see HOW YOU KEEP YOUR BALANCE, p.162) due to a viral infection, may be the cause. A stroke is a less likely possibility.

ACTION There is no specific treatment for labyrinthitis. However, your doctor may prescribe *antiemetic drugs* to relieve the vomiting. The condition should gradually improve but may last for 2–3 weeks. If your doctor is concerned about a possible stroke, you should be sent for immediate evaluation in an emergency department.

NO

Are you taking any prescribed drugs?

YES

SEE YOUR DOCTOR WITHIN 24 HOURS

POSSIBLE CAUSE AND ACTION Certain prescribed drugs may cause nausea and vomiting as a side effect. Do not stop taking your prescription drugs unless your doctor advises you to do so.

NO

Are you pregnant?

YES

NO

SELF-HELP Preventing dehydration in adults

Vomiting and diarrhea can cause dehydration as a result of the loss of large amounts of fluids and salts from the body. Elderly people are particularly vulnerable to dehydration, as are babies and children. The following self-help measures may be useful in reversing or preventing dehydration:

Drink plenty of clear fluids every 1–2 hours, while symptoms last. The fluids should contain salts and electrolytes and include broth or over-the-counter non-caffeinated sports drinks.

If you have vomiting and diarrhea for more than 24 hours or if you develop further symptoms, call your doctor.

Fluid intake
Make sure that you have frequent drinks, even if you are vomiting.

Go to chart **141** NAUSEA AND VOMITING IN PREGNANCY (p.278)

CALL YOUR DOCTOR IF YOU ARE UNABLE TO MAKE A DIAGNOSIS FROM THIS CHART AND VOMITING CONTINUES FOR MORE THAN 24 HOURS.

SELF-HELP Avoiding food poisoning

Food poisoning is usually caused by eating food contaminated with bacteria or toxins and may be avoided by taking the following measures:
- Regularly clean work surfaces with disinfectant and hot water.
- Wash your hands thoroughly before and after handling food.
- Use separate chopping boards for raw meat, cooked meat, and vegetables, and clean each board thoroughly after use.
- Make sure the refrigerator is set at the recommended temperature.
- Always use food by the expiration date.

- Put chilled food in the refrigerator as soon as possible after purchase.
- Store raw meat and fish away from other foods inside the refrigerator.
- Once leftover food has cooled, cover or wrap it properly and store it in the refrigerator.
- Defrost frozen food before cooking it, and never refreeze thawed food.

Safe food preparation
Always wash fresh fruit and vegetables before preparing them. Chopping boards should be washed in hot soapy water after use.

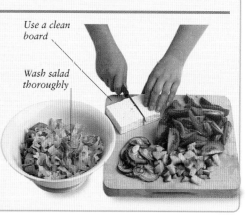

Use a clean board

Wash salad thoroughly

99 Recurrent nausea and vomiting

For isolated attacks of vomiting, see chart 98, VOMITING (p.210). For vomiting during pregnancy, see chart 141, NAUSEA AND VOMITING IN PREGNANCY (p.278). Consult this chart if you have vomited or felt nauseated repeatedly over a number of days or weeks. Recurrent

vomiting can be caused by inflammation of the stomach lining or by an ulcer. Lifestyle factors such as irregular meals or excess alcohol can make the symptoms worse. Recurrent vomiting associated with weight loss or abdominal pain may have a serious cause, and you should consult your doctor.

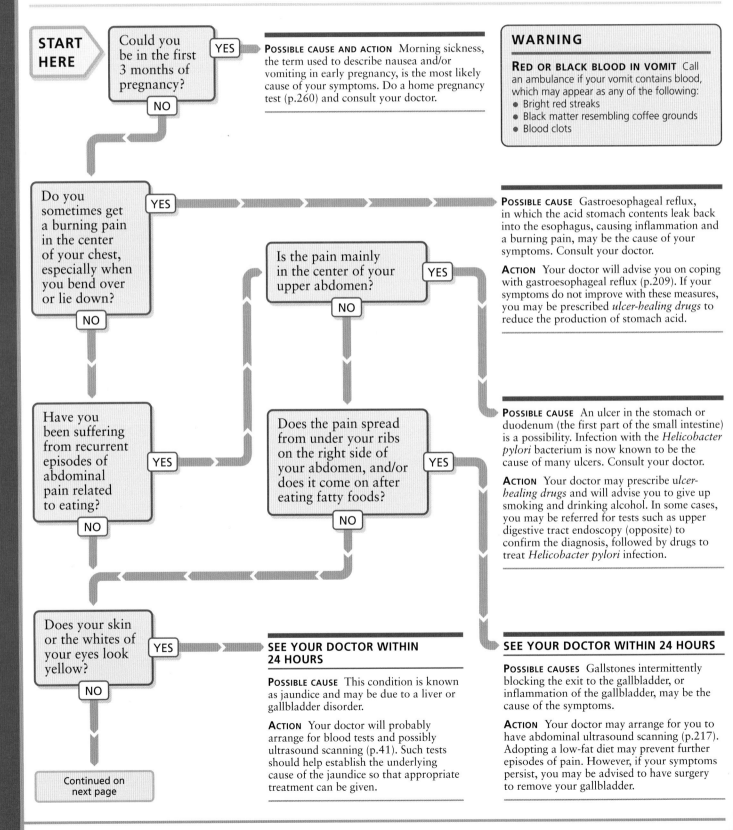

START HERE

Could you be in the first 3 months of pregnancy?

YES → **POSSIBLE CAUSE AND ACTION** Morning sickness, the term used to describe nausea and/or vomiting in early pregnancy, is the most likely cause of your symptoms. Do a home pregnancy test (p.260) and consult your doctor.

NO

WARNING

RED OR BLACK BLOOD IN VOMIT Call an ambulance if your vomit contains blood, which may appear as any of the following:
- Bright red streaks
- Black matter resembling coffee grounds
- Blood clots

Do you sometimes get a burning pain in the center of your chest, especially when you bend over or lie down?

YES → **Is the pain mainly in the center of your upper abdomen?**

YES → **POSSIBLE CAUSE** Gastroesophageal reflux, in which the acid stomach contents leak back into the esophagus, causing inflammation and a burning pain, may be the cause of your symptoms. Consult your doctor.

ACTION Your doctor will advise you on coping with gastroesophageal reflux (p.209). If your symptoms do not improve with these measures, you may be prescribed *ulcer-healing drugs* to reduce the production of stomach acid.

NO

NO

Have you been suffering from recurrent episodes of abdominal pain related to eating?

YES → **Does the pain spread from under your ribs on the right side of your abdomen, and/or does it come on after eating fatty foods?**

YES → **POSSIBLE CAUSE** An ulcer in the stomach or duodenum (the first part of the small intestine) is a possibility. Infection with the *Helicobacter pylori* bacterium is now known to be the cause of many ulcers. Consult your doctor.

ACTION Your doctor may prescribe u*lcer-healing drugs* and will advise you to give up smoking and drinking alcohol. In some cases, you may be referred for tests such as upper digestive tract endoscopy (opposite) to confirm the diagnosis, followed by drugs to treat *Helicobacter pylori* infection.

NO

NO

Does your skin or the whites of your eyes look yellow?

YES → **SEE YOUR DOCTOR WITHIN 24 HOURS**

POSSIBLE CAUSE This condition is known as jaundice and may be due to a liver or gallbladder disorder.

ACTION Your doctor will probably arrange for blood tests and possibly ultrasound scanning (p.41). Such tests should help establish the underlying cause of the jaundice so that appropriate treatment can be given.

SEE YOUR DOCTOR WITHIN 24 HOURS

POSSIBLE CAUSES Gallstones intermittently blocking the exit to the gallbladder, or inflammation of the gallbladder, may be the cause of the symptoms.

ACTION Your doctor may arrange for you to have abdominal ultrasound scanning (p.217). Adopting a low-fat diet may prevent further episodes of pain. However, if your symptoms persist, you may be advised to have surgery to remove your gallbladder.

NO

Continued on next page

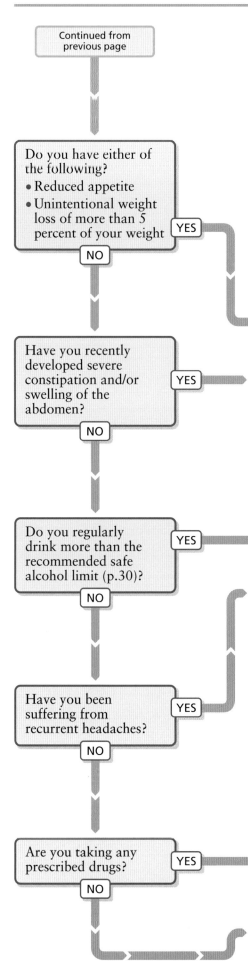

Continued from previous page

Do you have either of the following?
• Reduced appetite
• Unintentional weight loss of more than 5 percent of your weight

YES / **NO**

Have you recently developed severe constipation and/or swelling of the abdomen?

YES / **NO**

Do you regularly drink more than the recommended safe alcohol limit (p.30)?

YES / **NO**

Have you been suffering from recurrent headaches?

YES / **NO**

Are you taking any prescribed drugs?

YES / **NO**

Upper digestive tract endoscopy

Endoscopy of the upper digestive tract involves passing a flexible viewing tube through the mouth to examine the inside of the oesophagus, stomach, and duodenum (first part of the small intestine) to look for disorders such as ulcers. Your throat may be sprayed with a local anesthetic and/or you may be sedated. The procedure usually takes about 15 minutes. Samples for analysis can be taken during the procedure.

Viewing the digestive tract
The doctor can inspect the lining of the digestive tract, which is displayed on the monitor as the endoscope is moved around.

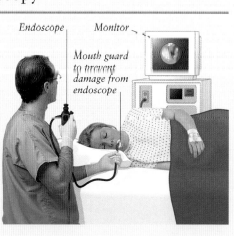

Endoscope   Monitor

Mouth guard to prevent damage from endoscope

CALL YOUR DOCTOR NOW

POSSIBLE CAUSE A blockage in the intestine could be the cause of your symptoms.

ACTION Your doctor will examine you and may send you to the hospital for tests such as X rays (p.39). If the vomiting is severe, you may be given fluids intravenously instead of by mouth. In some cases, surgery may be needed to relieve the blockage.

SEE YOUR DOCTOR WITHIN 24 HOURS

POSSIBLE CAUSE A condition that causes increased pressure on the brain, such as a tumor, may be the cause. However, such conditions are rare, and recurrent attacks of vomiting associated with headaches are more likely to be due to migraine.

ACTION If you have not previously been diagnosed as having migraine, your doctor will examine you to exclude other causes. He or she may also refer you for MRI scanning (p.41) of the brain. If migraine is the cause of your symptoms, follow the advice on relieving a headache (p.159) and reducing the frequency of migraine (p.159).

SEE YOUR DOCTOR WITHIN 24 HOURS

POSSIBLE CAUSES An ulcer in the stomach or duodenum (the first part of the small intestine) is the most likely cause of your symptoms, but there is a slight possibility of stomach cancer.

ACTION Your doctor will probably arrange for you to have upper digestive tract endoscopy (above). Ulcers may be treated with a course of *antibiotics* to kill the *Helicobacter pylori* bacteria that are responsible for the majority of these ulcers. Stomach cancer usually needs to be treated surgically.

POSSIBLE CAUSE Gastritis (persistent inflammation of the stomach lining) is a possibility. This disorder is aggravated by excessive alcohol intake. Consult your doctor.

ACTION Your doctor will advise you to cut down your alcohol intake to within the recommended limits. He or she may also prescribe *antacids*. Eat small, regular meals and, if you smoke, stop. If your symptoms persist, your doctor may refer you for upper digestive tract endoscopy (above).

SEE YOUR DOCTOR WITHIN 24 HOURS

POSSIBLE CAUSE AND ACTION Certain drugs can cause recurrent vomiting as a side effect. Do not stop taking your prescribed drugs without your doctor's advice. Remember that vomiting can reduce the effectiveness of certain drugs (*see* VOMITING AND DRUGS, p.210).

CONSULT YOUR DOCTOR IF YOU ARE UNABLE TO MAKE A DIAGNOSIS FROM THIS CHART.

100 Abdominal pain

For recurrent abdominal pain, see chart 101, RECURRENT
ABDOMINAL PAIN **(p.216).**
Many cases of abdominal pain are short-lived and are due
simply to eating or drinking too much or too quickly.

However, pain in the abdomen may also be due to a disorder
affecting the digestive system, urinary system, or, in women,
the reproductive system. Any abdominal pain that is severe
or persistent should receive prompt medical attention.

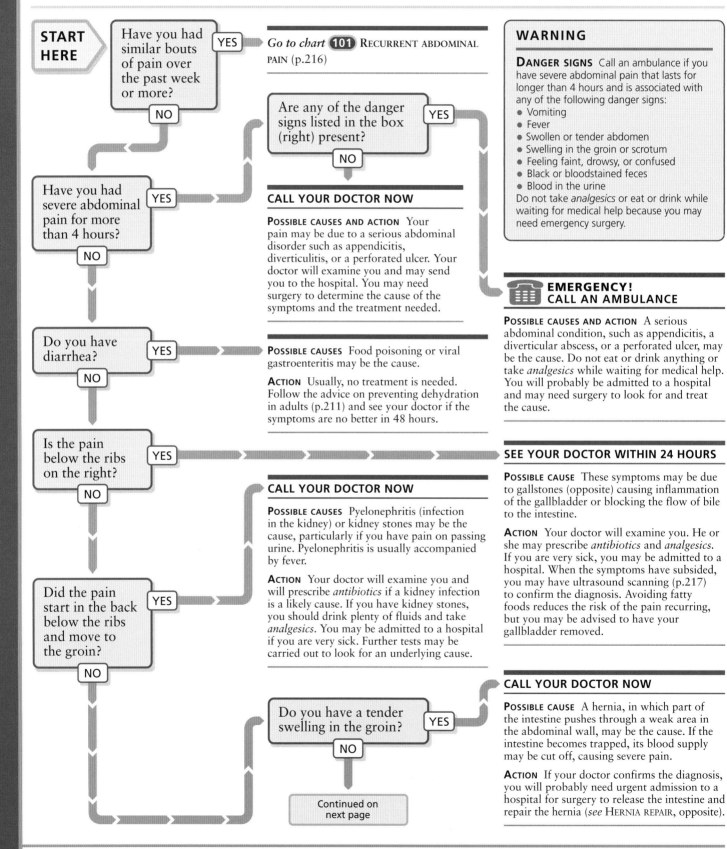

START HERE

Have you had similar bouts of pain over the past week or more?
— YES → *Go to chart* **101** RECURRENT ABDOMINAL PAIN (p.216)
— NO

Have you had severe abdominal pain for more than 4 hours?
— YES → **Are any of the danger signs listed in the box (right) present?**
  — YES → EMERGENCY! CALL AN AMBULANCE
  — NO → **CALL YOUR DOCTOR NOW**

    POSSIBLE CAUSES AND ACTION Your pain may be due to a serious abdominal disorder such as appendicitis, diverticulitis, or a perforated ulcer. Your doctor will examine you and may send you to the hospital. You may need surgery to determine the cause of the symptoms and the treatment needed.
— NO

Do you have diarrhea?
— YES → **POSSIBLE CAUSES** Food poisoning or viral gastroenteritis may be the cause.

  ACTION Usually, no treatment is needed. Follow the advice on preventing dehydration in adults (p.211) and see your doctor if the symptoms are no better in 48 hours.
— NO

Is the pain below the ribs on the right?
— YES → **SEE YOUR DOCTOR WITHIN 24 HOURS**
— NO

Did the pain start in the back below the ribs and move to the groin?
— YES → **CALL YOUR DOCTOR NOW**

  POSSIBLE CAUSES Pyelonephritis (infection in the kidney) or kidney stones may be the cause, particularly if you have pain on passing urine. Pyelonephritis is usually accompanied by fever.

  ACTION Your doctor will examine you and will prescribe *antibiotics* if a kidney infection is a likely cause. If you have kidney stones, you should drink plenty of fluids and take *analgesics*. You may be admitted to a hospital if you are very sick. Further tests may be carried out to look for an underlying cause.
— NO

Do you have a tender swelling in the groin?
— YES → **CALL YOUR DOCTOR NOW**
— NO → Continued on next page

WARNING

DANGER SIGNS Call an ambulance if you have severe abdominal pain that lasts for longer than 4 hours and is associated with any of the following danger signs:
- Vomiting
- Fever
- Swollen or tender abdomen
- Swelling in the groin or scrotum
- Feeling faint, drowsy, or confused
- Black or bloodstained feces
- Blood in the urine

Do not take *analgesics* or eat or drink while waiting for medical help because you may need emergency surgery.

☎ EMERGENCY! CALL AN AMBULANCE

POSSIBLE CAUSES AND ACTION A serious abdominal condition, such as appendicitis, a diverticular abscess, or a perforated ulcer, may be the cause. Do not eat or drink anything or take *analgesics* while waiting for medical help. You will probably be admitted to a hospital and may need surgery to look for and treat the cause.

SEE YOUR DOCTOR WITHIN 24 HOURS

POSSIBLE CAUSE These symptoms may be due to gallstones (opposite) causing inflammation of the gallbladder or blocking the flow of bile to the intestine.

ACTION Your doctor will examine you. He or she may prescribe *antibiotics* and *analgesics*. If you are very sick, you may be admitted to a hospital. When the symptoms have subsided, you may have ultrasound scanning (p.217) to confirm the diagnosis. Avoiding fatty foods reduces the risk of the pain recurring, but you may be advised to have your gallbladder removed.

CALL YOUR DOCTOR NOW

POSSIBLE CAUSE A hernia, in which part of the intestine pushes through a weak area in the abdominal wall, may be the cause. If the intestine becomes trapped, its blood supply may be cut off, causing severe pain.

ACTION If your doctor confirms the diagnosis, you will probably need urgent admission to a hospital for surgery to release the intestine and repair the hernia (*see* HERNIA REPAIR, opposite).

Continued from previous page

Is the pain in the center of the upper abdomen? **YES** → Does the pain become worse when you bend over or lie down? **YES** →

NO

NO

Is it worse after eating a large meal or drinking excessive alcohol? **YES** →

NO

POSSIBLE CAUSE Gastroesophageal reflux, in which the acid stomach contents leak back up the esophagus, may be the cause. This condition causes inflammation of the esophagus and a burning pain in the chest. Consult your doctor.

ACTION Your doctor will advise you on coping with gastroesophageal reflux (p.209). If your symptoms do not improve, you may be prescribed *ulcer-healing drugs* to reduce the production of stomach acid.

POSSIBLE CAUSES Gastritis (persistent inflammation of the lining of the stomach) or indigestion, often due to overeating, are the most likely causes. Gastritis may be aggravated by drinking alcohol.

ACTION Try to eat small, regular meals and cut down on your alcohol intake (see SAFE ALCOHOL LIMITS, p.30). *Antacids* may help to relieve the pain. Consult your doctor if antacids do not ease the pain, or if attacks of pain occur frequently.

POSSIBLE CAUSE Pain in the center of the upper abdomen may be due to a heart condition.

Go to chart **93** CHEST PAIN (p.202)

Are you passing urine more often than normal and/or is urination painful? **YES** →

NO

SEE YOUR DOCTOR WITHIN 24 HOURS

POSSIBLE CAUSE AND ACTION You may have cystitis, inflammation of the bladder lining (usually due to bacterial infection). Your doctor will arrange for urine tests to confirm the diagnosis, and you will probably be prescribed *antibiotics*. Follow the self-help measures for urinary tract infections (p.226). If the condition recurs, more tests may be arranged to exclude an underlying problem.

Are you male? **YES** →

NO

Go to chart **136** LOWER ABDOMINAL PAIN IN WOMEN (p.269)

Do you have a swollen or painful testis or scrotum? **YES** →

NO

CONSULT YOUR DOCTOR OR, IF PAIN IS SEVERE, CALL YOUR DOCTOR NOW.

Gallstones

About 1 in 10 people over the age of 40 has gallstones. The stones are formed in the gallbladder from bile (a liquid produced by the liver that aids in digestion). There is often no obvious cause for gallstone formation, although they are more common in people who are overweight and/or who eat a high-fat diet. Gallstones do not always result in symptoms, but they sometimes inflame the gallbladder or block its exit so that bile cannot be emptied into the intestine. In both these cases, the result may be episodes of abdominal pain, nausea, and vomiting. The frequency of these painful episodes may be reduced by eating a low-fat diet, but in some cases the gallbladder needs to be removed.

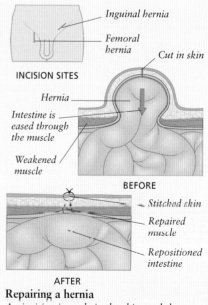

EMERGENCY! CALL AN AMBULANCE

POSSIBLE CAUSE AND ACTION You may have torsion of the testis (p.131), in which a testis is twisted in the scrotum, cutting off the blood supply. This can cause pain in the abdomen as well as in the scrotum. Torsion requires urgent surgery to untwist the testis and restore blood flow. Both testes are then stitched to the inside of the scrotum to prevent a recurrence.

Hernia repair

When part of an organ, usually the intestine, protrudes through a weakened muscle, it forms a hernia. Common types of hernia include inguinal and femoral hernias, both of which occur in the groin. Most hernias can be repaired by a simple operation, which is done under a local or general anesthetic. During the procedure, the contents of the hernia are eased back into place and the weakened muscle is repaired. In some cases a piece of synthetic mesh is sewn into the weakened muscle to strengthen it.

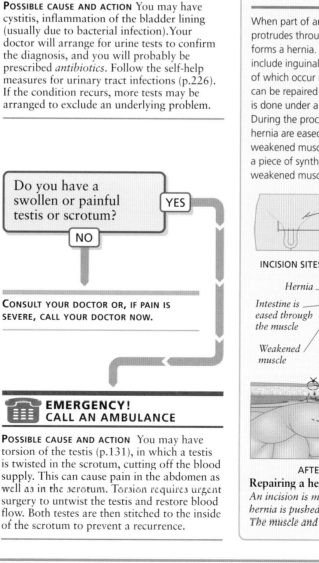

Inguinal hernia

Femoral hernia

INCISION SITES

Cut in skin

Hernia

Intestine is eased through the muscle

Weakened muscle

BEFORE

Stitched skin

Repaired muscle

Repositioned intestine

AFTER

Repairing a hernia
An incision is made in the skin, and the hernia is pushed back through the muscle. The muscle and skin are then stitched.

101 Recurrent abdominal pain

For an isolated attack of abdominal pain, see chart 100, ABDOMINAL PAIN **(p.214).**
Consult this chart if you have had several episodes of pain in the abdomen (between the rib cage and the groin) over a number of days or weeks. Most recurrent abdominal pain is the result of minor digestive disorders and can be relieved by a change in eating habits. If the pain persists, you should consult your doctor, even if you think you know what is causing the pain, so that he or she can eliminate the slight possibility of a serious underlying problem.

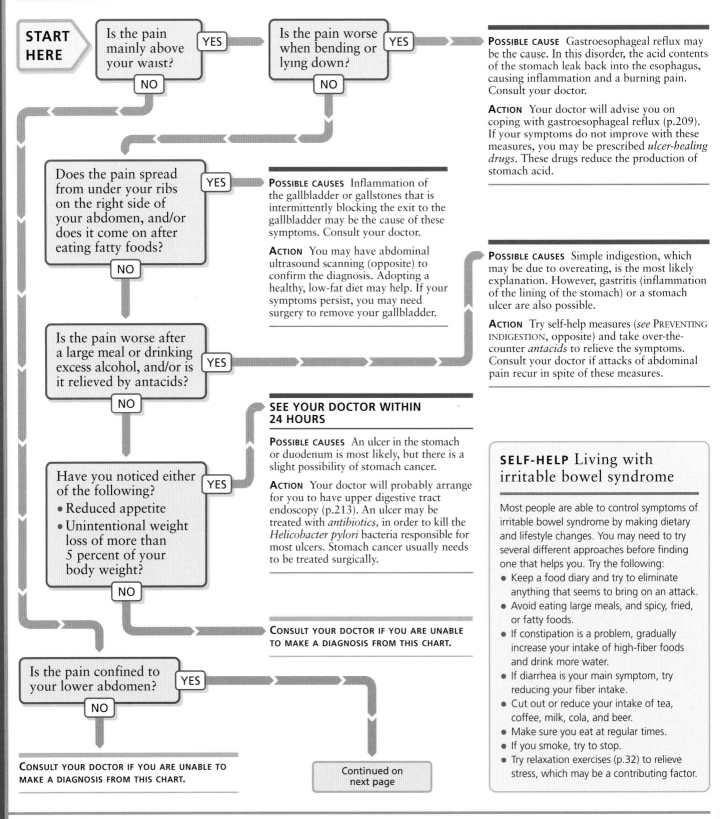

START HERE

Is the pain mainly above your waist? — YES → **Is the pain worse when bending or lying down?** — YES →

POSSIBLE CAUSE Gastroesophageal reflux may be the cause. In this disorder, the acid contents of the stomach leak back into the esophagus, causing inflammation and a burning pain. Consult your doctor.

ACTION Your doctor will advise you on coping with gastroesophageal reflux (p.209). If your symptoms do not improve with these measures, you may be prescribed *ulcer-healing drugs*. These drugs reduce the production of stomach acid.

Does the pain spread from under your ribs on the right side of your abdomen, and/or does it come on after eating fatty foods? — YES →

POSSIBLE CAUSES Inflammation of the gallbladder or gallstones that is intermittently blocking the exit to the gallbladder may be the cause of these symptoms. Consult your doctor.

ACTION You may have abdominal ultrasound scanning (opposite) to confirm the diagnosis. Adopting a healthy, low-fat diet may help. If your symptoms persist, you may need surgery to remove your gallbladder.

POSSIBLE CAUSES Simple indigestion, which may be due to overeating, is the most likely explanation. However, gastritis (inflammation of the lining of the stomach) or a stomach ulcer are also possible.

ACTION Try self-help measures (*see* PREVENTING INDIGESTION, opposite) and take over-the-counter *antacids* to relieve the symptoms. Consult your doctor if attacks of abdominal pain recur in spite of these measures.

Is the pain worse after a large meal or drinking excess alcohol, and/or is it relieved by antacids? — YES →

SEE YOUR DOCTOR WITHIN 24 HOURS

POSSIBLE CAUSES An ulcer in the stomach or duodenum is most likely, but there is a slight possibility of stomach cancer.

ACTION Your doctor will probably arrange for you to have upper digestive tract endoscopy (p.213). An ulcer may be treated with *antibiotics*, in order to kill the *Helicobacter pylori* bacteria responsible for most ulcers. Stomach cancer usually needs to be treated surgically.

Have you noticed either of the following?
• Reduced appetite
• Unintentional weight loss of more than 5 percent of your body weight? — YES →

CONSULT YOUR DOCTOR IF YOU ARE UNABLE TO MAKE A DIAGNOSIS FROM THIS CHART.

Is the pain confined to your lower abdomen? — YES →

CONSULT YOUR DOCTOR IF YOU ARE UNABLE TO MAKE A DIAGNOSIS FROM THIS CHART.

Continued on next page

SELF-HELP Living with irritable bowel syndrome

Most people are able to control symptoms of irritable bowel syndrome by making dietary and lifestyle changes. You may need to try several different approaches before finding one that helps you. Try the following:
• Keep a food diary and try to eliminate anything that seems to bring on an attack.
• Avoid eating large meals, and spicy, fried, or fatty foods.
• If constipation is a problem, gradually increase your intake of high-fiber foods and drink more water.
• If diarrhea is your main symptom, try reducing your fiber intake.
• Cut out or reduce your intake of tea, coffee, milk, cola, and beer.
• Make sure you eat at regular times.
• If you smoke, try to stop.
• Try relaxation exercises (p.32) to relieve stress, which may be a contributing factor.

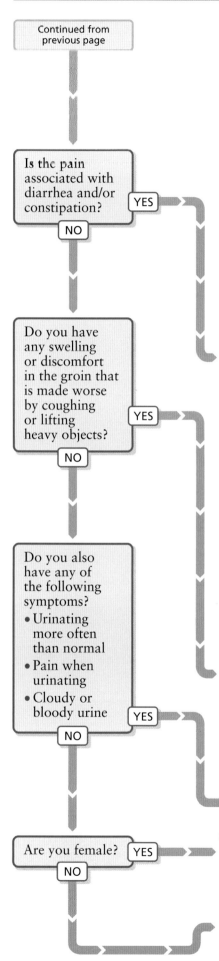

Continued from previous page

Is the pain associated with diarrhea and/or constipation? NO / YES

Do you have any swelling or discomfort in the groin that is made worse by coughing or lifting heavy objects? NO / YES

Do you also have any of the following symptoms?
- Urinating more often than normal
- Pain when urinating
- Cloudy or bloody urine

NO / YES

Are you female? NO / YES

Abdominal ultrasound scanning

In ultrasound scanning (p.41), a device called a transducer emits high frequency sound waves and receives their echoes to produce images of internal organs. Ultrasound scanning of the abdomen is often used to investigate the liver, the gallbladder, and the kidneys. To produce good contact between the transducer and the abdomen, gel is placed on the skin over the area to be examined. The technician or radiologist moves the transducer over the area, using gentle pressure, and images from it are displayed on a monitor. The procedure is painless and safe.

During the procedure
The hand-held transducer is moved over the skin of the abdomen. The images displayed on the monitor are continually updated.

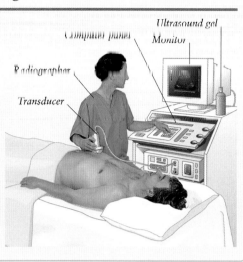

Computer panel *Ultrasound gel*
Monitor
Radiographer
Transducer

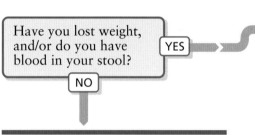

Have you lost weight, and/or do you have blood in your stool? NO / YES

POSSIBLE CAUSE You probably have irritable bowel syndrome, a disorder in which there is a combination of intermittent abdominal pain, constipation, and/or diarrhea. However, there is a slight possibility of cancer of the colon, especially in older people. Consult your doctor.

ACTION Your doctor will examine you and may arrange for tests such as colonoscopy (p.222) to rule out cancer of the colon. Most people are able to control the symptoms of irritable bowel syndrome using the self-help measures described (*see* LIVING WITH IRRITABLE BOWEL SYNDROME, opposite).

POSSIBLE CAUSE A hernia, in which part of the intestine pushes through a weak area in the abdominal wall, may be the cause of these symptoms. Consult your doctor.

ACTION If your doctor confirms the diagnosis, you may need to have an operation to repair the hernia (p.215).

Go to chart **136** LOWER ABDOMINAL PAIN IN WOMEN (p.269)

CONSULT YOUR DOCTOR IF YOU ARE UNABLE TO MAKE A DIAGNOSIS FROM THIS CHART.

SEE YOUR DOCTOR WITHIN 24 HOURS

POSSIBLE CAUSES Ulcerative colitis and Crohn's disease, disorders in which areas of the intestine become inflamed, are possible causes. There is also a possibility of cancer of the colon.

ACTION You will probably be referred to a hospital for tests such as colonoscopy (p.222) to establish the cause. Inflammation of the intestines may be treated with *corticosteroid* and other drugs. If cancer of the colon is the cause, it will be treated with surgery.

SEE YOUR DOCTOR WITHIN 24 HOURS

POSSIBLE CAUSES A urinary tract infection is likely. However, the possibility of a more serious condition, such as a bladder stone or a tumor, needs to be ruled out.

ACTION Your doctor will arrange for urine tests to confirm the diagnosis. If you have an infection, you will probably be prescribed *antibiotics*. Drink plenty of fluids and take *analgesics* to relieve the symptoms. If there is no infection, you will need ultrasound scanning (p.41), intravenous urography (p.227), or cystoscopy (p.224) to determine the correct treatment.

SELF-HELP Preventing indigestion

The following measures may be helpful in preventing bouts of indigestion:
- Eat at regular intervals without rushing.
- Avoid eating large meals late at night.
- Cut down on alcohol, coffee, and tea.
- Avoid eating rich, fatty foods.
- Keep a food diary and avoid foods that trigger indigestion.
- Avoid medicines that irritate the stomach, such as aspirin.

102 Swollen abdomen

An enlarged abdomen is most often due to excess weight that builds up over a period of years. Abdominal swelling that develops over a relatively short time is usually caused by excess gas in the intestines or by a distention of the bladder. In women, abdominal swelling may also be due to a disorder of the reproductive organs or to pregnancy.

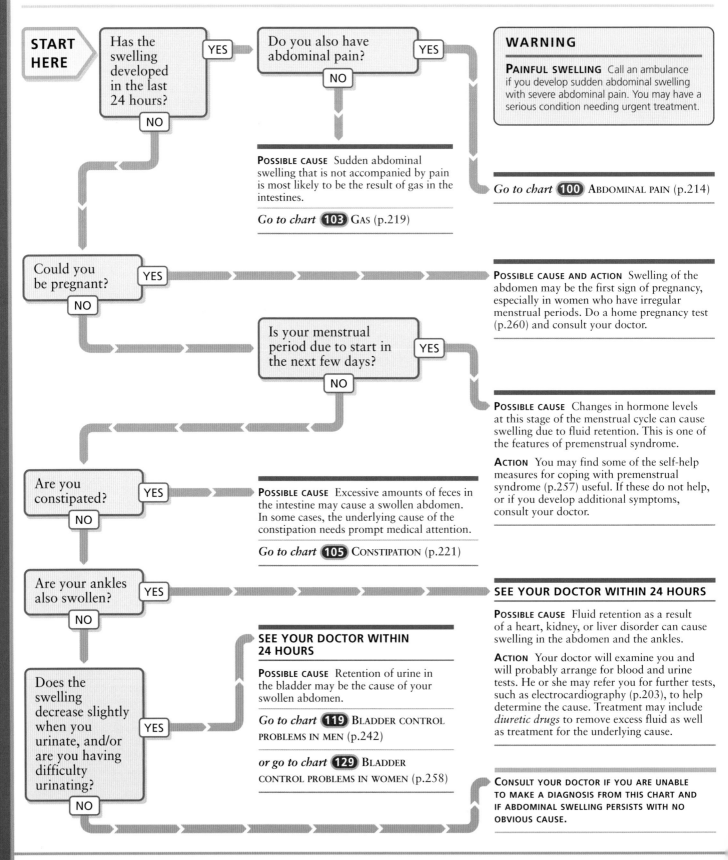

START HERE

Has the swelling developed in the last 24 hours? YES → **Do you also have abdominal pain?** YES →

NO (from abdominal pain) → **POSSIBLE CAUSE** Sudden abdominal swelling that is not accompanied by pain is most likely to be the result of gas in the intestines.

Go to chart **103** GAS (p.219)

YES (from abdominal pain) →

WARNING

PAINFUL SWELLING Call an ambulance if you develop sudden abdominal swelling with severe abdominal pain. You may have a serious condition needing urgent treatment.

Go to chart **100** ABDOMINAL PAIN (p.214)

NO (swelling developed) → **Could you be pregnant?** YES → **POSSIBLE CAUSE AND ACTION** Swelling of the abdomen may be the first sign of pregnancy, especially in women who have irregular menstrual periods. Do a home pregnancy test (p.260) and consult your doctor.

NO (pregnant) → **Is your menstrual period due to start in the next few days?** YES →

NO (menstrual period) → **POSSIBLE CAUSE** Changes in hormone levels at this stage of the menstrual cycle can cause swelling due to fluid retention. This is one of the features of premenstrual syndrome.

ACTION You may find some of the self-help measures for coping with premenstrual syndrome (p.257) useful. If these do not help, or if you develop additional symptoms, consult your doctor.

Are you constipated? YES → **POSSIBLE CAUSE** Excessive amounts of feces in the intestine may cause a swollen abdomen. In some cases, the underlying cause of the constipation needs prompt medical attention.

Go to chart **105** CONSTIPATION (p.221)

NO (constipated) → **Are your ankles also swollen?** YES →

SEE YOUR DOCTOR WITHIN 24 HOURS

POSSIBLE CAUSE Fluid retention as a result of a heart, kidney, or liver disorder can cause swelling in the abdomen and the ankles.

ACTION Your doctor will examine you and will probably arrange for blood and urine tests. He or she may refer you for further tests, such as electrocardiography (p.203), to help determine the cause. Treatment may include *diuretic drugs* to remove excess fluid as well as treatment for the underlying cause.

NO (ankles swollen) → **Does the swelling decrease slightly when you urinate, and/or are you having difficulty urinating?** YES →

SEE YOUR DOCTOR WITHIN 24 HOURS

POSSIBLE CAUSE Retention of urine in the bladder may be the cause of your swollen abdomen.

Go to chart **119** BLADDER CONTROL PROBLEMS IN MEN (p.242)

or go to chart **129** BLADDER CONTROL PROBLEMS IN WOMEN (p.258)

NO →

CONSULT YOUR DOCTOR IF YOU ARE UNABLE TO MAKE A DIAGNOSIS FROM THIS CHART AND IF ABDOMINAL SWELLING PERSISTS WITH NO OBVIOUS CAUSE.

103 Gas

Excess gas in the digestive system can cause discomfort and a bloated feeling. Expelling the gas through either the mouth (belching) or the anus generally relieves these symptoms. Gas is often caused by swallowing air while eating. It may also occur when certain foods are not broken down properly in the intestines; the food residues then ferment, producing gas. High-fiber foods such as cabbage are common causes of gas, although some people are affected by other types of food, such as dairy products. Usually, gas is nothing to worry about, but you should consult your doctor if you suddenly develop problems with gas without having had a change in your diet.

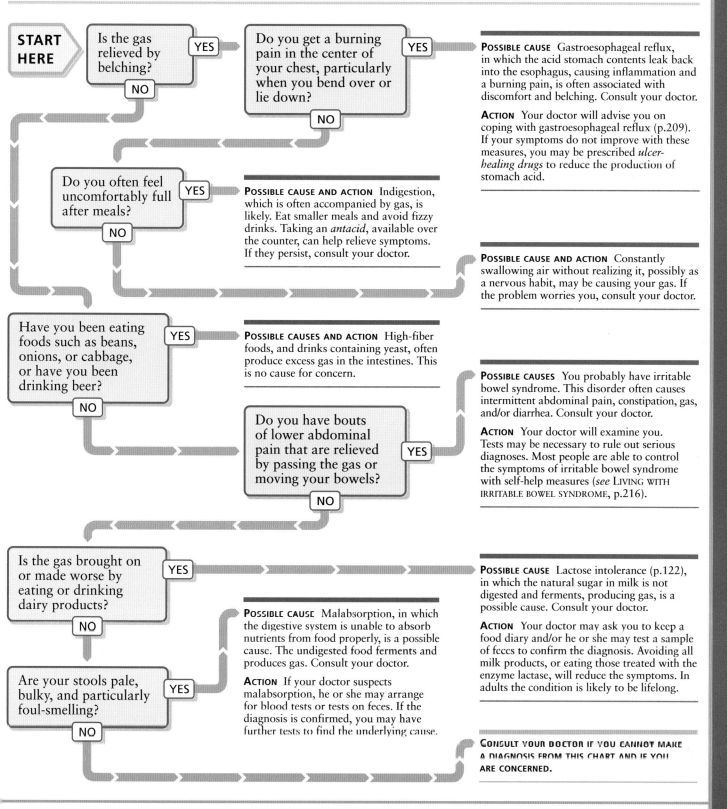

START HERE

Is the gas relieved by belching? YES → **Do you get a burning pain in the center of your chest, particularly when you bend over or lie down?** YES →

POSSIBLE CAUSE Gastroesophageal reflux, in which the acid stomach contents leak back into the esophagus, causing inflammation and a burning pain, is often associated with discomfort and belching. Consult your doctor.

ACTION Your doctor will advise you on coping with gastroesophageal reflux (p.209). If your symptoms do not improve with these measures, you may be prescribed *ulcer-healing drugs* to reduce the production of stomach acid.

NO

Do you often feel uncomfortably full after meals? YES →

POSSIBLE CAUSE AND ACTION Indigestion, which is often accompanied by gas, is likely. Eat smaller meals and avoid fizzy drinks. Taking an *antacid*, available over the counter, can help relieve symptoms. If they persist, consult your doctor.

NO

POSSIBLE CAUSE AND ACTION Constantly swallowing air without realizing it, possibly as a nervous habit, may be causing your gas. If the problem worries you, consult your doctor.

Have you been eating foods such as beans, onions, or cabbage, or have you been drinking beer? YES →

POSSIBLE CAUSES AND ACTION High-fiber foods, and drinks containing yeast, often produce excess gas in the intestines. This is no cause for concern.

NO

Do you have bouts of lower abdominal pain that are relieved by passing the gas or moving your bowels? YES →

POSSIBLE CAUSES You probably have irritable bowel syndrome. This disorder often causes intermittent abdominal pain, constipation, gas, and/or diarrhea. Consult your doctor.

ACTION Your doctor will examine you. Tests may be necessary to rule out serious diagnoses. Most people are able to control the symptoms of irritable bowel syndrome with self-help measures (*see* LIVING WITH IRRITABLE BOWEL SYNDROME, p.216).

NO

Is the gas brought on or made worse by eating or drinking dairy products? YES →

POSSIBLE CAUSE Lactose intolerance (p.122), in which the natural sugar in milk is not digested and ferments, producing gas, is a possible cause. Consult your doctor.

ACTION Your doctor may ask you to keep a food diary and/or he or she may test a sample of feces to confirm the diagnosis. Avoiding all milk products, or eating those treated with the enzyme lactase, will reduce the symptoms. In adults the condition is likely to be lifelong.

NO

Are your stools pale, bulky, and particularly foul-smelling? YES →

POSSIBLE CAUSE Malabsorption, in which the digestive system is unable to absorb nutrients from food properly, is a possible cause. The undigested food ferments and produces gas. Consult your doctor.

ACTION If your doctor suspects malabsorption, he or she may arrange for blood tests or tests on feces. If the diagnosis is confirmed, you may have further tests to find the underlying cause.

NO

CONSULT YOUR DOCTOR IF YOU CANNOT MAKE A DIAGNOSIS FROM THIS CHART AND IF YOU ARE CONCERNED.

104 Diarrhea

Diarrhea is the frequent passing of unusually loose or watery stools. It is often accompanied by cramping pains in the lower abdomen. Most attacks of diarrhea result from viral infections and last for less than 48 hours. Diarrhea is rarely serious, and usually no treatment is needed other than

ensuring that you drink plenty of fluids in order to avoid dehydration. However, you should see your doctor if diarrhea lasts more than 48 hours or if you have frequent episodes of diarrhea. Also see your doctor if you have diarrhea and your job involves handling food.

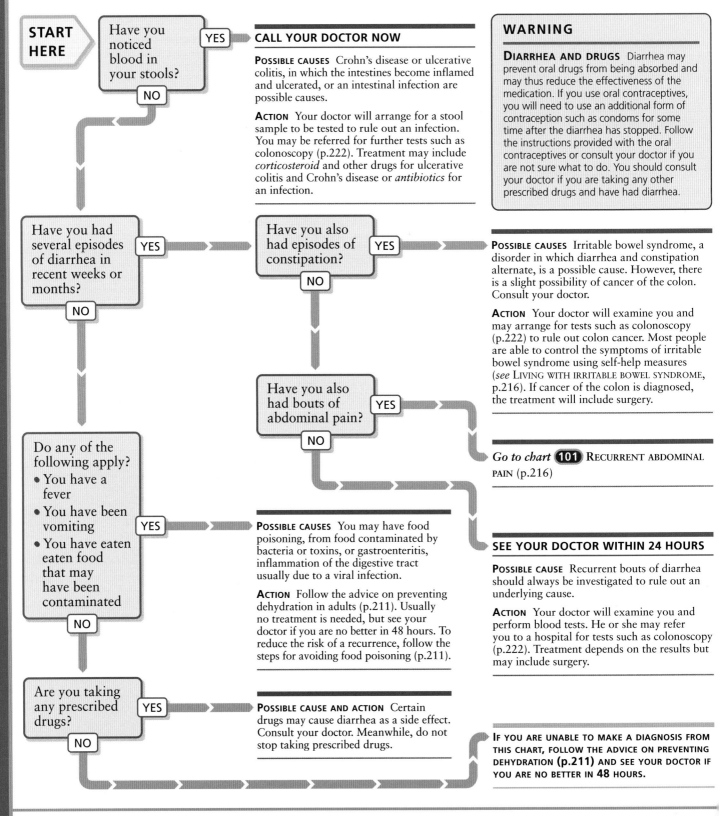

START HERE

Have you noticed blood in your stools? — YES

NO

CALL YOUR DOCTOR NOW

POSSIBLE CAUSES Crohn's disease or ulcerative colitis, in which the intestines become inflamed and ulcerated, or an intestinal infection are possible causes.

ACTION Your doctor will arrange for a stool sample to be tested to rule out an infection. You may be referred for further tests such as colonoscopy (p.222). Treatment may include *corticosteroid* and other drugs for ulcerative colitis and Crohn's disease or *antibiotics* for an infection.

WARNING

DIARRHEA AND DRUGS Diarrhea may prevent oral drugs from being absorbed and may thus reduce the effectiveness of the medication. If you use oral contraceptives, you will need to use an additional form of contraception such as condoms for some time after the diarrhea has stopped. Follow the instructions provided with the oral contraceptives or consult your doctor if you are not sure what to do. You should consult your doctor if you are taking any other prescribed drugs and have had diarrhea.

Have you had several episodes of diarrhea in recent weeks or months? — YES

NO

Have you also had episodes of constipation? — YES

NO

POSSIBLE CAUSES Irritable bowel syndrome, a disorder in which diarrhea and constipation alternate, is a possible cause. However, there is a slight possibility of cancer of the colon. Consult your doctor.

ACTION Your doctor will examine you and may arrange for tests such as colonoscopy (p.222) to rule out colon cancer. Most people are able to control the symptoms of irritable bowel syndrome using self-help measures (*see* LIVING WITH IRRITABLE BOWEL SYNDROME, p.216). If cancer of the colon is diagnosed, the treatment will include surgery.

Have you also had bouts of abdominal pain? — YES

NO

Go to chart **101** RECURRENT ABDOMINAL PAIN (p.216)

Do any of the following apply?
- You have a fever
- You have been vomiting
- You have eaten eaten food that may have been contaminated

YES

NO

POSSIBLE CAUSES You may have food poisoning, from food contaminated by bacteria or toxins, or gastroenteritis, inflammation of the digestive tract usually due to a viral infection.

ACTION Follow the advice on preventing dehydration in adults (p.211). Usually no treatment is needed, but see your doctor if you are no better in 48 hours. To reduce the risk of a recurrence, follow the steps for avoiding food poisoning (p.211).

SEE YOUR DOCTOR WITHIN 24 HOURS

POSSIBLE CAUSE Recurrent bouts of diarrhea should always be investigated to rule out an underlying cause.

ACTION Your doctor will examine you and perform blood tests. He or she may refer you to a hospital for tests such as colonoscopy (p.222). Treatment depends on the results but may include surgery.

Are you taking any prescribed drugs? — YES

NO

POSSIBLE CAUSE AND ACTION Certain drugs may cause diarrhea as a side effect. Consult your doctor. Meanwhile, do not stop taking prescribed drugs.

IF YOU ARE UNABLE TO MAKE A DIAGNOSIS FROM THIS CHART, FOLLOW THE ADVICE ON PREVENTING DEHYDRATION (p.211) AND SEE YOUR DOCTOR IF YOU ARE NO BETTER IN 48 HOURS.

105 Constipation

Some people have a bowel movement once or twice a day; others, less frequently. If you have fewer bowel movements than usual, or if your stools are small and hard, you are constipated. The cause is often a lack of fluid or fiber-rich foods in the diet. Constipation is also common in pregnancy because hormone changes cause intestinal muscles to relax. If you are constipated for longer than 2 weeks, consult your doctor so that serious causes can be ruled out.

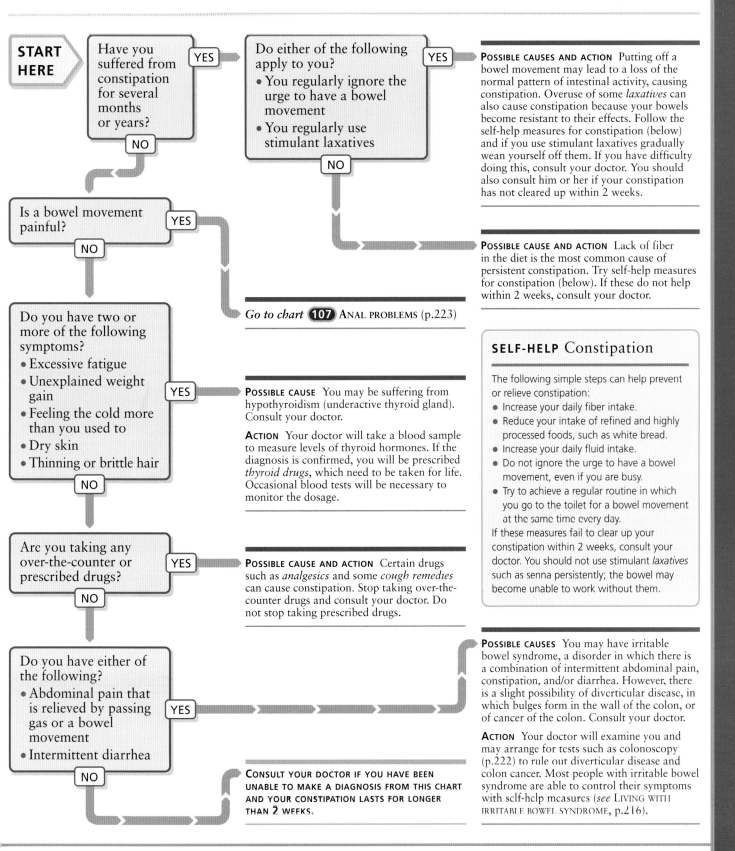

START HERE

Have you suffered from constipation for several months or years?
YES →

NO ↓

Do either of the following apply to you?
- You regularly ignore the urge to have a bowel movement
- You regularly use stimulant laxatives

YES →

NO ↓

POSSIBLE CAUSES AND ACTION Putting off a bowel movement may lead to a loss of the normal pattern of intestinal activity, causing constipation. Overuse of some *laxatives* can also cause constipation because your bowels become resistant to their effects. Follow the self-help measures for constipation (below) and if you use stimulant laxatives gradually wean yourself off them. If you have difficulty doing this, consult your doctor. You should also consult him or her if your constipation has not cleared up within 2 weeks.

POSSIBLE CAUSE AND ACTION Lack of fiber in the diet is the most common cause of persistent constipation. Try self-help measures for constipation (below). If these do not help within 2 weeks, consult your doctor.

Is a bowel movement painful?
YES →

NO ↓

Go to chart **107** ANAL PROBLEMS (p.223)

Do you have two or more of the following symptoms?
- Excessive fatigue
- Unexplained weight gain
- Feeling the cold more than you used to
- Dry skin
- Thinning or brittle hair

YES →

NO ↓

POSSIBLE CAUSE You may be suffering from hypothyroidism (underactive thyroid gland). Consult your doctor.

ACTION Your doctor will take a blood sample to measure levels of thyroid hormones. If the diagnosis is confirmed, you will be prescribed *thyroid drugs*, which need to be taken for life. Occasional blood tests will be necessary to monitor the dosage.

SELF-HELP Constipation

The following simple steps can help prevent or relieve constipation:
- Increase your daily fiber intake.
- Reduce your intake of refined and highly processed foods, such as white bread.
- Increase your daily fluid intake.
- Do not ignore the urge to have a bowel movement, even if you are busy.
- Try to achieve a regular routine in which you go to the toilet for a bowel movement at the same time every day.

If these measures fail to clear up your constipation within 2 weeks, consult your doctor. You should not use stimulant *laxatives* such as senna persistently; the bowel may become unable to work without them.

Are you taking any over-the-counter or prescribed drugs?
YES →

NO ↓

POSSIBLE CAUSE AND ACTION Certain drugs such as *analgesics* and some *cough remedies* can cause constipation. Stop taking over-the-counter drugs and consult your doctor. Do not stop taking prescribed drugs.

Do you have either of the following?
- Abdominal pain that is relieved by passing gas or a bowel movement
- Intermittent diarrhea

YES →

NO ↓

POSSIBLE CAUSES You may have irritable bowel syndrome, a disorder in which there is a combination of intermittent abdominal pain, constipation, and/or diarrhea. However, there is a slight possibility of diverticular disease, in which bulges form in the wall of the colon, or of cancer of the colon. Consult your doctor.

ACTION Your doctor will examine you and may arrange for tests such as colonoscopy (p.222) to rule out diverticular disease and colon cancer. Most people with irritable bowel syndrome are able to control their symptoms with self-help measures (*see* LIVING WITH IRRITABLE BOWEL SYNDROME, p.216).

CONSULT YOUR DOCTOR IF YOU HAVE BEEN UNABLE TO MAKE A DIAGNOSIS FROM THIS CHART AND YOUR CONSTIPATION LASTS FOR LONGER THAN 2 WEEKS.

106 Abnormal-looking stools

Most minor changes in the color and consistency of your stools are due to a recent change in diet or a temporary digestive upset. However, if the stools are significantly darker or lighter in color than usual, or if they are streaked with blood, this may indicate a potentially serious disorder of the digestive system that requires medical attention.

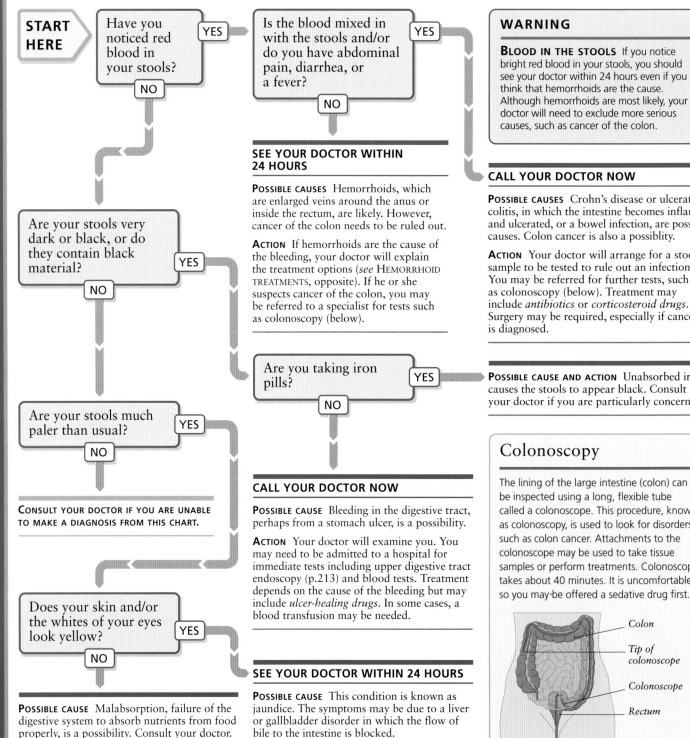

START HERE

Have you noticed red blood in your stools? — YES → **Is the blood mixed in with the stools and/or do you have abdominal pain, diarrhea, or a fever?** — YES →

NO ↓ / NO ↓

Are your stools very dark or black, or do they contain black material? — YES →

NO ↓

Are your stools much paler than usual? — YES →

NO ↓

Are you taking iron pills? — YES →

NO ↓

Does your skin and/or the whites of your eyes look yellow? — YES →

NO ↓

WARNING

BLOOD IN THE STOOLS If you notice bright red blood in your stools, you should see your doctor within 24 hours even if you think that hemorrhoids are the cause. Although hemorrhoids are most likely, your doctor will need to exclude more serious causes, such as cancer of the colon.

SEE YOUR DOCTOR WITHIN 24 HOURS

POSSIBLE CAUSES Hemorrhoids, which are enlarged veins around the anus or inside the rectum, are likely. However, cancer of the colon needs to be ruled out.

ACTION If hemorrhoids are the cause of the bleeding, your doctor will explain the treatment options (*see* HEMORRHOID TREATMENTS, opposite). If he or she suspects cancer of the colon, you may be referred to a specialist for tests such as colonoscopy (below).

CALL YOUR DOCTOR NOW

POSSIBLE CAUSES Crohn's disease or ulcerative colitis, in which the intestine becomes inflamed and ulcerated, or a bowel infection, are possible causes. Colon cancer is also a possiblity.

ACTION Your doctor will arrange for a stool sample to be tested to rule out an infection. You may be referred for further tests, such as colonoscopy (below). Treatment may include *antibiotics* or *corticosteroid drugs*. Surgery may be required, especially if cancer is diagnosed.

POSSIBLE CAUSE AND ACTION Unabsorbed iron causes the stools to appear black. Consult your doctor if you are particularly concerned.

CONSULT YOUR DOCTOR IF YOU ARE UNABLE TO MAKE A DIAGNOSIS FROM THIS CHART.

CALL YOUR DOCTOR NOW

POSSIBLE CAUSE Bleeding in the digestive tract, perhaps from a stomach ulcer, is a possibility.

ACTION Your doctor will examine you. You may need to be admitted to a hospital for immediate tests including upper digestive tract endoscopy (p.213) and blood tests. Treatment depends on the cause of the bleeding but may include *ulcer-healing drugs*. In some cases, a blood transfusion may be needed.

SEE YOUR DOCTOR WITHIN 24 HOURS

POSSIBLE CAUSE This condition is known as jaundice. The symptoms may be due to a liver or gallbladder disorder in which the flow of bile to the intestine is blocked.

ACTION Your doctor will probably arrange for blood tests and possibly for abdominal ultrasound scanning (p.217). Such tests should help establish the underlying cause so that appropriate treatment can be given.

POSSIBLE CAUSE Malabsorption, failure of the digestive system to absorb nutrients from food properly, is a possibility. Consult your doctor.

ACTION If your doctor suspects malabsorption, he or she may arrange for tests on blood and stools. If the diagnosis is confirmed, you may have further tests to determine the cause of the malabsorption so that treatment can be given.

Colonoscopy

The lining of the large intestine (colon) can be inspected using a long, flexible tube called a colonoscope. This procedure, known as colonoscopy, is used to look for disorders such as colon cancer. Attachments to the colonoscope may be used to take tissue samples or perform treatments. Colonoscopy takes about 40 minutes. It is uncomfortable, so you may be offered a sedative drug first.

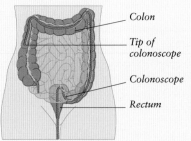

Colon

Tip of colonoscope

Colonoscope

Rectum

During the procedure
The colonoscope is passed through the rectum up into the colon. Air is passed in to give a clearer view of the colon.

107 Anal and rectal problems

The rectum is the last part of the digestive tract, and is linked to the outside of the body by the anus. The anus contains a ring of muscles that keep it closed except when passing stools. The most common symptoms affecting the anus are itching and pain, which are not usually signs of a serious disorder. Bleeding should always be assessed by your doctor.

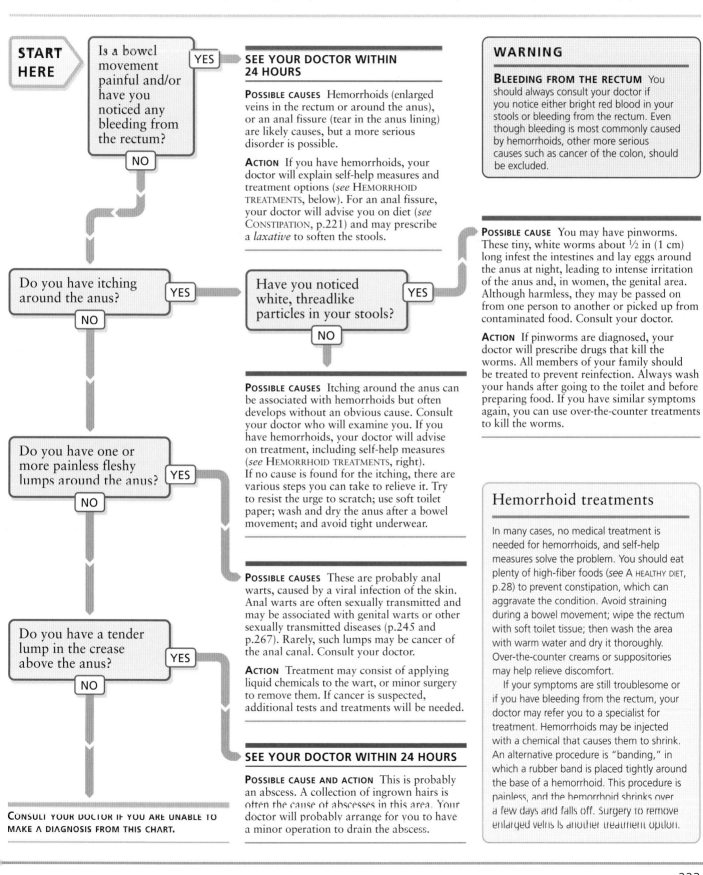

START HERE

Is a bowel movement painful and/or have you noticed any bleeding from the rectum? — YES

Do you have itching around the anus? — YES

Do you have one or more painless fleshy lumps around the anus? — YES

Do you have a tender lump in the crease above the anus? — YES

SEE YOUR DOCTOR WITHIN 24 HOURS

POSSIBLE CAUSES Hemorrhoids (enlarged veins in the rectum or around the anus), or an anal fissure (tear in the anus lining) are likely causes, but a more serious disorder is possible.

ACTION If you have hemorrhoids, your doctor will explain self-help measures and treatment options (see HEMORRHOID TREATMENTS, below). For an anal fissure, your doctor will advise you on diet (see CONSTIPATION, p.221) and may prescribe a *laxative* to soften the stools.

Have you noticed white, threadlike particles in your stools? — YES

POSSIBLE CAUSES Itching around the anus can be associated with hemorrhoids but often develops without an obvious cause. Consult your doctor who will examine you. If you have hemorrhoids, your doctor will advise on treatment, including self-help measures (see HEMORRHOID TREATMENTS, right). If no cause is found for the itching, there are various steps you can take to relieve it. Try to resist the urge to scratch; use soft toilet paper; wash and dry the anus after a bowel movement; and avoid tight underwear.

POSSIBLE CAUSES These are probably anal warts, caused by a viral infection of the skin. Anal warts are often sexually transmitted and may be associated with genital warts or other sexually transmitted diseases (p.245 and p.267). Rarely, such lumps may be cancer of the anal canal. Consult your doctor.

ACTION Treatment may consist of applying liquid chemicals to the wart, or minor surgery to remove them. If cancer is suspected, additional tests and treatments will be needed.

SEE YOUR DOCTOR WITHIN 24 HOURS

POSSIBLE CAUSE AND ACTION This is probably an abscess. A collection of ingrown hairs is often the cause of abscesses in this area. Your doctor will probably arrange for you to have a minor operation to drain the abscess.

CONSULT YOUR DOCTOR IF YOU ARE UNABLE TO MAKE A DIAGNOSIS FROM THIS CHART.

WARNING

BLEEDING FROM THE RECTUM You should always consult your doctor if you notice either bright red blood in your stools or bleeding from the rectum. Even though bleeding is most commonly caused by hemorrhoids, other more serious causes such as cancer of the colon, should be excluded.

POSSIBLE CAUSE You may have pinworms. These tiny, white worms about 1/2 in (1 cm) long infest the intestines and lay eggs around the anus at night, leading to intense irritation of the anus and, in women, the genital area. Although harmless, they may be passed on from one person to another or picked up from contaminated food. Consult your doctor.

ACTION If pinworms are diagnosed, your doctor will prescribe drugs that kill the worms. All members of your family should be treated to prevent reinfection. Always wash your hands after going to the toilet and before preparing food. If you have similar symptoms again, you can use over-the-counter treatments to kill the worms.

Hemorrhoid treatments

In many cases, no medical treatment is needed for hemorrhoids, and self-help measures solve the problem. You should eat plenty of high-fiber foods (see A HEALTHY DIET, p.28) to prevent constipation, which can aggravate the condition. Avoid straining during a bowel movement; wipe the rectum with soft toilet tissue; then wash the area with warm water and dry it thoroughly. Over-the-counter creams or suppositories may help relieve discomfort.

If your symptoms are still troublesome or if you have bleeding from the rectum, your doctor may refer you to a specialist for treatment. Hemorrhoids may be injected with a chemical that causes them to shrink. An alternative procedure is "banding," in which a rubber band is placed tightly around the base of a hemorrhoid. This procedure is painless, and the hemorrhoid shrinks over a few days and falls off. Surgery to remove enlarged veins is another treatment option.

108 General urinary problems

Consult this chart for problems such as a change in the number of times you need to urinate or the amount of urine you produce. In some cases, these variations may be due simply to drinking large amounts of coffee or tea or to anxiety. However, a change may be caused by a bladder or kidney problem or a disorder of the nerves to the urinary tract.

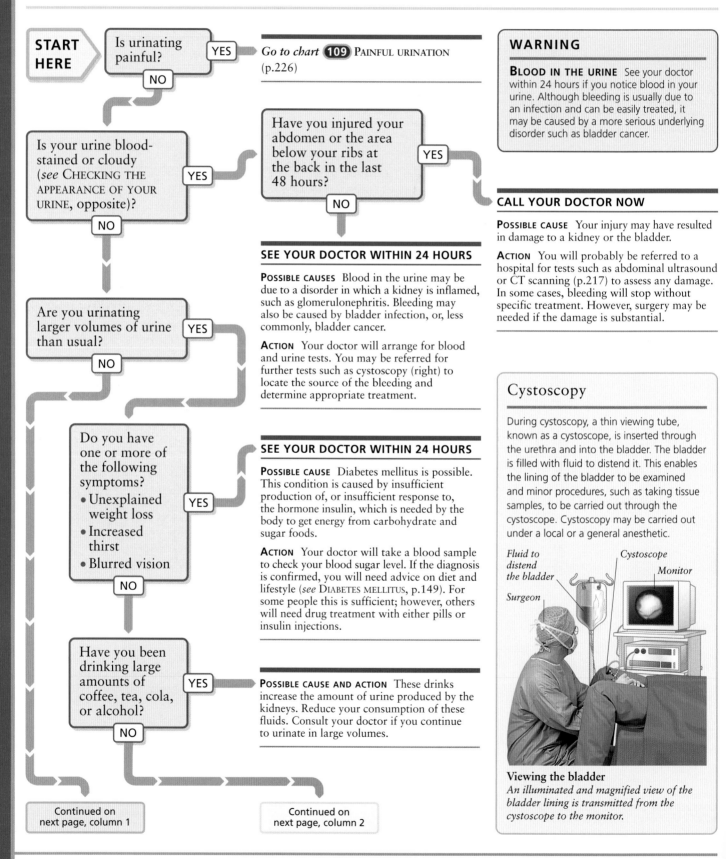

START HERE

Is urinating painful?

YES → *Go to chart* **109** PAINFUL URINATION (p.226)

NO ↓

Is your urine blood-stained or cloudy (*see* CHECKING THE APPEARANCE OF YOUR URINE, opposite)?

YES → **Have you injured your abdomen or the area below your ribs at the back in the last 48 hours?**

  YES → (see CALL YOUR DOCTOR NOW)

  NO ↓

SEE YOUR DOCTOR WITHIN 24 HOURS

POSSIBLE CAUSES Blood in the urine may be due to a disorder in which a kidney is inflamed, such as glomerulonephritis. Bleeding may also be caused by bladder infection, or, less commonly, bladder cancer.

ACTION Your doctor will arrange for blood and urine tests. You may be referred for further tests such as cystoscopy (right) to locate the source of the bleeding and determine appropriate treatment.

NO ↓

Are you urinating larger volumes of urine than usual?

YES → (go to Diabetes section below)

NO ↓

Do you have one or more of the following symptoms?
- Unexplained weight loss
- Increased thirst
- Blurred vision

YES →

SEE YOUR DOCTOR WITHIN 24 HOURS

POSSIBLE CAUSE Diabetes mellitus is possible. This condition is caused by insufficient production of, or insufficient response to, the hormone insulin, which is needed by the body to get energy from carbohydrate and sugar foods.

ACTION Your doctor will take a blood sample to check your blood sugar level. If the diagnosis is confirmed, you will need advice on diet and lifestyle (*see* DIABETES MELLITUS, p.149). For some people this is sufficient; however, others will need drug treatment with either pills or insulin injections.

NO ↓

Have you been drinking large amounts of coffee, tea, cola, or alcohol?

YES → **POSSIBLE CAUSE AND ACTION** These drinks increase the amount of urine produced by the kidneys. Reduce your consumption of these fluids. Consult your doctor if you continue to urinate in large volumes.

NO ↓

Continued on next page, column 1

Continued on next page, column 2

WARNING

BLOOD IN THE URINE See your doctor within 24 hours if you notice blood in your urine. Although bleeding is usually due to an infection and can be easily treated, it may be caused by a more serious underlying disorder such as bladder cancer.

CALL YOUR DOCTOR NOW

POSSIBLE CAUSE Your injury may have resulted in damage to a kidney or the bladder.

ACTION You will probably be referred to a hospital for tests such as abdominal ultrasound or CT scanning (p.217) to assess any damage. In some cases, bleeding will stop without specific treatment. However, surgery may be needed if the damage is substantial.

Cystoscopy

During cystoscopy, a thin viewing tube, known as a cystoscope, is inserted through the urethra and into the bladder. The bladder is filled with fluid to distend it. This enables the lining of the bladder to be examined and minor procedures, such as taking tissue samples, to be carried out through the cystoscope. Cystoscopy may be carried out under a local or a general anesthetic.

Fluid to distend the bladder

Cystoscope

Monitor

Surgeon

Viewing the bladder
An illuminated and magnified view of the bladder lining is transmitted from the cystoscope to the monitor.

Continued from previous page, column 1

Continued from previous page, column 2

Are you urinating more frequently than usual? — YES / NO

Are you currently taking any over-the-counter or prescribed drugs? — YES / NO

POSSIBLE CAUSE AND ACTION Drugs such as *diuretics* are prescribed for conditions such as heart failure to increase the amount of urine passed. Other drugs can also cause you to urinate more than usual as a side effect. Stop taking any over-the-counter drugs, and consult your doctor. Meanwhile, do not stop taking any prescribed drugs.

POSSIBLE CAUSE If you are not drinking excessive amounts of liquids, a kidney or hormone disorder may be the cause. Consult your doctor.

ACTION Your doctor will examine you and arrange for blood and urine tests. You may be referred for further tests, such as ultrasound scanning (p.41) of the kidneys, which will help confirm the cause and determine the appropriate treatment.

Could you be or are you pregnant? — YES / NO

POSSIBLE CAUSE AND ACTION Urinating frequently is a common symptom in early pregnancy and is nothing to worry about. If you are not sure whether you are pregnant, do a home pregnancy test (p.260) and consult your doctor.

Do you have a strong urge to urinate but urinate a small amount? — YES / NO

POSSIBLE CAUSES You may have a small or oversensitive bladder. Alternatively, the exit from the bladder may be partially blocked by a bladder stone. In men, an enlarged prostate gland may be the cause. Consult your doctor.

ACTION Your doctor will test your urine and may arrange for ultrasound scanning (p.41), cystoscopy (opposite), or tests to study the pressures in your bladder (see URODYNAMIC STUDIES, p.258). If you have an oversensitive or small bladder, your doctor may advise you on self-help measures to control your symptoms, or prescribe drugs. Surgery may be necessary to remove bladder stones. An enlarged prostate gland may be treated with either drugs or surgery (see PROSTATECTOMY, p.243).

Do you feel particularly anxious, or do your symptoms occur when you are under stress? — YES / NO

POSSIBLE CAUSE Anxiety commonly causes an urge to urinate, even when the bladder is not completely full.

Go to chart **73** ANXIETY (p.172)

Are you male? — YES / NO

Go to chart **119** BLADDER CONTROL PROBLEMS IN MEN (p.242)

Go to chart **129** BLADDER CONTROL PROBLEMS IN WOMEN (p.258)

Do you have difficulty controlling your bladder? — YES / NO

Checking the appearance of your urine

The appearance of urine varies. It is often darker in the morning than later in the day. A temporary color change may be due to some drugs and foods. However, a change in your urine may indicate a disorder. Very dark urine may be a sign of liver disease, and red or cloudy urine may be due to bleeding or infection in the kidney or bladder. If you are not sure whether a change in the appearance of your urine is normal, consult your doctor.

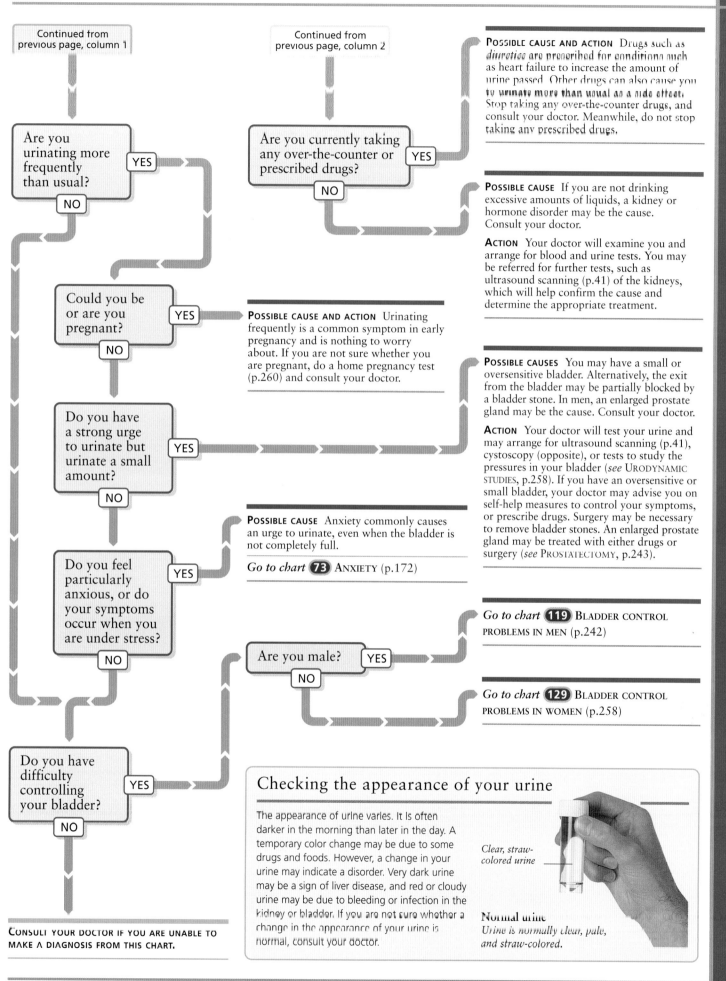

Clear, straw-colored urine

Normal urine
Urine is normally clear, pale, and straw-colored.

CONSULT YOUR DOCTOR IF YOU ARE UNABLE TO MAKE A DIAGNOSIS FROM THIS CHART.

109 Painful urination

Pain or discomfort while urinating is usually caused by inflammation of the lower urinary tract, often due to infection. In women, pain while urinating may be due to inflammation in the genital area. Painful urination may sometimes be accompanied by cloudy or blood-stained urine (*see* CHECKING THE APPEARANCE OF YOUR URINE, p.225).

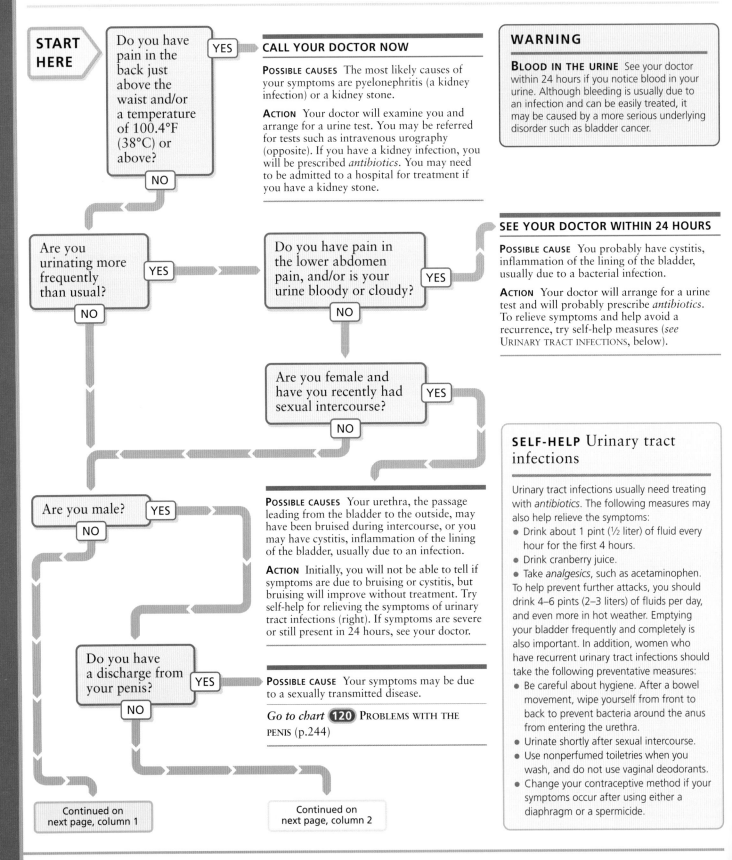

START HERE

Do you have pain in the back just above the waist and/or a temperature of 100.4°F (38°C) or above? — YES →

CALL YOUR DOCTOR NOW

POSSIBLE CAUSES The most likely causes of your symptoms are pyelonephritis (a kidney infection) or a kidney stone.

ACTION Your doctor will examine you and arrange for a urine test. You may be referred for tests such as intravenous urography (opposite). If you have a kidney infection, you will be prescribed *antibiotics*. You may need to be admitted to a hospital for treatment if you have a kidney stone.

NO ↓

Are you urinating more frequently than usual? — YES →

Do you have pain in the lower abdomen pain, and/or is your urine bloody or cloudy? — YES →

SEE YOUR DOCTOR WITHIN 24 HOURS

POSSIBLE CAUSE You probably have cystitis, inflammation of the lining of the bladder, usually due to a bacterial infection.

ACTION Your doctor will arrange for a urine test and will probably prescribe *antibiotics*. To relieve symptoms and help avoid a recurrence, try self-help measures (*see* URINARY TRACT INFECTIONS, below).

NO (Are you urinating more frequently) ↓

NO (Do you have pain in the lower abdomen) ↓

Are you female and have you recently had sexual intercourse? — YES →

NO ↓

Are you male? — YES →

POSSIBLE CAUSES Your urethra, the passage leading from the bladder to the outside, may have been bruised during intercourse, or you may have cystitis, inflammation of the lining of the bladder, usually due to an infection.

ACTION Initially, you will not be able to tell if symptoms are due to bruising or cystitis, but bruising will improve without treatment. Try self-help for relieving the symptoms of urinary tract infections (right). If symptoms are severe or still present in 24 hours, see your doctor.

NO ↓

Do you have a discharge from your penis? — YES →

POSSIBLE CAUSE Your symptoms may be due to a sexually transmitted disease.

Go to chart **120** PROBLEMS WITH THE PENIS (p.244)

NO ↓

Continued on next page, column 1

Continued on next page, column 2

WARNING

BLOOD IN THE URINE See your doctor within 24 hours if you notice blood in your urine. Although bleeding is usually due to an infection and can be easily treated, it may be caused by a more serious underlying disorder such as bladder cancer.

SELF-HELP Urinary tract infections

Urinary tract infections usually need treating with *antibiotics*. The following measures may also help relieve the symptoms:
- Drink about 1 pint (½ liter) of fluid every hour for the first 4 hours.
- Drink cranberry juice.
- Take *analgesics*, such as acetaminophen.

To help prevent further attacks, you should drink 4–6 pints (2–3 liters) of fluids per day, and even more in hot weather. Emptying your bladder frequently and completely is also important. In addition, women who have recurrent urinary tract infections should take the following preventative measures:
- Be careful about hygiene. After a bowel movement, wipe yourself from front to back to prevent bacteria around the anus from entering the urethra.
- Urinate shortly after sexual intercourse.
- Use nonperfumed toiletries when you wash, and do not use vaginal deodorants.
- Change your contraceptive method if your symptoms occur after using either a diaphragm or a spermicide.

Continued from previous page, column 1

Continued from previous page, column 2

Do you have pain in the rectal area and behind the scrotum?
YES →

POSSIBLE CAUSE Prostatitis, inflammation of the prostate gland, usually as a result of a bacterial infection, is a likely cause. In some cases, the infection may be sexually transmitted (*see* SEXUALLY TRANSMITTED DISEASES IN MEN, p.245). Consult your doctor.

ACTION Your doctor will examine you and, if a sexually transmitted disease is likely, may refer you to a specialist. You will probably be prescribed *antibiotics* and advised to drink plenty of fluids.

NO ↓

Have you noticed soreness or itching in the genital area?
YES →

NO ↓

Do you have blisters or shallow ulcers on your penis?
YES →

POSSIBLE CAUSE You may have genital herpes (*see* SEXUALLY TRANSMITTED DISEASES IN MEN, p.245). This condition can cause pain if urine comes into contact with the ulcers. Consult your doctor.

ACTION Your doctor will examine you, and, if genital herpes is a possibility, he or she may refer you to a specialist. If the diagnosis is confirmed, you may be prescribed *antiviral drugs*. Over-the-counter *analgesics* may help relieve the pain. This condition can sometimes recur, but subsequent attacks are usually less severe.

NO ↓

CONSULT YOUR DOCTOR IF YOU ARE UNABLE TO MAKE A DIAGNOSIS FROM THIS CHART.

CONSULT YOUR DOCTOR IF YOU ARE UNABLE TO MAKE A DIAGNOSIS FROM THIS CHART.

Do you have an abnormal vaginal discharge?
YES →

POSSIBLE CAUSE A vulval or vaginal infection can cause pain when urine is passed.

Go to chart **134** ABNORMAL VAGINAL DISCHARGE (p.266)

NO ↓

Do you have blisters or shallow ulcers in the genital area?
YES →

NO ↓

CONSULT YOUR DOCTOR IF YOU ARE UNABLE TO MAKE A DIAGNOSIS FROM THIS CHART.

POSSIBLE CAUSE You may have genital herpes (*see* SEXUALLY TRANSMITTED DISEASES IN WOMEN, p.267). This condition can cause pain if urine comes into contact with the ulcers. Consult your doctor.

ACTION Your doctor will examine you, and, if genital herpes is a possibility, he or she may refer you to a specialist. If the diagnosis is confirmed, you may be prescribed *antiviral drugs*. Over-the-counter *analgesics* may help relieve the pain. This condition can sometimes recur, but subsequent attacks are usually less severe.

Intravenous urography

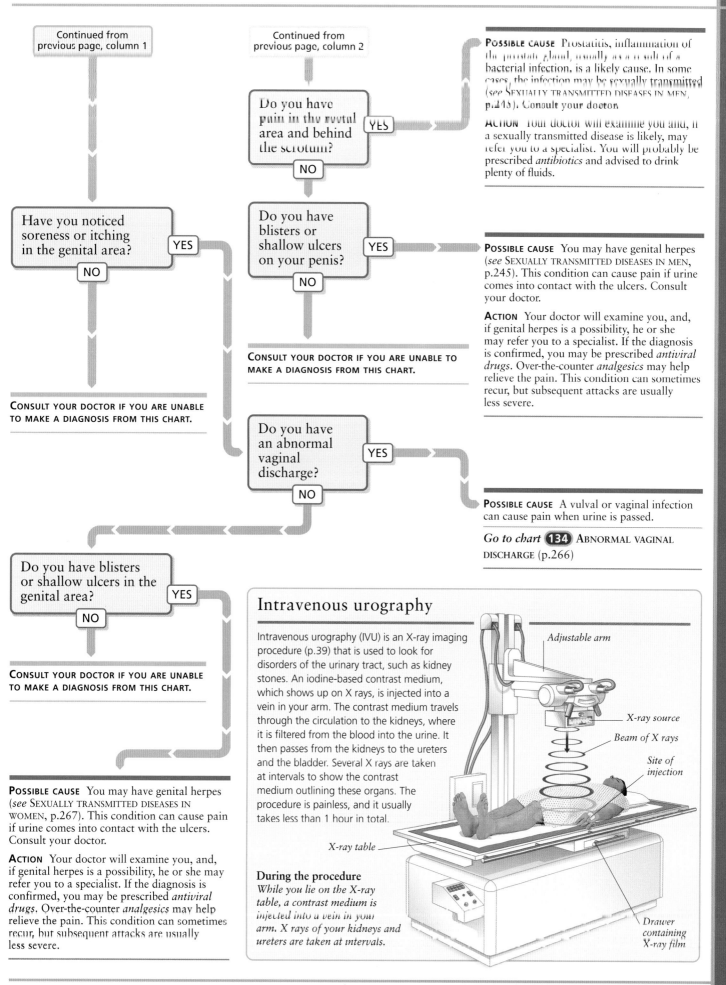

Intravenous urography (IVU) is an X-ray imaging procedure (p.39) that is used to look for disorders of the urinary tract, such as kidney stones. An iodine-based contrast medium, which shows up on X rays, is injected into a vein in your arm. The contrast medium travels through the circulation to the kidneys, where it is filtered from the blood into the urine. It then passes from the kidneys to the ureters and the bladder. Several X rays are taken at intervals to show the contrast medium outlining these organs. The procedure is painless, and it usually takes less than 1 hour in total.

Adjustable arm
X-ray source
Beam of X rays
Site of injection
X-ray table
Drawer containing X-ray film

During the procedure
While you lie on the X-ray table, a contrast medium is injected into a vein in your arm. X rays of your kidneys and ureters are taken at intervals.

227

110 Painful joints

For swelling of the ankles with no associated pain, see chart 115, SWOLLEN ANKLES (p.235).

A joint is the junction of two or more bones. Most joints are designed to allow some movement, but the range and type of movement depend on the structure of the joint. Aches and pains in joints are common and are most often the result of overuse or of a minor injury. Such symptoms are usually short-lived and do not need medical treatment. However, persistent pain in a joint implies a potentially serious underlying disorder and should be investigated. The major weight-bearing joints, such as the hips and the knees, undergo constant wear and tear and are particularly prone to disorders such as osteoarthritis. Consult this chart if you have one or more painful joints.

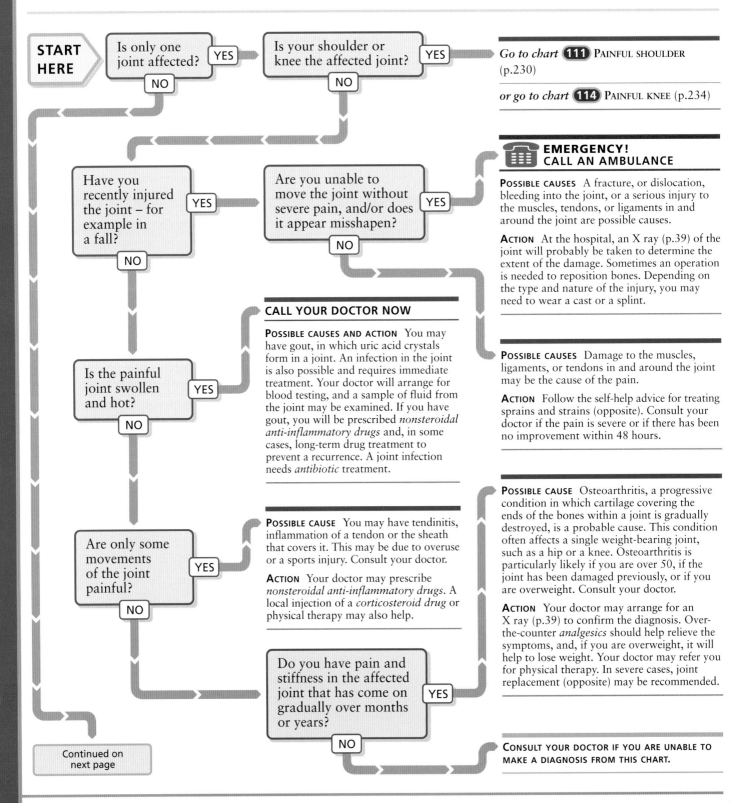

START HERE

Is only one joint affected? — YES → **Is your shoulder or knee the affected joint?** — YES → *Go to chart* **111** PAINFUL SHOULDER (p.230)

or go to chart **114** PAINFUL KNEE (p.234)

NO ↓ (from "Is only one joint affected?")

NO ↓ (from "Is your shoulder or knee the affected joint?")

Have you recently injured the joint – for example in a fall? — YES → **Are you unable to move the joint without severe pain, and/or does it appear misshapen?** — YES →

☎ EMERGENCY! CALL AN AMBULANCE

POSSIBLE CAUSES A fracture, or dislocation, bleeding into the joint, or a serious injury to the muscles, tendons, or ligaments in and around the joint are possible causes.

ACTION At the hospital, an X ray (p.39) of the joint will probably be taken to determine the extent of the damage. Sometimes an operation is needed to reposition bones. Depending on the type and nature of the injury, you may need to wear a cast or a splint.

NO ↓ (from "Are you unable to move the joint...")

POSSIBLE CAUSES Damage to the muscles, ligaments, or tendons in and around the joint may be the cause of the pain.

ACTION Follow the self-help advice for treating sprains and strains (opposite). Consult your doctor if the pain is severe or if there has been no improvement within 48 hours.

NO ↓ (from "Have you recently injured the joint...")

Is the painful joint swollen and hot? — YES →

CALL YOUR DOCTOR NOW

POSSIBLE CAUSES AND ACTION You may have gout, in which uric acid crystals form in a joint. An infection in the joint is also possible and requires immediate treatment. Your doctor will arrange for blood testing, and a sample of fluid from the joint may be examined. If you have gout, you will be prescribed *nonsteroidal anti-inflammatory drugs* and, in some cases, long-term drug treatment to prevent a recurrence. A joint infection needs *antibiotic* treatment.

NO ↓ (from "Is the painful joint swollen and hot?")

Are only some movements of the joint painful? — YES →

POSSIBLE CAUSE You may have tendinitis, inflammation of a tendon or the sheath that covers it. This may be due to overuse or a sports injury. Consult your doctor.

ACTION Your doctor may prescribe *nonsteroidal anti-inflammatory drugs*. A local injection of a *corticosteroid drug* or physical therapy may also help.

NO ↓ (from "Are only some movements of the joint painful?")

Do you have pain and stiffness in the affected joint that has come on gradually over months or years? — YES →

POSSIBLE CAUSE Osteoarthritis, a progressive condition in which cartilage covering the ends of the bones within a joint is gradually destroyed, is a probable cause. This condition often affects a single weight-bearing joint, such as a hip or a knee. Osteoarthritis is particularly likely if you are over 50, if the joint has been damaged previously, or if you are overweight. Consult your doctor.

ACTION Your doctor may arrange for an X ray (p.39) to confirm the diagnosis. Over-the-counter *analgesics* should help relieve the symptoms, and, if you are overweight, it will help to lose weight. Your doctor may refer you for physical therapy. In severe cases, joint replacement (opposite) may be recommended.

NO ↓ (from "Do you have pain and stiffness...")

CONSULT YOUR DOCTOR IF YOU ARE UNABLE TO MAKE A DIAGNOSIS FROM THIS CHART.

Continued on next page

Continued from previous page

Are several of your joints hot and swollen? **NO** / **YES**

Do you have pain and stiffness in your joints that has come on gradually over several months or years? **YES** / **NO**

CONSULT YOUR DOCTOR IF YOU ARE UNABLE TO MAKE A DIAGNOSIS FROM THIS CHART.

POSSIBLE CAUSE Osteoarthritis, a progressive condition in which cartilage covering the ends of the bones within a joint is gradually destroyed, is a probable cause. This condition may run in families, particularly if the small joints at the ends of the fingers are affected. Consult your doctor.

ACTION Your doctor may arrange for blood tests or an X ray (p.39) to exclude other types of arthritis. Over-the-counter *analgesics* should help relieve the symptoms. Your doctor may refer you for physical therapy.

SELF-HELP Treating sprains and strains

Treat sprains and strains by following the RICE procedure: Rest, Ice, Compression, and Elevation. Apply a cold compress or wrapped ice pack for 10–20 minutes. Then wrap a bandage firmly over a thick layer of cotton to provide compression. Try to rest with the injury elevated for at least 24 hours. If it is no better in 48 hours, consult your doctor.

Treating sprains
Apply an ice pack to the affected area, and keep the limb raised.

Ice pack

Have you recently had an infection such as a genital tract infection or gastroenteritis? **YES** / **NO**

Do you have psoriasis or an inflammatory bowel disease, such as Crohn's disease or ulcerative colitis? **YES** / **NO**

Do you have any of the following?
- Pain and swelling affecting the small joints of both hands
- Generalized stiffness lasting at least 20 minutes in the morning
- Fatigue and feeling generally ill

YES / **NO**

SEE YOUR DOCTOR WITHIN 24 HOURS IF YOU ARE UNABLE TO MAKE A DIAGNOSIS FROM THIS CHART.

SEE YOUR DOCTOR WITHIN 24 HOURS

POSSIBLE CAUSE Rheumatoid arthritis, an autoimmune disorder, in which the body attacks its own tissues, is the most likely cause of your symptoms.

ACTION Your doctor may arrange for a blood test and X rays (p.39) to confirm the diagnosis. He or she will probably prescribe *nonsteroidal anti-inflammatory drugs* to relieve the pain. In most cases, you will be referred for further treatment with drugs that suppress the immune system and for physical therapy.

SEE YOUR DOCTOR WITHIN 24 HOURS

POSSIBLE CAUSE Reactive arthritis, which is inflammation of the joints in response to an infection elsewhere, may be the cause.

ACTION Your doctor may arrange for tests to confirm that the infection has cleared up. He or she will probably prescribe *nonsteroidal anti-inflammatory drugs* and sometimes *antibiotics*. Reactive arthritis often clears up promptly but in rare cases may persist for months or even years.

SEE YOUR DOCTOR WITHIN 24 HOURS

POSSIBLE CAUSE These conditions may be associated with a type of arthritis affecting the lower spine and pelvis. In many cases, other joints are also involved.

ACTION Further treatment of your underlying condition may improve your joint symptoms. Your doctor may prescribe *nonsteroidal anti-inflammatory drugs* to relieve joint pain.

Joint replacement

Joints that have been severely damaged by a disorder such as arthritis or by an injury may be surgically replaced with artificial joints made of metal, ceramic, or plastic. Joint replacement is most commonly performed for hips, knees, and shoulders, but most joints in the body can now be replaced, even tiny finger joints. During the operation, the ends of the damaged bones are removed, and the artificial components are fixed in place. The procedure usually relieves pain and increases the range of movement possible in the affected joint.

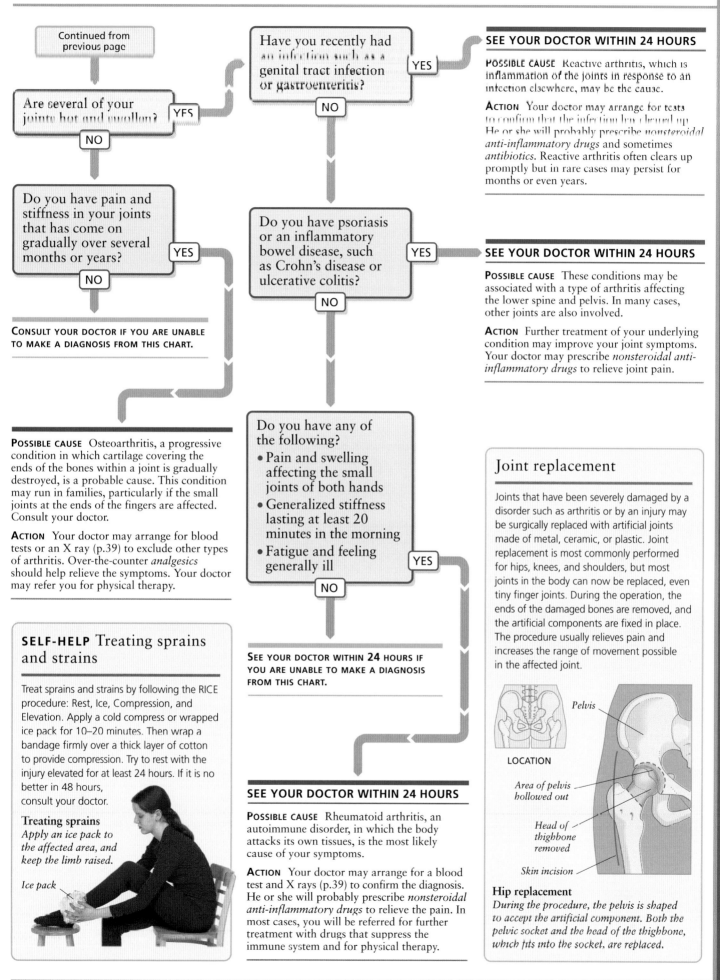

Pelvis

LOCATION

Area of pelvis hollowed out

Head of thighbone removed

Skin incision

Hip replacement
During the procedure, the pelvis is shaped to accept the artificial component. Both the pelvic socket and the head of the thighbone, which fits into the socket, are replaced.

111 Painful shoulder

The shoulder is one of the most complex joints in the body and has a very wide range of movements. If you play sports that involve strenuous arm movements, such as tennis, or regularly lift heavy weights, you are more likely to suffer shoulder injuries. Shoulder pain and/or stiffness without any obvious cause occurs most commonly in elderly people.

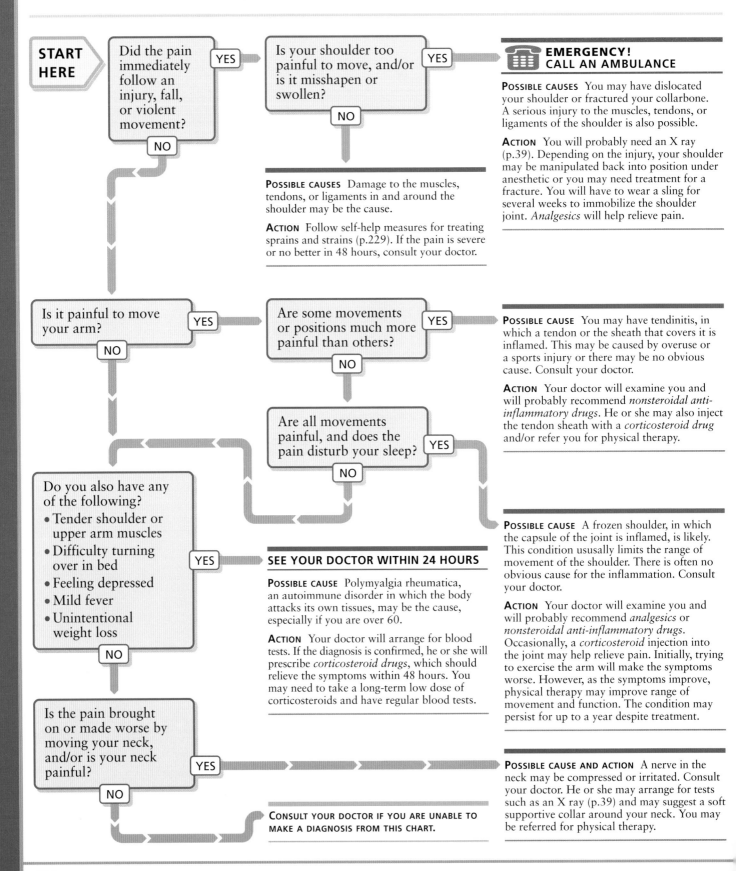

START HERE

Did the pain immediately follow an injury, fall, or violent movement?
— YES → **Is your shoulder too painful to move, and/or is it misshapen or swollen?**
— YES → **EMERGENCY! CALL AN AMBULANCE**

POSSIBLE CAUSES You may have dislocated your shoulder or fractured your collarbone. A serious injury to the muscles, tendons, or ligaments of the shoulder is also possible.

ACTION You will probably need an X ray (p.39). Depending on the injury, your shoulder may be manipulated back into position under anesthetic or you may need treatment for a fracture. You will have to wear a sling for several weeks to immobilize the shoulder joint. *Analgesics* will help relieve pain.

(from "Is your shoulder too painful to move...") — NO ↓

POSSIBLE CAUSES Damage to the muscles, tendons, or ligaments in and around the shoulder may be the cause.

ACTION Follow self-help measures for treating sprains and strains (p.229). If the pain is severe or no better in 48 hours, consult your doctor.

(from START question) — NO ↓

Is it painful to move your arm?
— YES → **Are some movements or positions much more painful than others?**
— YES → **POSSIBLE CAUSE** You may have tendinitis, in which a tendon or the sheath that covers it is inflamed. This may be caused by overuse or a sports injury or there may be no obvious cause. Consult your doctor.

ACTION Your doctor will examine you and will probably recommend *nonsteroidal anti-inflammatory drugs*. He or she may also inject the tendon sheath with a *corticosteroid drug* and/or refer you for physical therapy.

(from "Are some movements...") — NO ↓

Are all movements painful, and does the pain disturb your sleep?
— YES → **POSSIBLE CAUSE** A frozen shoulder, in which the capsule of the joint is inflamed, is likely. This condition ususally limits the range of movement of the shoulder. There is often no obvious cause for the inflammation. Consult your doctor.

ACTION Your doctor will examine you and will probably recommend *analgesics* or *nonsteroidal anti-inflammatory drugs*. Occasionally, a *corticosteroid* injection into the joint may help relieve pain. Initially, trying to exercise the arm will make the symptoms worse. However, as the symptoms improve, physical therapy may improve range of movement and function. The condition may persist for up to a year despite treatment.

(from "Are all movements painful...") — NO ↓

(from "Is it painful to move your arm?") — NO ↓

Do you also have any of the following?
- Tender shoulder or upper arm muscles
- Difficulty turning over in bed
- Feeling depressed
- Mild fever
- Unintentional weight loss

— YES → **SEE YOUR DOCTOR WITHIN 24 HOURS**

POSSIBLE CAUSE Polymyalgia rheumatica, an autoimmune disorder in which the body attacks its own tissues, may be the cause, especially if you are over 60.

ACTION Your doctor will arrange for blood tests. If the diagnosis is confirmed, he or she will prescribe *corticosteroid drugs*, which should relieve the symptoms within 48 hours. You may need to take a long-term low dose of corticosteroids and have regular blood tests.

(from "Do you also have any of the following?") — NO ↓

Is the pain brought on or made worse by moving your neck, and/or is your neck painful?
— YES → **POSSIBLE CAUSE AND ACTION** A nerve in the neck may be compressed or irritated. Consult your doctor. He or she may arrange for tests such as an X ray (p.39) and may suggest a soft supportive collar around your neck. You may be referred for physical therapy.

— NO ↓

CONSULT YOUR DOCTOR IF YOU ARE UNABLE TO MAKE A DIAGNOSIS FROM THIS CHART.

112 Painful arm

Pain in the arm may result from injury or straining of the muscles, tendons, or ligaments that hold the various bones and joints in place. Such injuries are particularly likely to occur after any unaccustomed, strenuous physical activity, such as playing a sport for the first time in many years. Arm pain that develops gradually may originate from problems in the neck. In some cases, pain may be related to repetitive movements such as typing or playing a musical instrument.

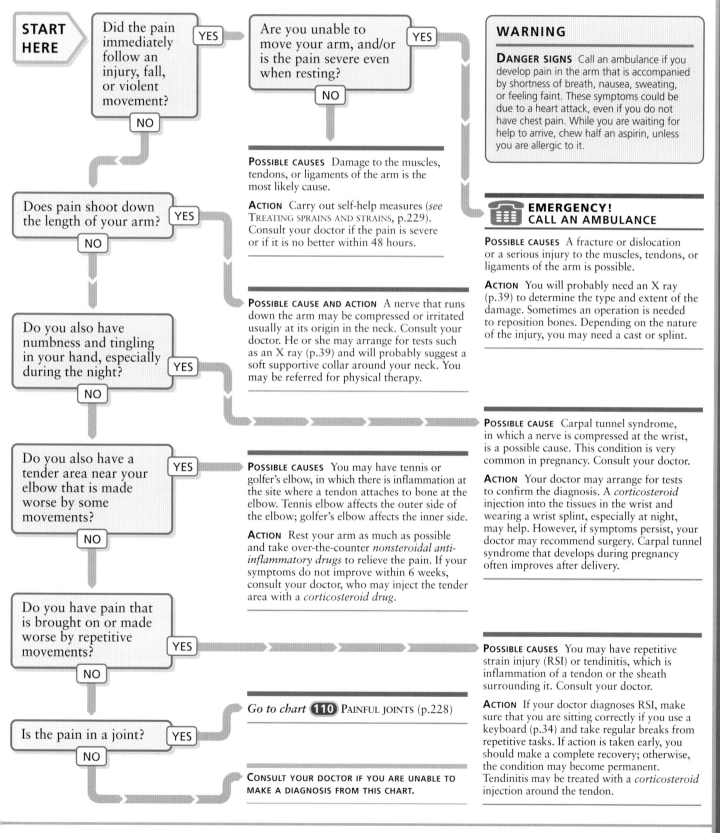

START HERE

Did the pain immediately follow an injury, fall, or violent movement? — YES → **Are you unable to move your arm, and/or is the pain severe even when resting?** — YES →

WARNING

DANGER SIGNS Call an ambulance if you develop pain in the arm that is accompanied by shortness of breath, nausea, sweating, or feeling faint. These symptoms could be due to a heart attack, even if you do not have chest pain. While you are waiting for help to arrive, chew half an aspirin, unless you are allergic to it.

Did the pain immediately follow an injury, fall, or violent movement? — NO ↓

Are you unable to move your arm, and/or is the pain severe even when resting? — NO ↓

POSSIBLE CAUSES Damage to the muscles, tendons, or ligaments of the arm is the most likely cause.

ACTION Carry out self-help measures (*see* TREATING SPRAINS AND STRAINS, p.229). Consult your doctor if the pain is severe or if it is no better within 48 hours.

EMERGENCY! CALL AN AMBULANCE

POSSIBLE CAUSES A fracture or dislocation or a serious injury to the muscles, tendons, or ligaments of the arm is possible.

ACTION You will probably need an X ray (p.39) to determine the type and extent of the damage. Sometimes an operation is needed to reposition bones. Depending on the nature of the injury, you may need a cast or splint.

Does pain shoot down the length of your arm? — YES →

POSSIBLE CAUSE AND ACTION A nerve that runs down the arm may be compressed or irritated usually at its origin in the neck. Consult your doctor. He or she may arrange for tests such as an X ray (p.39) and will probably suggest a soft supportive collar around your neck. You may be referred for physical therapy.

Does pain shoot down the length of your arm? — NO ↓

Do you also have numbness and tingling in your hand, especially during the night? — YES →

POSSIBLE CAUSE Carpal tunnel syndrome, in which a nerve is compressed at the wrist, is a possible cause. This condition is very common in pregnancy. Consult your doctor.

ACTION Your doctor may arrange for tests to confirm the diagnosis. A *corticosteroid* injection into the tissues in the wrist and wearing a wrist splint, especially at night, may help. However, if symptoms persist, your doctor may recommend surgery. Carpal tunnel syndrome that develops during pregnancy often improves after delivery.

Do you also have numbness and tingling in your hand, especially during the night? — NO ↓

Do you also have a tender area near your elbow that is made worse by some movements? — YES →

POSSIBLE CAUSES You may have tennis or golfer's elbow, in which there is inflammation at the site where a tendon attaches to bone at the elbow. Tennis elbow affects the outer side of the elbow; golfer's elbow affects the inner side.

ACTION Rest your arm as much as possible and take over-the-counter *nonsteroidal anti-inflammatory drugs* to relieve the pain. If your symptoms do not improve within 6 weeks, consult your doctor, who may inject the tender area with a *corticosteroid drug*.

Do you also have a tender area near your elbow that is made worse by some movements? — NO ↓

Do you have pain that is brought on or made worse by repetitive movements? — YES →

POSSIBLE CAUSES You may have repetitive strain injury (RSI) or tendinitis, which is inflammation of a tendon or the sheath surrounding it. Consult your doctor.

ACTION If your doctor diagnoses RSI, make sure that you are sitting correctly if you use a keyboard (p.34) and take regular breaks from repetitive tasks. If action is taken early, you should make a complete recovery; otherwise, the condition may become permanent. Tendinitis may be treated with a *corticosteroid* injection around the tendon.

Do you have pain that is brought on or made worse by repetitive movements? — NO ↓

Go to chart **110** PAINFUL JOINTS (p.228)

Is the pain in a joint? — YES →

Is the pain in a joint? — NO ↓

CONSULT YOUR DOCTOR IF YOU ARE UNABLE TO MAKE A DIAGNOSIS FROM THIS CHART.

113 Painful leg

For pain in the foot, see chart 116, FOOT PROBLEMS (p.236). Pain in the leg is often the result of minor damage to muscles, tendons, or ligaments. Such injuries are likely to be the cause of pain that comes on after unaccustomed strenuous exercise or playing a sport for the first time in years. However, pain in the leg may also have a more serious cause such as a disorder affecting the blood vessels that supply the leg. If you are in any doubt about the cause of a painful leg, consult your doctor.

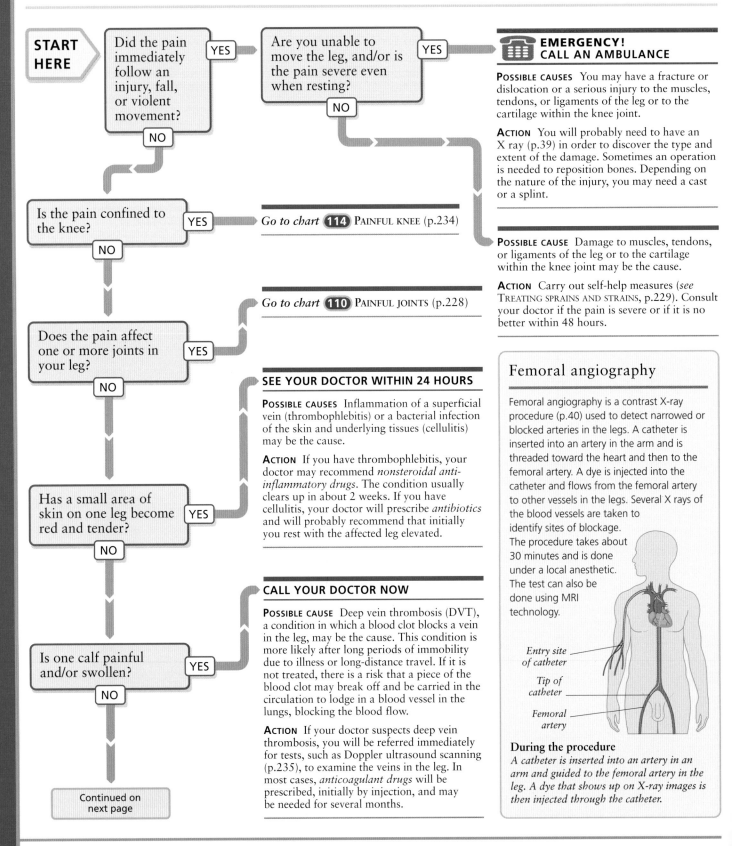

START HERE

Did the pain immediately follow an injury, fall, or violent movement? — YES → **Are you unable to move the leg, and/or is the pain severe even when resting?** — YES → 📞 **EMERGENCY! CALL AN AMBULANCE**

NO ↓ (from first question)

NO ↓ (from second question)

Is the pain confined to the knee? — YES → *Go to chart* **114** PAINFUL KNEE (p.234)

NO ↓

Does the pain affect one or more joints in your leg? — YES → *Go to chart* **110** PAINFUL JOINTS (p.228)

NO ↓

Has a small area of skin on one leg become red and tender? — YES → **SEE YOUR DOCTOR WITHIN 24 HOURS**

NO ↓

Is one calf painful and/or swollen? — YES → **CALL YOUR DOCTOR NOW**

NO ↓

Continued on next page

EMERGENCY! CALL AN AMBULANCE

POSSIBLE CAUSES You may have a fracture or dislocation or a serious injury to the muscles, tendons, or ligaments of the leg or to the cartilage within the knee joint.

ACTION You will probably need to have an X ray (p.39) in order to discover the type and extent of the damage. Sometimes an operation is needed to reposition bones. Depending on the nature of the injury, you may need a cast or a splint.

POSSIBLE CAUSE Damage to muscles, tendons, or ligaments of the leg or to the cartilage within the knee joint may be the cause.

ACTION Carry out self-help measures (*see* TREATING SPRAINS AND STRAINS, p.229). Consult your doctor if the pain is severe or if it is no better within 48 hours.

SEE YOUR DOCTOR WITHIN 24 HOURS

POSSIBLE CAUSES Inflammation of a superficial vein (thrombophlebitis) or a bacterial infection of the skin and underlying tissues (cellulitis) may be the cause.

ACTION If you have thrombophlebitis, your doctor may recommend *nonsteroidal anti-inflammatory drugs*. The condition usually clears up in about 2 weeks. If you have cellulitis, your doctor will prescribe *antibiotics* and will probably recommend that initially you rest with the affected leg elevated.

CALL YOUR DOCTOR NOW

POSSIBLE CAUSE Deep vein thrombosis (DVT), a condition in which a blood clot blocks a vein in the leg, may be the cause. This condition is more likely after long periods of immobility due to illness or long-distance travel. If it is not treated, there is a risk that a piece of the blood clot may break off and be carried in the circulation to lodge in a blood vessel in the lungs, blocking the blood flow.

ACTION If your doctor suspects deep vein thrombosis, you will be referred immediately for tests, such as Doppler ultrasound scanning (p.235), to examine the veins in the leg. In most cases, *anticoagulant drugs* will be prescribed, initially by injection, and may be needed for several months.

Femoral angiography

Femoral angiography is a contrast X-ray procedure (p.40) used to detect narrowed or blocked arteries in the legs. A catheter is inserted into an artery in the arm and is threaded toward the heart and then to the femoral artery. A dye is injected into the catheter and flows from the femoral artery to other vessels in the legs. Several X rays of the blood vessels are taken to identify sites of blockage. The procedure takes about 30 minutes and is done under a local anesthetic. The test can also be done using MRI technology.

Entry site of catheter

Tip of catheter

Femoral artery

During the procedure
A catheter is inserted into an artery in an arm and guided to the femoral artery in the leg. A dye that shows up on X-ray images is then injected through the catheter.

Continued from
previous page

Did the pain come on a few hours after unaccustomed or unusually strenuous exercise? YES

NO

POSSIBLE CAUSE Damage to a muscle, tendon, or ligament is the likely cause of your pain.

ACTION Carry out self help measures (see TREATING SPRAINS AND STRAINS, p.229). Do not exercise until the pain has gone completely. When you do start exercising again, always include warmup and cool down exercises (see EXERCISING SAFELY, p.29). Consult your doctor if the pain is severe or no better within 48 hours.

Does the pain always develop after the same amount of exercise, such as walking a given distance, and does it disappear with rest? YES

NO

POSSIBLE CAUSE Impaired blood flow to the legs as a result of narrowing of the arteries can cause this type of pain and may result in serious complications. Consult your doctor.

ACTION Your doctor will examine you and may refer you for tests such as specialized blood pressure measurements or femoral angiography (opposite) to assess the blood vessels in your legs. You may also need other tests to see if blood vessels elsewhere are affected. If you smoke, you should stop. You will be advised to cut down the amount of fat in your diet and to exercise regularly. In some cases, surgery will be required to widen or bypass the affected arteries.

Do you have episodes of pain in the muscles of one or both calves? YES

NO

POSSIBLE CAUSE These are probably muscle cramps – uncontrollable, painful contractions of a muscle that occur without warning. Cramp often has no obvious cause but may develop during exercise or while lying in bed.

ACTION Stretch and rub the affected muscle to relieve the pain. If you have frequent attacks of cramp, consult your doctor.

Do one or both legs ache and feel heavy, especially after prolonged standing? YES

NO

POSSIBLE CAUSE Sciatica is likely. In this condition, the sciatic nerve, which runs down the entire length of the leg, is compressed or irritated where it leaves the spine. The compression or irritation may be due to a slipped disk. Consult your doctor.

ACTION Your doctor may suggest physical therapy or manipulation of the spine. If the pain is severe, you may have MRI (p.41) to establish the cause and determine the appropriate treatment.

POSSIBLE CAUSE Varicose veins, swollen and distorted veins in the legs, may be the cause. If varicose veins are severe, they increase the risk of a leg ulcer developing in the future. Consult your doctor.

ACTION Your doctor will examine you to confirm the diagnosis. Symptoms can usually be controlled by following self-help advice on coping with varicose veins (above). If your symptoms are severe or you are at risk of developing a leg ulcer, your doctor may recommend treatment such as surgery (see TREATMENTS FOR VARICOSE VEINS, below).

Does the pain shoot down the back or side of the leg from the buttock? YES

NO

Treatments for varicose veins

If they are severe, varicose veins, which are swollen, distorted veins in the leg, may be treated by injection therapy or by surgery. Injection therapy is mainly used to treat varicose veins below the knee. In this procedure, a chemical is injected into the vein, causing the walls to stick together and thereby preventing blood from entering the vein. Surgical treatment may involve tying off small veins called perforating veins, which prevents blood pooling in the affected vein. Alternatively, the entire varicose vein may be surgically removed.

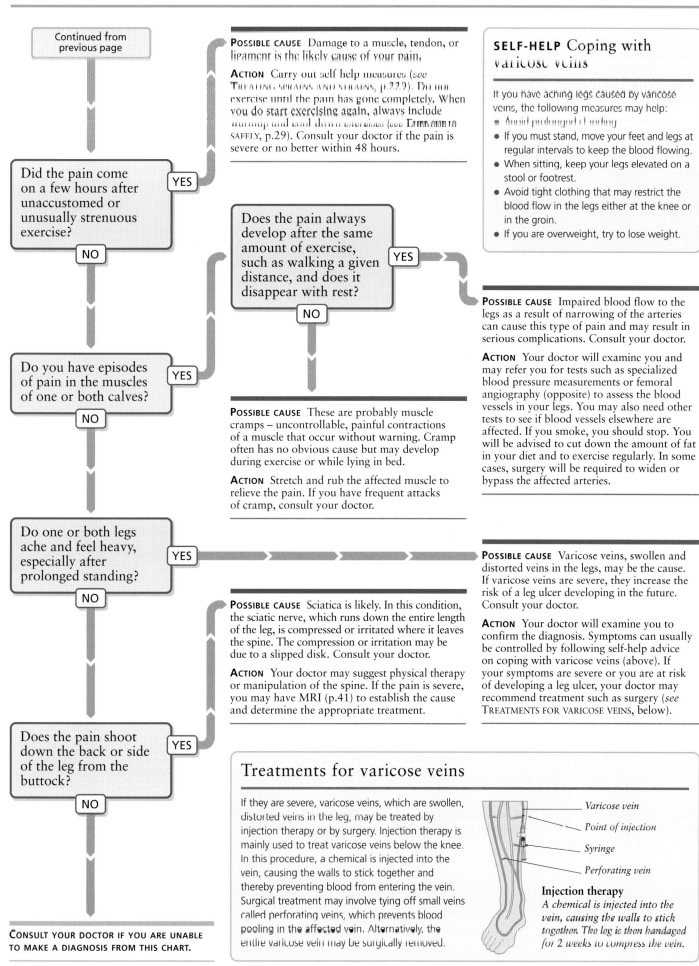

Varicose vein
Point of injection
Syringe
Perforating vein

Injection therapy
A chemical is injected into the vein, causing the walls to stick together. The leg is then bandaged for 2 weeks to compress the vein.

CONSULT YOUR DOCTOR IF YOU ARE UNABLE TO MAKE A DIAGNOSIS FROM THIS CHART.

114 Painful knee

The knee is one of the principal weight-bearing joints in the body and is subject to much wear and tear. Its stability largely depends on the muscles and ligaments around it.

Doing work that involves a lot of bending or kneeling, or playing certain sports, increases the risk of damaging your knees. Consult this chart if one or both knees are painful.

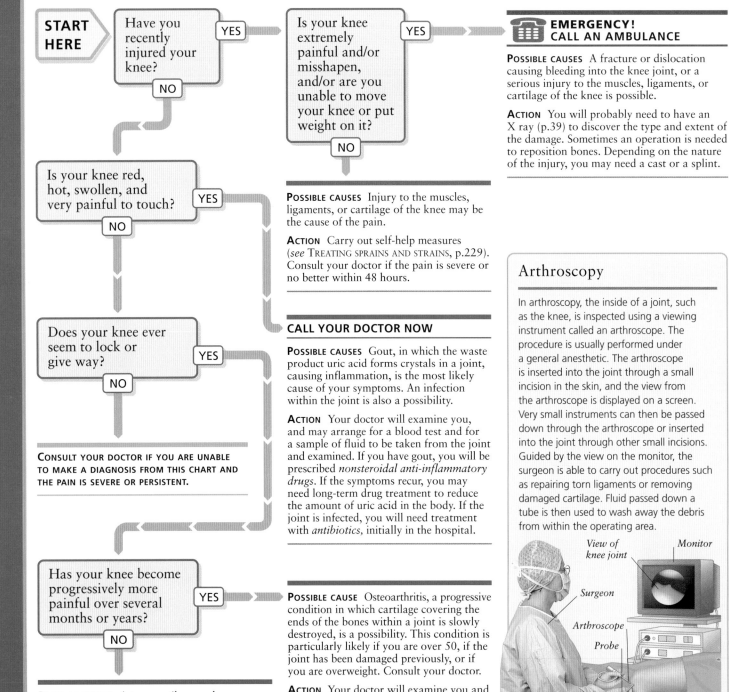

START HERE

Have you recently injured your knee? — YES → **Is your knee extremely painful and/or misshapen, and/or are you unable to move your knee or put weight on it?** — YES →

NO

NO

Is your knee red, hot, swollen, and very painful to touch? — YES

NO

Does your knee ever seem to lock or give way? — YES

NO

CONSULT YOUR DOCTOR IF YOU ARE UNABLE TO MAKE A DIAGNOSIS FROM THIS CHART AND THE PAIN IS SEVERE OR PERSISTENT.

Has your knee become progressively more painful over several months or years? — YES

NO

POSSIBLE CAUSES A torn cartilage or damage to a ligament within the knee joint may be the cause. Such injuries are commonly caused by twisting the joint while it is supporting your weight. Consult your doctor.

ACTION You doctor may refer you to specialist for tests such as arthroscopy (right). Damage may be repaired during the arthroscopy, or you may require surgery at a later date.

EMERGENCY! CALL AN AMBULANCE

POSSIBLE CAUSES A fracture or dislocation causing bleeding into the knee joint, or a serious injury to the muscles, ligaments, or cartilage of the knee is possible.

ACTION You will probably need to have an X ray (p.39) to discover the type and extent of the damage. Sometimes an operation is needed to reposition bones. Depending on the nature of the injury, you may need a cast or a splint.

POSSIBLE CAUSES Injury to the muscles, ligaments, or cartilage of the knee may be the cause of the pain.

ACTION Carry out self-help measures (*see* TREATING SPRAINS AND STRAINS, p.229). Consult your doctor if the pain is severe or no better within 48 hours.

CALL YOUR DOCTOR NOW

POSSIBLE CAUSES Gout, in which the waste product uric acid forms crystals in a joint, causing inflammation, is the most likely cause of your symptoms. An infection within the joint is also a possibility.

ACTION Your doctor will examine you, and may arrange for a blood test and for a sample of fluid to be taken from the joint and examined. If you have gout, you will be prescribed *nonsteroidal anti-inflammatory drugs*. If the symptoms recur, you may need long-term drug treatment to reduce the amount of uric acid in the body. If the joint is infected, you will need treatment with *antibiotics*, initially in the hospital.

POSSIBLE CAUSE Osteoarthritis, a progressive condition in which cartilage covering the ends of the bones within a joint is slowly destroyed, is a possibility. This condition is particularly likely if you are over 50, if the joint has been damaged previously, or if you are overweight. Consult your doctor.

ACTION Your doctor will examine you and may arrange for you to have blood tests and an X ray (p.39) to confirm the diagnosis. Over-the-counter *analgesics* should help relieve your symptoms. If you are also overweight, it will help if you lose weight. In some cases, your doctor may refer you for physical therapy to strengthen the muscles around the joint. In severe cases, a joint replacement (p.229) may be needed.

Arthroscopy

In arthroscopy, the inside of a joint, such as the knee, is inspected using a viewing instrument called an arthroscope. The procedure is usually performed under a general anesthetic. The arthroscope is inserted into the joint through a small incision in the skin, and the view from the arthroscope is displayed on a screen. Very small instruments can then be passed down through the arthroscope or inserted into the joint through other small incisions. Guided by the view on the monitor, the surgeon is able to carry out procedures such as repairing torn ligaments or removing damaged cartilage. Fluid passed down a tube is then used to wash away the debris from within the operating area.

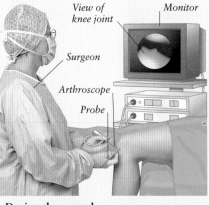

View of knee joint   *Monitor*

Surgeon

Arthroscope

Probe

During the procedure
An arthroscope and a probe are inserted into the joint, allowing the surgeon to inspect the joint. The probe can be used to manipulate the cartilage and improve the view.

115 Swollen ankles

If you are pregnant, see chart 146, SWOLLEN ANKLES IN PREGNANCY (p.283). For painful swelling of one or both ankles, see chart 110, PAINFUL JOINTS (p.228). Painless swelling of the ankles is most often caused by fluid accumulating in the tissues after long periods of sitting or standing still. It is also common in pregnancy due to increased pressure on blood vessels in the abdomen. However, swelling of the ankles may be due to a potentially serious heart, liver, or kidney disorder. If you frequently have swollen ankles, consult your doctor.

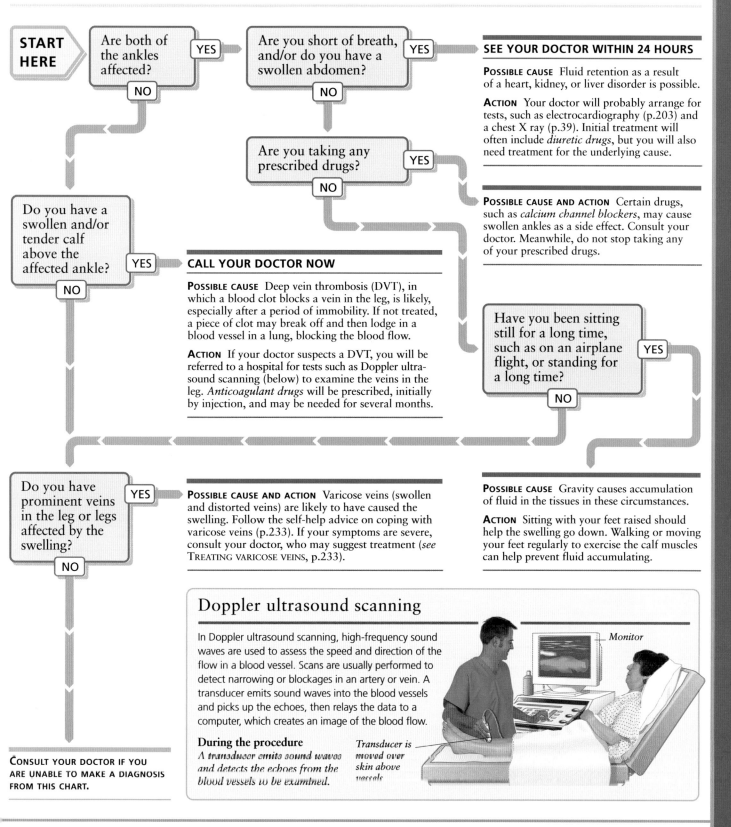

START HERE → **Are both of the ankles affected?** — YES → **Are you short of breath, and/or do you have a swollen abdomen?** — YES →

NO ↓ (from both ankles)

Are you taking any prescribed drugs? — YES →

NO ↓

SEE YOUR DOCTOR WITHIN 24 HOURS

POSSIBLE CAUSE Fluid retention as a result of a heart, kidney, or liver disorder is possible.

ACTION Your doctor will probably arrange for tests, such as electrocardiography (p.203) and a chest X ray (p.39). Initial treatment will often include *diuretic drugs*, but you will also need treatment for the underlying cause.

POSSIBLE CAUSE AND ACTION Certain drugs, such as *calcium channel blockers*, may cause swollen ankles as a side effect. Consult your doctor. Meanwhile, do not stop taking any of your prescribed drugs.

Do you have a swollen and/or tender calf above the affected ankle? — YES →

NO ↓

Have you been sitting still for a long time, such as on an airplane flight, or standing for a long time? — YES →

NO ↓

CALL YOUR DOCTOR NOW

POSSIBLE CAUSE Deep vein thrombosis (DVT), in which a blood clot blocks a vein in the leg, is likely, especially after a period of immobility. If not treated, a piece of clot may break off and then lodge in a blood vessel in a lung, blocking the blood flow.

ACTION If your doctor suspects a DVT, you will be referred to a hospital for tests such as Doppler ultrasound scanning (below) to examine the veins in the leg. *Anticoagulant drugs* will be prescribed, initially by injection, and may be needed for several months.

Do you have prominent veins in the leg or legs affected by the swelling? — YES →

NO ↓

POSSIBLE CAUSE AND ACTION Varicose veins (swollen and distorted veins) are likely to have caused the swelling. Follow the self-help advice on coping with varicose veins (p.233). If your symptoms are severe, consult your doctor, who may suggest treatment (*see* TREATING VARICOSE VEINS, p.233).

POSSIBLE CAUSE Gravity causes accumulation of fluid in the tissues in these circumstances.

ACTION Sitting with your feet raised should help the swelling go down. Walking or moving your feet regularly to exercise the calf muscles can help prevent fluid accumulating.

Doppler ultrasound scanning

In Doppler ultrasound scanning, high-frequency sound waves are used to assess the speed and direction of the flow in a blood vessel. Scans are usually performed to detect narrowing or blockages in an artery or vein. A transducer emits sound waves into the blood vessels and picks up the echoes, then relays the data to a computer, which creates an image of the blood flow.

During the procedure
A transducer emits sound waves and detects the echoes from the blood vessels to be examined.

Monitor

Transducer is moved over skin above vessels

CONSULT YOUR DOCTOR IF YOU ARE UNABLE TO MAKE A DIAGNOSIS FROM THIS CHART.

116 Foot problems

For ankles that are swollen but not painful, see chart 115,
SWOLLEN ANKLES **(p.235).**
Most foot problems are the result of an injury or infections of the skin or nails and are usually minor, except in people

whose feet are affected by poor circulation, such as those who have diabetes mellitus. Consult this chart if you have any pain, irritation, or itching in your feet or if your feet become misshapen in any way.

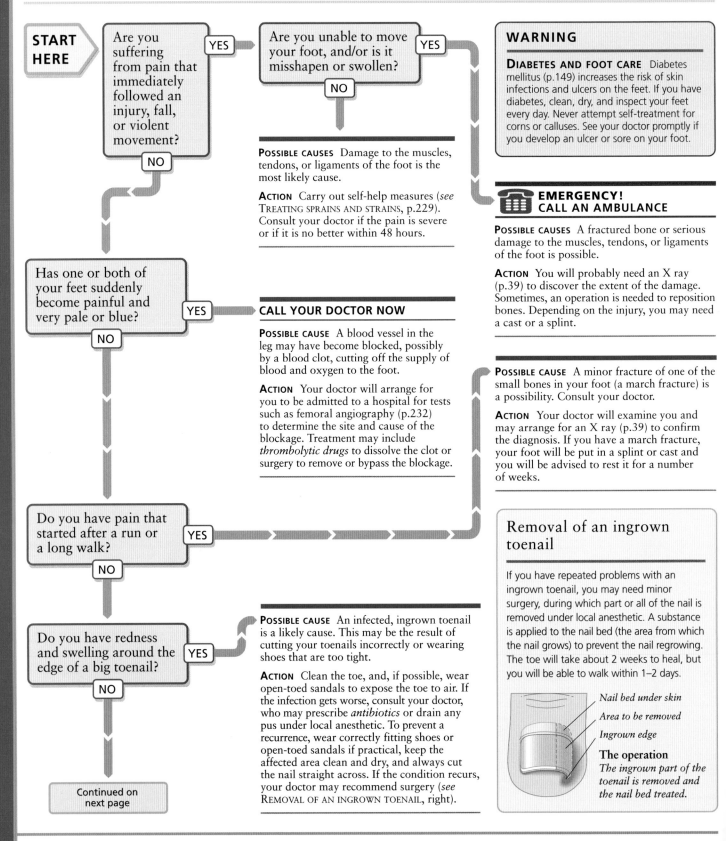

START HERE

Are you suffering from pain that immediately followed an injury, fall, or violent movement?
— YES → **Are you unable to move your foot, and/or is it misshapen or swollen?** — YES →
NO

Are you unable to move your foot, and/or is it misshapen or swollen?
NO

POSSIBLE CAUSES Damage to the muscles, tendons, or ligaments of the foot is the most likely cause.

ACTION Carry out self-help measures (*see* TREATING SPRAINS AND STRAINS, p.229). Consult your doctor if the pain is severe or if it is no better within 48 hours.

Has one or both of your feet suddenly become painful and very pale or blue?
— YES →
NO

CALL YOUR DOCTOR NOW

POSSIBLE CAUSE A blood vessel in the leg may have become blocked, possibly by a blood clot, cutting off the supply of blood and oxygen to the foot.

ACTION Your doctor will arrange for you to be admitted to a hospital for tests such as femoral angiography (p.232) to determine the site and cause of the blockage. Treatment may include *thrombolytic drugs* to dissolve the clot or surgery to remove or bypass the blockage.

Do you have pain that started after a run or a long walk?
— YES →
NO

Do you have redness and swelling around the edge of a big toenail?
— YES →
NO

POSSIBLE CAUSE An infected, ingrown toenail is a likely cause. This may be the result of cutting your toenails incorrectly or wearing shoes that are too tight.

ACTION Clean the toe, and, if possible, wear open-toed sandals to expose the toe to air. If the infection gets worse, consult your doctor, who may prescribe *antibiotics* or drain any pus under local anesthetic. To prevent a recurrence, wear correctly fitting shoes or open-toed sandals if practical, keep the affected area clean and dry, and always cut the nail straight across. If the condition recurs, your doctor may recommend surgery (*see* REMOVAL OF AN INGROWN TOENAIL, right).

Continued on next page

WARNING

DIABETES AND FOOT CARE Diabetes mellitus (p.149) increases the risk of skin infections and ulcers on the feet. If you have diabetes, clean, dry, and inspect your feet every day. Never attempt self-treatment for corns or calluses. See your doctor promptly if you develop an ulcer or sore on your foot.

☎ EMERGENCY! CALL AN AMBULANCE

POSSIBLE CAUSES A fractured bone or serious damage to the muscles, tendons, or ligaments of the foot is possible.

ACTION You will probably need an X ray (p.39) to discover the extent of the damage. Sometimes, an operation is needed to reposition bones. Depending on the injury, you may need a cast or a splint.

POSSIBLE CAUSE A minor fracture of one of the small bones in your foot (a march fracture) is a possibility. Consult your doctor.

ACTION Your doctor will examine you and may arrange for an X ray (p.39) to confirm the diagnosis. If you have a march fracture, your foot will be put in a splint or cast and you will be advised to rest it for a number of weeks.

Removal of an ingrown toenail

If you have repeated problems with an ingrown toenail, you may need minor surgery, during which part or all of the nail is removed under local anesthetic. A substance is applied to the nail bed (the area from which the nail grows) to prevent the nail regrowing. The toe will take about 2 weeks to heal, but you will be able to walk within 1–2 days.

Nail bed under skin

Area to be removed

Ingrown edge

The operation
The ingrown part of the toenail is removed and the nail bed treated.

Continued from previous page

Is the skin of the heel thickened, and are there painful cracks?
YES → **POSSIBLE CAUSE** Thickened skin on the heels tends to crack over time, causing pain.

ACTION Avoid thickened skin building up by soaking your feet and then using a pumice stone or foot file on the skin. Use moisturizing cream regularly. If these measures do not help, consult your doctor or a podiatrist. If you have diabetes mellitus (p.149), consult your doctor before removing thickened skin.

NO ↓

Do you have pain in a heel when you put weight on it?
YES → **POSSIBLE CAUSE** You may have plantar fasciitis, in which fibrous tissues in the heel are inflamed. This condition may be associated with certain types of arthritis or an overgrowth of bone under the heel. Consult your doctor.

ACTION Your doctor may arrange for blood tests or X rays (p.39) to look for associated conditions. He or she may recommend you wear inserts in your shoes to cushion your feet. You may be given an injection of a *corticosteroid drug* into the heel.

NO ↓

Do you have one or more lumps of hard skin on your feet?
YES → **Are the lumps on the toes or the sides of the feet?**
YES → **POSSIBLE CAUSE** These are probably areas of abnormally thickened skin that are known as calluses (or corns if they are on a toe). Calluses and corns form to protect the foot in areas where there is excessive pressure, such as that caused by badly fitting shoes.

ACTION Soak your feet to soften the skin, and rub the lumps with a pumice stone. Adhesive sponge padding, available over the counter, can be stuck over tender areas to protect them from pressure. If this does not help, consult your doctor or a podiatrist. If you have diabetes, consult your doctor before removing any thickened skin. To prevent a recurrence, always wear correctly fitting shoes.

NO ↓ (Are the lumps)

POSSIBLE CAUSE A wart caused by a viral infection of the skin, is a possibility, especially if the lump is on the sole of the foot. A plantar wart may be tender because it grows into the sole of the foot.

ACTION Most warts disappear without treatment, but this may take months or years. Several preparations for treating warts are available over the counter. If a wart persists after self-treatment and is painful, consult your doctor. He or she may remove the wart by freezing or scraping it off.

NO ↓

Is the skin between your toes peeling, sore, and itchy?
YES → **POSSIBLE CAUSE** Athlete's foot, a fungal infection, is the likeliest cause.

ACTION Wash and dry your feet carefully, particularly between your toes, and apply an over-the-counter *antifungal* preparation. When indoors, wear open-toed sandals or go without shoes whenever possible. If the symptoms persist for more than 2 weeks, consult your doctor. If redness and swelling develop, see your doctor within 24 hours.

NO ↓

Is the joint at the base of the big toe painful and swollen?
YES → **Did the pain come on suddenly, and is the area red, hot, and tender?**
YES → **CALL YOUR DOCTOR NOW**

POSSIBLE CAUSES Gout, in which uric acid accumulates in the bloodstream, causing crystals to form in the joints, is the most likely cause of these symptoms. Alternatively, you may have an infection in the joint.

ACTION Your doctor will examine you. He or she may arrange for a blood test and may withdraw a sample of fluid from the joint for testing. If you have gout, your doctor will prescribe *nonsteroidal anti-inflammatory drugs*. If your symptoms recur, you may need long-term drug treatment. A joint infection usually needs to be initally treated in the hospital with *antibiotics*.

NO ↓

POSSIBLE CAUSE You may have a bunion, in which inflamed, thickened tissue develops over a misaligned joint. The condition tends to run in families and may be made worse by wearing shoes with pointed toes.

ACTION Although a bunion may look unsightly and cause discomfort, it is not a serious medical problem. Wearing well-fitting shoes should help reduce discomfort. If you are still concerned, consult your doctor, who may suggest surgery to correct the underlying misalignment.

NO ↓

CONSULT YOUR DOCTOR IF YOU ARE UNABLE TO MAKE A DIAGNOSIS FROM THIS CHART.

117 Back pain

Most people have at least one episode of back pain during their lives, and they usually recover without needing medical help. Back pain is often due to poor posture. However, it may be a sign of damage to the joints, ligaments, or disks of cartilage in the spine, in many cases as a result of tasks such as lifting excessively heavy objects. Severe back pain may be due to pressure on a nerve or rarely to a problem with an internal organ such as a kidney.

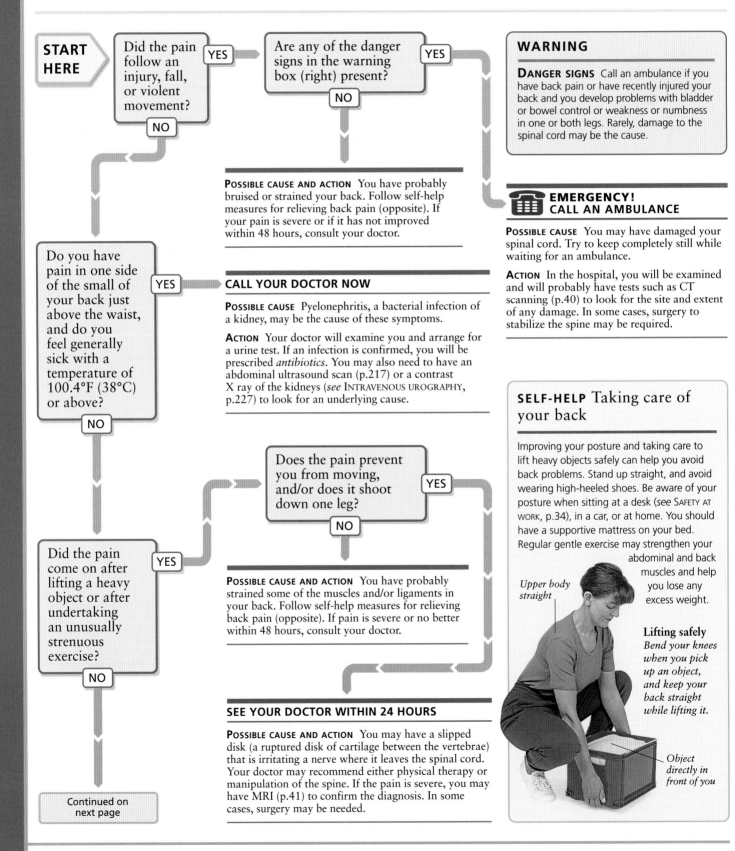

START HERE

Did the pain follow an injury, fall, or violent movement? — YES / NO

Are any of the danger signs in the warning box (right) present? — YES / NO

POSSIBLE CAUSE AND ACTION You have probably bruised or strained your back. Follow self-help measures for relieving back pain (opposite). If your pain is severe or if it has not improved within 48 hours, consult your doctor.

Do you have pain in one side of the small of your back just above the waist, and do you feel generally sick with a temperature of 100.4°F (38°C) or above? — YES / NO

CALL YOUR DOCTOR NOW

POSSIBLE CAUSE Pyelonephritis, a bacterial infection of a kidney, may be the cause of these symptoms.

ACTION Your doctor will examine you and arrange for a urine test. If an infection is confirmed, you will be prescribed *antibiotics*. You may also need to have an abdominal ultrasound scan (p.217) or a contrast X ray of the kidneys (*see* INTRAVENOUS UROGRAPHY, p.227) to look for an underlying cause.

Does the pain prevent you from moving, and/or does it shoot down one leg? — YES / NO

Did the pain come on after lifting a heavy object or after undertaking an unusually strenuous exercise? — YES / NO

POSSIBLE CAUSE AND ACTION You have probably strained some of the muscles and/or ligaments in your back. Follow self-help measures for relieving back pain (opposite). If pain is severe or no better within 48 hours, consult your doctor.

SEE YOUR DOCTOR WITHIN 24 HOURS

POSSIBLE CAUSE AND ACTION You may have a slipped disk (a ruptured disk of cartilage between the vertebrae) that is irritating a nerve where it leaves the spinal cord. Your doctor may recommend either physical therapy or manipulation of the spine. If the pain is severe, you may have MRI (p.41) to confirm the diagnosis. In some cases, surgery may be needed.

Continued on next page

WARNING

DANGER SIGNS Call an ambulance if you have back pain or have recently injured your back and you develop problems with bladder or bowel control or weakness or numbness in one or both legs. Rarely, damage to the spinal cord may be the cause.

EMERGENCY! CALL AN AMBULANCE

POSSIBLE CAUSE You may have damaged your spinal cord. Try to keep completely still while waiting for an ambulance.

ACTION In the hospital, you will be examined and will probably have tests such as CT scanning (p.40) to look for the site and extent of any damage. In some cases, surgery to stabilize the spine may be required.

SELF-HELP Taking care of your back

Improving your posture and taking care to lift heavy objects safely can help you avoid back problems. Stand up straight, and avoid wearing high-heeled shoes. Be aware of your posture when sitting at a desk (*see* SAFETY AT WORK, p.34), in a car, or at home. You should have a supportive mattress on your bed. Regular gentle exercise may strengthen your abdominal and back muscles and help you lose any excess weight.

Upper body straight

Lifting safely
Bend your knees when you pick up an object, and keep your back straight while lifting it.

Object directly in front of you

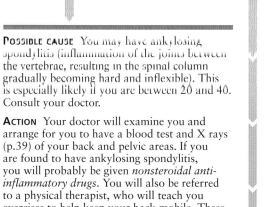

Continued from previous page

Has your back gradually become stiff as well as painful over a period of months or years? **YES** / **NO**

Did the pain come on suddenly after an extended stay in bed or confinement to a wheelchair, or are you over 60? **YES** / **NO**

Are you female and pregnant? **YES** / **NO**

CONSULT YOUR DOCTOR IF YOU ARE UNABLE TO MAKE A DIAGNOSIS FROM THIS CHART AND YOUR BACK PAIN IS SEVERE OR IF THE NATURE OF LONG-STANDING BACK PAIN SUDDENLY CHANGES.

Go to chart **147** BACK PAIN IN PREGNANCY (p.284)

Are you over 50? **YES** / **NO**

POSSIBLE CAUSE You may have ankylosing spondylitis (inflammation of the joints between the vertebrae, resulting in the spinal column gradually becoming hard and inflexible). This is especially likely if you are between 20 and 40. Consult your doctor.

ACTION Your doctor will examine you and arrange for you to have a blood test and X rays (p.39) of your back and pelvic areas. If you are found to have ankylosing spondylitis, you will probably be given *nonsteroidal anti-inflammatory drugs*. You will also be referred to a physical therapist, who will teach you exercises to help keep your back mobile. These mobility exercises are an essential part of the treatment for this disorder and can be supplemented by other physical activities, such as swimming.

SEE YOUR DOCTOR WITHIN 24 HOURS

POSSIBLE CAUSE You may have a compression fracture of a vertebra as a result of osteoporosis, in which bones throughout the body become thin and weak. Osteoporosis is symptomless unless a fracture occurs. The disorder is most common in women who have passed menopause. A prolonged period of immobility may also lead to the development of osteoporosis.

ACTION Initial treatment for the pain is with *analgesics*. Your doctor may also request bone densitometry (below). Specific treatment for osteoporosis depends on the underlying cause. However, in all cases, it is important that you try to remain active and do weight-bearing exercise, such as walking.

SELF-HELP Relieving back pain

Most back pain is the result of minor sprains or strains and can usually be helped by simple measures. Try the following:
- If possible, keep moving and carry out your normal daily activities.
- Rest in bed if the pain is severe, but do not stay in bed for more than 2 days.
- Take over-the-counter *nonsteroidal anti-inflammatory drugs*.
- Place a heating pad or wrapped hot-water bottle against the painful area.
- If heat does not provide relief, try using an ice pack (or a wrapped pack of frozen peas); place it over the painful area for 15 minutes every 2–3 hours.

If your backache is severe or is no better within 2 days, consult your doctor.

Once your back pain has cleared up, you should take steps to prevent a recurrence by following the self-help advice for taking care of your back (opposite).

POSSIBLE CAUSE Osteoarthritis of the spine is probably the cause of your symptoms. In this condition, joints between the vertebrae in the spine are progressively damaged. This is particularly likely if you are over 50 and you are overweight. Consult your doctor.

ACTION Your doctor may arrange for blood tests and an X ray (p.39) to confirm the diagnosis. Over-the-counter *analgesics* should help relieve your symptoms. If you are overweight, it will help to lose weight (*see* HOW TO LOSE WEIGHT SAFELY, p.151). Your doctor may refer you for physical therapy to help you strengthen the muscles that support the spine.

Bone densitometry

This technique uses low-intensity X rays (p.39) to measure the density of bone. X rays are passed through the body, and their absorption is interpreted by a computer and displayed as an image. The computer calculates the average bone density and compares it with the normal range for the person's age and sex. The procedure takes about 20 minutes and is painless.

During the procedure
The X-ray generator and detector move along the length of the spine, and information is displayed on a monitor.

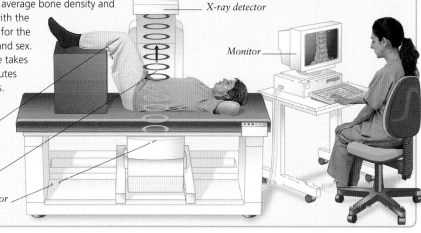

Knees raised to keep the spine flat / X-ray beam / X-ray generator / X-ray detector / Monitor

118 Painful or stiff neck

A painful or stiff neck is most often the result of a muscle spasm brought on by sitting or sleeping in an uncomfortable position or by doing unaccustomed exercise or activity.

Although the symptoms are uncomfortable, they usually improve within 48 hours without medical attention. If the pain and/or stiffness persist or become severe, consult your doctor.

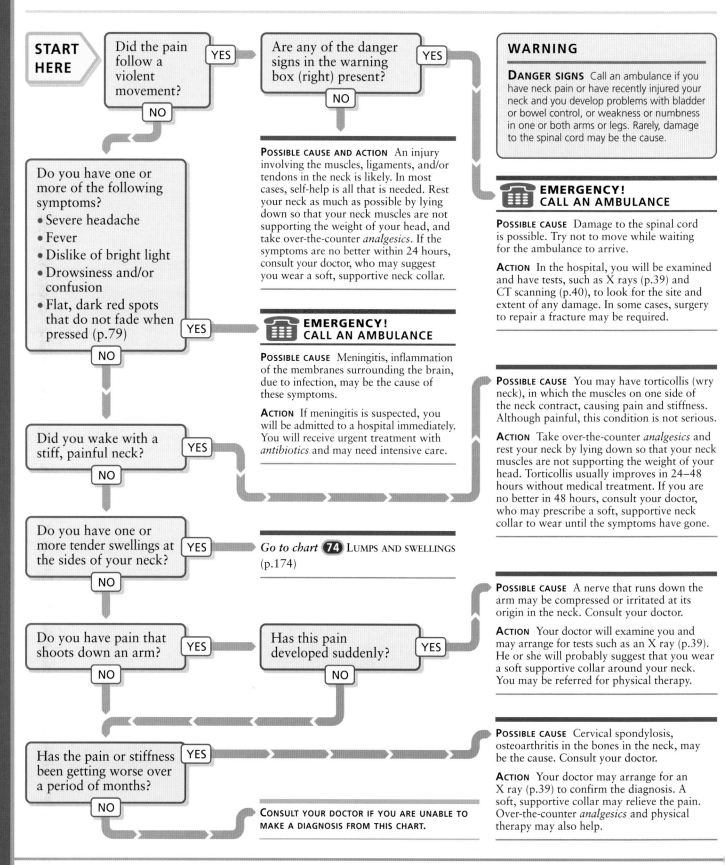

START HERE

Did the pain follow a violent movement? — **YES** → **Are any of the danger signs in the warning box (right) present?** — **YES** →

NO ↓

NO ↓

WARNING

DANGER SIGNS Call an ambulance if you have neck pain or have recently injured your neck and you develop problems with bladder or bowel control, or weakness or numbness in one or both arms or legs. Rarely, damage to the spinal cord may be the cause.

Do you have one or more of the following symptoms?
- Severe headache
- Fever
- Dislike of bright light
- Drowsiness and/or confusion
- Flat, dark red spots that do not fade when pressed (p.79)

— **YES** →

NO ↓

POSSIBLE CAUSE AND ACTION An injury involving the muscles, ligaments, and/or tendons in the neck is likely. In most cases, self-help is all that is needed. Rest your neck as much as possible by lying down so that your neck muscles are not supporting the weight of your head, and take over-the-counter *analgesics*. If the symptoms are no better within 24 hours, consult your doctor, who may suggest you wear a soft, supportive neck collar.

EMERGENCY! CALL AN AMBULANCE

POSSIBLE CAUSE Damage to the spinal cord is possible. Try not to move while waiting for the ambulance to arrive.

ACTION In the hospital, you will be examined and have tests, such as X rays (p.39) and CT scanning (p.40), to look for the site and extent of any damage. In some cases, surgery to repair a fracture may be required.

EMERGENCY! CALL AN AMBULANCE

POSSIBLE CAUSE Meningitis, inflammation of the membranes surrounding the brain, due to infection, may be the cause of these symptoms.

ACTION If meningitis is suspected, you will be admitted to a hospital immediately. You will receive urgent treatment with *antibiotics* and may need intensive care.

POSSIBLE CAUSE You may have torticollis (wry neck), in which the muscles on one side of the neck contract, causing pain and stiffness. Although painful, this condition is not serious.

ACTION Take over-the-counter *analgesics* and rest your neck by lying down so that your neck muscles are not supporting the weight of your head. Torticollis usually improves in 24–48 hours without medical treatment. If you are no better in 48 hours, consult your doctor, who may prescribe a soft, supportive neck collar to wear until the symptoms have gone.

Did you wake with a stiff, painful neck? — **YES** →

NO ↓

Do you have one or more tender swellings at the sides of your neck? — **YES** → *Go to chart* **74** LUMPS AND SWELLINGS (p.174)

NO ↓

Do you have pain that shoots down an arm? — **YES** → **Has this pain developed suddenly?** — **YES** →

NO ↓　　　　　　　　　　　　　　**NO** ↓

POSSIBLE CAUSE A nerve that runs down the arm may be compressed or irritated at its origin in the neck. Consult your doctor.

ACTION Your doctor will examine you and may arrange for tests such as an X ray (p.39). He or she will probably suggest that you wear a soft supportive collar around your neck. You may be referred for physical therapy.

Has the pain or stiffness been getting worse over a period of months? — **YES** →

NO ↓

POSSIBLE CAUSE Cervical spondylosis, osteoarthritis in the bones in the neck, may be the cause. Consult your doctor.

ACTION Your doctor may arrange for an X ray (p.39) to confirm the diagnosis. A soft, supportive collar may relieve the pain. Over-the-counter *analgesics* and physical therapy may also help.

CONSULT YOUR DOCTOR IF YOU ARE UNABLE TO MAKE A DIAGNOSIS FROM THIS CHART.

CHARTS FOR MEN

119 Bladder control problems in men

For other urinary problems, see chart 108, GENERAL
URINARY PROBLEMS *(p.224).*
Problems with bladder control may range from a complete
inability to urinate to incontinence, in which urine is passed
involuntarily. These problems can be due to various
underlying conditions, including an enlarged prostate gland,
which can block the outflow of urine from the bladder, and
disorders affecting the nerves that supply the bladder.

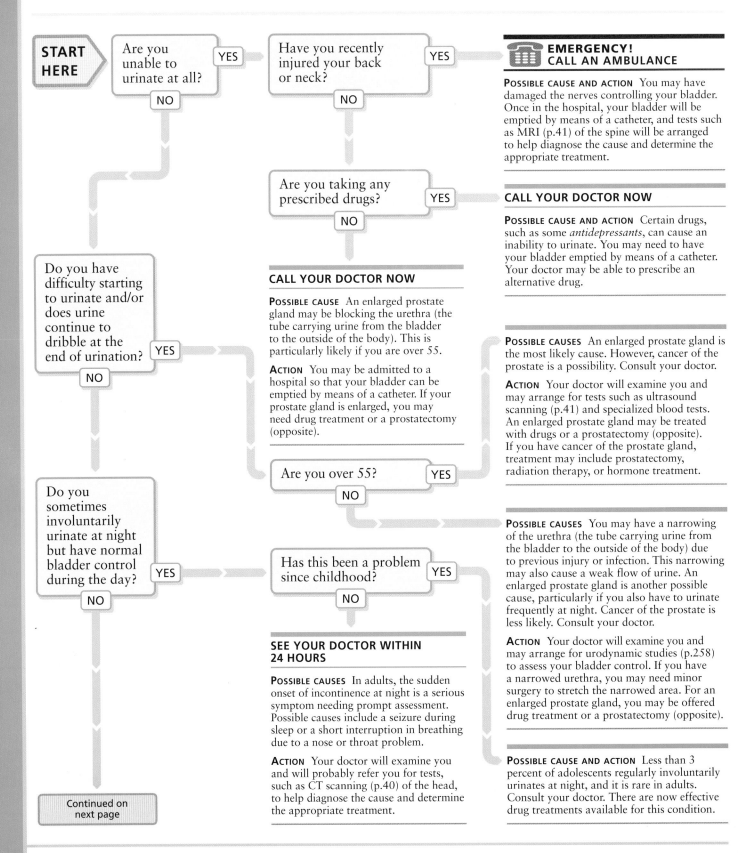

START HERE

Are you unable to urinate at all? — YES → **Have you recently injured your back or neck?** — YES →

☎ **EMERGENCY! CALL AN AMBULANCE**

POSSIBLE CAUSE AND ACTION You may have damaged the nerves controlling your bladder. Once in the hospital, your bladder will be emptied by means of a catheter, and tests such as MRI (p.41) of the spine will be arranged to help diagnose the cause and determine the appropriate treatment.

Have you recently injured your back or neck? — NO → **Are you taking any prescribed drugs?** — YES →

CALL YOUR DOCTOR NOW

POSSIBLE CAUSE AND ACTION Certain drugs, such as some *antidepressants*, can cause an inability to urinate. You may need to have your bladder emptied by means of a catheter. Your doctor may be able to prescribe an alternative drug.

Are you unable to urinate at all? — NO → **Do you have difficulty starting to urinate and/or does urine continue to dribble at the end of urination?** — YES →

Are you taking any prescribed drugs? — NO →

CALL YOUR DOCTOR NOW

POSSIBLE CAUSE An enlarged prostate gland may be blocking the urethra (the tube carrying urine from the bladder to the outside of the body). This is particularly likely if you are over 55.

ACTION You may be admitted to a hospital so that your bladder can be emptied by means of a catheter. If your prostate gland is enlarged, you may need drug treatment or a prostatectomy (opposite).

Do you have difficulty starting to urinate and/or does urine continue to dribble at the end of urination? — YES → **Are you over 55?** — YES →

POSSIBLE CAUSES An enlarged prostate gland is the most likely cause. However, cancer of the prostate is a possibility. Consult your doctor.

ACTION Your doctor will examine you and may arrange for tests such as ultrasound scanning (p.41) and specialized blood tests. An enlarged prostate gland may be treated with drugs or a prostatectomy (opposite). If you have cancer of the prostate gland, treatment may include prostatectomy, radiation therapy, or hormone treatment.

Are you over 55? — NO →

Do you sometimes involuntarily urinate at night but have normal bladder control during the day? — YES → **Has this been a problem since childhood?** — YES →

POSSIBLE CAUSES You may have a narrowing of the urethra (the tube carrying urine from the bladder to the outside of the body) due to previous injury or infection. This narrowing may also cause a weak flow of urine. An enlarged prostate gland is another possible cause, particularly if you also have to urinate frequently at night. Cancer of the prostate is less likely. Consult your doctor.

ACTION Your doctor will examine you and may arrange for urodynamic studies (p.258) to assess your bladder control. If you have a narrowed urethra, you may need minor surgery to stretch the narrowed area. For an enlarged prostate gland, you may be offered drug treatment or a prostatectomy (opposite).

Has this been a problem since childhood? — NO →

SEE YOUR DOCTOR WITHIN 24 HOURS

POSSIBLE CAUSES In adults, the sudden onset of incontinence at night is a serious symptom needing prompt assessment. Possible causes include a seizure during sleep or a short interruption in breathing due to a nose or throat problem.

ACTION Your doctor will examine you and will probably refer you for tests, such as CT scanning (p.40) of the head, to help diagnose the cause and determine the appropriate treatment.

POSSIBLE CAUSE AND ACTION Less than 3 percent of adolescents regularly involuntarily urinate at night, and it is rare in adults. Consult your doctor. There are now effective drug treatments available for this condition.

Do you sometimes involuntarily urinate at night but have normal bladder control during the day? — NO →

Continued on next page

Continued from previous page

Do you have problems with incontinence during the daytime? **YES** / **NO**

Do any of the following apply to you?
• You have had a stroke
• You have diabetes
• You have multiple sclerosis or another long-standing nervous system disorder
YES / **NO**

POSSIBLE CAUSE In some cases, damage to the brain, spinal cord, or nerves controlling the bladder can cause continence problems. Consult your doctor.

ACTION Your doctor will examine you and may request a urine test to exclude an additional problem such as a urine infection. In some cases, drug treatment may help. Alternatively, you may be referred to a urologist, who will help you manage the problem.

POSSIBLE CAUSE In some cases, constipation can prevent the bladder from emptying normally, resulting in the bladder becoming overfilled and sometimes leaking urine. Consult your doctor.

ACTION Your doctor will examine you in order to confirm the diagnosis. He or she may prescribe *laxatives* and may arrange for tests to investigate the cause of the constipation.

CONSULT YOUR DOCTOR IF YOU ARE UNABLE TO MAKE A DIAGNOSIS FROM THIS CHART.

Is the incontinence associated with swelling of the abdomen, and/or do you pass only small volumes of urine when you try to empty your bladder? **YES** / **NO**

Are you constipated? **YES** / **NO**

POSSIBLE CAUSE You may have an enlarged prostate gland that is blocking the flow of urine out of the bladder. This results in the bladder becoming overfilled and possibly leaking urine. Consult your doctor.

ACTION Your doctor will examine you and may arrange for tests, including ultrasound scanning (p.41) and specialized blood tests, to establish the cause. If the blockage is due to an enlarged prostate, treatment will be with either drugs or a prostatectomy (right).

Are you taking any prescribed drugs? **YES** / **NO**

POSSIBLE CAUSE AND ACTION Drugs such as *diuretics*, which result in a sudden increase in the amount of urine produced, may cause episodes of incontinence. Consult your doctor about the problem. He or she may be able to adjust your drug treatment or give you advice on coping with the effects of the drugs.

Are you over 65, and have you become increasingly forgetful? **YES** / **NO**

POSSIBLE CAUSE A decline in mental function that occurs with many neurological diseases associated with increasing age can sometimes result in problems with bladder control. Consult your doctor.

ACTION Your doctor will examine you and may arrange for tests to exclude other causes. A urologist may be able to advise you on ways of coping with your symptoms.

CONSULT YOUR DOCTOR IF YOU ARE UNABLE TO MAKE A DIAGNOSIS FROM THIS CHART.

Prostatectomy

Prostatectomy is a surgical procedure in which part or all of the prostate gland is removed. Partial prostatectomy is usually performed to relieve urinary symptoms, such as leakage of urine, caused by an enlarged prostate gland. The most common procedure is transurethral prostatectomy (TURP), in which the excess tissue is removed through the urethra. Total prostatectomy may be performed to treat prostate cancer. It involves removing the entire gland through an incision in the abdomen and requires a longer stay in the hospital than TURP. Both types of prostatectomy can cause fertility problems because sperm may pass into the bladder on ejaculation. Other complications such as incontinence or erectile dysfunction are rare with TURP but can occur after total prostatectomy.

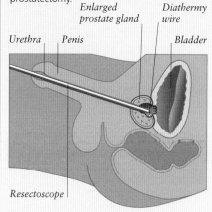

Transurethral prostatectomy (TURP)
An instrument called a resectoscope is passed along the urethra. A heated wire (diathermy wire) introduced through the resectoscope is used to cut away excess tissue.

120 Problems with the penis

For ejaculation problems or blood in the semen, see chart 122, EJACULATION PROBLEMS (p.247). For pain when urinating, see chart 109, PAINFUL URINATION (p.226). Pain in the penis or soreness of the skin can signal a variety of disorders affecting the penis itself or the urinary tract.

Many painful conditions are the result of minor injuries, such as bruising or abrasion (perhaps sustained in activities such as playing sports), or are caused by infections, some of which can be sexually transmitted. Good genital hygiene is essential to avoid problems, particularly in uncircumcised men.

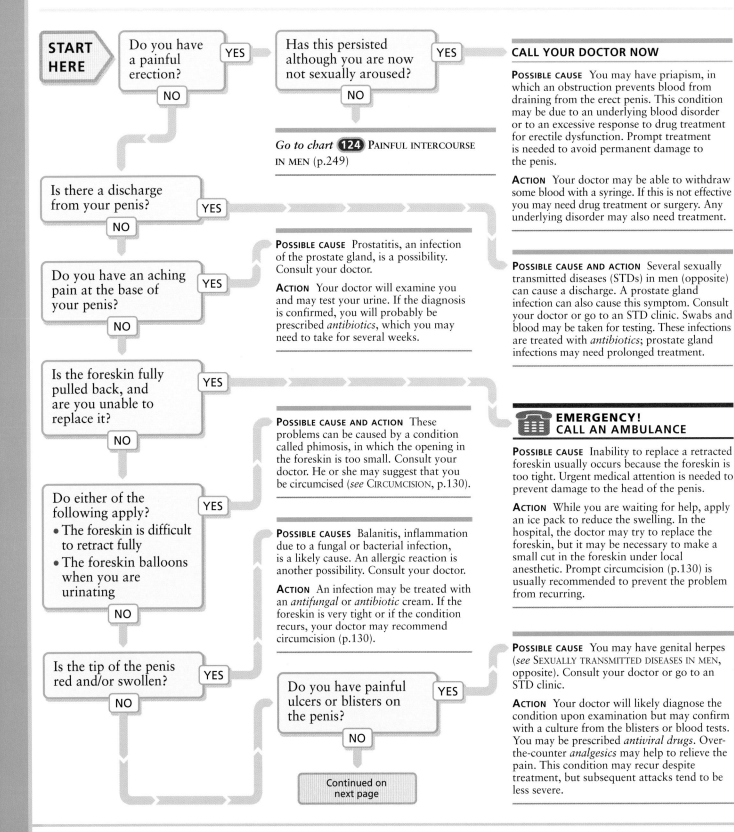

START HERE

Do you have a painful erection? — YES → **Has this persisted although you are now not sexually aroused?** — YES →

NO / NO

Go to chart **124** PAINFUL INTERCOURSE IN MEN (p.249)

Is there a discharge from your penis? — YES →

NO

Do you have an aching pain at the base of your penis? — YES →

POSSIBLE CAUSE Prostatitis, an infection of the prostate gland, is a possibility. Consult your doctor.

ACTION Your doctor will examine you and may test your urine. If the diagnosis is confirmed, you will probably be prescribed *antibiotics*, which you may need to take for several weeks.

NO

Is the foreskin fully pulled back, and are you unable to replace it? — YES →

NO

Do either of the following apply?
- The foreskin is difficult to retract fully
- The foreskin balloons when you are urinating

— YES →

POSSIBLE CAUSE AND ACTION These problems can be caused by a condition called phimosis, in which the opening in the foreskin is too small. Consult your doctor. He or she may suggest that you be circumcised (*see* CIRCUMCISION, p.130).

NO

POSSIBLE CAUSES Balanitis, inflammation due to a fungal or bacterial infection, is a likely cause. An allergic reaction is another possibility. Consult your doctor.

ACTION An infection may be treated with an *antifungal* or *antibiotic* cream. If the foreskin is very tight or if the condition recurs, your doctor may recommend circumcision (p.130).

Is the tip of the penis red and/or swollen? — YES →

NO

Do you have painful ulcers or blisters on the penis? — YES →

NO

Continued on next page

CALL YOUR DOCTOR NOW

POSSIBLE CAUSE You may have priapism, in which an obstruction prevents blood from draining from the erect penis. This condition may be due to an underlying blood disorder or to an excessive response to drug treatment for erectile dysfunction. Prompt treatment is needed to avoid permanent damage to the penis.

ACTION Your doctor may be able to withdraw some blood with a syringe. If this is not effective you may need drug treatment or surgery. Any underlying disorder may also need treatment.

POSSIBLE CAUSE AND ACTION Several sexually transmitted diseases (STDs) in men (opposite) can cause a discharge. A prostate gland infection can also cause this symptom. Consult your doctor or go to an STD clinic. Swabs and blood may be taken for testing. These infections are treated with *antibiotics*; prostate gland infections may need prolonged treatment.

EMERGENCY! CALL AN AMBULANCE

POSSIBLE CAUSE Inability to replace a retracted foreskin usually occurs because the foreskin is too tight. Urgent medical attention is needed to prevent damage to the head of the penis.

ACTION While you are waiting for help, apply an ice pack to reduce the swelling. In the hospital, the doctor may try to replace the foreskin, but it may be necessary to make a small cut in the foreskin under local anesthetic. Prompt circumcision (p.130) is usually recommended to prevent the problem from recurring.

POSSIBLE CAUSE You may have genital herpes (*see* SEXUALLY TRANSMITTED DISEASES IN MEN, opposite). Consult your doctor or go to an STD clinic.

ACTION Your doctor will likely diagnose the condition upon examination but may confirm with a culture from the blisters or blood tests. You may be prescribed *antiviral drugs*. Over-the-counter *analgesics* may help to relieve the pain. This condition may recur despite treatment, but subsequent attacks tend to be less severe.

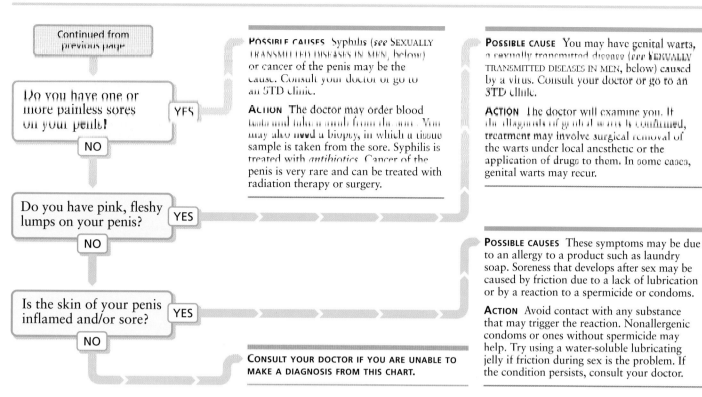

Continued from previous page

Do you have one or more painless sores on your penis? YES / NO

POSSIBLE CAUSES Syphilis (see SEXUALLY TRANSMITTED DISEASES IN MEN, below) or cancer of the penis may be the cause. Consult your doctor or go to an STD clinic.

ACTION The doctor may order blood tests and take a swab from the sore. You may also need a biopsy, in which a tissue sample is taken from the sore. Syphilis is treated with *antibiotics*. Cancer of the penis is very rare and can be treated with radiation therapy or surgery.

Do you have pink, fleshy lumps on your penis? YES / NO

POSSIBLE CAUSE You may have genital warts, a sexually transmitted disease (see SEXUALLY TRANSMITTED DISEASES IN MEN, below) caused by a virus. Consult your doctor or go to an STD clinic.

ACTION The doctor will examine you. If the diagnosis of genital warts is confirmed, treatment may involve surgical removal of the warts under local anesthetic or the application of drugs to them. In some cases, genital warts may recur.

Is the skin of your penis inflamed and/or sore? YES / NO

POSSIBLE CAUSES These symptoms may be due to an allergy to a product such as laundry soap. Soreness that develops after sex may be caused by friction due to a lack of lubrication or by a reaction to a spermicide or condoms.

ACTION Avoid contact with any substance that may trigger the reaction. Nonallergenic condoms or ones without spermicide may help. Try using a water-soluble lubricating jelly if friction during sex is the problem. If the condition persists, consult your doctor.

CONSULT YOUR DOCTOR IF YOU ARE UNABLE TO MAKE A DIAGNOSIS FROM THIS CHART.

Sexually transmitted diseases in men

Infections passed from one person to another during sexual intercourse (vaginal, anal, or oral) are known as sexually transmitted diseases (STDs). Although these infections affect both men and women, the symptoms are often different (see SEXUALLY TRANSMITTED DISEASES IN WOMEN, p.245). The symptoms may also vary depending on the type of sexual contact you have had; for example, in homosexual men, rectal symptoms are often more common. Even if there are few symptoms, some infections can be serious and may cause permanent damage if left untreated. If you think that you or your partner has an STD, you should consult your doctor or go to an STD clinic, where you will be treated in confidence. It is common to have more than one STD at a time, and tests will be arranged to look for several diseases. You should avoid sex until your doctor confirms that the infection has completely cleared up. The risk of contracting an STD can be reduced by practicing safe sex (p.32).

Infection	Incubation period*	Symptoms in men	Diagnosis and treatment
Genital herpes	4–7 days	Initial symptoms include soreness or itching on the shaft of the penis or, in some cases, on the thighs. A crop of small, painful blisters then appears. These burst to produce shallow, painful ulcers, which heal after 10–21 days. Some people may also have a fever during the attack. The condition tends to be recurrent.	The diagnosis is usually made according to the appearance of the skin. Oral antiviral drugs taken early shorten the episodes but do not eradicate the virus. Genital herpes is most infectious while the ulcers are present, but in some cases can remain infectious after the ulcers have healed.
Genital warts	1–20 months	Pink, fleshy lumps on the penis and, in some cases, around the anus. A rectal infection may cause pain on passing stools.	Treatment may be by surgical removal under local anesthetic or by applying topical drugs to the warts. In some cases, the warts may recur after treatment.
Gonorrhea	2–10 days	There may be pain on passing urine and, in some cases, a discharge from the penis.	The doctor will take a swab from the rectum or the urethra (the tube that carries urine out of the body) to identify the infectious organism. Treatment is with *antibiotics*.
HIV infection	6–8 weeks	There may be no initial symptoms, but some people may have a brief flulike illness, sometimes with a rash and swollen lymph nodes. After years without symptoms, AIDS may develop (see HIV INFECTION AND AIDS, p.148). HIV can be passed on whether or not you have symptoms.	Diagnosis is made by a blood test taken 3 or more months after the initial infection. People with HIV infection may be referred to a specialist for treatment. Combinations of *antiviral drugs* are given that may be effective in delaying the progression of HIV to AIDS.
Nongonococcal urethritis	1–6 weeks	Pain on passing urine, especially first thing in the morning. There may also be a discharge from the penis.	The doctor will take a swab from the urethra (the tube that carries urine out of the body) to find the cause, often a chlamydial infection. Treatment is usually with antibiotics.
Pubic lice	0–17 days	Usually there is intense itching in the pubic region, particularly at night. Lice are 1–2 mm long and may be visible.	Treatment is with a lotion that kills the lice and their eggs. Such lotions can be bought over the counter.
Syphilis	1–12 weeks	A highly infectious, painless sore develops in the genital area, usually on the penis or in the rectum. If untreated, the condition can progress to involve internal organs, and rash, fever, and swollen lymph nodes will develop.	The disease is diagnosed by blood tests and tests on swabs taken from any sores. The usual treatment is a course of *antibiotic* injections, followed by blood tests to check for a recurrence of the condition.

*Time between contact with the disease and the appearance of symptoms

121 Erection difficulties

If you have a painful erection, see chart 120, PROBLEMS WITH THE PENIS **(p.244).**

From time to time, most men have problems with achieving or maintaining an erection. Although distressing, occasional erection difficulties are normal and are usually caused by stress, fatigue, anxiety, or alcohol. If you frequently have difficulty achieving an erection, consult your doctor. Safe and effective treatments for erectile dysfunction are available.

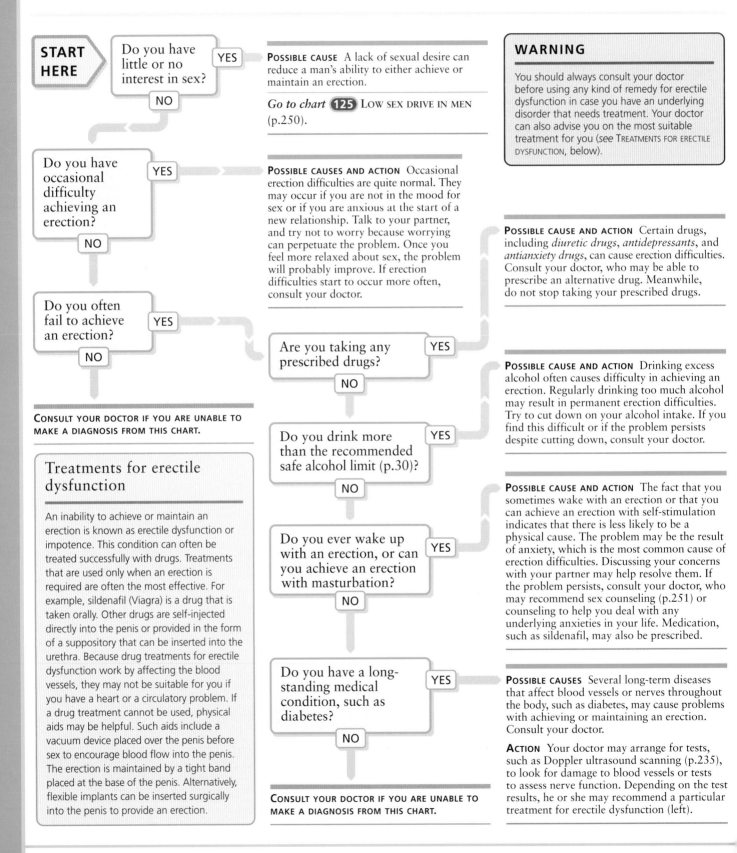

START HERE

Do you have little or no interest in sex? — YES

POSSIBLE CAUSE A lack of sexual desire can reduce a man's ability to either achieve or maintain an erection.

Go to chart **125** LOW SEX DRIVE IN MEN (p.250).

NO

Do you have occasional difficulty achieving an erection? — YES

POSSIBLE CAUSES AND ACTION Occasional erection difficulties are quite normal. They may occur if you are not in the mood for sex or if you are anxious at the start of a new relationship. Talk to your partner, and try not to worry because worrying can perpetuate the problem. Once you feel more relaxed about sex, the problem will probably improve. If erection difficulties start to occur more often, consult your doctor.

NO

Do you often fail to achieve an erection? — YES

NO

CONSULT YOUR DOCTOR IF YOU ARE UNABLE TO MAKE A DIAGNOSIS FROM THIS CHART.

Are you taking any prescribed drugs? — YES

NO

Do you drink more than the recommended safe alcohol limit (p.30)? — YES

NO

Do you ever wake up with an erection, or can you achieve an erection with masturbation? — YES

NO

Do you have a long-standing medical condition, such as diabetes? — YES

NO

CONSULT YOUR DOCTOR IF YOU ARE UNABLE TO MAKE A DIAGNOSIS FROM THIS CHART.

WARNING

You should always consult your doctor before using any kind of remedy for erectile dysfunction in case you have an underlying disorder that needs treatment. Your doctor can also advise you on the most suitable treatment for you (*see* TREATMENTS FOR ERECTILE DYSFUNCTION, below).

POSSIBLE CAUSE AND ACTION Certain drugs, including *diuretic drugs, antidepressants,* and *antianxiety drugs,* can cause erection difficulties. Consult your doctor, who may be able to prescribe an alternative drug. Meanwhile, do not stop taking your prescribed drugs.

POSSIBLE CAUSE AND ACTION Drinking excess alcohol often causes difficulty in achieving an erection. Regularly drinking too much alcohol may result in permanent erection difficulties. Try to cut down on your alcohol intake. If you find this difficult or if the problem persists despite cutting down, consult your doctor.

POSSIBLE CAUSE AND ACTION The fact that you sometimes wake with an erection or that you can achieve an erection with self-stimulation indicates that there is less likely to be a physical cause. The problem may be the result of anxiety, which is the most common cause of erection difficulties. Discussing your concerns with your partner may help resolve them. If the problem persists, consult your doctor, who may recommend sex counseling (p.251) or counseling to help you deal with any underlying anxieties in your life. Medication, such as sildenafil, may also be prescribed.

POSSIBLE CAUSES Several long-term diseases that affect blood vessels or nerves throughout the body, such as diabetes, may cause problems with achieving or maintaining an erection. Consult your doctor.

ACTION Your doctor may arrange for tests, such as Doppler ultrasound scanning (p.235), to look for damage to blood vessels or tests to assess nerve function. Depending on the test results, he or she may recommend a particular treatment for erectile dysfunction (left).

Treatments for erectile dysfunction

An inability to achieve or maintain an erection is known as erectile dysfunction or impotence. This condition can often be treated successfully with drugs. Treatments that are used only when an erection is required are often the most effective. For example, sildenafil (Viagra) is a drug that is taken orally. Other drugs are self-injected directly into the penis or provided in the form of a suppository that can be inserted into the urethra. Because drug treatments for erectile dysfunction work by affecting the blood vessels, they may not be suitable for you if you have a heart or a circulatory problem. If a drug treatment cannot be used, physical aids may be helpful. Such aids include a vacuum device placed over the penis before sex to encourage blood flow into the penis. The erection is maintained by a tight band placed at the base of the penis. Alternatively, flexible implants can be inserted surgically into the penis to provide an erection.

122 Ejaculation problems

If you are unable to achieve an erection, see chart 121,
ERECTION DIFFICULTIES (p.246).
Consult this chart if ejaculation (the moment at which semen
is released at orgasm) occurs sooner than you and your
partner would like, or, if despite having a normal erection,
ejaculation is delayed or does not occur. Ejaculation problems
are common and can be made worse by the resulting anxiety.
Discussing your sexual needs with your partner can help relieve
many of these problems. Premature ejaculation rarely has a
physical cause. Absence of delayed ejaculation may result from
a physical cause or an emotional problem. Orgasm without
ejaculation is usually the result of previous prostate surgery

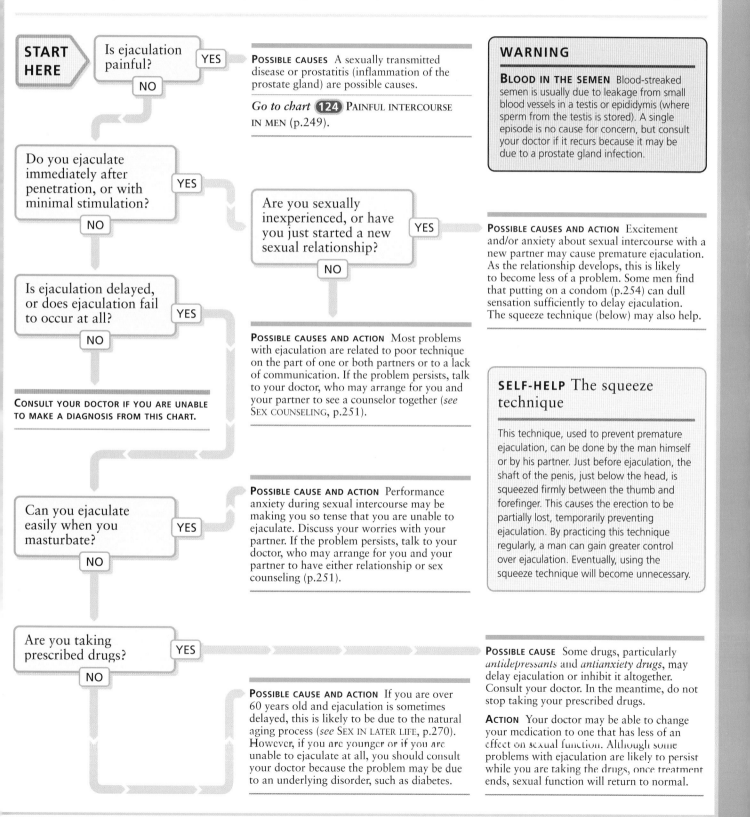

START HERE

Is ejaculation painful?
— YES → **POSSIBLE CAUSES** A sexually transmitted disease or prostatitis (inflammation of the prostate gland) are possible causes.

Go to chart **124** PAINFUL INTERCOURSE IN MEN (p.249).

— NO ↓

Do you ejaculate immediately after penetration, or with minimal stimulation?
— YES → **Are you sexually inexperienced, or have you just started a new sexual relationship?**
— YES → **POSSIBLE CAUSES AND ACTION** Excitement and/or anxiety about sexual intercourse with a new partner may cause premature ejaculation. As the relationship develops, this is likely to become less of a problem. Some men find that putting on a condom (p.254) can dull sensation sufficiently to delay ejaculation. The squeeze technique (below) may also help.

— NO ↓ (from "Are you sexually inexperienced...")
POSSIBLE CAUSES AND ACTION Most problems with ejaculation are related to poor technique on the part of one or both partners or to a lack of communication. If the problem persists, talk to your doctor, who may arrange for you and your partner to see a counselor together (*see* SEX COUNSELING, p.251).

— NO ↓ (from "Do you ejaculate immediately...")

Is ejaculation delayed, or does ejaculation fail to occur at all?
— YES → **POSSIBLE CAUSE AND ACTION** Performance anxiety during sexual intercourse may be making you so tense that you are unable to ejaculate. Discuss your worries with your partner. If the problem persists, talk to your doctor, who may arrange for you and your partner to have either relationship or sex counseling (p.251).

— NO ↓

CONSULT YOUR DOCTOR IF YOU ARE UNABLE TO MAKE A DIAGNOSIS FROM THIS CHART.

Can you ejaculate easily when you masturbate?
— YES →
— NO ↓

Are you taking prescribed drugs?
— YES → **POSSIBLE CAUSE** Some drugs, particularly *antidepressants* and *antianxiety drugs*, may delay ejaculation or inhibit it altogether. Consult your doctor. In the meantime, do not stop taking your prescribed drugs.

ACTION Your doctor may be able to change your medication to one that has less of an effect on sexual function. Although some problems with ejaculation are likely to persist while you are taking the drugs, once treatment ends, sexual function will return to normal.

— NO ↓
POSSIBLE CAUSE AND ACTION If you are over 60 years old and ejaculation is sometimes delayed, this is likely to be due to the natural aging process (*see* SEX IN LATER LIFE, p.270). However, if you are younger or if you are unable to ejaculate at all, you should consult your doctor because the problem may be due to an underlying disorder, such as diabetes.

WARNING

BLOOD IN THE SEMEN Blood-streaked semen is usually due to leakage from small blood vessels in a testis or epididymis (where sperm from the testis is stored). A single episode is no cause for concern, but consult your doctor if it recurs because it may be due to a prostate gland infection.

SELF-HELP The squeeze technique

This technique, used to prevent premature ejaculation, can be done by the man himself or by his partner. Just before ejaculation, the shaft of the penis, just below the head, is squeezed firmly between the thumb and forefinger. This causes the erection to be partially lost, temporarily preventing ejaculation. By practicing this technique regularly, a man can gain greater control over ejaculation. Eventually, using the squeeze technique will become unnecessary.

123 Testes and scrotum problems

All men should examine their testes regularly (*see* EXAMINING THE TESTES, below) because there is a small possibility that a change could indicate cancer of the testis. Cancer treatment is most likely to be successful if the diagnosis is made early.

If you have pain or notice a lump or swelling in or around the testes or elsewhere in the scrotum, consult this chart to determine how soon you should seek medical advice. In some cases, prompt treatment is essential to preserve fertility.

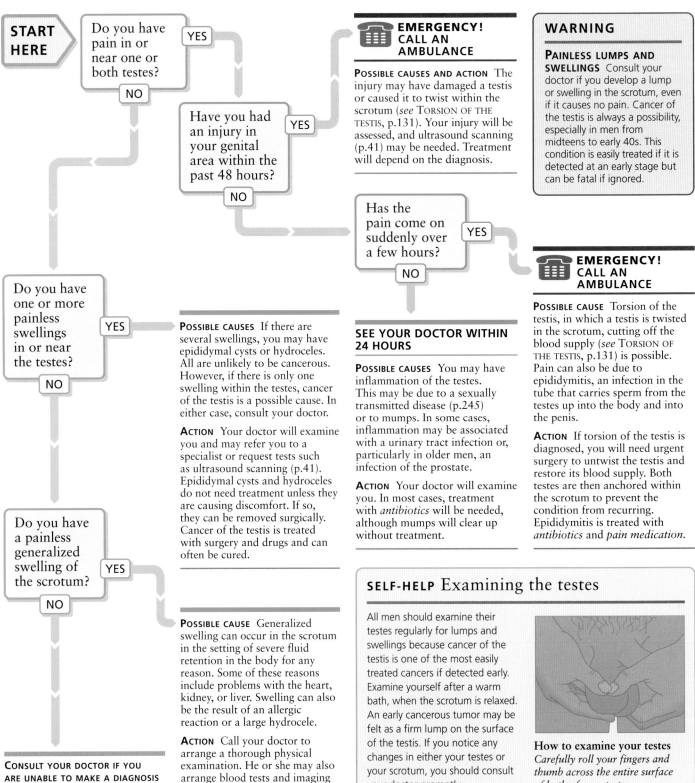

START HERE

Do you have pain in or near one or both testes? — YES / NO

Have you had an injury in your genital area within the past 48 hours? — YES / NO

EMERGENCY! CALL AN AMBULANCE

POSSIBLE CAUSES AND ACTION The injury may have damaged a testis or caused it to twist within the scrotum (*see* TORSION OF THE TESTIS, p.131). Your injury will be assessed, and ultrasound scanning (p.41) may be needed. Treatment will depend on the diagnosis.

WARNING

PAINLESS LUMPS AND SWELLINGS Consult your doctor if you develop a lump or swelling in the scrotum, even if it causes no pain. Cancer of the testis is always a possibility, especially in men from midteens to early 40s. This condition is easily treated if it is detected at an early stage but can be fatal if ignored.

Has the pain come on suddenly over a few hours? — YES / NO

EMERGENCY! CALL AN AMBULANCE

POSSIBLE CAUSE Torsion of the testis, in which a testis is twisted in the scrotum, cutting off the blood supply (*see* TORSION OF THE TESTIS, p.131) is possible. Pain can also be due to epididymitis, an infection in the tube that carries sperm from the testes up into the body and into the penis.

ACTION If torsion of the testis is diagnosed, you will need urgent surgery to untwist the testis and restore its blood supply. Both testes are then anchored within the scrotum to prevent the condition from recurring. Epididymitis is treated with *antibiotics* and *pain medication*.

Do you have one or more painless swellings in or near the testes? — YES / NO

POSSIBLE CAUSES If there are several swellings, you may have epididymal cysts or hydroceles. All are unlikely to be cancerous. However, if there is only one swelling within the testes, cancer of the testis is a possible cause. In either case, consult your doctor.

ACTION Your doctor will examine you and may refer you to a specialist or request tests such as ultrasound scanning (p.41). Epididymal cysts and hydroceles do not need treatment unless they are causing discomfort. If so, they can be removed surgically. Cancer of the testis is treated with surgery and drugs and can often be cured.

SEE YOUR DOCTOR WITHIN 24 HOURS

POSSIBLE CAUSES You may have inflammation of the testes. This may be due to a sexually transmitted disease (p.245) or to mumps. In some cases, inflammation may be associated with a urinary tract infection or, particularly in older men, an infection of the prostate.

ACTION Your doctor will examine you. In most cases, treatment with *antibiotics* will be needed, although mumps will clear up without treatment.

Do you have a painless generalized swelling of the scrotum? — YES / NO

POSSIBLE CAUSE Generalized swelling can occur in the scrotum in the setting of severe fluid retention in the body for any reason. Some of these reasons include problems with the heart, kidney, or liver. Swelling can also be the result of an allergic reaction or a large hydrocele.

ACTION Call your doctor to arrange a thorough physical examination. He or she may also arrange blood tests and imaging studies to determine the cause.

CONSULT YOUR DOCTOR IF YOU ARE UNABLE TO MAKE A DIAGNOSIS FROM THIS CHART.

SELF-HELP Examining the testes

All men should examine their testes regularly for lumps and swellings because cancer of the testis is one of the most easily treated cancers if detected early. Examine yourself after a warm bath, when the scrotum is relaxed. An early cancerous tumor may be felt as a firm lump on the surface of the testis. If you notice any changes in either your testes or your scrotum, you should consult your doctor promptly.

How to examine your testes
Carefully roll your fingers and thumb across the entire surface of both of your testes.

124 Painful intercourse in men

Consult this chart if sexual intercourse is painful. If the cause of the pain is not treated, erection difficulties and ejaculation problems may develop. There are several different possible causes of painful intercourse in men, including a disorder affecting the surface of the penis, a tight foreskin, an infection, or lack of lubrication.

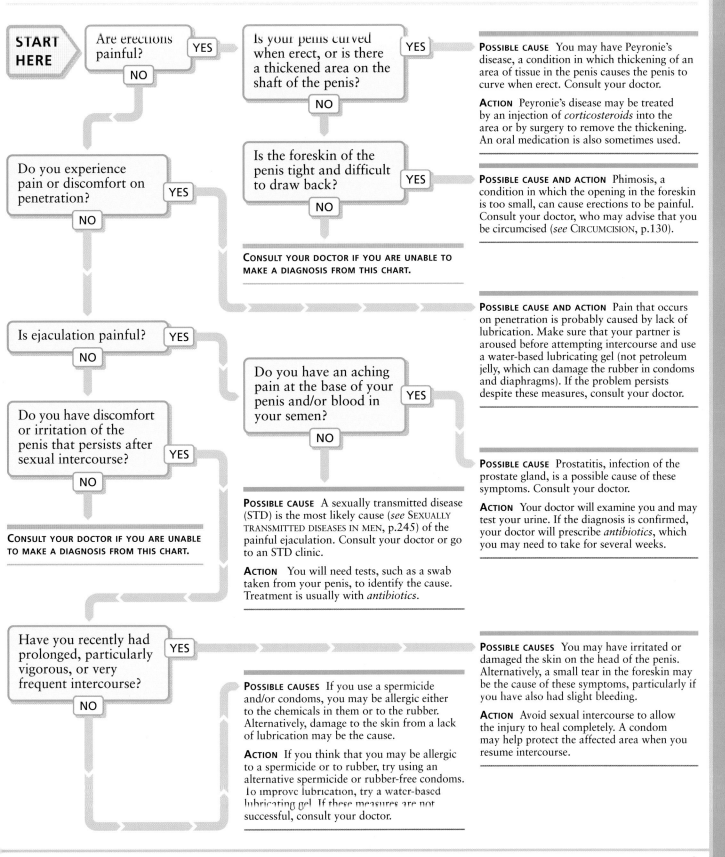

START HERE

Are erections painful? YES / NO

Is your penis curved when erect, or is there a thickened area on the shaft of the penis? YES / NO

POSSIBLE CAUSE You may have Peyronie's disease, a condition in which thickening of an area of tissue in the penis causes the penis to curve when erect. Consult your doctor.

ACTION Peyronie's disease may be treated by an injection of *corticosteroids* into the area or by surgery to remove the thickening. An oral medication is also sometimes used.

Do you experience pain or discomfort on penetration? YES / NO

Is the foreskin of the penis tight and difficult to draw back? YES / NO

POSSIBLE CAUSE AND ACTION Phimosis, a condition in which the opening in the foreskin is too small, can cause erections to be painful. Consult your doctor, who may advise that you be circumcised (*see* CIRCUMCISION, p.130).

CONSULT YOUR DOCTOR IF YOU ARE UNABLE TO MAKE A DIAGNOSIS FROM THIS CHART.

POSSIBLE CAUSE AND ACTION Pain that occurs on penetration is probably caused by lack of lubrication. Make sure that your partner is aroused before attempting intercourse and use a water-based lubricating gel (not petroleum jelly, which can damage the rubber in condoms and diaphragms). If the problem persists despite these measures, consult your doctor.

Is ejaculation painful? YES / NO

Do you have an aching pain at the base of your penis and/or blood in your semen? YES / NO

Do you have discomfort or irritation of the penis that persists after sexual intercourse? YES / NO

POSSIBLE CAUSE Prostatitis, infection of the prostate gland, is a possible cause of these symptoms. Consult your doctor.

ACTION Your doctor will examine you and may test your urine. If the diagnosis is confirmed, your doctor will prescribe *antibiotics*, which you may need to take for several weeks.

CONSULT YOUR DOCTOR IF YOU ARE UNABLE TO MAKE A DIAGNOSIS FROM THIS CHART.

POSSIBLE CAUSE A sexually transmitted disease (STD) is the most likely cause (*see* SEXUALLY TRANSMITTED DISEASES IN MEN, p.245) of the painful ejaculation. Consult your doctor or go to an STD clinic.

ACTION You will need tests, such as a swab taken from your penis, to identify the cause. Treatment is usually with *antibiotics*.

Have you recently had prolonged, particularly vigorous, or very frequent intercourse? YES / NO

POSSIBLE CAUSES You may have irritated or damaged the skin on the head of the penis. Alternatively, a small tear in the foreskin may be the cause of these symptoms, particularly if you have also had slight bleeding.

ACTION Avoid sexual intercourse to allow the injury to heal completely. A condom may help protect the affected area when you resume intercourse.

POSSIBLE CAUSES If you use a spermicide and/or condoms, you may be allergic either to the chemicals in them or to the rubber. Alternatively, damage to the skin from a lack of lubrication may be the cause.

ACTION If you think that you may be allergic to a spermicide or to rubber, try using an alternative spermicide or rubber-free condoms. To improve lubrication, try a water-based lubricating gel. If these measures are not successful, consult your doctor.

125 Low sex drive in men

Normal levels of interest in sex vary from person to person. If you have always had little interest in a sexual relationship or rarely masturbate or feel sexually aroused, you may simply have a naturally low sex drive. Consult this chart if you are concerned about your low sex drive or if your sex drive has decreased recently. A decrease in sex drive often has a psychological cause but can also be the result of a disorder affecting levels of the sex hormone testosterone.

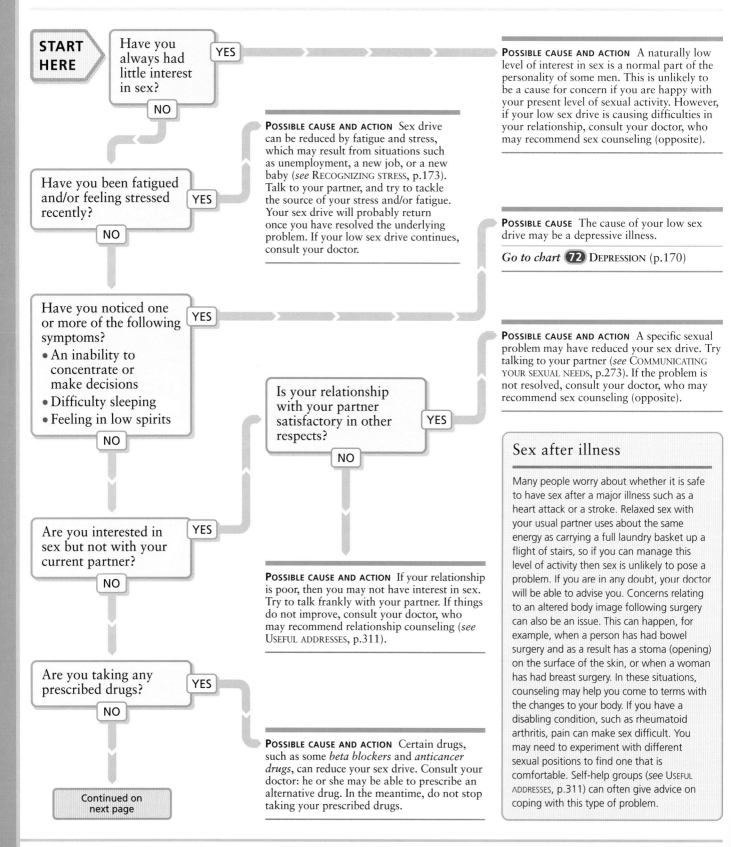

START HERE

Have you always had little interest in sex?

YES → **POSSIBLE CAUSE AND ACTION** A naturally low level of interest in sex is a normal part of the personality of some men. This is unlikely to be a cause for concern if you are happy with your present level of sexual activity. However, if your low sex drive is causing difficulties in your relationship, consult your doctor, who may recommend sex counseling (opposite).

NO ↓

Have you been fatigued and/or feeling stressed recently?

YES → **POSSIBLE CAUSE AND ACTION** Sex drive can be reduced by fatigue and stress, which may result from situations such as unemployment, a new job, or a new baby (*see* RECOGNIZING STRESS, p.173). Talk to your partner, and try to tackle the source of your stress and/or fatigue. Your sex drive will probably return once you have resolved the underlying problem. If your low sex drive continues, consult your doctor.

NO ↓

Have you noticed one or more of the following symptoms?
- An inability to concentrate or make decisions
- Difficulty sleeping
- Feeling in low spirits

YES → **POSSIBLE CAUSE** The cause of your low sex drive may be a depressive illness.

Go to chart **72** DEPRESSION (p.170)

NO ↓

Is your relationship with your partner satisfactory in other respects?

YES → **POSSIBLE CAUSE AND ACTION** A specific sexual problem may have reduced your sex drive. Try talking to your partner (*see* COMMUNICATING YOUR SEXUAL NEEDS, p.273). If the problem is not resolved, consult your doctor, who may recommend sex counseling (opposite).

NO ↓

POSSIBLE CAUSE AND ACTION If your relationship is poor, then you may not have interest in sex. Try to talk frankly with your partner. If things do not improve, consult your doctor, who may recommend relationship counseling (*see* USEFUL ADDRESSES, p.311).

Are you interested in sex but not with your current partner?

YES →

NO ↓

Are you taking any prescribed drugs?

YES → **POSSIBLE CAUSE AND ACTION** Certain drugs, such as some *beta blockers* and *anticancer drugs*, can reduce your sex drive. Consult your doctor: he or she may be able to prescribe an alternative drug. In the meantime, do not stop taking your prescribed drugs.

NO ↓

Continued on next page

Sex after illness

Many people worry about whether it is safe to have sex after a major illness such as a heart attack or a stroke. Relaxed sex with your usual partner uses about the same energy as carrying a full laundry basket up a flight of stairs, so if you can manage this level of activity then sex is unlikely to pose a problem. If you are in any doubt, your doctor will be able to advise you. Concerns relating to an altered body image following surgery can also be an issue. This can happen, for example, when a person has had bowel surgery and as a result has a stoma (opening) on the surface of the skin, or when a woman has had breast surgery. In these situations, counseling may help you come to terms with the changes to your body. If you have a disabling condition, such as rheumatoid arthritis, pain can make sex difficult. You may need to experiment with different sexual positions to find one that is comfortable. Self-help groups (*see* USEFUL ADDRESSES, p.311) can often give advice on coping with this type of problem.

Continued from
previous page

Have you recently
recovered from a major
illness or operation? **YES**
NO

Have you noticed any
of the following?
• Loss of body hair
• Reduced testes size
• Development
  of breasts **YES**
NO

Do you often drink
more than the
recommended safe
alcohol limit (p.30)? **YES**
NO

Are you generally
anxious, and/or do you
have specific anxieties
about sex? **YES**
NO

Are you over 50? **YES**
NO

CONSULT YOUR DOCTOR IF YOU ARE UNABLE TO
MAKE A DIAGNOSIS FROM THIS CHART.

Sex counseling

Counseling with a sex therapist or counselor is often helpful when there is a psychological basis for a sexual problem. The sessions usually last about 1 hour and a course of treatment may last for several weeks or months. Both partners need to attend the therapy sessions so that the therapist can help them to understand their sexual needs and communicate them honestly. A therapist may also suggest exercises to do at home. One such exercise is a technique called sensate focus. In this exercise, a couple touch and stimulate each other's bodies but agree not to have full sexual intercourse for several weeks. Sensate focus can be helpful for problems that stem from anxiety about sexual performance.

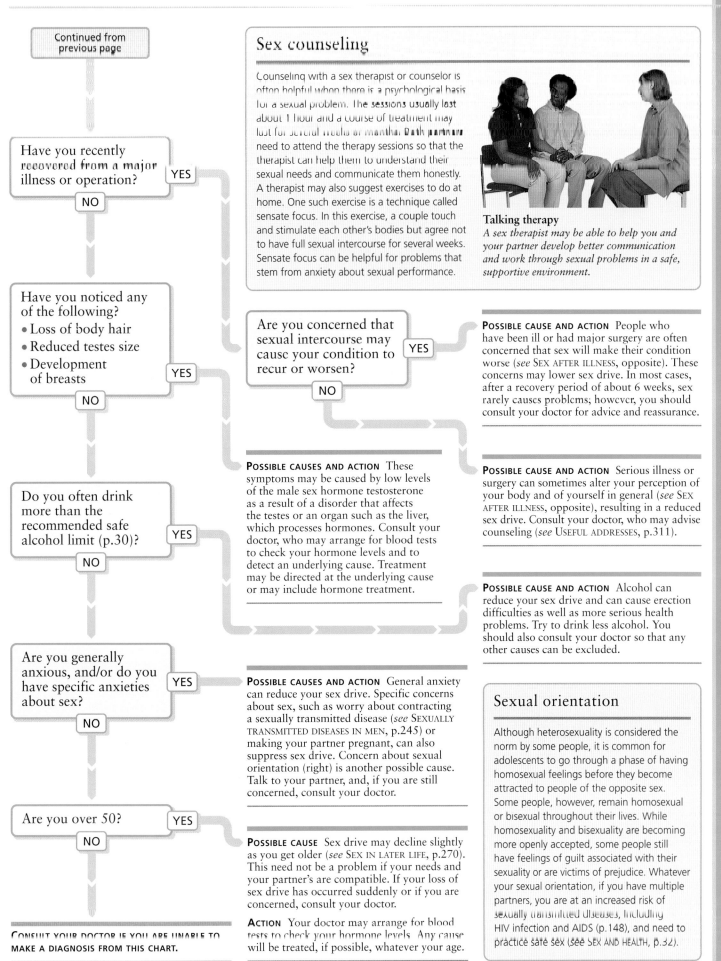

Talking therapy
A sex therapist may be able to help you and your partner develop better communication and work through sexual problems in a safe, supportive environment.

Are you concerned that
sexual intercourse may
cause your condition to
recur or worsen? **YES**
NO

POSSIBLE CAUSES AND ACTION These symptoms may be caused by low levels of the male sex hormone testosterone as a result of a disorder that affects the testes or an organ such as the liver, which processes hormones. Consult your doctor, who may arrange for blood tests to check your hormone levels and to detect an underlying cause. Treatment may be directed at the underlying cause or may include hormone treatment.

POSSIBLE CAUSES AND ACTION General anxiety can reduce your sex drive. Specific concerns about sex, such as worry about contracting a sexually transmitted disease (*see* SEXUALLY TRANSMITTED DISEASES IN MEN, p.245) or making your partner pregnant, can also suppress sex drive. Concern about sexual orientation (right) is another possible cause. Talk to your partner, and, if you are still concerned, consult your doctor.

POSSIBLE CAUSE Sex drive may decline slightly as you get older (*see* SEX IN LATER LIFE, p.270). This need not be a problem if your needs and your partner's are compatible. If your loss of sex drive has occurred suddenly or if you are concerned, consult your doctor.

ACTION Your doctor may arrange for blood tests to check your hormone levels. Any cause will be treated, if possible, whatever your age.

POSSIBLE CAUSE AND ACTION People who have been ill or had major surgery are often concerned that sex will make their condition worse (*see* SEX AFTER ILLNESS, opposite). These concerns may lower sex drive. In most cases, after a recovery period of about 6 weeks, sex rarely causes problems; however, you should consult your doctor for advice and reassurance.

POSSIBLE CAUSE AND ACTION Serious illness or surgery can sometimes alter your perception of your body and of yourself in general (*see* SEX AFTER ILLNESS, opposite), resulting in a reduced sex drive. Consult your doctor, who may advise counseling (*see* USEFUL ADDRESSES, p.311).

POSSIBLE CAUSE AND ACTION Alcohol can reduce your sex drive and can cause erection difficulties as well as more serious health problems. Try to drink less alcohol. You should also consult your doctor so that any other causes can be excluded.

Sexual orientation

Although heterosexuality is considered the norm by some people, it is common for adolescents to go through a phase of having homosexual feelings before they become attracted to people of the opposite sex. Some people, however, remain homosexual or bisexual throughout their lives. While homosexuality and bisexuality are becoming more openly accepted, some people still have feelings of guilt associated with their sexuality or are victims of prejudice. Whatever your sexual orientation, if you have multiple partners, you are at an increased risk of sexually transmitted diseases, including HIV infection and AIDS (p.148), and need to practice safe sex (*see* SEX AND HEALTH, p.32).

126 Fertility problems in men

See also chart 139, FERTILITY PROBLEMS IN WOMEN **(p.274).** Fertility problems affect 1 in 7 couples who want children, and, in many cases, a cause is not found. Failure to conceive may be the result of a problem affecting either one or both partners; this chart deals only with possible problems in men. The two main causes of infertility in men are insufficient sperm production and a blockage of the vas deferens, the tubes that transport the sperm to the penis during ejaculation.

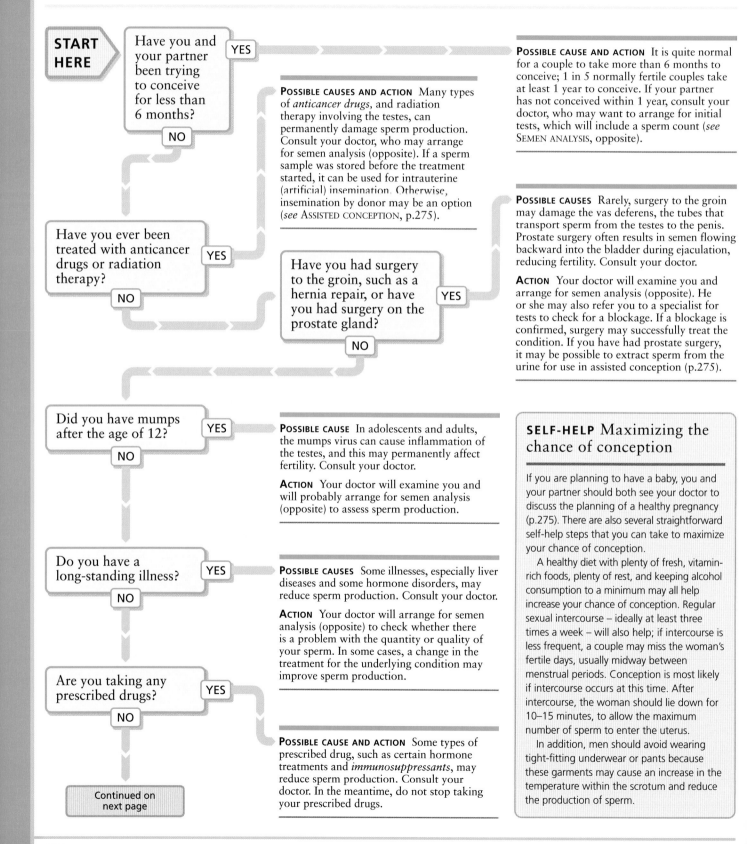

START HERE → **Have you and your partner been trying to conceive for less than 6 months?** YES / NO

POSSIBLE CAUSE AND ACTION It is quite normal for a couple to take more than 6 months to conceive; 1 in 5 normally fertile couples take at least 1 year to conceive. If your partner has not conceived within 1 year, consult your doctor, who may want to arrange for initial tests, which will include a sperm count (*see* SEMEN ANALYSIS, opposite).

Have you ever been treated with anticancer drugs or radiation therapy? YES / NO

POSSIBLE CAUSES AND ACTION Many types of *anticancer drugs*, and radiation therapy involving the testes, can permanently damage sperm production. Consult your doctor, who may arrange for semen analysis (opposite). If a sperm sample was stored before the treatment started, it can be used for intrauterine (artificial) insemination. Otherwise, insemination by donor may be an option (*see* ASSISTED CONCEPTION, p.275).

Have you had surgery to the groin, such as a hernia repair, or have you had surgery on the prostate gland? YES / NO

POSSIBLE CAUSES Rarely, surgery to the groin may damage the vas deferens, the tubes that transport sperm from the testes to the penis. Prostate surgery often results in semen flowing backward into the bladder during ejaculation, reducing fertility. Consult your doctor.

ACTION Your doctor will examine you and arrange for semen analysis (opposite). He or she may also refer you to a specialist for tests to check for a blockage. If a blockage is confirmed, surgery may successfully treat the condition. If you have had prostate surgery, it may be possible to extract sperm from the urine for use in assisted conception (p.275).

Did you have mumps after the age of 12? YES / NO

POSSIBLE CAUSE In adolescents and adults, the mumps virus can cause inflammation of the testes, and this may permanently affect fertility. Consult your doctor.

ACTION Your doctor will examine you and will probably arrange for semen analysis (opposite) to assess sperm production.

Do you have a long-standing illness? YES / NO

POSSIBLE CAUSES Some illnesses, especially liver diseases and some hormone disorders, may reduce sperm production. Consult your doctor.

ACTION Your doctor will arrange for semen analysis (opposite) to check whether there is a problem with the quantity or quality of your sperm. In some cases, a change in the treatment for the underlying condition may improve sperm production.

Are you taking any prescribed drugs? YES / NO

POSSIBLE CAUSE AND ACTION Some types of prescribed drug, such as certain hormone treatments and *immunosuppressants*, may reduce sperm production. Consult your doctor. In the meantime, do not stop taking your prescribed drugs.

Continued on next page

SELF-HELP Maximizing the chance of conception

If you are planning to have a baby, you and your partner should both see your doctor to discuss the planning of a healthy pregnancy (p.275). There are also several straightforward self-help steps that you can take to maximize your chance of conception.

A healthy diet with plenty of fresh, vitamin-rich foods, plenty of rest, and keeping alcohol consumption to a minimum may all help increase your chance of conception. Regular sexual intercourse – ideally at least three times a week – will also help; if intercourse is less frequent, a couple may miss the woman's fertile days, usually midway between menstrual periods. Conception is most likely if intercourse occurs at this time. After intercourse, the woman should lie down for 10–15 minutes, to allow the maximum number of sperm to enter the uterus.

In addition, men should avoid wearing tight-fitting underwear or pants because these garments may cause an increase in the temperature within the scrotum and reduce the production of sperm.

Continued from
previous page

Have you had a sexually transmitted disease in the past?
YES →

POSSIBLE CAUSE Sexually transmitted diseases (see SEXUALLY TRANSMITTED DISEASES IN MEN, p.245) can result in a blockage of the vas deferens, the tubes that transport sperm from the testes to the penis. Consult your doctor.

ACTION Your doctor will examine you, and he or she may refer you to a specialist for tests to establish whether the tubes leading from your testes are blocked. In some cases, surgery to relieve the blockage may be possible.

NO ↓

Do you have sex less often than three times a week on average?
YES →

POSSIBLE CAUSE AND ACTION Infrequent intercourse is a common cause of failure to conceive. If you have sex less than three times a week, the chance of sperm being present to fertilize an egg when it is released is reduced. If possible, try to have intercourse with your partner more often (see MAXIMIZING THE CHANCE OF CONCEPTION, opposite). If your partner has still not conceived within a further 3–6 months, consult your doctor.

NO ↓

Do you regularly drink more than the recommended safe alcohol limit (p.30)?
YES →

NO ↓

Are you outside the healthy weight range for your height (see ASSESSING YOUR WEIGHT, p.29), or has there been a sudden change in your weight?
YES →

POSSIBLE CAUSES AND ACTION If you are substantially overweight or underweight your fertility may be reduced. Consult your doctor, who may arrange for semen analysis (above). Make sure that you eat a healthy diet. If you are overweight, you should try to lose weight (see HOW TO LOSE WEIGHT SAFELY, p.151). If you are underweight, follow the advice on gaining weight safely (p.149).

NO ↓

Do you smoke or use recreational drugs?
YES →

POSSIBLE CAUSES Smoking and/or using recreational drugs can impair sperm function or reduce the production of sperm in the testes. Consult your doctor.

ACTION Your doctor may arrange for semen analysis (above). Try to stop smoking and/or using recreational drugs.

NO ↓

Do you wear underpants that are fit tightly, or do you take hot baths, saunas, or use hot tubs frequently?
YES →

NO ↓

CONSULT YOUR DOCTOR IF YOU ARE UNABLE TO MAKE A DIAGNOSIS FROM THIS CHART.

Semen analysis

If a couple has fertility problems, semen analysis is usually one of the first tests that is carried out. The man is asked to ejaculate into a clean container (semen collected from a condom is not suitable). The volume of semen is measured, and a sample is then viewed under a microscope to assess the shape and activity levels of the sperm and to count the number of sperm. Each milliliter of semen normally contains at least 50 million sperm, the majority of which are healthy. A low sperm count is defined as fewer than 20 million sperm per milliliter. If the test shows any abnormality, it will be repeated for confirmation.

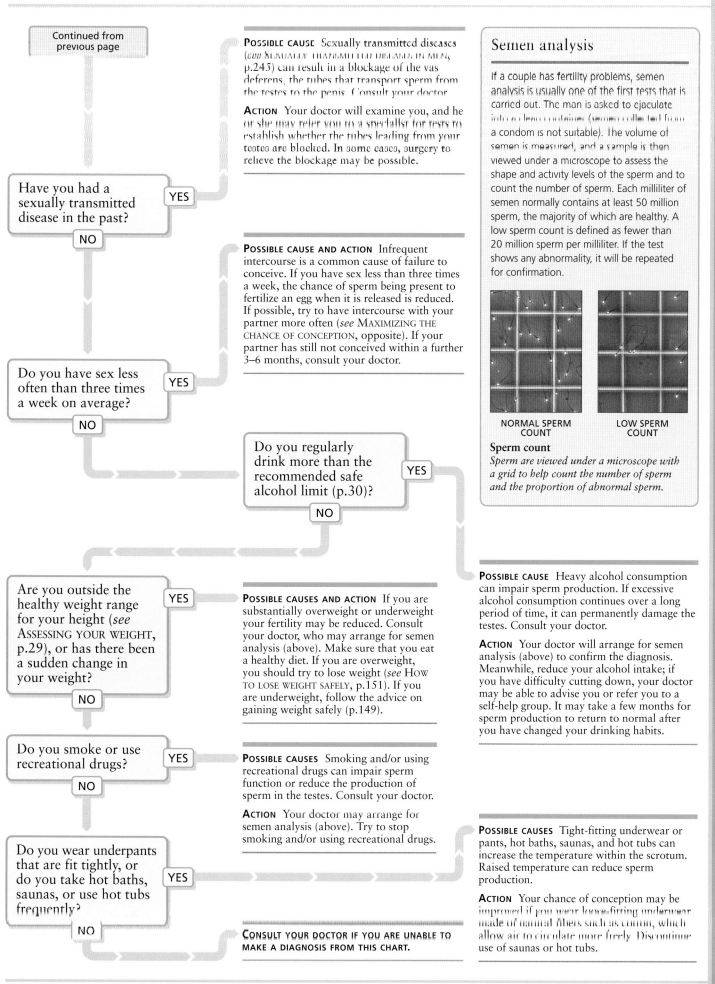

NORMAL SPERM COUNT   LOW SPERM COUNT

Sperm count
Sperm are viewed under a microscope with a grid to help count the number of sperm and the proportion of abnormal sperm.

POSSIBLE CAUSE Heavy alcohol consumption can impair sperm production. If excessive alcohol consumption continues over a long period of time, it can permanently damage the testes. Consult your doctor.

ACTION Your doctor will arrange for semen analysis (above) to confirm the diagnosis. Meanwhile, reduce your alcohol intake; if you have difficulty cutting down, your doctor may be able to advise you or refer you to a self-help group. It may take a few months for sperm production to return to normal after you have changed your drinking habits.

POSSIBLE CAUSES Tight-fitting underwear or pants, hot baths, saunas, and hot tubs can increase the temperature within the scrotum. Raised temperature can reduce sperm production.

ACTION Your chance of conception may be improved if you wear loose-fitting underwear made of natural fibers such as cotton, which allow air to circulate more freely. Discontinue use of saunas or hot tubs.

127 Contraception choices for men

For women's contraception choices, see chart 140, Contraception choices for women (p.276).
The two main methods of contraception currently available for men are condoms and vasectomy. There is no hormonal method of contraception for men. Your choice of contraceptive method will depend on various factors, including your sexual lifestyle and age. If you have a regular partner, the decision is best shared. Condoms have the advantages of being 95 percent effective and of helping to provide protection against sexually transmitted diseases for both the user and his sexual partner. Many men choose to have a vasectomy (male sterilization) when they are certain they will not want children in the future. Vasectomy is a simple procedure, but it must be considered irreversible.

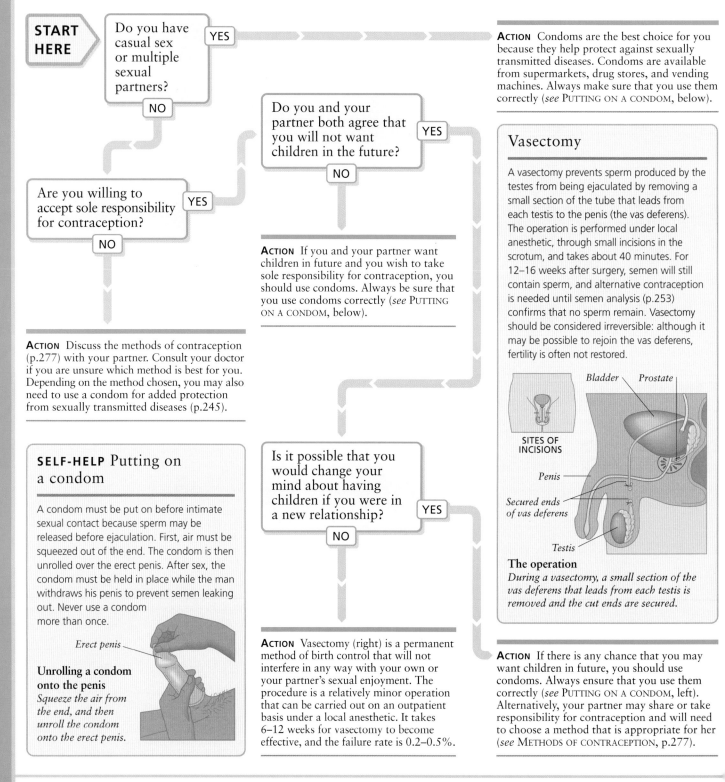

START HERE

Do you have casual sex or multiple sexual partners? — **YES**

NO

Are you willing to accept sole responsibility for contraception? — **YES**

NO

ACTION Discuss the methods of contraception (p.277) with your partner. Consult your doctor if you are unsure which method is best for you. Depending on the method chosen, you may also need to use a condom for added protection from sexually transmitted diseases (p.245).

Do you and your partner both agree that you will not want children in the future? — **YES**

NO

ACTION If you and your partner want children in future and you wish to take sole responsibility for contraception, you should use condoms. Always be sure that you use condoms correctly (*see* Putting on a condom, below).

Is it possible that you would change your mind about having children if you were in a new relationship? — **YES**

NO

ACTION Vasectomy (right) is a permanent method of birth control that will not interfere in any way with your own or your partner's sexual enjoyment. The procedure is a relatively minor operation that can be carried out on an outpatient basis under a local anesthetic. It takes 6–12 weeks for vasectomy to become effective, and the failure rate is 0.2–0.5%.

ACTION Condoms are the best choice for you because they help protect against sexually transmitted diseases. Condoms are available from supermarkets, drug stores, and vending machines. Always make sure that you use them correctly (*see* Putting on a condom, below).

Vasectomy

A vasectomy prevents sperm produced by the testes from being ejaculated by removing a small section of the tube that leads from each testis to the penis (the vas deferens). The operation is performed under local anesthetic, through small incisions in the scrotum, and takes about 40 minutes. For 12–16 weeks after surgery, semen will still contain sperm, and alternative contraception is needed until semen analysis (p.253) confirms that no sperm remain. Vasectomy should be considered irreversible: although it may be possible to rejoin the vas deferens, fertility is often not restored.

Bladder   Prostate

SITES OF INCISIONS

Penis

Secured ends of vas deferens

Testis

The operation
During a vasectomy, a small section of the vas deferens that leads from each testis is removed and the cut ends are secured.

ACTION If there is any chance that you may want children in future, you should use condoms. Always ensure that you use them correctly (*see* Putting on a condom, left). Alternatively, your partner may share or take responsibility for contraception and will need to choose a method that is appropriate for her (*see* Methods of contraception, p.277).

SELF-HELP Putting on a condom

A condom must be put on before intimate sexual contact because sperm may be released before ejaculation. First, air must be squeezed out of the end. The condom is then unrolled over the erect penis. After sex, the condom must be held in place while the man withdraws his penis to prevent semen leaking out. Never use a condom more than once.

Erect penis

Unrolling a condom onto the penis
Squeeze the air from the end, and then unroll the condom onto the erect penis.

CHARTS FOR WOMEN

128 Breast problems

For breast problems during pregnancy or after giving birth, see chart 149, BREAST PROBLEMS AND PREGNANCY *(p.286).* Although the majority of breast problems are not serious, breast cancer is one of the most common cancers in women. Rarely, it also occurs in men. If diagnosed early enough, breast cancer can often be successfully treated. It is therefore important to familiarize yourself with the look and feel of your breasts (*see* BREAST SELF-AWARENESS, below) so that you will be able to detect any changes. If you do find a change in your breast, you should seek medical advice immediately.

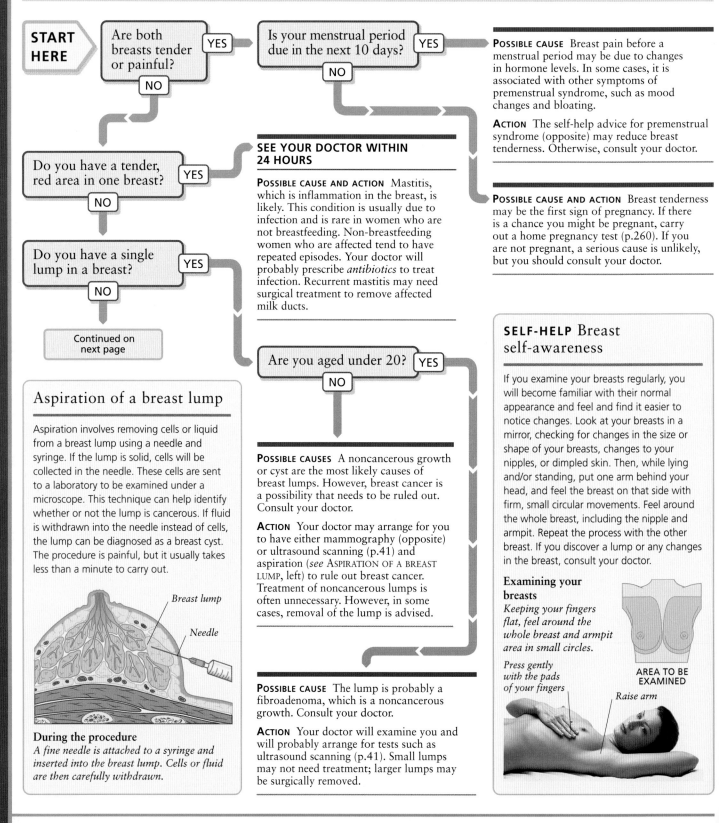

START HERE → **Are both breasts tender or painful?** — YES → **Is your menstrual period due in the next 10 days?** — YES →

NO

NO

Do you have a tender, red area in one breast? — YES →

NO

Do you have a single lump in a breast? — YES →

NO

Continued on next page

Are you aged under 20? — YES →

NO

SEE YOUR DOCTOR WITHIN 24 HOURS

POSSIBLE CAUSE AND ACTION Mastitis, which is inflammation in the breast, is likely. This condition is usually due to infection and is rare in women who are not breastfeeding. Non-breastfeeding women who are affected tend to have repeated episodes. Your doctor will probably prescribe *antibiotics* to treat infection. Recurrent mastitis may need surgical treatment to remove affected milk ducts.

POSSIBLE CAUSE Breast pain before a menstrual period may be due to changes in hormone levels. In some cases, it is associated with other symptoms of premenstrual syndrome, such as mood changes and bloating.

ACTION The self-help advice for premenstrual syndrome (opposite) may reduce breast tenderness. Otherwise, consult your doctor.

POSSIBLE CAUSE AND ACTION Breast tenderness may be the first sign of pregnancy. If there is a chance you might be pregnant, carry out a home pregnancy test (p.260). If you are not pregnant, a serious cause is unlikely, but you should consult your doctor.

Aspiration of a breast lump

Aspiration involves removing cells or liquid from a breast lump using a needle and syringe. If the lump is solid, cells will be collected in the needle. These cells are sent to a laboratory to be examined under a microscope. This technique can help identify whether or not the lump is cancerous. If fluid is withdrawn into the needle instead of cells, the lump can be diagnosed as a breast cyst. The procedure is painful, but it usually takes less than a minute to carry out.

Breast lump

Needle

During the procedure
A fine needle is attached to a syringe and inserted into the breast lump. Cells or fluid are then carefully withdrawn.

POSSIBLE CAUSES A noncancerous growth or cyst are the most likely causes of breast lumps. However, breast cancer is a possibility that needs to be ruled out. Consult your doctor.

ACTION Your doctor may arrange for you to have either mammography (opposite) or ultrasound scanning (p.41) and aspiration (*see* ASPIRATION OF A BREAST LUMP, left) to rule out breast cancer. Treatment of noncancerous lumps is often unnecessary. However, in some cases, removal of the lump is advised.

POSSIBLE CAUSE The lump is probably a fibroadenoma, which is a noncancerous growth. Consult your doctor.

ACTION Your doctor will examine you and will probably arrange for tests such as ultrasound scanning (p.41). Small lumps may not need treatment; larger lumps may be surgically removed.

SELF-HELP Breast self-awareness

If you examine your breasts regularly, you will become familiar with their normal appearance and feel and find it easier to notice changes. Look at your breasts in a mirror, checking for changes in the size or shape of your breasts, changes to your nipples, or dimpled skin. Then, while lying and/or standing, put one arm behind your head, and feel the breast on that side with firm, small circular movements. Feel around the whole breast, including the nipple and armpit. Repeat the process with the other breast. If you discover a lump or any changes in the breast, consult your doctor.

Examining your breasts
Keeping your fingers flat, feel around the whole breast and armpit area in small circles.

Press gently with the pads of your fingers

AREA TO BE EXAMINED

Raise arm

Mammography

Mammography uses X rays (p. 39) to detect abnormal areas of breast tissue. It is used as a screening test to detect signs of breast cancer and is also carried out to investigate breast lumps. Mammography is recommended every 1–3 years from age 40 or 50 to 70. The breast is positioned on the X-ray plate and compressed so that the breast tissue can be seen on the X ray. Two X rays are usually taken of each breast. The procedure is uncomfortable but lasts only a few seconds. If an abnormality is detected, you will need further tests such as aspiration (see ASPIRATION OF A BREAST LUMP, opposite) to determine the cause of the abnormality.

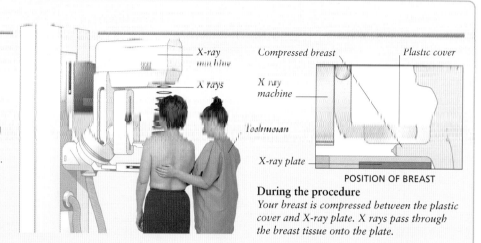

X-ray machine
X rays
Technician
Compressed breast
Plastic cover
X-ray machine
X-ray plate

POSITION OF BREAST

During the procedure
Your breast is compressed between the plastic cover and X-ray plate. X rays pass through the breast tissue onto the plate.

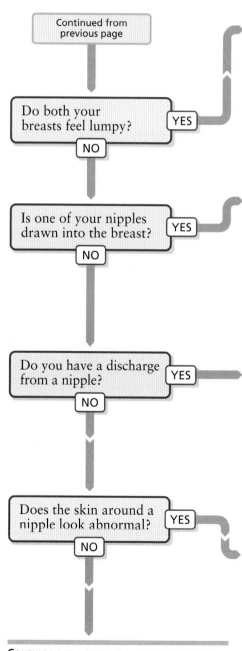

Continued from previous page

Do both your breasts feel lumpy? — NO / YES

POSSIBLE CAUSE AND ACTION Some women have lumpier breasts than others. Lumps are usually more obvious before a menstrual period. If you are worried, consult your doctor, who will examine your breasts to make sure that there are no lumps that require investigation. Naturally lumpy breasts do not require treatment and do not increase the risk of breast cancer.

Is one of your nipples drawn into the breast? — NO / YES

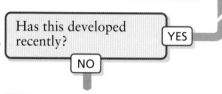

Has this developed recently? — NO / YES

POSSIBLE CAUSES A change in a nipple may be a sign of breast cancer. However, normal aging may also cause a nipple to become indrawn. Consult your doctor.

ACTION Your doctor will examine your breasts and will probably arrange for tests such as mammography (above) to exclude a problem deeper in the breast.

POSSIBLE CAUSE AND ACTION If your nipple has always been drawn in, this is not a cause for concern, although it may make breastfeeding difficult. Wearing a nipple shell inside your bra during pregnancy may help draw the nipple out in preparation for breastfeeding.

Do you have a discharge from a nipple? — NO / YES

POSSIBLE CAUSES AND ACTION Milky nipple discharge is usually due to hormone changes and is no cause for concern. In rare cases, a cancerous or noncancerous growth affecting a milk duct is the cause, especially if the discharge is not milky or appears bloody. Consult your doctor, who will examine your breasts and may arrange for mammography (above) to exclude an abnormality in the underlying breast tissue. Treatment is often not necessary, but occasionally affected milk ducts may need to be removed surgically.

Does the skin around a nipple look abnormal? — NO / YES

POSSIBLE CAUSES AND ACTION You may have a skin condition, such as eczema. However, Paget's disease, a rare form of breast cancer, is a possibility. Consult your doctor, who will examine your breasts. If you have a skin condition, *corticosteroid* creams may be prescribed. If your doctor suspects Paget's disease, you will probably be referred for tests such as mammography (above) or a biopsy of the abnormal area.

CONSULT YOUR DOCTOR IF YOU ARE UNABLE TO MAKE A DIAGNOSIS FROM THIS CHART.

SELF-HELP Premenstrual syndrome

Premenstrual syndrome is a group of symptoms, often including bloating, mood swings, and breast tenderness, that some women experience in the days leading up to a menstrual period. The following measures may help prevent or relieve your symptoms:

- If possible, keep stress to a minimum.
- Try relaxation exercises (p.32) or an exercise such as yoga.
- Eat little and often, including plenty of carbohydrates and fiber.
- Reduce your salt intake.
- Do not eat fried foods or excessive amounts of chocolate.
- Avoid drinks containing large amounts of caffeine, such as coffee, tea, and cola.
- Take the recommended daily allowance of a vitamin B_6 supplement.
- Consider trying evening primrose oil, particularly in the days before your menstrual period.
- When PMS is very severe, treatment should be discussed with your doctor.

129 Bladder control problems in women

For other urinary problems, see chart 108, GENERAL URINARY PROBLEMS (p.224).

Bladder control problems affect 1 in 10 women. Incontinence, or urinating involuntarily, is the most common problem. This is often related to childbirth, but it may have other causes. Many effective treatments for incontinence are now available. Inability to urinate is a less common problem but always needs immediate medical attention.

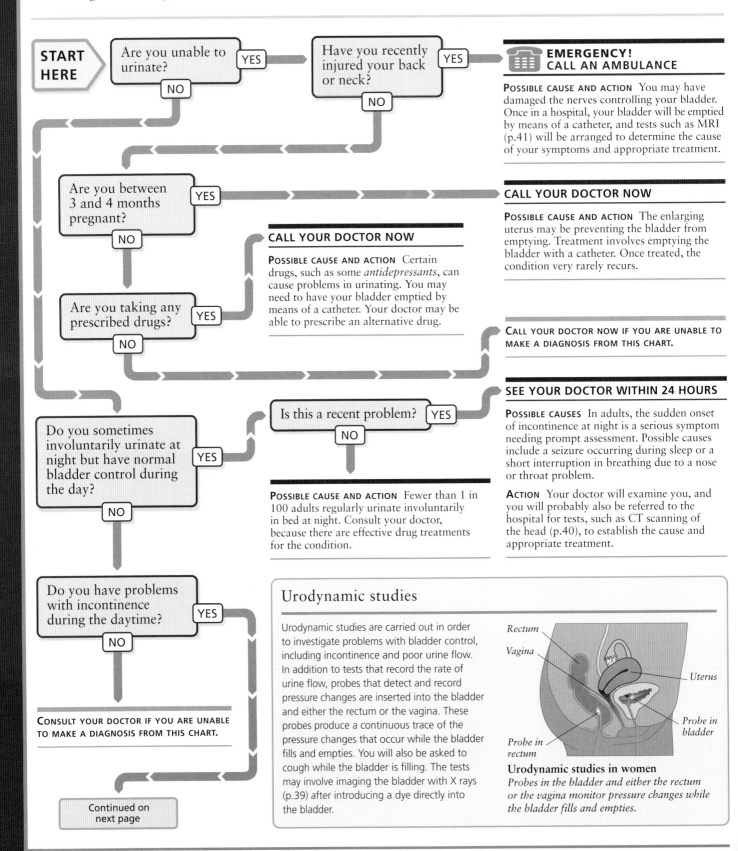

START HERE

Are you unable to urinate? — YES → **Have you recently injured your back or neck?** — YES → 📞 **EMERGENCY! CALL AN AMBULANCE**

POSSIBLE CAUSE AND ACTION You may have damaged the nerves controlling your bladder. Once in a hospital, your bladder will be emptied by means of a catheter, and tests such as MRI (p.41) will be arranged to determine the cause of your symptoms and appropriate treatment.

NO ↓ (Are you unable to urinate?)

NO ↓ (Have you recently injured your back or neck?)

Are you between 3 and 4 months pregnant? — YES → **CALL YOUR DOCTOR NOW**

POSSIBLE CAUSE AND ACTION The enlarging uterus may be preventing the bladder from emptying. Treatment involves emptying the bladder with a catheter. Once treated, the condition very rarely recurs.

NO ↓

Are you taking any prescribed drugs? — YES → **CALL YOUR DOCTOR NOW**

POSSIBLE CAUSE AND ACTION Certain drugs, such as some *antidepressants*, can cause problems in urinating. You may need to have your bladder emptied by means of a catheter. Your doctor may be able to prescribe an alternative drug.

CALL YOUR DOCTOR NOW IF YOU ARE UNABLE TO MAKE A DIAGNOSIS FROM THIS CHART.

NO ↓

Do you sometimes involuntarily urinate at night but have normal bladder control during the day? — YES → **Is this a recent problem?** — YES → **SEE YOUR DOCTOR WITHIN 24 HOURS**

POSSIBLE CAUSES In adults, the sudden onset of incontinence at night is a serious symptom needing prompt assessment. Possible causes include a seizure occurring during sleep or a short interruption in breathing due to a nose or throat problem.

ACTION Your doctor will examine you, and you will probably also be referred to the hospital for tests, such as CT scanning of the head (p.40), to establish the cause and appropriate treatment.

NO ↓ (Is this a recent problem?)

POSSIBLE CAUSE AND ACTION Fewer than 1 in 100 adults regularly urinate involuntarily in bed at night. Consult your doctor, because there are effective drug treatments for the condition.

NO ↓ (Do you sometimes involuntarily urinate at night...)

Do you have problems with incontinence during the daytime? — YES →

CONSULT YOUR DOCTOR IF YOU ARE UNABLE TO MAKE A DIAGNOSIS FROM THIS CHART.

NO ↓

Continued on next page

Urodynamic studies

Urodynamic studies are carried out in order to investigate problems with bladder control, including incontinence and poor urine flow. In addition to tests that record the rate of urine flow, probes that detect and record pressure changes are inserted into the bladder and either the rectum or the vagina. These probes produce a continuous trace of the pressure changes that occur while the bladder fills and empties. You will also be asked to cough while the bladder is filling. The tests may involve imaging the bladder with X rays (p.39) after introducing a dye directly into the bladder.

Rectum
Vagina
Uterus
Probe in bladder
Probe in rectum

Urodynamic studies in women
Probes in the bladder and either the rectum or the vagina monitor pressure changes while the bladder fills and empties.

Continued from previous page

Do you leak urine when you sneeze, cough, or run? — YES →

Have you recently had a baby? — YES →

NO ↓

POSSIBLE CAUSE You probably have stress incontinence as a result of weak muscles supporting the neck of the bladder. This is a common problem. Consult your doctor.

ACTION Your doctor will examine you to exclude a prolapse of the uterus, which is sometimes associated with this condition. He or she may arrange for urodynamic studies (opposite). You may be advised to do pelvic-floor exercises (right). In severe cases, surgery may be needed.

NO ↓

Do you often have a sudden urge to urinate that is difficult to control? — YES →

POSSIBLE CAUSE AND ACTION Childbirth has probably weakened the muscles that support the neck of the bladder. This is very common. Regular Kegel exercises (right) should restore control. Consult your doctor if bladder control does not return within 2 months.

NO ↓

Do any of the following apply to you?
- You have had a stroke recently
- You have diabetes
- You have a chronic nervous system disorder such as multiple sclerosis

— YES →

POSSIBLE CAUSE In some cases, damage to the brain, spinal cord, or nerves controlling the bladder can cause continence problems. Consult your doctor.

ACTION Your doctor will examine you and may request a urine test to exclude an additional problem such as a urine infection. In some cases, drug treatment may help. Alternatively, you may be referred to a urologist, who will help you manage the problem.

NO ↓

Is incontinence associated with swelling of the abdomen, and do you urinate only in small volumes when you try to empty your bladder? — YES →

NO ↓

Are you taking any prescribed drugs? — YES →

POSSIBLE CAUSE AND ACTION Drugs such as *diuretics*, which result in a sudden increase in the amount of urine produced, may precipitate incontinence. Talk to your doctor about the problem. He or she may be able to alter your drugs or give advice on coping with their effects.

NO ↓

Are you over 65, and have you become increasingly forgetful? — YES →

NO ↓

CONSULT YOUR DOCTOR IF YOU ARE UNABLE TO MAKE A DIAGNOSIS FROM THIS CHART.

SELF-HELP Kegel exercises

Kegel exercises can help strengthen the pelvic-floor muscles, which support the bladder, uterus, and rectum. If done regularly, they can help prevent and treat urinary incontinence.

You can perform Kegel exercises lying down, sitting, or standing. In order to identify the pelvic-floor muscles, imagine that you are passing urine and have to stop suddenly midstream. The muscles that you feel tighten around the vagina, urethra, and rectum are the pelvic-floor muscles.

To strengthen the pelvic-floor muscles, contract them and hold them contracted for 10 seconds. Then relax the muscles slowly. Repeat this contraction and relaxation cycle 10 times. Practice your Kegel exercises at least every hour during the day.

If you have been doing the exercises to treat bladder control problems, you should see an improvement within 2 weeks, but you will need to continue doing the exercises regularly to maintain the improvement.

POSSIBLE CAUSE You may have an irritable bladder, in which there is a strong urge to urinate even when the bladder contains little urine. Consult your doctor.

ACTION Your doctor will examine you and test your urine to rule out an infection, which can cause similar symptoms. He or she may also arrange for bladder function tests (*see* URODYNAMIC STUDIES, opposite). In most cases, drug treatment to reduce the sensitivity of the bladder combined with exercises to increase the amount of urine that the bladder can hold without triggering the urge to urinate will help improve the symptoms.

POSSIBLE CAUSE AND ACTION You may have an obstruction to the outflow of the bladder, which is preventing the bladder from emptying normally. This causes the bladder to become overfull and results in urine leaking from the bladder. Constipation is a possible cause of the obstruction. Consult your doctor, who will probably arrange for tests to determine the underlying cause. He or she may refer you to a specialist so that your bladder can be drained and for treatment of the blockage.

POSSIBLE CAUSE A decline in mental function that occurs with several neurological diseases associated with increasing age can sometimes result in problems with bladder control. Consult your doctor.

ACTION Your doctor will examine you and may arrange for tests to exclude other causes. You may be referred to a urologist, who can advise you on ways of managing the problem.

130 Absent menstrual periods

Menstruation normally starts between the ages of 11 and 14, although in girls who are below average height and/or weight it may not start until some time later. Once menstrual periods start, they may be irregular for the first few years and become regular in a monthly cycle in the late teens. Once the menstrual cycle is established, it varies in length among individual women from as little as 24 days between periods to about 35 days. Absence of menstrual periods (amenorrhea) may occur in healthy women for several reasons, the most common of which is pregnancy. Other factors that may affect your monthly cycle include illness, stress, and strenuous physical activity. It is normal for menstrual periods to cease permanently as you approach middle age. Only rarely is absence of periods a sign of an underlying disorder. Consult this chart if you have never had a menstrual period, or if your period is more than 2 weeks late.

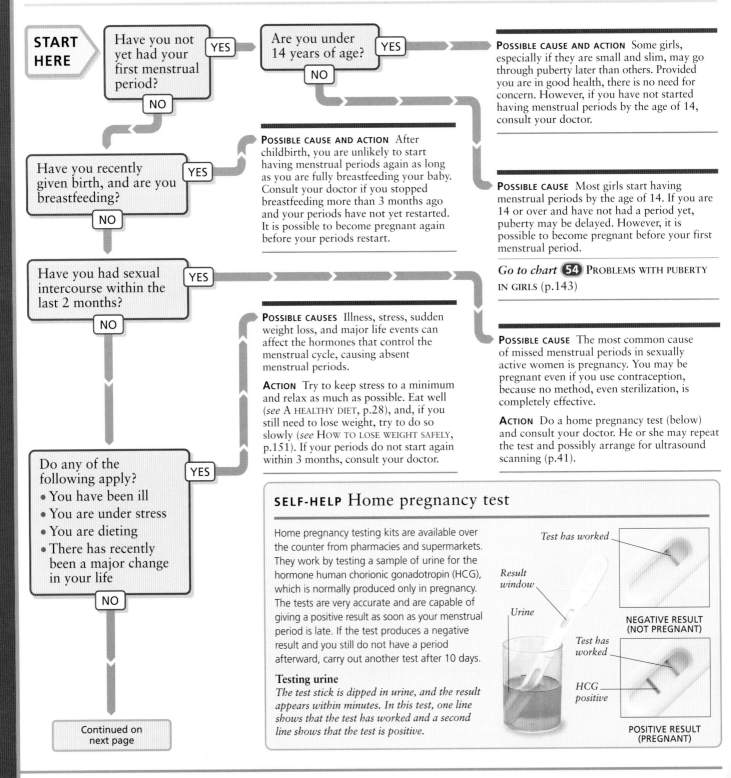

START HERE

Have you not yet had your first menstrual period? — YES → **Are you under 14 years of age?** — YES →

POSSIBLE CAUSE AND ACTION Some girls, especially if they are small and slim, may go through puberty later than others. Provided you are in good health, there is no need for concern. However, if you have not started having menstrual periods by the age of 14, consult your doctor.

NO (under 14 years of age)

POSSIBLE CAUSE Most girls start having menstrual periods by the age of 14. If you are 14 or over and have not had a period yet, puberty may be delayed. However, it is possible to become pregnant before your first menstrual period.

Go to chart **54** PROBLEMS WITH PUBERTY IN GIRLS (p.143)

NO →

Have you recently given birth, and are you breastfeeding? — YES →

POSSIBLE CAUSE AND ACTION After childbirth, you are unlikely to start having menstrual periods again as long as you are fully breastfeeding your baby. Consult your doctor if you stopped breastfeeding more than 3 months ago and your periods have not yet restarted. It is possible to become pregnant again before your periods restart.

NO →

Have you had sexual intercourse within the last 2 months? — YES →

POSSIBLE CAUSE The most common cause of missed menstrual periods in sexually active women is pregnancy. You may be pregnant even if you use contraception, because no method, even sterilization, is completely effective.

ACTION Do a home pregnancy test (below) and consult your doctor. He or she may repeat the test and possibly arrange for ultrasound scanning (p.41).

NO →

Do any of the following apply?
- You have been ill
- You are under stress
- You are dieting
- There has recently been a major change in your life

— YES →

POSSIBLE CAUSES Illness, stress, sudden weight loss, and major life events can affect the hormones that control the menstrual cycle, causing absent menstrual periods.

ACTION Try to keep stress to a minimum and relax as much as possible. Eat well (*see* A HEALTHY DIET, p.28), and, if you still need to lose weight, try to do so slowly (*see* HOW TO LOSE WEIGHT SAFELY, p.151). If your periods do not start again within 3 months, consult your doctor.

NO →

Continued on next page

SELF-HELP Home pregnancy test

Home pregnancy testing kits are available over the counter from pharmacies and supermarkets. They work by testing a sample of urine for the hormone human chorionic gonadotropin (HCG), which is normally produced only in pregnancy. The tests are very accurate and are capable of giving a positive result as soon as your menstrual period is late. If the test produces a negative result and you still do not have a period afterward, carry out another test after 10 days.

Testing urine
The test stick is dipped in urine, and the result appears within minutes. In this test, one line shows that the test has worked and a second line shows that the test is positive.

Test has worked

Result window

Urine

NEGATIVE RESULT (NOT PREGNANT)

Test has worked

HCG positive

POSITIVE RESULT (PREGNANT)

Continued from previous page

Are you underweight (*see* ASSESSING YOUR WEIGHT, p.29), and/or do you have a rigorous exercise program?

YES →

POSSIBLE CAUSES Being underweight and/or following a rigorous exercise program can cause menstrual periods to stop temporarily.

ACTION Eat a healthy diet (p.28), and cut down on the amount of exercise you do. If your menstrual periods do not start again within 3 months, consult your doctor.

NO ↓

Have you recently started or stopped taking oral contraceptives?

YES →

POSSIBLE CAUSE AND ACTION Oral contraceptives alter your normal hormone levels and may affect your menstrual periods. Some pills intentionally stop periods from occurring. If your periods do not return after stopping the pill, carry out a home pregnancy test (opposite). If the result is negative and your menstrual periods have not restarted within 3 months, consult your doctor.

NO ↓

Have you recently been fitted with a progestin intrauterine contraceptive device?

YES →

POSSIBLE CAUSE AND ACTION Progestin intrauterine contraceptive devices can reduce the amount of bleeding during menstrual periods or stop menstrual periods altogether. Many women consider this an advantage, but if you are worried, consult your doctor. He or she may suggest an alternative method of contraception (*see* METHODS OF CONTRACEPTION, p.277).

NO ↓

Have you had chemotherapy and/or radiation therapy to the lower abdomen?

YES →

POSSIBLE CAUSES Both chemotherapy and radiation therapy may damage the ovaries, causing premature menopause and absent menstrual periods. Consult your doctor.

ACTION Your doctor may arrange for a blood test to confirm that you are menopausal. He or she may want to discuss with you the possibility of hormone replacement therapy (*see* A HEALTHY MENOPAUSE, right).

NO ↓

Are you over 45?

YES →

POSSIBLE CAUSE You may be approaching menopause. Consult your doctor.

ACTION Your doctor may arrange for a blood test to confirm that you are menopausal. He or she may discuss hormone replacement therapy with you (*see* A HEALTHY MENOPAUSE, right).

NO ↓

Have you noticed an increase in facial or body hair and/or deepening of the voice?

YES →

POSSIBLE CAUSES You may have polycystic ovary syndrome, a condition in which there are multiple fluid-filled cysts on both of the ovaries and ovulation does not occur normally. Alternatively, a hormonal disorder is a possibility. Consult your doctor.

ACTION Your doctor will probably arrange for tests, such as blood tests to measure hormone levels and ultrasound scanning (p.41) of your pelvis to detect ovarian cysts. Treatment depends on the cause but will probably include drug treatment.

NO ↓

CONSULT YOUR DOCTOR IF YOU ARE UNABLE TO MAKE A DIAGNOSIS FROM THIS CHART.

A healthy menopause

Menopause is the stage in a woman's life when menstrual periods stop, the ovaries no longer produce eggs, and the amount of the sex hormone estrogen declines. It normally occurs between the ages of 45 and 55. Around 8 in 10 women have mild symptoms at menopause, but some may develop more severe problems, including hot flashes, mood swings, and night sweats. The decline in estrogen levels also increases the risk of osteoporosis and heart disease in later life.

Lifestyle changes
An adequate intake of calcium and regular weight-bearing exercise will help reduce the risk of osteoporosis. Exercise also helps protect against heart disease, as does stopping smoking and eating a healthy diet (p.28). If you are having symptoms such as sweating, hot flashes, or dryness, it may be worth adding soy products to your diet because they have a natural estrogen-boosting effect. If you suffer from mood swings, talk to your partner or to friends going through menopause. Relaxation techniques may also be helpful.

Drug treatment
Talk to your doctor about hormone replacement therapy (HRT), which replaces diminishing estrogen and may help prevent heart disease and osteoporosis but may increase the risk of breast cancer. It is suitable for many, but not all, women.

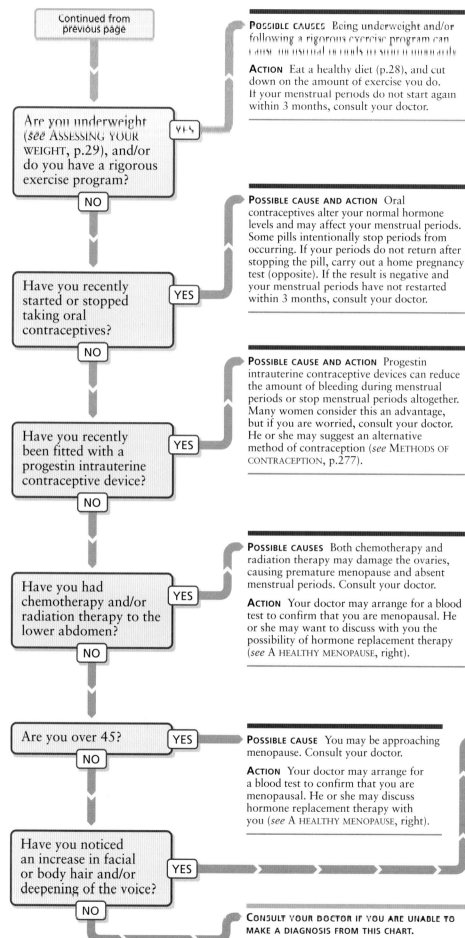

Keeping active
Weight-bearing exercise, such as jogging, may help reduce the chances of osteoporosis after menopause. Exercise is also good for the heart and has a positive effect on mood.

131 Heavy menstrual periods

Heavy menstrual periods, also known as menorrhagia, are periods in which an excessive amount of blood is lost due to heavy or prolonged bleeding. For most women, bleeding lasts about 5 days. Consult this chart if your periods last longer than this, if normal sanitary protection is insufficient, if you pass clots, or if your periods suddenly become heavier than usual. In most cases, the cause is not serious, but heavy periods can cause iron deficiency and lead to anemia.

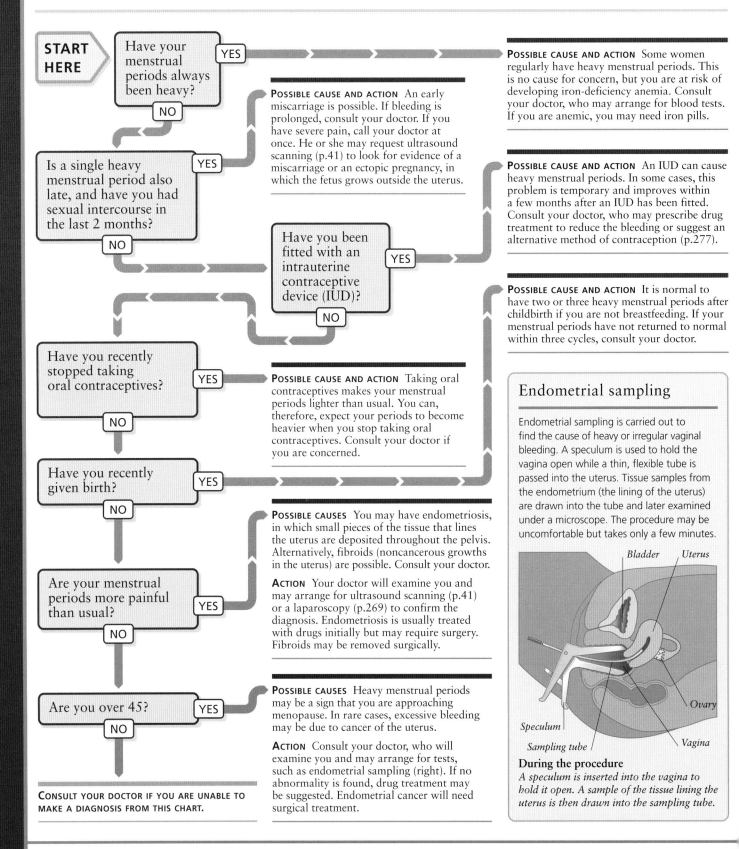

START HERE

Have your menstrual periods always been heavy?
YES → **POSSIBLE CAUSE AND ACTION** Some women regularly have heavy menstrual periods. This is no cause for concern, but you are at risk of developing iron-deficiency anemia. Consult your doctor, who may arrange for blood tests. If you are anemic, you may need iron pills.

NO ↓

Is a single heavy menstrual period also late, and have you had sexual intercourse in the last 2 months?
YES → **POSSIBLE CAUSE AND ACTION** An early miscarriage is possible. If bleeding is prolonged, consult your doctor. If you have severe pain, call your doctor at once. He or she may request ultrasound scanning (p.41) to look for evidence of a miscarriage or an ectopic pregnancy, in which the fetus grows outside the uterus.

NO ↓

Have you been fitted with an intrauterine contraceptive device (IUD)?
YES → **POSSIBLE CAUSE AND ACTION** An IUD can cause heavy menstrual periods. In some cases, this problem is temporary and improves within a few months after an IUD has been fitted. Consult your doctor, who may prescribe drug treatment to reduce the bleeding or suggest an alternative method of contraception (p.277).

NO ↓

Have you recently stopped taking oral contraceptives?
YES → **POSSIBLE CAUSE AND ACTION** Taking oral contraceptives makes your menstrual periods lighter than usual. You can, therefore, expect your periods to become heavier when you stop taking oral contraceptives. Consult your doctor if you are concerned.

NO ↓

Have you recently given birth?
YES → **POSSIBLE CAUSE AND ACTION** It is normal to have two or three heavy menstrual periods after childbirth if you are not breastfeeding. If your menstrual periods have not returned to normal within three cycles, consult your doctor.

NO ↓

Are your menstrual periods more painful than usual?
YES → **POSSIBLE CAUSES** You may have endometriosis, in which small pieces of the tissue that lines the uterus are deposited throughout the pelvis. Alternatively, fibroids (noncancerous growths in the uterus) are possible. Consult your doctor.

ACTION Your doctor will examine you and may arrange for ultrasound scanning (p.41) or a laparoscopy (p.269) to confirm the diagnosis. Endometriosis is usually treated with drugs initially but may require surgery. Fibroids may be removed surgically.

NO ↓

Are you over 45?
YES → **POSSIBLE CAUSES** Heavy menstrual periods may be a sign that you are approaching menopause. In rare cases, excessive bleeding may be due to cancer of the uterus.

ACTION Consult your doctor, who will examine you and may arrange for tests, such as endometrial sampling (right). If no abnormality is found, drug treatment may be suggested. Endometrial cancer will need surgical treatment.

NO

CONSULT YOUR DOCTOR IF YOU ARE UNABLE TO MAKE A DIAGNOSIS FROM THIS CHART.

Endometrial sampling

Endometrial sampling is carried out to find the cause of heavy or irregular vaginal bleeding. A speculum is used to hold the vagina open while a thin, flexible tube is passed into the uterus. Tissue samples from the endometrium (the lining of the uterus) are drawn into the tube and later examined under a microscope. The procedure may be uncomfortable but takes only a few minutes.

Bladder — Uterus
Ovary
Speculum
Vagina
Sampling tube

During the procedure
A speculum is inserted into the vagina to hold it open. A sample of the tissue lining the uterus is then drawn into the sampling tube.

132 Painful menstrual periods

Many women experience some degree of pain or discomfort during their menstrual periods. The pain – sometimes known as dysmenorrhea – is usually cramping and is felt in the lower abdomen or back. In most cases, painful periods are not due to an underlying disorder and do not disrupt everyday activities. However, if you suffer from severe pain or if your periods suddenly become much more painful than usual, you should consult your doctor.

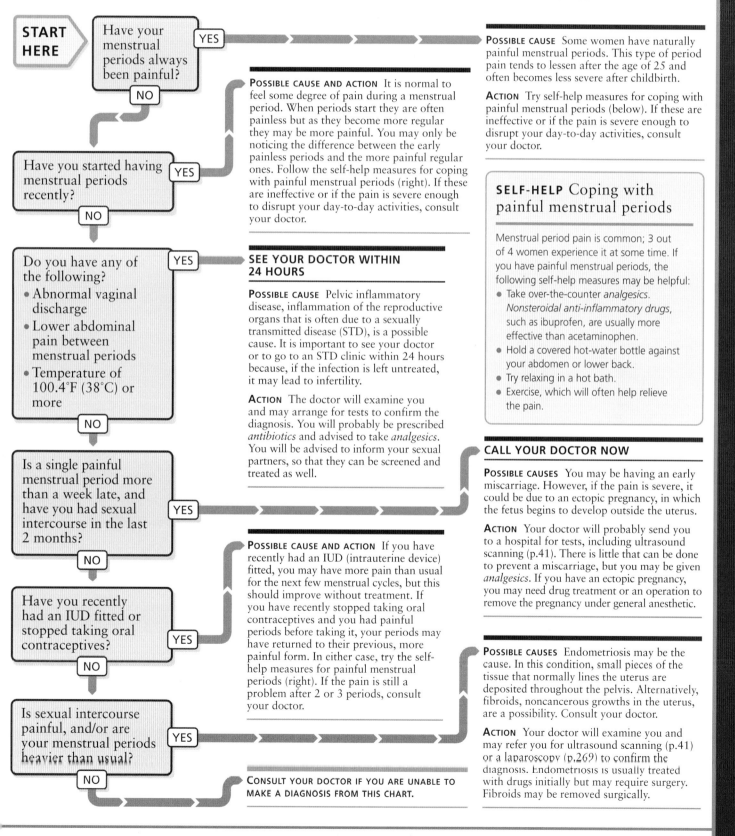

START HERE

Have your menstrual periods always been painful?
— YES ➤➤➤

— NO

Have you started having menstrual periods recently?
— YES

— NO

Do you have any of the following?
- Abnormal vaginal discharge
- Lower abdominal pain between menstrual periods
- Temperature of 100.4°F (38°C) or more

— YES

— NO

Is a single painful menstrual period more than a week late, and have you had sexual intercourse in the last 2 months?
— YES

— NO

Have you recently had an IUD fitted or stopped taking oral contraceptives?
— YES

— NO

Is sexual intercourse painful, and/or are your menstrual periods heavier than usual?
— YES ➤➤➤

— NO

POSSIBLE CAUSE AND ACTION It is normal to feel some degree of pain during a menstrual period. When periods start they are often painless but as they become more regular they may be more painful. You may only be noticing the difference between the early painless periods and the more painful regular ones. Follow the self-help measures for coping with painful menstrual periods (right). If these are ineffective or if the pain is severe enough to disrupt your day-to-day activities, consult your doctor.

SEE YOUR DOCTOR WITHIN 24 HOURS

POSSIBLE CAUSE Pelvic inflammatory disease, inflammation of the reproductive organs that is often due to a sexually transmitted disease (STD), is a possible cause. It is important to see your doctor or to go to an STD clinic within 24 hours because, if the infection is left untreated, it may lead to infertility.

ACTION The doctor will examine you and may arrange for tests to confirm the diagnosis. You will probably be prescribed *antibiotics* and advised to take *analgesics*. You will be advised to inform your sexual partners, so that they can be screened and treated as well.

POSSIBLE CAUSE AND ACTION If you have recently had an IUD (intrauterine device) fitted, you may have more pain than usual for the next few menstrual cycles, but this should improve without treatment. If you have recently stopped taking oral contraceptives and you had painful periods before taking it, your periods may have returned to their previous, more painful form. In either case, try the self-help measures for painful menstrual periods (right). If the pain is still a problem after 2 or 3 periods, consult your doctor.

CONSULT YOUR DOCTOR IF YOU ARE UNABLE TO MAKE A DIAGNOSIS FROM THIS CHART.

POSSIBLE CAUSE Some women have naturally painful menstrual periods. This type of period pain tends to lessen after the age of 25 and often becomes less severe after childbirth.

ACTION Try self-help measures for coping with painful menstrual periods (below). If these are ineffective or if the pain is severe enough to disrupt your day-to-day activities, consult your doctor.

SELF-HELP Coping with painful menstrual periods

Menstrual period pain is common; 3 out of 4 women experience it at some time. If you have painful menstrual periods, the following self-help measures may be helpful:
- Take over-the-counter *analgesics*. *Nonsteroidal anti-inflammatory drugs*, such as ibuprofen, are usually more effective than acetaminophen.
- Hold a covered hot-water bottle against your abdomen or lower back.
- Try relaxing in a hot bath.
- Exercise, which will often help relieve the pain.

CALL YOUR DOCTOR NOW

POSSIBLE CAUSES You may be having an early miscarriage. However, if the pain is severe, it could be due to an ectopic pregnancy, in which the fetus begins to develop outside the uterus.

ACTION Your doctor will probably send you to a hospital for tests, including ultrasound scanning (p.41). There is little that can be done to prevent a miscarriage, but you may be given *analgesics*. If you have an ectopic pregnancy, you may need drug treatment or an operation to remove the pregnancy under general anesthetic.

POSSIBLE CAUSES Endometriosis may be the cause. In this condition, small pieces of the tissue that normally lines the uterus are deposited throughout the pelvis. Alternatively, fibroids, noncancerous growths in the uterus, are a possibility. Consult your doctor.

ACTION Your doctor will examine you and may refer you for ultrasound scanning (p.41) or a laparoscopy (p.269) to confirm the diagnosis. Endometriosis is usually treated with drugs initially but may require surgery. Fibroids may be removed surgically.

133 Irregular vaginal bleeding

Irregular vaginal bleeding includes any bleeding outside the normal menstrual cycle or after menopause. The bleeding may consist of occasional light "spotting," or it may be heavier. Although there is often a simple explanation, you should always consult your doctor if you have any abnormal vaginal bleeding. Bleeding between menstrual periods or after sexual intercourse may be a sign of a serious underlying disorder and should be investigated by your doctor.

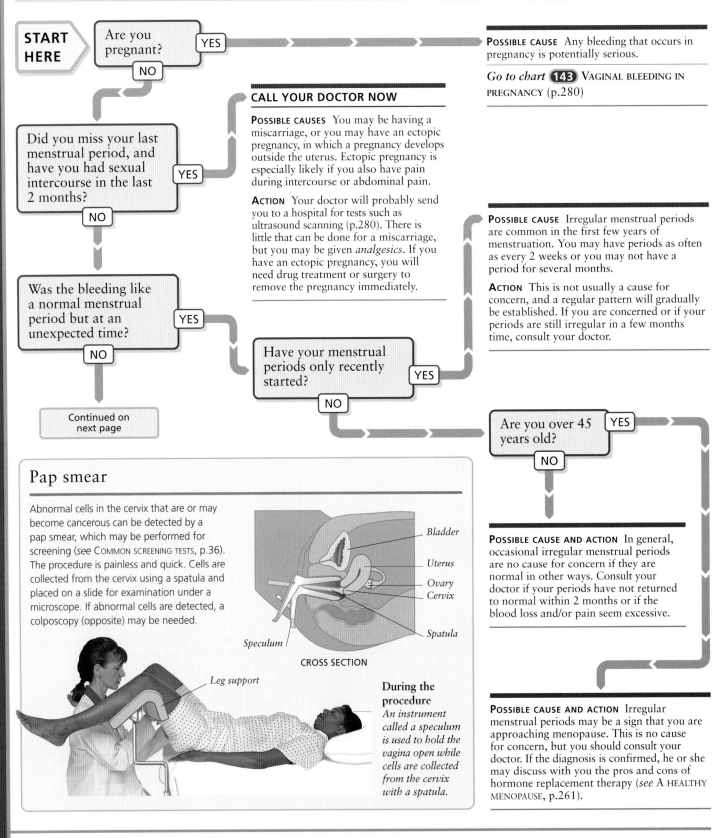

START HERE

Are you pregnant? — YES →

POSSIBLE CAUSE Any bleeding that occurs in pregnancy is potentially serious.

Go to chart **143** VAGINAL BLEEDING IN PREGNANCY (p.280)

NO ↓

Did you miss your last menstrual period, and have you had sexual intercourse in the last 2 months? — YES →

CALL YOUR DOCTOR NOW

POSSIBLE CAUSES You may be having a miscarriage, or you may have an ectopic pregnancy, in which a pregnancy develops outside the uterus. Ectopic pregnancy is especially likely if you also have pain during intercourse or abdominal pain.

ACTION Your doctor will probably send you to a hospital for tests such as ultrasound scanning (p.280). There is little that can be done for a miscarriage, but you may be given *analgesics*. If you have an ectopic pregnancy, you will need drug treatment or surgery to remove the pregnancy immediately.

NO ↓

Was the bleeding like a normal menstrual period but at an unexpected time? — YES →

Have your menstrual periods only recently started? — YES →

POSSIBLE CAUSE Irregular menstrual periods are common in the first few years of menstruation. You may have periods as often as every 2 weeks or you may not have a period for several months.

ACTION This is not usually a cause for concern, and a regular pattern will gradually be established. If you are concerned or if your periods are still irregular in a few months time, consult your doctor.

NO ↓

NO ↓

Continued on next page

Are you over 45 years old? — YES →

NO ↓

POSSIBLE CAUSE AND ACTION In general, occasional irregular menstrual periods are no cause for concern if they are normal in other ways. Consult your doctor if your periods have not returned to normal within 2 months or if the blood loss and/or pain seem excessive.

POSSIBLE CAUSE AND ACTION Irregular menstrual periods may be a sign that you are approaching menopause. This is no cause for concern, but you should consult your doctor. If the diagnosis is confirmed, he or she may discuss with you the pros and cons of hormone replacement therapy (*see* A HEALTHY MENOPAUSE, p.261).

Pap smear

Abnormal cells in the cervix that are or may become cancerous can be detected by a pap smear, which may be performed for screening (*see* COMMON SCREENING TESTS, p.36). The procedure is painless and quick. Cells are collected from the cervix using a spatula and placed on a slide for examination under a microscope. If abnormal cells are detected, a colposcopy (opposite) may be needed.

Bladder

Uterus

Ovary

Cervix

Speculum

Spatula

CROSS SECTION

Leg support

During the procedure
An instrument called a speculum is used to hold the vagina open while cells are collected from the cervix with a spatula.

Continued from previous page

Does the unexpected bleeding occur only in the first few hours after sexual intercourse?

NO **YES**

Are you over 45, and is it more than 6 months since your last menstrual period?

NO **YES**

Colposcopy

A colposcope is a microscope that gives a magnified view of the cervix from outside the body. It is used if a cervical smear test (opposite) has detected abnormal cells. During the procedure, the doctor may apply a substance to the cervix that distinguishes between normal and abnormal tissue. Samples can then be taken from abnormal areas for examination in a laboratory. Various treatments can also be carried out during colposcopy. For example, abnormal tissue can be destroyed using a laser or by freezing tissue with a probe. The whole procedure usually takes less than 40 minutes.

During the procedure
The vagina is held open by a speculum, and the doctor inspects the cervix through the colposcope. A monitor may display the image.

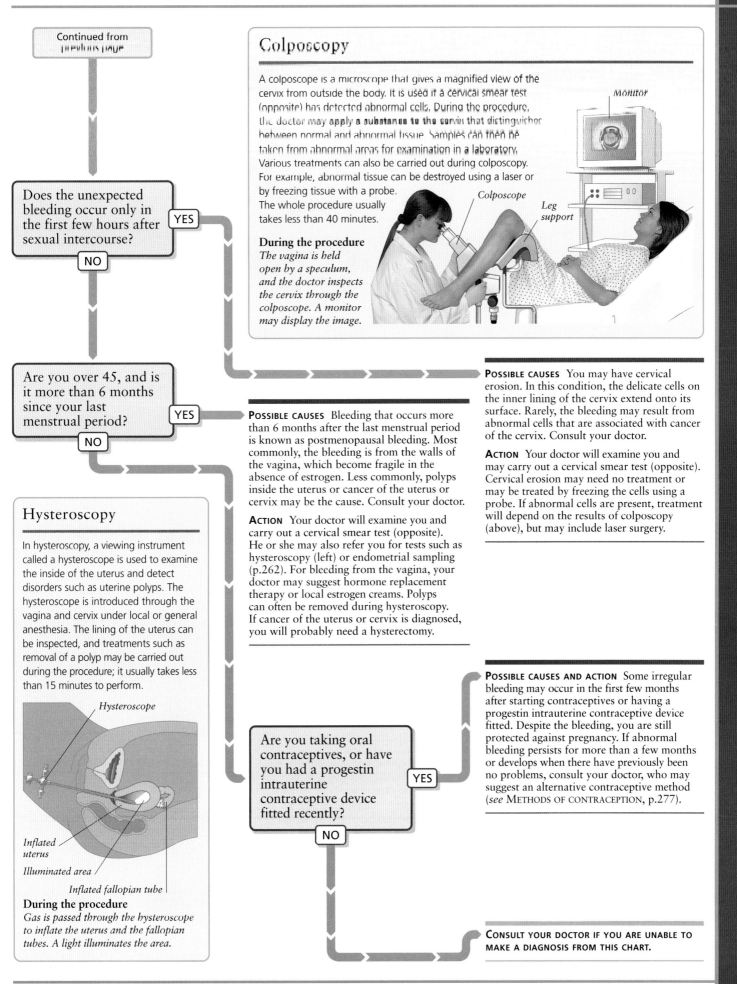

Monitor

Colposcope

Leg support

Hysteroscopy

In hysteroscopy, a viewing instrument called a hysteroscope is used to examine the inside of the uterus and detect disorders such as uterine polyps. The hysteroscope is introduced through the vagina and cervix under local or general anesthesia. The lining of the uterus can be inspected, and treatments such as removal of a polyp may be carried out during the procedure; it usually takes less than 15 minutes to perform.

Hysteroscope

Inflated uterus

Illuminated area

Inflated fallopian tube

During the procedure
Gas is passed through the hysteroscope to inflate the uterus and the fallopian tubes. A light illuminates the area.

POSSIBLE CAUSES Bleeding that occurs more than 6 months after the last menstrual period is known as postmenopausal bleeding. Most commonly, the bleeding is from the walls of the vagina, which become fragile in the absence of estrogen. Less commonly, polyps inside the uterus or cancer of the uterus or cervix may be the cause. Consult your doctor.

ACTION Your doctor will examine you and carry out a cervical smear test (opposite). He or she may also refer you for tests such as hysteroscopy (left) or endometrial sampling (p.262). For bleeding from the vagina, your doctor may suggest hormone replacement therapy or local estrogen creams. Polyps can often be removed during hysteroscopy. If cancer of the uterus or cervix is diagnosed, you will probably need a hysterectomy.

POSSIBLE CAUSES You may have cervical erosion. In this condition, the delicate cells on the inner lining of the cervix extend onto its surface. Rarely, the bleeding may result from abnormal cells that are associated with cancer of the cervix. Consult your doctor.

ACTION Your doctor will examine you and may carry out a cervical smear test (opposite). Cervical erosion may need no treatment or may be treated by freezing the cells using a probe. If abnormal cells are present, treatment will depend on the results of colposcopy (above), but may include laser surgery.

POSSIBLE CAUSES AND ACTION Some irregular bleeding may occur in the first few months after starting contraceptives or having a progestin intrauterine contraceptive device fitted. Despite the bleeding, you are still protected against pregnancy. If abnormal bleeding persists for more than a few months or develops when there have previously been no problems, consult your doctor, who may suggest an alternative contraceptive method (*see* METHODS OF CONTRACEPTION, p.277).

Are you taking oral contraceptives, or have you had a progestin intrauterine contraceptive device fitted recently?

NO **YES**

CONSULT YOUR DOCTOR IF YOU ARE UNABLE TO MAKE A DIAGNOSIS FROM THIS CHART.

134 Abnormal vaginal discharge

Consult this chart if you notice an increase in your vaginal discharge or a change in its color, consistency, or smell. Secretions from the walls of the vagina and the cervix keep the vagina moist and clean. The secretions usually produce a thin yellowish white discharge that varies in quantity and consistency during the menstrual cycle. The volume of secretions increases at times of sexual arousal and during

pregnancy. This is completely normal and is no cause for concern. However, a sudden increase in the amount of vaginal discharge for no obvious reason or vaginal discharge that looks abnormal or smells unpleasant may be a sign of an infection. If the abnormal discharge is accompanied by abdominal pain and/or fever, the infection may involve the reproductive organs and needs urgent treatment.

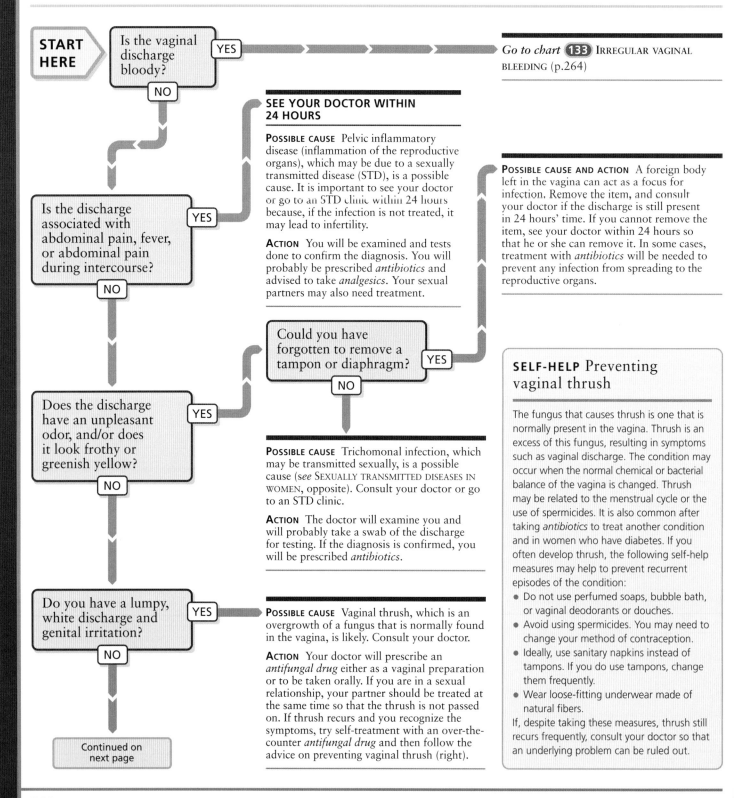

START HERE

Is the vaginal discharge bloody?

YES → *Go to chart* **133** IRREGULAR VAGINAL BLEEDING (p.264)

NO

Is the discharge associated with abdominal pain, fever, or abdominal pain during intercourse?

YES →

SEE YOUR DOCTOR WITHIN 24 HOURS

POSSIBLE CAUSE Pelvic inflammatory disease (inflammation of the reproductive organs), which may be due to a sexually transmitted disease (STD), is a possible cause. It is important to see your doctor or go to an STD clinic within 24 hours because, if the infection is not treated, it may lead to infertility.

ACTION You will be examined and tests done to confirm the diagnosis. You will probably be prescribed *antibiotics* and advised to take *analgesics*. Your sexual partners may also need treatment.

NO

Does the discharge have an unpleasant odor, and/or does it look frothy or greenish yellow?

YES →

Could you have forgotten to remove a tampon or diaphragm?

YES →

POSSIBLE CAUSE AND ACTION A foreign body left in the vagina can act as a focus for infection. Remove the item, and consult your doctor if the discharge is still present in 24 hours' time. If you cannot remove the item, see your doctor within 24 hours so that he or she can remove it. In some cases, treatment with *antibiotics* will be needed to prevent any infection from spreading to the reproductive organs.

NO

POSSIBLE CAUSE Trichomonal infection, which may be transmitted sexually, is a possible cause (see SEXUALLY TRANSMITTED DISEASES IN WOMEN, opposite). Consult your doctor or go to an STD clinic.

ACTION The doctor will examine you and will probably take a swab of the discharge for testing. If the diagnosis is confirmed, you will be prescribed *antibiotics*.

NO

Do you have a lumpy, white discharge and genital irritation?

YES →

POSSIBLE CAUSE Vaginal thrush, which is an overgrowth of a fungus that is normally found in the vagina, is likely. Consult your doctor.

ACTION Your doctor will prescribe an *antifungal drug* either as a vaginal preparation or to be taken orally. If you are in a sexual relationship, your partner should be treated at the same time so that the thrush is not passed on. If thrush recurs and you recognize the symptoms, try self-treatment with an over-the-counter *antifungal drug* and then follow the advice on preventing vaginal thrush (right).

NO

Continued on next page

SELF-HELP Preventing vaginal thrush

The fungus that causes thrush is one that is normally present in the vagina. Thrush is an excess of this fungus, resulting in symptoms such as vaginal discharge. The condition may occur when the normal chemical or bacterial balance of the vagina is changed. Thrush may be related to the menstrual cycle or the use of spermicides. It is also common after taking *antibiotics* to treat another condition and in women who have diabetes. If you often develop thrush, the following self-help measures may help to prevent recurrent episodes of the condition:

- Do not use perfumed soaps, bubble bath, or vaginal deodorants or douches.
- Avoid using spermicides. You may need to change your method of contraception.
- Ideally, use sanitary napkins instead of tampons. If you do use tampons, change them frequently.
- Wear loose-fitting underwear made of natural fibers.

If, despite taking these measures, thrush still recurs frequently, consult your doctor so that an underlying problem can be ruled out.

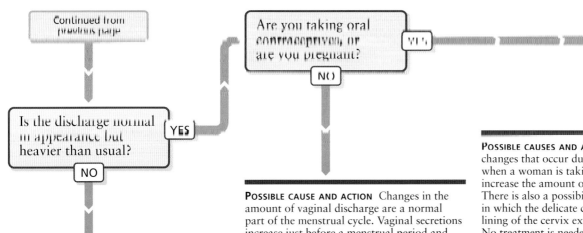

Continued from previous page

Is the discharge normal in appearance but heavier than usual? → YES

NO

CONSULT YOUR DOCTOR IF YOU ARE UNABLE TO MAKE A DIAGNOSIS FROM THIS CHART.

Are you taking oral contraceptives, or are you pregnant? → YES

NO

POSSIBLE CAUSE AND ACTION Changes in the amount of vaginal discharge are a normal part of the menstrual cycle. Vaginal secretions increase just before a menstrual period and when you are sexually aroused. Your symptoms are unlikely to be due to a disorder, but consult your doctor if you are concerned.

POSSIBLE CAUSES AND ACTION The hormonal changes that occur during pregnancy or when a woman is taking oral contraceptives increase the amount of vaginal secretions. There is also a possibility of cervical erosion, in which the delicate cells on the inner lining of the cervix extend onto its surface. No treatment is needed, but if you are not pregnant, your doctor may recommend a cervical smear test (p.264) to check for cervical erosion.

Sexually transmitted diseases in women

Infections passed from one person to another during sexual intercourse (vaginal, anal, or oral) are known as sexually transmitted diseases (STDs). Although these infections affect both men and women, the symptoms are often different (see SEXUALLY TRANSMITTED DISEASES IN MEN, p.245). The symptoms may also affect different areas of the body depending on which type of sexual contact you have had. Even when there are few symptoms, infection can spread from the vagina to all of the reproductive organs and may cause permanent damage if left untreated. An STD contracted during pregnancy may affect the fetus before birth, or the baby may acquire the infection during delivery. If you think you or your partner has an STD, you should consult your doctor or go to an STD clinic, where you will be treated in confidence. You should avoid sex until your doctor confirms that the infection has cleared up. The risk of contracting an STD can be reduced by practicing safe sex (p.32).

Infection	Incubation period*	Symptoms in women	Diagnosis and treatment
Chlamydial infection	14–21 days	Often causes few or no symptoms. There may be an abnormal vaginal discharge or pain on urinating. If the infection affects the fallopian tubes, there may be fever, abdominal pain, or pain on intercourse.	The doctor will take a swab from the cervix to identify the infectious organism. Treatment is usually with *antibiotics*.
Genital herpes	4–7 days	There is usually soreness or itching in the genital area or on the thighs, followed by the appearance of a crop of small, painful blisters. The blisters burst to produce shallow ulcers, which are painful when urinating. The ulcers heal after 10–21 days. The condition may recur.	The diagnosis is usually made according to the appearance of the skin. Oral *antiviral drugs* taken early shorten episodes but do not eradicate the virus. Genital herpes is most infectious while the ulcers are present, but in some cases can remain infectious after the ulcers heal.
Genital warts	1–20 months	Pink, fleshy lumps on the vulva, and in some cases, inside the vagina, on the cervix, and around the anus. Warts may go unnoticed if they occur internally.	Warts may be removed by surgery or by applying drugs to them. In some cases, they recur after treatment. Regular cervical smear tests (p.264) are needed because some types of genital wart may be associated with cervical cancer.
Gonorrhea	7–21 days	May be symptomless in women. It may cause abnormal vaginal discharge, pain in the lower abdomen, and fever. If there is rectal infection, there may be pain when passing feces.	The doctor will take a swab from the vagina or the rectum to identify the infectious organism. Treatment is with *antibiotics*.
HIV infection	6–8 weeks	May be no initial symptoms, but some people may have a brief flulike illness, sometimes with a rash and swollen lymph nodes. After years without symptoms, AIDS may develop (see HIV INFECTION AND AIDS, p.148). HIV can be passed on whether or not you have symptoms.	Diagnosis is made by a blood test taken 3 or more months after the initial infection. People with HIV infection are usually referred to a specialist for treatment. Combinations of *antiviral drugs* are often effective in delaying the progression of HIV to AIDS.
Pubic lice	0–17 days	Usually there is intense itching in the pubic region, particularly at night. The lice are 1–2 mm long and may be visible.	Treatment is with a lotion that kills the lice and their eggs. Such lotions can be bought over the counter.
Syphilis	1–12 weeks	In the first stage, a highly infectious, painless sore called a chancre develops in the genital area or inside the vagina. In some cases, the sores go unnoticed. If the condition is left untreated, it can progress to involve internal organs, causing a rash, fever, and swollen lymph nodes.	The disease is diagnosed by blood tests and tests on swabs taken from any sores. The usual treatment is a course of *antibiotic* injections. You will need to have regular blood tests for 2 years after the treatment to check that the disease has not recurred.
Trichomonal infection	Variable	An unpleasant-smelling, greenish yellow vaginal discharge, associated with irritation and soreness around the vagina. Pain on intercourse.	The diagnosis is confirmed by examination of a sample of discharge taken from the vagina. The usual treatment is with oral *antibiotics*.

Time between contact with the disease and the appearance of symptoms

135 Genital irritation

Consult this chart if you are suffering from itching and/or discomfort in the vagina or around the vulva (the external genital area). Such irritation may also cause stinging when you urinate and may make sexual intercourse uncomfortable. In many cases, these symptoms are the result of an infection, but an allergic reaction is another common cause. Scented soaps, vaginal deodorants, and douches can often cause irritation, and you should avoid using them.

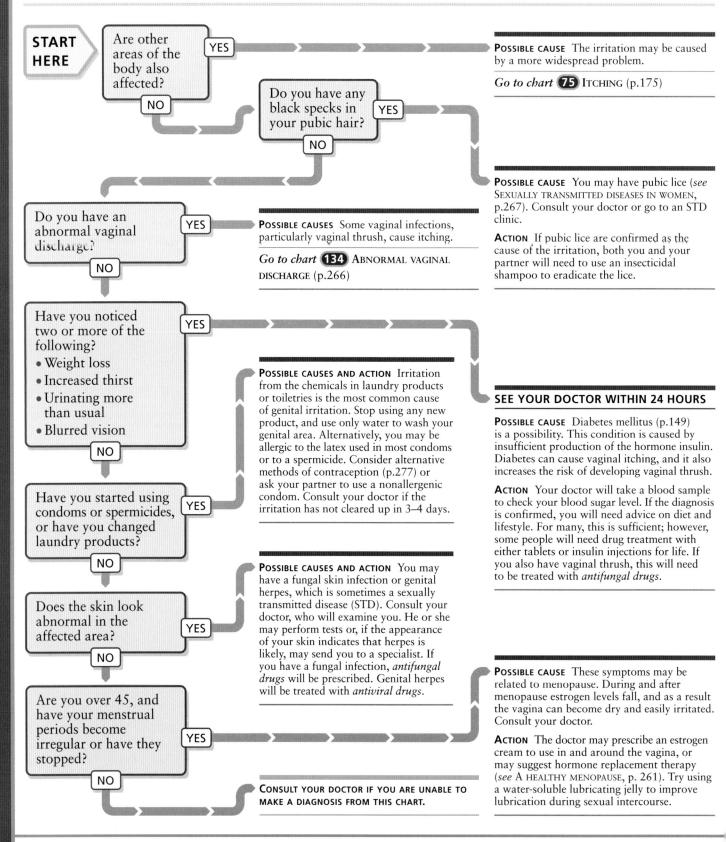

START HERE

Are other areas of the body also affected?
YES →

POSSIBLE CAUSE The irritation may be caused by a more widespread problem.

Go to chart **75** ITCHING (p.175)

NO ↓

Do you have any black specks in your pubic hair?
YES →

NO ↓

POSSIBLE CAUSE You may have pubic lice (*see* SEXUALLY TRANSMITTED DISEASES IN WOMEN, p.267). Consult your doctor or go to an STD clinic.

ACTION If pubic lice are confirmed as the cause of the irritation, both you and your partner will need to use an insecticidal shampoo to eradicate the lice.

Do you have an abnormal vaginal discharge?
YES →

POSSIBLE CAUSES Some vaginal infections, particularly vaginal thrush, cause itching.

Go to chart **134** ABNORMAL VAGINAL DISCHARGE (p.266)

NO ↓

Have you noticed two or more of the following?
• Weight loss
• Increased thirst
• Urinating more than usual
• Blurred vision
YES →

NO ↓

SEE YOUR DOCTOR WITHIN 24 HOURS

POSSIBLE CAUSE Diabetes mellitus (p.149) is a possibility. This condition is caused by insufficient production of the hormone insulin. Diabetes can cause vaginal itching, and it also increases the risk of developing vaginal thrush.

ACTION Your doctor will take a blood sample to check your blood sugar level. If the diagnosis is confirmed, you will need advice on diet and lifestyle. For many, this is sufficient; however, some people will need drug treatment with either tablets or insulin injections for life. If you also have vaginal thrush, this will need to be treated with *antifungal drugs*.

Have you started using condoms or spermicides, or have you changed laundry products?
YES →

POSSIBLE CAUSES AND ACTION Irritation from the chemicals in laundry products or toiletries is the most common cause of genital irritation. Stop using any new product, and use only water to wash your genital area. Alternatively, you may be allergic to the latex used in most condoms or to a spermicide. Consider alternative methods of contraception (p.277) or ask your partner to use a nonallergenic condom. Consult your doctor if the irritation has not cleared up in 3–4 days.

NO ↓

Does the skin look abnormal in the affected area?
YES →

POSSIBLE CAUSES AND ACTION You may have a fungal skin infection or genital herpes, which is sometimes a sexually transmitted disease (STD). Consult your doctor, who will examine you. He or she may perform tests or, if the appearance of your skin indicates that herpes is likely, may send you to a specialist. If you have a fungal infection, *antifungal drugs* will be prescribed. Genital herpes will be treated with *antiviral drugs*.

NO ↓

Are you over 45, and have your menstrual periods become irregular or have they stopped?
YES →

POSSIBLE CAUSE These symptoms may be related to menopause. During and after menopause estrogen levels fall, and as a result the vagina can become dry and easily irritated. Consult your doctor.

ACTION The doctor may prescribe an estrogen cream to use in and around the vagina, or may suggest hormone replacement therapy (*see* A HEALTHY MENOPAUSE, p. 261). Try using a water-soluble lubricating jelly to improve lubrication during sexual intercourse.

NO ↓

CONSULT YOUR DOCTOR IF YOU ARE UNABLE TO MAKE A DIAGNOSIS FROM THIS CHART.

136 Lower abdominal pain in women

Consult this chart only after reading chart 100,
ABDOMINAL PAIN (p.214).
Disorders affecting the urinary tract or the intestine may cause abdominal pain in both men and women but there are

also several disorders causing lower abdominal pain that are specific to women. These disorders affect the female reproductive organs, such as the ovaries, uterus, and the fallopian tubes. Some of them may need medical attention.

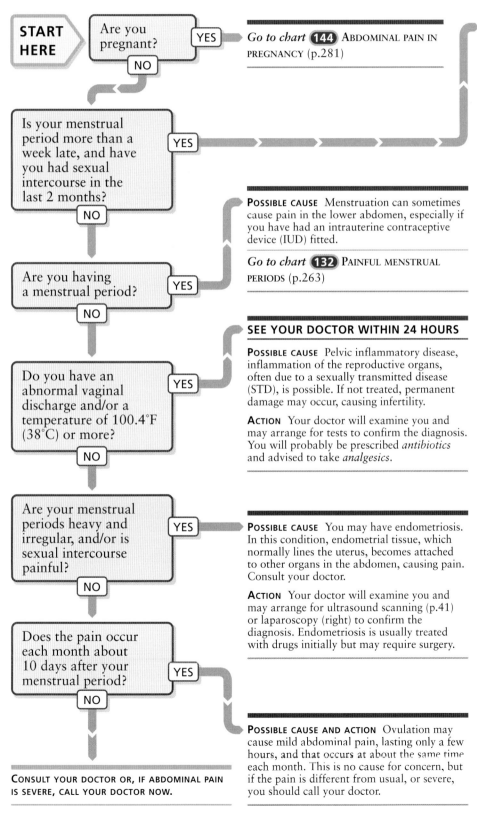

START HERE → **Are you pregnant?** — YES → *Go to chart* **144** ABDOMINAL PAIN IN PREGNANCY (p.281)

NO ↓

Is your menstrual period more than a week late, and have you had sexual intercourse in the last 2 months? — YES →

NO ↓

Are you having a menstrual period? — YES → **POSSIBLE CAUSE** Menstruation can sometimes cause pain in the lower abdomen, especially if you have had an intrauterine contraceptive device (IUD) fitted.

Go to chart **132** PAINFUL MENSTRUAL PERIODS (p.263)

NO ↓

Do you have an abnormal vaginal discharge and/or a temperature of 100.4°F (38°C) or more? — YES →

SEE YOUR DOCTOR WITHIN 24 HOURS

POSSIBLE CAUSE Pelvic inflammatory disease, inflammation of the reproductive organs, often due to a sexually transmitted disease (STD), is possible. If not treated, permanent damage may occur, causing infertility.

ACTION Your doctor will examine you and may arrange for tests to confirm the diagnosis. You will probably be prescribed *antibiotics* and advised to take *analgesics*.

NO ↓

Are your menstrual periods heavy and irregular, and/or is sexual intercourse painful? — YES →

POSSIBLE CAUSE You may have endometriosis. In this condition, endometrial tissue, which normally lines the uterus, becomes attached to other organs in the abdomen, causing pain. Consult your doctor.

ACTION Your doctor will examine you and may arrange for ultrasound scanning (p.41) or laparoscopy (right) to confirm the diagnosis. Endometriosis is usually treated with drugs initially but may require surgery.

NO ↓

Does the pain occur each month about 10 days after your menstrual period? — YES →

POSSIBLE CAUSE AND ACTION Ovulation may cause mild abdominal pain, lasting only a few hours, and that occurs at about the same time each month. This is no cause for concern, but if the pain is different from usual, or severe, you should call your doctor.

NO ↓

CONSULT YOUR DOCTOR OR, IF ABDOMINAL PAIN IS SEVERE, CALL YOUR DOCTOR NOW.

CALL YOUR DOCTOR NOW

POSSIBLE CAUSES You may be pregnant and having a miscarriage, or you may have an ectopic pregnancy, in which a pregnancy develops outside the uterus.

ACTION Your doctor will probably send you to a hospital for ultrasound scanning (p.41). There is little that can be done to prevent a miscarriage, but you may be given *analgesics*. If you have an ectopic pregnancy, you may need drug treatment or an operation immediately.

Laparoscopy

Laparoscopy is a procedure in which a rigid, tubelike viewing instrument is introduced into the abdomen through a small incision. It may be performed to look for disorders of the female reproductive organs, such as endometriosis, or to investigate other abdominal disorders, such as appendicitis. It is also used to take tissue samples or carry out surgery. Before the laparoscope is inserted, gas is pumped through the incision to make viewing easier. Tools for performing procedures may be introduced through another small incision in the abdomen or through the vagina. The procedure is done under general anesthetic.

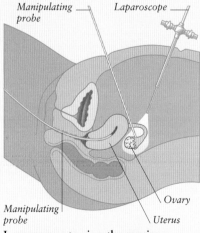

Manipulating probe   *Laparoscope*

Manipulating probe   *Ovary*   *Uterus*

Laparoscopy to view the ovaries
The laparoscope is inserted through a small incision to give an illuminated view of the ovaries. Probes are used to move organs or manipulate the ovaries for better viewing.

137 Painful intercourse in women

Consult this chart if sexual intercourse is painful. Feeling pain or discomfort in or around the vagina at the time of penetration or during or following intercourse is a relatively common problem in women. It may occur for a variety of physical or emotional reasons. Whatever the reason, you should seek medical advice. Persistent pain during intercourse will affect your desire for sex and may damage your relationship with your partner.

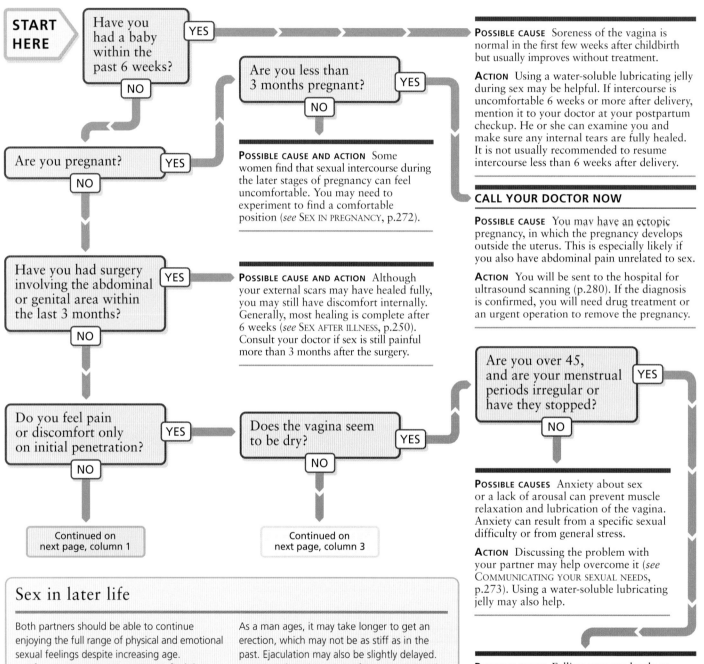

START HERE

Have you had a baby within the past 6 weeks? — YES
NO

Are you pregnant? — YES
NO

Are you less than 3 months pregnant? — YES
NO

POSSIBLE CAUSE AND ACTION Some women find that sexual intercourse during the later stages of pregnancy can feel uncomfortable. You may need to experiment to find a comfortable position (*see* SEX IN PREGNANCY, p.272).

Have you had surgery involving the abdominal or genital area within the last 3 months? — YES
NO

POSSIBLE CAUSE AND ACTION Although your external scars may have healed fully, you may still have discomfort internally. Generally, most healing is complete after 6 weeks (*see* SEX AFTER ILLNESS, p.250). Consult your doctor if sex is still painful more than 3 months after the surgery.

Do you feel pain or discomfort only on initial penetration? — YES
NO

Does the vagina seem to be dry? — YES
NO

Are you over 45, and are your menstrual periods irregular or have they stopped? — YES
NO

POSSIBLE CAUSE Soreness of the vagina is normal in the first few weeks after childbirth but usually improves without treatment.

ACTION Using a water-soluble lubricating jelly during sex may be helpful. If intercourse is uncomfortable 6 weeks or more after delivery, mention it to your doctor at your postpartum checkup. He or she can examine you and make sure any internal tears are fully healed. It is not usually recommended to resume intercourse less than 6 weeks after delivery.

CALL YOUR DOCTOR NOW

POSSIBLE CAUSE You may have an ectopic pregnancy, in which the pregnancy develops outside the uterus. This is especially likely if you also have abdominal pain unrelated to sex.

ACTION You will be sent to the hospital for ultrasound scanning (p.280). If the diagnosis is confirmed, you will need drug treatment or an urgent operation to remove the pregnancy.

POSSIBLE CAUSES Anxiety about sex or a lack of arousal can prevent muscle relaxation and lubrication of the vagina. Anxiety can result from a specific sexual difficulty or from general stress.

ACTION Discussing the problem with your partner may help overcome it (*see* COMMUNICATING YOUR SEXUAL NEEDS, p.273). Using a water-soluble lubricating jelly may also help.

POSSIBLE CAUSE Falling estrogen levels at menopause cause the vagina to become drier and more fragile, which can make intercourse uncomfortable (*see* MENOPAUSE, p.21). Consult your doctor to exclude other causes.

ACTION Your doctor may recommend a water-soluble lubricating jelly and may discuss with you the pros and cons of hormone replacement therapy (*see* A HEALTHY MENOPAUSE, p.261), which can help to relieve the symptoms.

Continued on next page, column 1

Continued on next page, column 3

Sex in later life

Both partners should be able to continue enjoying the full range of physical and emotional sexual feelings despite increasing age.

After menopause, some women find that sexual intercourse is uncomfortable as a result of reduced vaginal lubrication due to a fall in levels of estrogen. In the short term, using a water-soluble lubricant jelly and adapting sexual techniques are often the best solutions. In the long term, vaginal dryness can sometimes be helped by hormone replacement therapy (*see* A HEALTHY MENOPAUSE, p.261).

As a man ages, it may take longer to get an erection, which may not be as stiff as in the past. Ejaculation may also be slightly delayed. However, these issues are often compensated for by increased experience and confidence.

If either partner has a disabling disease, experimenting with different positions and forms of sexual contact may help. Some people who have had sexual problems in the past use age as an excuse to avoid sex, but it is never too late to seek counseling for a problem and age is not an obstacle to receiving treatment.

Continued from
previous page, column 1

Do you have a fever and/or an abnormal vaginal discharge?

NO → (continues down)

YES →

SEE YOUR DOCTOR WITHIN 24 HOURS

POSSIBLE CAUSE You may have pelvic inflammatory disease, inflammation of the reproductive organs due to an infection.

ACTION Your doctor will examine you and may arrange for tests to confirm the diagnosis. You will probably be prescribed *antibiotics* and advised to take *analgesics*.

Are menstrual periods irregular, heavy, and/or painful?

NO → (continues down)

YES →

POSSIBLE CAUSE You may have endometriosis, in which small pieces of the tissue normally lining the uterus become attached to organs in the pelvic cavity. Consult your doctor.

ACTION Your doctor will examine you and may arrange for a laparoscopy (p.269) to confirm the diagnosis. Treatment is usually with drugs and/or surgery.

Do you feel pain only when having intercourse in certain positions?

NO → (continues down)

YES →

POSSIBLE CAUSES The pain may be caused by pressure on an ovary during intercourse. However, an ovarian cyst is also a possibility. Consult your doctor.

ACTION Your doctor will examine you and may arrange for you to have ultrasound scanning (p.41) or a laparoscopy (p.269), which will determine what treatment, if any, you will need.

CONSULT YOUR DOCTOR IF YOU ARE UNABLE TO MAKE A DIAGNOSIS FROM THIS CHART.

Treatments for vaginismus

Vaginismus is a condition in which the muscles around the vagina go into spasm, preventing penetration. In one method of treatment, the woman inserts dilators of gradually increasing diameter into her vagina. This can help allay fears about the ability of the vagina to stretch sufficiently to allow penetration. Vaginismus and some other sexual problems that affect women often have a psychological basis. Sexual counseling can often help resolve fears or unreconciled past sexual traumas and thus treat the condition.

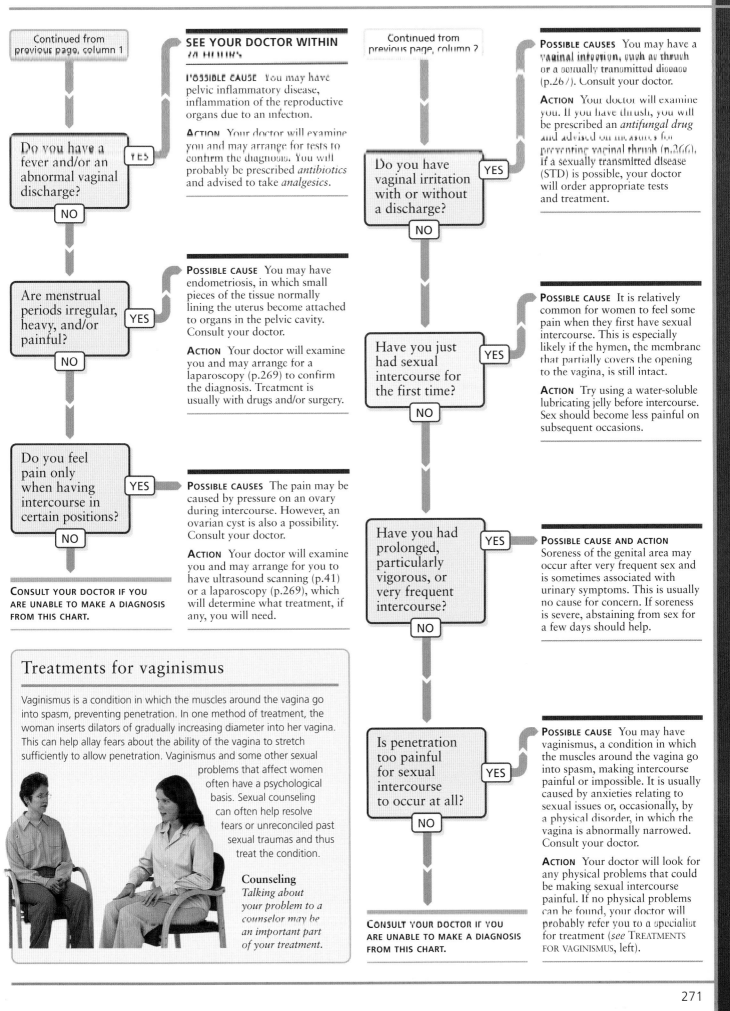

Counseling
Talking about your problem to a counselor may be an important part of your treatment.

Continued from
previous page, column 2

Do you have vaginal irritation with or without a discharge?

NO → (continues down)

YES →

POSSIBLE CAUSES You may have a vaginal infection, such as thrush or a sexually transmitted disease (p.267). Consult your doctor.

ACTION Your doctor will examine you. If you have thrush, you will be prescribed an *antifungal drug* and advised on measures for preventing vaginal thrush (p.260). If a sexually transmitted disease (STD) is possible, your doctor will order appropriate tests and treatment.

Have you just had sexual intercourse for the first time?

NO → (continues down)

YES →

POSSIBLE CAUSE It is relatively common for women to feel some pain when they first have sexual intercourse. This is especially likely if the hymen, the membrane that partially covers the opening to the vagina, is still intact.

ACTION Try using a water-soluble lubricating jelly before intercourse. Sex should become less painful on subsequent occasions.

Have you had prolonged, particularly vigorous, or very frequent intercourse?

NO → (continues down)

YES →

POSSIBLE CAUSE AND ACTION Soreness of the genital area may occur after very frequent sex and is sometimes associated with urinary symptoms. This is usually no cause for concern. If soreness is severe, abstaining from sex for a few days should help.

Is penetration too painful for sexual intercourse to occur at all?

NO → (continues down)

YES →

POSSIBLE CAUSE You may have vaginismus, a condition in which the muscles around the vagina go into spasm, making intercourse painful or impossible. It is usually caused by anxieties relating to sexual issues or, occasionally, by a physical disorder, in which the vagina is abnormally narrowed. Consult your doctor.

ACTION Your doctor will look for any physical problems that could be making sexual intercourse painful. If no physical problems can be found, your doctor will probably refer you to a specialist for treatment (*see* TREATMENTS FOR VAGINISMUS, left).

CONSULT YOUR DOCTOR IF YOU ARE UNABLE TO MAKE A DIAGNOSIS FROM THIS CHART.

138 Low sex drive in women

Some women feel the need for sex once or twice a week or less, others every day. All points in this range are normal; however, a sudden decrease in your normal level of sexual desire may be a sign of a problem. There may be a physical cause, such as an infection that makes intercourse uncomfortable and reduces your sex drive. In many cases, low sex drive has a psychological cause, such as stress, depression, or anxiety about a specific sexual difficulty. Consult this chart if you are concerned that your interest in sex is abnormally low or you notice that you are not as easily aroused as you used to be. A delay in seeking help could damage the relationship with your partner.

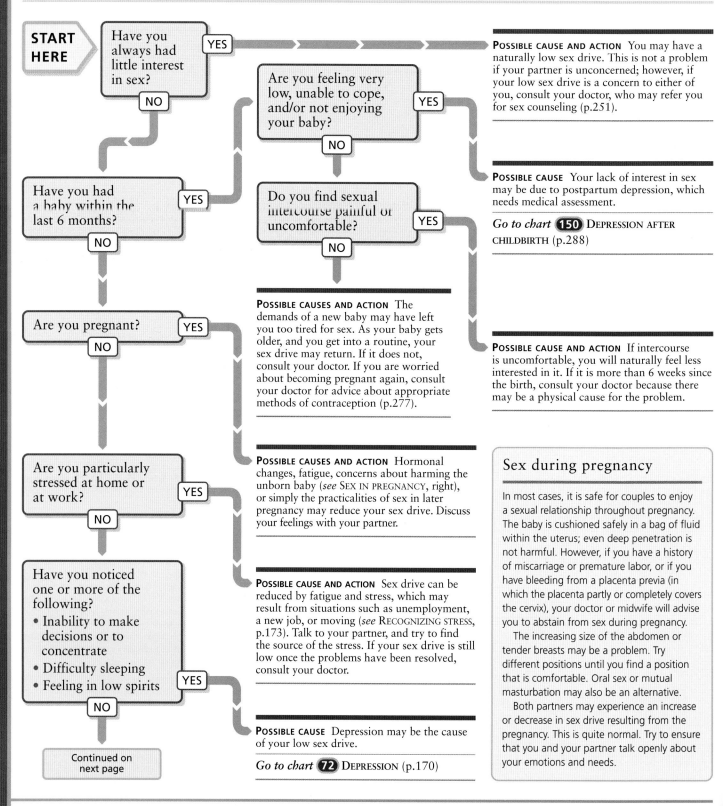

START HERE

Have you always had little interest in sex? — **YES** →

POSSIBLE CAUSE AND ACTION You may have a naturally low sex drive. This is not a problem if your partner is unconcerned; however, if your low sex drive is a concern to either of you, consult your doctor, who may refer you for sex counseling (p.251).

NO ↓

Are you feeling very low, unable to cope, and/or not enjoying your baby? — **YES** →

POSSIBLE CAUSE Your lack of interest in sex may be due to postpartum depression, which needs medical assessment.

Go to chart **150** DEPRESSION AFTER CHILDBIRTH (p.288)

NO ↓

Have you had a baby within the last 6 months? — **YES** →

Do you find sexual intercourse painful or uncomfortable? — **YES** →

POSSIBLE CAUSE AND ACTION If intercourse is uncomfortable, you will naturally feel less interested in it. If it is more than 6 weeks since the birth, consult your doctor because there may be a physical cause for the problem.

NO ↓

POSSIBLE CAUSES AND ACTION The demands of a new baby may have left you too tired for sex. As your baby gets older, and you get into a routine, your sex drive may return. If it does not, consult your doctor. If you are worried about becoming pregnant again, consult your doctor for advice about appropriate methods of contraception (p.277).

NO ↓

Are you pregnant? — **YES** →

POSSIBLE CAUSES AND ACTION Hormonal changes, fatigue, concerns about harming the unborn baby (*see* SEX IN PREGNANCY, right), or simply the practicalities of sex in later pregnancy may reduce your sex drive. Discuss your feelings with your partner.

NO ↓

Are you particularly stressed at home or at work? — **YES** →

POSSIBLE CAUSE AND ACTION Sex drive can be reduced by fatigue and stress, which may result from situations such as unemployment, a new job, or moving (*see* RECOGNIZING STRESS, p.173). Talk to your partner, and try to find the source of the stress. If your sex drive is still low once the problems have been resolved, consult your doctor.

NO ↓

Have you noticed one or more of the following?
- **Inability to make decisions or to concentrate**
- **Difficulty sleeping**
- **Feeling in low spirits**

— **YES** →

POSSIBLE CAUSE Depression may be the cause of your low sex drive.

Go to chart **72** DEPRESSION (p.170)

NO ↓

Continued on next page

Sex during pregnancy

In most cases, it is safe for couples to enjoy a sexual relationship throughout pregnancy. The baby is cushioned safely in a bag of fluid within the uterus; even deep penetration is not harmful. However, if you have a history of miscarriage or premature labor, or if you have bleeding from a placenta previa (in which the placenta partly or completely covers the cervix), your doctor or midwife will advise you to abstain from sex during pregnancy.

The increasing size of the abdomen or tender breasts may be a problem. Try different positions until you find a position that is comfortable. Oral sex or mutual masturbation may also be an alternative.

Both partners may experience an increase or decrease in sex drive resulting from the pregnancy. This is quite normal. Try to ensure that you and your partner talk openly about your emotions and needs.

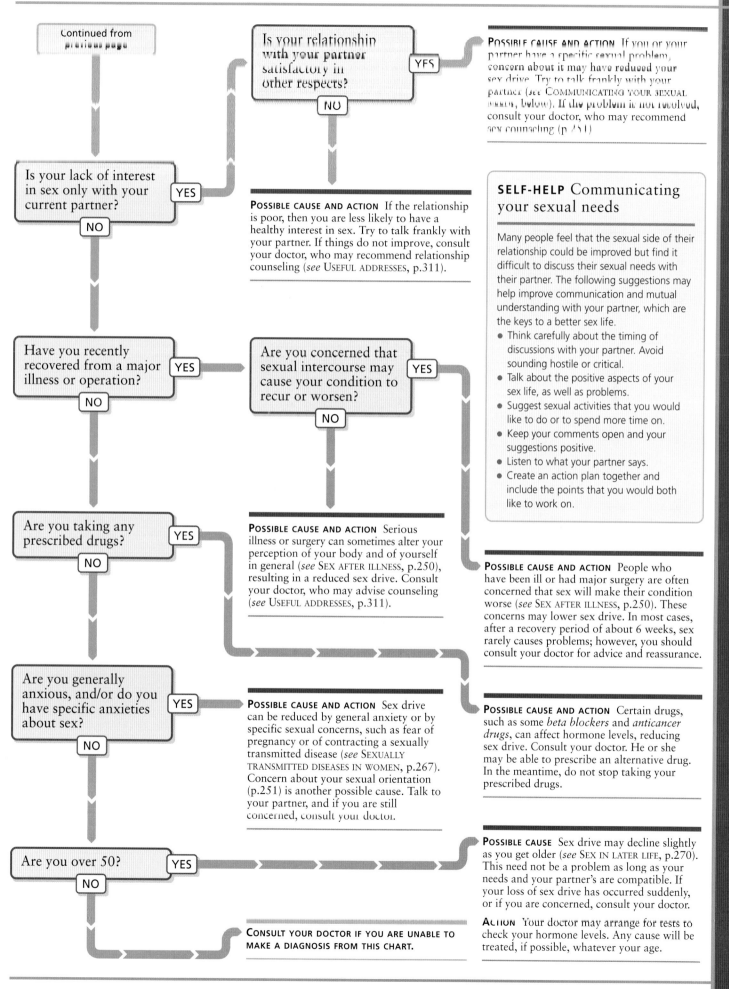

Continued from previous page

Is your relationship with your partner satisfactory in other respects?
YES

NO

POSSIBLE CAUSE AND ACTION If you or your partner have a specific sexual problem, concern about it may have reduced your sex drive. Try to talk frankly with your partner (see COMMUNICATING YOUR SEXUAL NEEDS, below). If the problem is not resolved, consult your doctor, who may recommend sex counseling (p.251).

Is your lack of interest in sex only with your current partner?
YES

NO

POSSIBLE CAUSE AND ACTION If the relationship is poor, then you are less likely to have a healthy interest in sex. Try to talk frankly with your partner. If things do not improve, consult your doctor, who may recommend relationship counseling (see USEFUL ADDRESSES, p.311).

SELF-HELP Communicating your sexual needs

Many people feel that the sexual side of their relationship could be improved but find it difficult to discuss their sexual needs with their partner. The following suggestions may help improve communication and mutual understanding with your partner, which are the keys to a better sex life.

- Think carefully about the timing of discussions with your partner. Avoid sounding hostile or critical.
- Talk about the positive aspects of your sex life, as well as problems.
- Suggest sexual activities that you would like to do or to spend more time on.
- Keep your comments open and your suggestions positive.
- Listen to what your partner says.
- Create an action plan together and include the points that you would both like to work on.

Have you recently recovered from a major illness or operation?
YES

NO

Are you concerned that sexual intercourse may cause your condition to recur or worsen?
YES

NO

POSSIBLE CAUSE AND ACTION Serious illness or surgery can sometimes alter your perception of your body and of yourself in general (see SEX AFTER ILLNESS, p.250), resulting in a reduced sex drive. Consult your doctor, who may advise counseling (see USEFUL ADDRESSES, p.311).

POSSIBLE CAUSE AND ACTION People who have been ill or had major surgery are often concerned that sex will make their condition worse (see SEX AFTER ILLNESS, p.250). These concerns may lower sex drive. In most cases, after a recovery period of about 6 weeks, sex rarely causes problems; however, you should consult your doctor for advice and reassurance.

Are you taking any prescribed drugs?
YES

NO

POSSIBLE CAUSE AND ACTION Certain drugs, such as some *beta blockers* and *anticancer drugs*, can affect hormone levels, reducing sex drive. Consult your doctor. He or she may be able to prescribe an alternative drug. In the meantime, do not stop taking your prescribed drugs.

Are you generally anxious, and/or do you have specific anxieties about sex?
YES

NO

POSSIBLE CAUSE AND ACTION Sex drive can be reduced by general anxiety or by specific sexual concerns, such as fear of pregnancy or of contracting a sexually transmitted disease (see SEXUALLY TRANSMITTED DISEASES IN WOMEN, p.267). Concern about your sexual orientation (p.251) is another possible cause. Talk to your partner, and if you are still concerned, consult your doctor.

Are you over 50?
YES

NO

POSSIBLE CAUSE Sex drive may decline slightly as you get older (see SEX IN LATER LIFE, p.270). This need not be a problem as long as your needs and your partner's are compatible. If your loss of sex drive has occurred suddenly, or if you are concerned, consult your doctor.

ACTION Your doctor may arrange for tests to check your hormone levels. Any cause will be treated, if possible, whatever your age.

CONSULT YOUR DOCTOR IF YOU ARE UNABLE TO MAKE A DIAGNOSIS FROM THIS CHART.

139 Fertility problems in women

See also chart 126, FERTILITY PROBLEMS IN MEN *(p.252).*
Fertility problems affect about 1 in 10 couples, and in about
one-third of these cases, a cause is not found. Failure to
conceive may be the result of a problem affecting either one
or both partners. This chart deals only with possible
problems in women that may be responsible. How soon you
should consult your doctor depends to some extent on your
age, since fertility begins to fall after age 25 to 30.

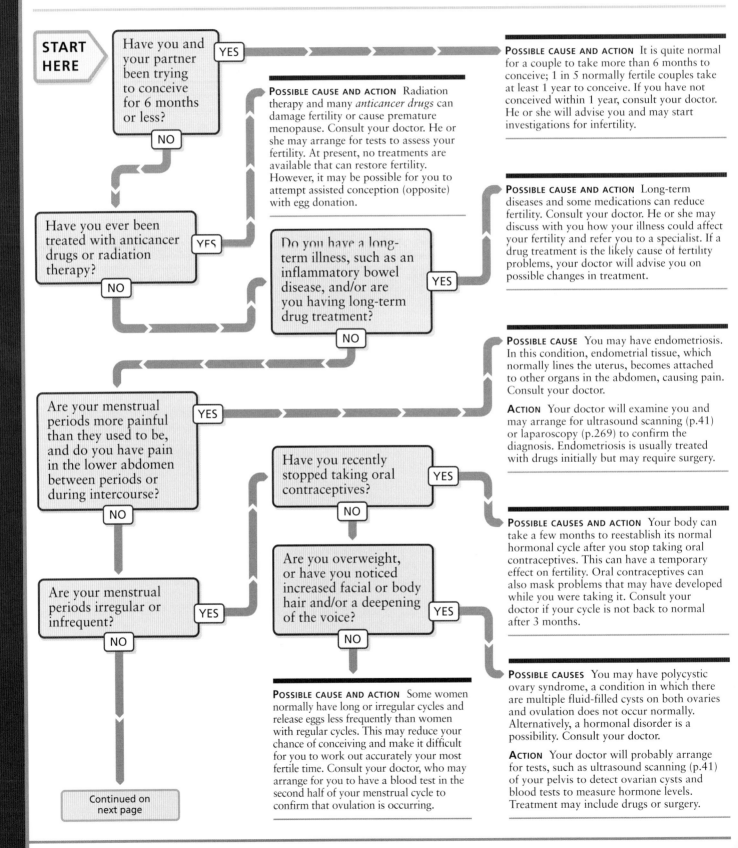

START HERE

Have you and your partner been trying to conceive for 6 months or less? — YES

> **POSSIBLE CAUSE AND ACTION** It is quite normal for a couple to take more than 6 months to conceive; 1 in 5 normally fertile couples take at least 1 year to conceive. If you have not conceived within 1 year, consult your doctor. He or she will advise you and may start investigations for infertility.

NO

Have you ever been treated with anticancer drugs or radiation therapy? — YES

> **POSSIBLE CAUSE AND ACTION** Radiation therapy and many *anticancer drugs* can damage fertility or cause premature menopause. Consult your doctor. He or she may arrange for tests to assess your fertility. At present, no treatments are available that can restore fertility. However, it may be possible for you to attempt assisted conception (opposite) with egg donation.

NO

Do you have a long-term illness, such as an inflammatory bowel disease, and/or are you having long-term drug treatment? — YES

> **POSSIBLE CAUSE AND ACTION** Long-term diseases and some medications can reduce fertility. Consult your doctor. He or she may discuss with you how your illness could affect your fertility and refer you to a specialist. If a drug treatment is the likely cause of fertility problems, your doctor will advise you on possible changes in treatment.

NO

Are your menstrual periods more painful than they used to be, and do you have pain in the lower abdomen between periods or during intercourse? — YES

> **POSSIBLE CAUSE** You may have endometriosis. In this condition, endometrial tissue, which normally lines the uterus, becomes attached to other organs in the abdomen, causing pain. Consult your doctor.
>
> **ACTION** Your doctor will examine you and may arrange for ultrasound scanning (p.41) or laparoscopy (p.269) to confirm the diagnosis. Endometriosis is usually treated with drugs initially but may require surgery.

NO

Have you recently stopped taking oral contraceptives? — YES

> **POSSIBLE CAUSES AND ACTION** Your body can take a few months to reestablish its normal hormonal cycle after you stop taking oral contraceptives. This can have a temporary effect on fertility. Oral contraceptives can also mask problems that may have developed while you were taking it. Consult your doctor if your cycle is not back to normal after 3 months.

NO

Are you overweight, or have you noticed increased facial or body hair and/or a deepening of the voice? — YES

> **POSSIBLE CAUSES** You may have polycystic ovary syndrome, a condition in which there are multiple fluid-filled cysts on both ovaries and ovulation does not occur normally. Alternatively, a hormonal disorder is a possibility. Consult your doctor.
>
> **ACTION** Your doctor will probably arrange for tests, such as ultrasound scanning (p.41) of your pelvis to detect ovarian cysts and blood tests to measure hormone levels. Treatment may include drugs or surgery.

NO

Are your menstrual periods irregular or infrequent? — YES

> **POSSIBLE CAUSE AND ACTION** Some women normally have long or irregular cycles and release eggs less frequently than women with regular cycles. This may reduce your chance of conceiving and make it difficult for you to work out accurately your most fertile time. Consult your doctor, who may arrange for you to have a blood test in the second half of your menstrual cycle to confirm that ovulation is occurring.

NO

Continued on next page

Continued from previous page

Have you ever had an infection of the reproductive tract or a pregnancy outside the uterus (ectopic pregnancy)? — YES / NO

POSSIBLE CAUSES Infection of the reproductive tract or a previous ectopic pregnancy may have damaged or blocked the fallopian tubes. Consult your doctor.

ACTION Your doctor will probably arrange for you to have a laparoscopy (p.269) to inspect the ovaries and establish whether the fallopian tubes are healthy. Surgery may be done to open damaged fallopian tubes. If surgery is not successful, you may be referred for IVF (see ASSISTED CONCEPTION, below).

Do you have sexual intercourse less often than three times a week on average? — YES / NO

POSSIBLE CAUSE AND ACTION Infrequent intercourse is a common cause of failure to conceive. If you have sex less than three times a week, the chance of sperm being present to fertilize an egg when it is released are reduced. If possible, try to have sexual intercourse with your partner more often. If, despite this, you have still not conceived within a further 3–6 months, consult your doctor.

Do you exercise frequently and/or play competitive sports? — YES / NO

POSSIBLE CAUSE AND ACTION Vigorous training may alter your hormone levels, affecting ovulation. Reducing your amount of exercise may improve your fertility. If you have not conceived 3–6 months after lowering your activity level, consult your doctor.

Planning for a healthy pregnancy

Whether or not you are having problems conceiving, it is worth taking steps to ensure that if or when you do conceive, you have the best chance of a healthy pregnancy. Ideally, you and your partner should see your doctor at least 3 months before you start trying to conceive so that any problems can be dealt with in advance. Your doctor will probably do the following:
- Ensure that any preexisting disease, such as diabetes, is well controlled.
- Review prescription drugs to avoid potential harm to the fetus.
- Ask about inherited conditions in your and your partner's families so that genetic counseling can be arranged if needed.
- Check that you are immune to rubella (German measles), which if contracted in early pregnancy can cause birth defects.
- Advise you to take a daily supplement of folic acid, starting at least 3 months before trying to conceive, to reduce the risk of neural tube defects such as spina bifida.
- Give you and your partner general health advice about factors that could affect fertility such as diet, smoking, and alcohol consumption (see MAXIMIZING THE CHANCE OF CONCEPTION, p.252).

Are you underweight (see ASSESSING YOUR WEIGHT, p.29), or have you recently lost a lot of weight? — YES / NO

CONSULT YOUR DOCTOR IF YOU ARE UNABLE TO MAKE A DIAGNOSIS FROM THIS CHART.

POSSIBLE CAUSES AND ACTION Being below a healthy weight for your height or losing weight rapidly can affect the menstrual cycle and reduce fertility. Try to eat sensibly; if you are trying to lose weight, aim to lose no more than 1 lb (0.5 kg) per week. If you are worried about your weight, consult your doctor.

Assisted conception

The most common techniques that are used to aid conception are intrauterine (artificial) insemination (IUI) and in vitro fertilization (IVF). IUI is the simplest technique. In this procedure, timed to coincide with ovulation, semen from the partner or a donor is introduced into the uterus through a flexible tube passed through the vagina and cervix. IVF involves combining eggs and sperm outside the body and can be done using donated eggs and/or sperm if necessary. Drugs are given to stimulate the ovary to produce several eggs, which are then collected during laparoscopy (p.269). In the laboratory, sperm are combined with the eggs to allow fertilization to take place. Two or three fertilized eggs are introduced into the uterus to ensure the best chance of successful implantation into the uterus. The success rate of assisted conception is variable; on average, one in six or seven attempts results in a pregnancy.

In vitro fertilization
In IVF, fertilization occurs in a laboratory. Two or three fertilized eggs are introduced into the uterus via a thin tube passed through the cervix.

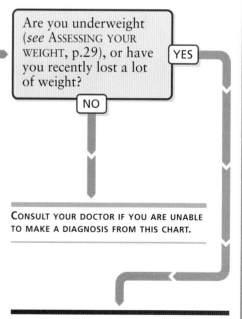
LOCATION
Uterus — Fallopian tube — Ovary — Fluid containing fertilized eggs — Thin tube — Cervix — Vagina

140 Contraception choices for women

For contraception choices for men, see chart 127, Contraception choices for men (p.254).
Deciding which method of contraception to use is partly a matter of personal choice; your age, lifestyle, state of health, and personal beliefs will all affect your choice. If you have a regular partner, the decision regarding contraceptive choice is best shared. This chart is intended as a guide to help you work out which methods might be

most suitable for you, so that you will be able to discuss them with your doctor. If you have had unprotected sex within the last 5 days, this chart will advise you on the actions you can take to reduce the risk of becoming pregnant. Most methods of contraception do not provide you with protection from sexually transmitted diseases (STDs); however, male and female condoms are thought to be 95 percent effective.

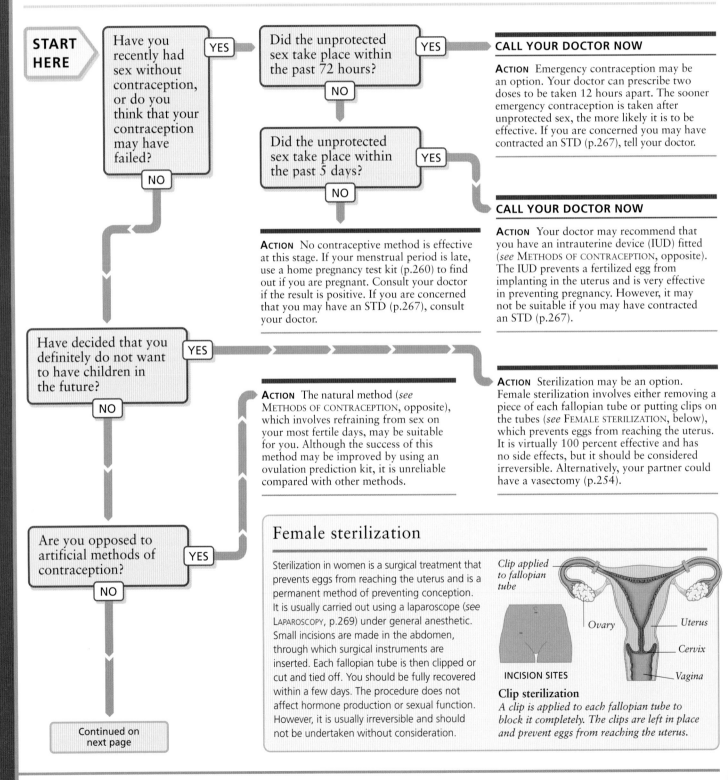

START HERE

Have you recently had sex without contraception, or do you think that your contraception may have failed? **NO** / **YES**

Did the unprotected sex take place within the past 72 hours? **NO** / **YES**

Did the unprotected sex take place within the past 5 days? **NO** / **YES**

CALL YOUR DOCTOR NOW

ACTION Emergency contraception may be an option. Your doctor can prescribe two doses to be taken 12 hours apart. The sooner emergency contraception is taken after unprotected sex, the more likely it is to be effective. If you are concerned you may have contracted an STD (p.267), tell your doctor.

ACTION No contraceptive method is effective at this stage. If your menstrual period is late, use a home pregnancy test kit (p.260) to find out if you are pregnant. Consult your doctor if the result is positive. If you are concerned that you may have an STD (p.267), consult your doctor.

CALL YOUR DOCTOR NOW

ACTION Your doctor may recommend that you have an intrauterine device (IUD) fitted (*see* METHODS OF CONTRACEPTION, opposite). The IUD prevents a fertilized egg from implanting in the uterus and is very effective in preventing pregnancy. However, it may not be suitable if you may have contracted an STD (p.267).

Have decided that you definitely do not want to have children in the future? **NO** / **YES**

ACTION The natural method (*see* METHODS OF CONTRACEPTION, opposite), which involves refraining from sex on your most fertile days, may be suitable for you. Although the success of this method may be improved by using an ovulation prediction kit, it is unreliable compared with other methods.

ACTION Sterilization may be an option. Female sterilization involves either removing a piece of each fallopian tube or putting clips on the tubes (*see* FEMALE STERILIZATION, below), which prevents eggs from reaching the uterus. It is virtually 100 percent effective and has no side effects, but it should be considered irreversible. Alternatively, your partner could have a vasectomy (p.254).

Are you opposed to artificial methods of contraception? **NO** / **YES**

Female sterilization

Sterilization in women is a surgical treatment that prevents eggs from reaching the uterus and is a permanent method of preventing conception. It is usually carried out using a laparoscope (*see* LAPAROSCOPY, p.269) under general anesthetic. Small incisions are made in the abdomen, through which surgical instruments are inserted. Each fallopian tube is then clipped or cut and tied off. You should be fully recovered within a few days. The procedure does not affect hormone production or sexual function. However, it is usually irreversible and should not be undertaken without consideration.

Clip applied to fallopian tube

INCISION SITES

Ovary — *Uterus* — *Cervix* — *Vagina*

Clip sterilization
A clip is applied to each fallopian tube to block it completely. The clips are left in place and prevent eggs from reaching the uterus.

Continued on next page

Methods of contraception

A wide choice of contraceptive methods is available, although the majority are for use by the woman. Pregnancy can be prevented in different ways, including using a barrier to sperm or altering the woman's hormone balance. Choose a method that is safe and effective for you and also suits your lifestyle and preferences. If you have decided you definitely do not want children in the future, male sterilization (see Vasectomy, p.254) or female sterilization (opposite) may be suitable.

Barrier methods
These methods prevent sperm entering the uterus. They include the cervical cap, the diaphragm (right), and male and female condoms. Barrier methods are more effective when used with a spermicide, already present in many condoms.

Hormonal methods
The combined oral contraceptive pill (COCP) contains the hormones estrogen and progestin and prevents the release of eggs. COCPs are effective and safe in women who do not have risk factors such as smoking, obesity, or a history of blood clots. The progestin-only pill (POP) works mainly by thickening the mucus at the entrance to the cervix, preventing penetration by sperm, and is suitable for most women. However, to be effective, POPs must be taken at exactly the same time each day. Progestins can also be given as 3-monthly injections or as an implant lasting up to 5 years.

Mechanical methods
The intrauterine device, or IUD, (right) is placed in the uterus by a doctor to prevent fertilized eggs implanting. The intrauterine system (IUS), a progestogen-releasing IUD, also reduces blood loss during periods and helps prevent pelvic infection.

Natural method
The most commonly used natural method involves monitoring body temperature and mucus from the cervix in order to predict ovulation. Sex is then avoided around this time.

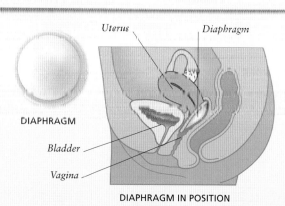
DIAPHRAGM
DIAPHRAGM IN POSITION
Uterus / Diaphragm / Bladder / Vagina

Combined oral contraceptive pills
These pills contain the hormones estrogen and progestin. They are usually taken, one a day, for 21 days, followed by 7 pill-free days, during which you will have your period. On the 29th day, you begin another pack.

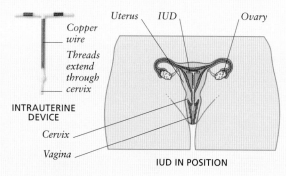
INTRAUTERINE DEVICE
Copper wire / Threads extend through cervix
IUD IN POSITION
Uterus / IUD / Ovary / Cervix / Vagina

The diaphragm
Before sex, the diaphragm is coated with spermicidal gel or cream and then inserted into the vagina so that it covers the cervix. During sex, it should not be felt by either partner. It must be left in place for at least 6 hours after sex and then removed and washed.

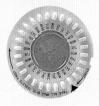

The intrauterine device (IUD)
Once fitted, many IUDs can be left in place for up to 5 years. Some IUDs contain copper, which kills sperm, but the main effect of all IUDs is to prevent fertilized eggs from implanting in the uterus.

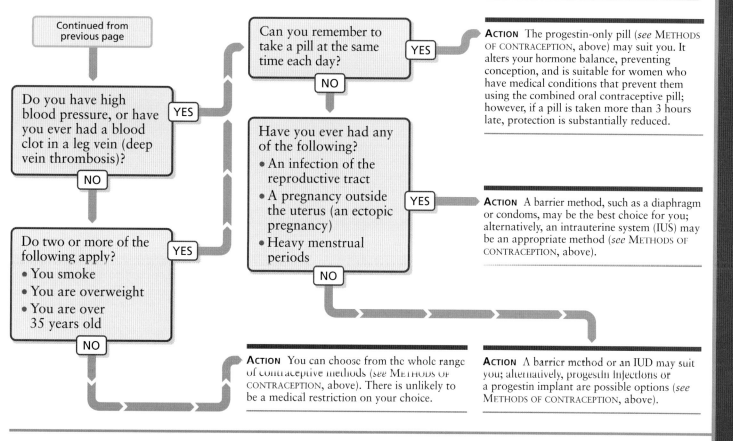

141 Nausea and vomiting in pregnancy

Consult this chart only after reading chart 98, VOMITING *(p.210).*

Most women experience some nausea and vomiting during the first 3 months of pregnancy. These symptoms are known as morning sickness, although they can occur at any time of day, especially when a woman is tired or hungry. Morning sickness is probably caused by the dramatic hormone changes of early pregnancy. Symptoms may be relieved by self-help measures, and usually improve around the 12th week of pregnancy. Vomiting that begins later in pregnancy may be due to a urinary tract infection or to a problem unrelated to the pregnancy, such as food poisoning.

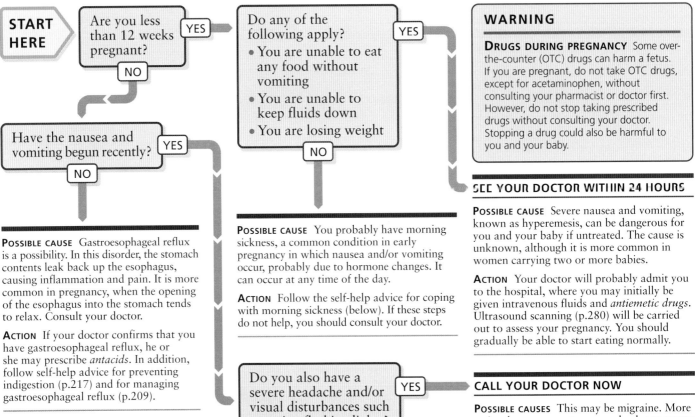

START HERE

Are you less than 12 weeks pregnant? — **YES**

NO

Have the nausea and vomiting begun recently? — **YES**

NO

Do any of the following apply?
- You are unable to eat any food without vomiting
- You are unable to keep fluids down
- You are losing weight

YES

NO

POSSIBLE CAUSE Gastroesophageal reflux is a possibility. In this disorder, the stomach contents leak back up the esophagus, causing inflammation and pain. It is more common in pregnancy, when the opening of the esophagus into the stomach tends to relax. Consult your doctor.

ACTION If your doctor confirms that you have gastroesophageal reflux, he or she may prescribe *antacids*. In addition, follow self-help advice for preventing indigestion (p.217) and for managing gastroesophageal reflux (p.209).

POSSIBLE CAUSE You probably have morning sickness, a common condition in early pregnancy in which nausea and/or vomiting occur, probably due to hormone changes. It can occur at any time of the day.

ACTION Follow the self-help advice for coping with morning sickness (below). If these steps do not help, you should consult your doctor.

WARNING

DRUGS DURING PREGNANCY Some over-the-counter (OTC) drugs can harm a fetus. If you are pregnant, do not take OTC drugs, except for acetaminophen, without consulting your pharmacist or doctor first. However, do not stop taking prescribed drugs without consulting your doctor. Stopping a drug could also be harmful to you and your baby.

SEE YOUR DOCTOR WITHIN 24 HOURS

POSSIBLE CAUSE Severe nausea and vomiting, known as hyperemesis, can be dangerous for you and your baby if untreated. The cause is unknown, although it is more common in women carrying two or more babies.

ACTION Your doctor will probably admit you to the hospital, where you may initially be given intravenous fluids and *antiemetic drugs*. Ultrasound scanning (p.280) will be carried out to assess your pregnancy. You should gradually be able to start eating normally.

SELF-HELP Coping with morning sickness

Nausea and vomiting are common in early pregnancy. Symptoms tend to be worse if you are tired or hungry. The following measures may help:
- If you usually feel nauseous first thing in the morning, keep dry foods, such as plain crackers, by your bedside and eat something before getting out of bed.
- Eat little and often throughout the day.
- Avoid rich or fatty foods.
- Make sure you drink plenty of fluids.
- Try drinks containing ginger or peppermint.
- Try using motion sickness wristbands, which press on acupressure points.

Do not take any drugs or medicines unless they are prescribed by your doctor. If you are unable to keep any food or fluids down, you should see your doctor within 24 hours.

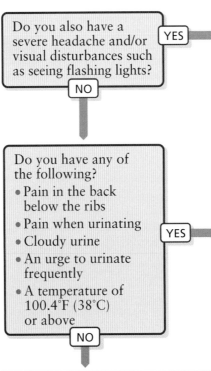

Do you also have a severe headache and/or visual disturbances such as seeing flashing lights? — **YES**

NO

Do you have any of the following?
- Pain in the back below the ribs
- Pain when urinating
- Cloudy urine
- An urge to urinate frequently
- A temperature of 100.4°F (38°C) or above

YES

NO

CONSULT YOUR DOCTOR IF YOU ARE UNABLE TO MAKE A DIAGNOSIS FROM THIS CHART.

CALL YOUR DOCTOR NOW

POSSIBLE CAUSES This may be migraine. More seriously, your symptoms may be due to severe preeclampsia (p.283), particularly if you are more than 28 weeks pregnant. This condition may threaten your life and that of your baby.

ACTION Your doctor will measure your blood pressure and test your urine for signs of preeclampsia. If migraine is the cause, it can be treated by resting in a dark room and taking *analgesics*. If you have preeclampsia, you will be admitted to the hospital immediately for monitoring and to control your blood pressure. Your baby may need to be delivered early.

CALL YOUR DOCTOR NOW

POSSIBLE CAUSE Pyelonephritis, inflammation of a kidney due to a bacterial infection, can result in nausea and vomiting. It is more common in pregnancy and may cause labor to begin prematurely.

ACTION Your doctor will test a sample of your urine and will probably prescribe *antibiotics*. If you are very sick, you may be admitted to the hospital for treatment.

142 Weight problems and pregnancy

It is normal to put on weight during pregnancy. This weight gain comes from the growing fetus, its surrounding amniotic fluid, extra fat stores, the growth of the breasts and uterus, and an increase in blood volume. Most women have gained 24–35 lb (11–16 kg) by the time their baby is born, most of it during the last 4 months. However, gaining more or less is not usually a cause for concern. Consult this chart only if you are concerned about your weight during or after pregnancy.

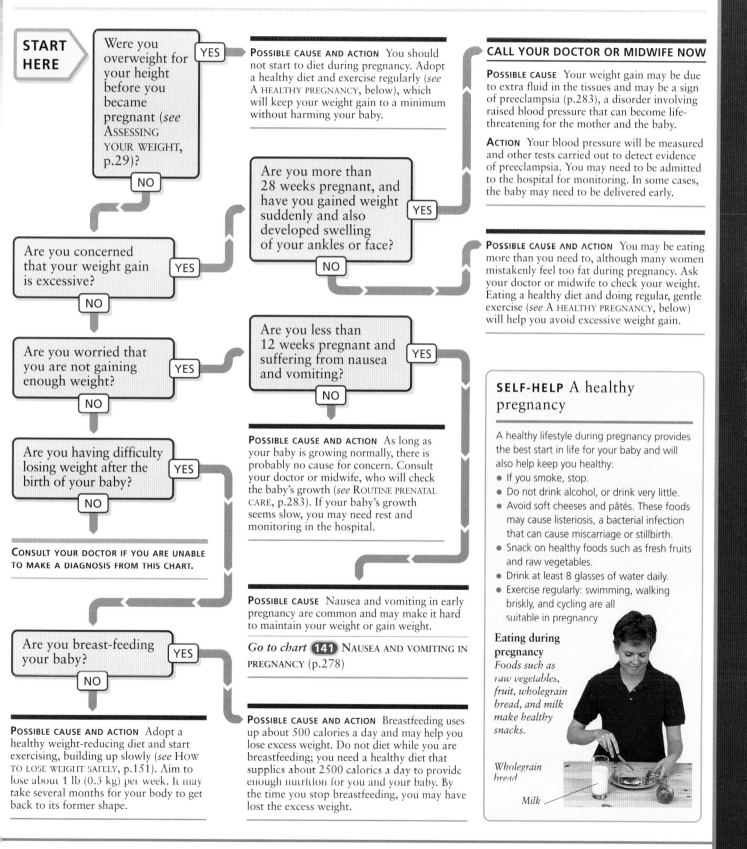

START HERE

Were you overweight for your height before you became pregnant (see ASSESSING YOUR WEIGHT, p.29)?

YES → **POSSIBLE CAUSE AND ACTION** You should not start to diet during pregnancy. Adopt a healthy diet and exercise regularly (see A HEALTHY PREGNANCY, below), which will keep your weight gain to a minimum without harming your baby.

NO

Are you concerned that your weight gain is excessive?

YES → **Are you more than 28 weeks pregnant, and have you gained weight suddenly and also developed swelling of your ankles or face?**

NO

YES → **CALL YOUR DOCTOR OR MIDWIFE NOW**
POSSIBLE CAUSE Your weight gain may be due to extra fluid in the tissues and may be a sign of preeclampsia (p.283), a disorder involving raised blood pressure that can become life-threatening for the mother and the baby.
ACTION Your blood pressure will be measured and other tests carried out to detect evidence of preeclampsia. You may need to be admitted to the hospital for monitoring. In some cases, the baby may need to be delivered early.

NO → **POSSIBLE CAUSE AND ACTION** You may be eating more than you need to, although many women mistakenly feel too fat during pregnancy. Ask your doctor or midwife to check your weight. Eating a healthy diet and doing regular, gentle exercise (see A HEALTHY PREGNANCY, below) will help you avoid excessive weight gain.

Are you worried that you are not gaining enough weight?

YES → **Are you less than 12 weeks pregnant and suffering from nausea and vomiting?**

NO

YES →

NO → **POSSIBLE CAUSE AND ACTION** As long as your baby is growing normally, there is probably no cause for concern. Consult your doctor or midwife, who will check the baby's growth (see ROUTINE PRENATAL CARE, p.283). If your baby's growth seems slow, you may need rest and monitoring in the hospital.

Are you having difficulty losing weight after the birth of your baby?

YES →

NO

CONSULT YOUR DOCTOR IF YOU ARE UNABLE TO MAKE A DIAGNOSIS FROM THIS CHART.

POSSIBLE CAUSE Nausea and vomiting in early pregnancy are common and may make it hard to maintain your weight or gain weight.
Go to chart **141** NAUSEA AND VOMITING IN PREGNANCY (p.278)

Are you breast-feeding your baby?

YES → **POSSIBLE CAUSE AND ACTION** Breastfeeding uses up about 500 calories a day and may help you lose excess weight. Do not diet while you are breastfeeding; you need a healthy diet that supplies about 2500 calories a day to provide enough nutrition for you and your baby. By the time you stop breastfeeding, you may have lost the excess weight.

NO

POSSIBLE CAUSE AND ACTION Adopt a healthy weight-reducing diet and start exercising, building up slowly (see HOW TO LOSE WEIGHT SAFELY, p.151). Aim to lose about 1 lb (0.5 kg) per week. It may take several months for your body to get back to its former shape.

SELF-HELP A healthy pregnancy

A healthy lifestyle during pregnancy provides the best start in life for your baby and will also help keep you healthy:
- If you smoke, stop.
- Do not drink alcohol, or drink very little.
- Avoid soft cheeses and pâtés. These foods may cause listeriosis, a bacterial infection that can cause miscarriage or stillbirth.
- Snack on healthy foods such as fresh fruits and raw vegetables.
- Drink at least 8 glasses of water daily.
- Exercise regularly: swimming, walking briskly, and cycling are all suitable in pregnancy.

Eating during pregnancy
Foods such as raw vegetables, fruit, wholegrain bread, and milk make healthy snacks.

Wholegrain bread

Milk

143 Vaginal bleeding during pregnancy

If you have any vaginal bleeding during pregnancy, consult this chart to determine how quickly you should seek medical advice. While in most cases there is no danger to you or the fetus, this is a potentially serious symptom and should always receive medical attention whether you have only slight spotting or more profuse blood loss. If the bleeding is from the placenta, emergency treatment may be necessary. In other cases, rest and regular monitoring may be all that is needed.

START HERE

Are you less than 12 weeks pregnant? YES → **Do you have pain in the lower abdomen or backache?** YES →

NO ↓   NO ↓

Are you more than 28 weeks pregnant? YES →

NO ↓

WARNING

HEAVY BLEEDING IN PREGNANCY Call an ambulance if you have heavy vaginal bleeding during pregnancy. There may be a problem affecting the placenta that may be life-threatening for you and your baby.

POSSIBLE CAUSES Some minor bleeding is common in early pregnancy, particularly as the placenta begins to develop. Heavy or persistent bleeding, however, may be due to a miscarriage. Consult your doctor.

ACTION Your doctor may recommend that you rest until the bleeding stops. If bleeding continues, you may be admitted to the hospital, where your pregnancy will be monitored (see ULTRASOUND SCANNING IN PREGNANCY, below).

CALL YOUR DOCTOR NOW

POSSIBLE CAUSE A serious complication, such as a miscarriage or an ectopic pregnancy, in which the pregnancy develops outside the uterus, is a possibility.

ACTION Your doctor will probably send you to a hospital for tests including ultrasound scanning (p.41). There is little that can be done to prevent a miscarriage, but you may be given *analgesics*. If you have an ectopic pregnancy, you may need drug treatment or an operation to remove the pregnancy.

CALL YOUR DOCTOR NOW

POSSIBLE CAUSE Bleeding that occurs at 12–28 weeks of pregnancy is uncommon, but a miscarriage or a problem with the placenta may be the cause.

ACTION Your doctor will probably send you to the hospital for ultrasound scanning (below). This will establish the site of the placenta and exclude other possible causes. Admission to a hospital for observation and bed rest may be necessary until the bleeding stops.

Is the vaginal bleeding accompanied by constant pain in the abdomen? YES →

NO ↓

📞 EMERGENCY! CALL AN AMBULANCE

POSSIBLE CAUSE You may have a placental abruption, in which the placenta partially separates from the wall of the uterus. This condition may be life-threatening for both you and your baby.

ACTION In the hospital, you will have ultrasound scanning (see ULTRASOUND SCANNING IN PREGNANCY, left) to confirm the diagnosis. Treatment depends on the severity of the condition. If bleeding is heavy, your baby may need to be delivered urgently by a cesarean section. In other cases, rest and observation in a hospital may be sufficient.

CALL YOUR DOCTOR NOW

POSSIBLE CAUSE Bleeding from a placenta previa, in which the placenta partly or completely covers the opening of the cervix, may be the cause.

ACTION Your doctor will arrange for you to be admitted to the hospital immediately. Once in the hospital, you will have ultrasound scanning (see ULTRASOUND SCANNING IN PREGNANCY, left) to determine the position of the placenta. If the bleeding is light, you may be closely observed in the hospital. If bleeding is heavy, you may need an emergency cesarean section.

Ultrasound scanning in pregnancy

Ultrasound scanning is a safe and painless procedure. A device called a transducer is moved over the skin, sending out ultrasound waves (high-frequency, inaudible sound waves). The sound waves are reflected off internal tissues and organs and are then picked up and passed to a computer, which creates an image on a monitor. During pregnancy, ultrasound scanning is used to produce detailed images of the fetus. Most women have at least one scan during pregnancy. A routine scan will detect multiple pregnancies, the site of the placenta, and the amount of amniotic fluid, which is the fluid that surrounds the baby in the uterus. Detailed scans after 20 weeks may detect abnormalities such as heart defects or a cleft palate. Ultrasound scanning is also used to investigate problems such as bleeding during pregnancy. The procedure usually takes less than 30 minutes.

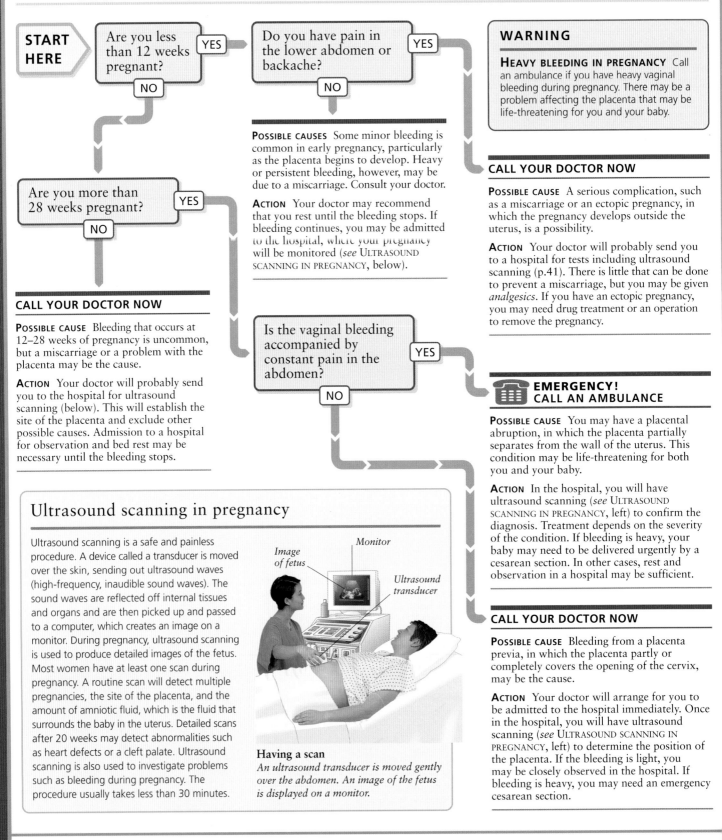

Monitor   *Image of fetus*   *Ultrasound transducer*

Having a scan
An ultrasound transducer is moved gently over the abdomen. An image of the fetus is displayed on a monitor.

144 Abdominal pain in pregnancy

Consult this chart only after reading chart 100, ABDOMINAL PAIN (p.214).
Conditions that cause abdominal pain in nonpregnant women, such as appendicitis, can also occur during pregnancy.

However, conditions specific to pregnancy can also cause abdominal pain. These may be the result of compression of the internal organs by the growing baby, hormone changes, or problems with the placenta or the uterus.

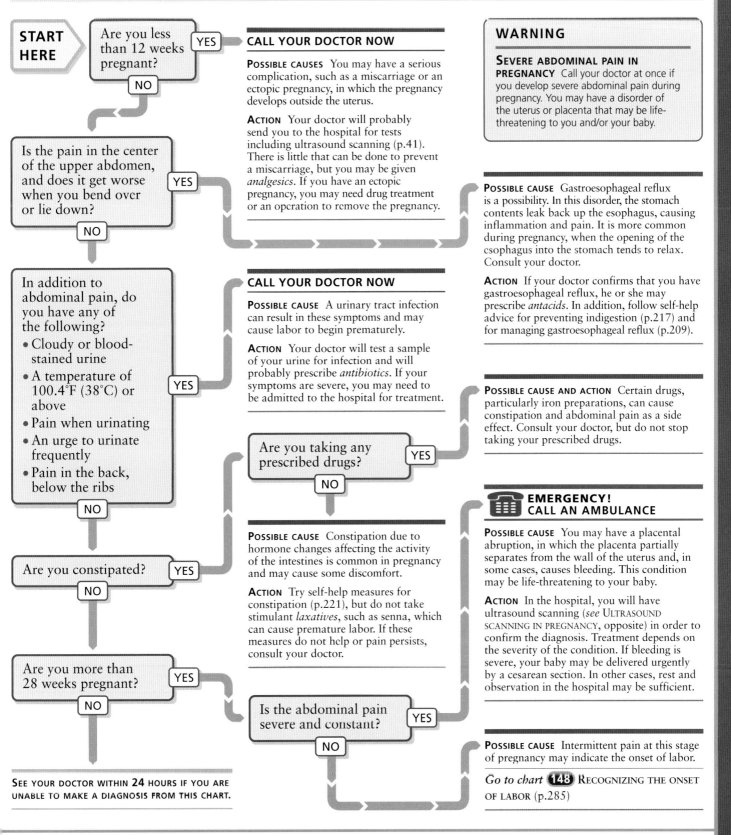

START HERE

Are you less than 12 weeks pregnant? — YES →

CALL YOUR DOCTOR NOW

POSSIBLE CAUSES You may have a serious complication, such as a miscarriage or an ectopic pregnancy, in which the pregnancy develops outside the uterus.

ACTION Your doctor will probably send you to the hospital for tests including ultrasound scanning (p.41). There is little that can be done to prevent a miscarriage, but you may be given *analgesics*. If you have an ectopic pregnancy, you may need drug treatment or an operation to remove the pregnancy.

NO ↓

Is the pain in the center of the upper abdomen, and does it get worse when you bend over or lie down? — YES →

POSSIBLE CAUSE Gastroesophageal reflux is a possibility. In this disorder, the stomach contents leak back up the esophagus, causing inflammation and pain. It is more common during pregnancy, when the opening of the esophagus into the stomach tends to relax. Consult your doctor.

ACTION If your doctor confirms that you have gastroesophageal reflux, he or she may prescribe *antacids*. In addition, follow self-help advice for preventing indigestion (p.217) and for managing gastroesophageal reflux (p.209).

NO ↓

In addition to abdominal pain, do you have any of the following?
- Cloudy or blood-stained urine
- A temperature of 100.4°F (38°C) or above
- Pain when urinating
- An urge to urinate frequently
- Pain in the back, below the ribs

— YES →

CALL YOUR DOCTOR NOW

POSSIBLE CAUSE A urinary tract infection can result in these symptoms and may cause labor to begin prematurely.

ACTION Your doctor will test a sample of your urine for infection and will probably prescribe *antibiotics*. If your symptoms are severe, you may need to be admitted to the hospital for treatment.

NO ↓

Are you constipated? — YES →

POSSIBLE CAUSE Constipation due to hormone changes affecting the activity of the intestines is common in pregnancy and may cause some discomfort.

ACTION Try self-help measures for constipation (p.221), but do not take stimulant *laxatives*, such as senna, which can cause premature labor. If these measures do not help or pain persists, consult your doctor.

NO ↓

Are you taking any prescribed drugs? — YES →

POSSIBLE CAUSE AND ACTION Certain drugs, particularly iron preparations, can cause constipation and abdominal pain as a side effect. Consult your doctor, but do not stop taking your prescribed drugs.

NO ↓

Are you more than 28 weeks pregnant? — YES →

Is the abdominal pain severe and constant? — YES →

EMERGENCY! CALL AN AMBULANCE

POSSIBLE CAUSE You may have a placental abruption, in which the placenta partially separates from the wall of the uterus and, in some cases, causes bleeding. This condition may be life-threatening to your baby.

ACTION In the hospital, you will have ultrasound scanning (*see* ULTRASOUND SCANNING IN PREGNANCY, opposite) in order to confirm the diagnosis. Treatment depends on the severity of the condition. If bleeding is severe, your baby may be delivered urgently by a cesarean section. In other cases, rest and observation in the hospital may be sufficient.

NO ↓

POSSIBLE CAUSE Intermittent pain at this stage of pregnancy may indicate the onset of labor.

Go to chart **148** RECOGNIZING THE ONSET OF LABOR (p.285)

> **WARNING**
>
> **SEVERE ABDOMINAL PAIN IN PREGNANCY** Call your doctor at once if you develop severe abdominal pain during pregnancy. You may have a disorder of the uterus or placenta that may be life-threatening to you and/or your baby.

SEE YOUR DOCTOR WITHIN 24 HOURS IF YOU ARE UNABLE TO MAKE A DIAGNOSIS FROM THIS CHART.

145 Skin changes during pregnancy

Hormone changes during pregnancy may affect the skin in a variety of ways. Most women find that their skin becomes more oily, but others may find it becomes drier. The skin often becomes darker due to an increase in pigment. If you had a skin condition before you became pregnant you may find that it improves during pregnancy but gets worse again after delivery. The exact effects of pregnancy on the skin depend on the woman's individual hormone balance and skin type.

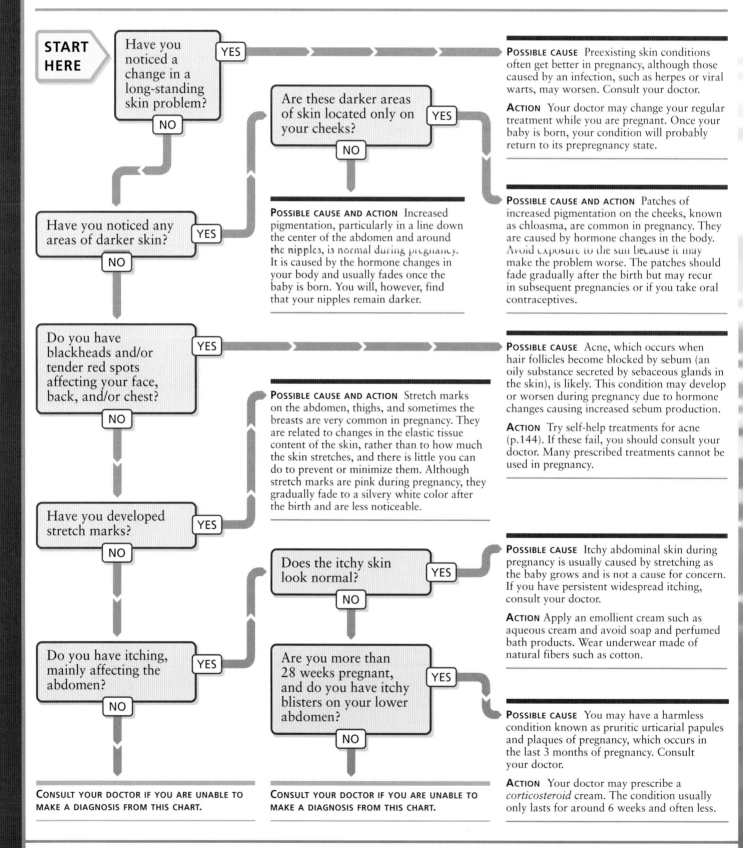

START HERE

Have you noticed a change in a long-standing skin problem? — YES

POSSIBLE CAUSE Preexisting skin conditions often get better in pregnancy, although those caused by an infection, such as herpes or viral warts, may worsen. Consult your doctor.

ACTION Your doctor may change your regular treatment while you are pregnant. Once your baby is born, your condition will probably return to its prepregnancy state.

NO

Are these darker areas of skin located only on your cheeks? — YES

POSSIBLE CAUSE AND ACTION Patches of increased pigmentation on the cheeks, known as chloasma, are common in pregnancy. They are caused by hormone changes in the body. Avoid exposure to the sun because it may make the problem worse. The patches should fade gradually after the birth but may recur in subsequent pregnancies or if you take oral contraceptives.

NO

Have you noticed any areas of darker skin? — YES

POSSIBLE CAUSE AND ACTION Increased pigmentation, particularly in a line down the center of the abdomen and around the nipples, is normal during pregnancy. It is caused by the hormone changes in your body and usually fades once the baby is born. You will, however, find that your nipples remain darker.

NO

Do you have blackheads and/or tender red spots affecting your face, back, and/or chest? — YES

POSSIBLE CAUSE Acne, which occurs when hair follicles become blocked by sebum (an oily substance secreted by sebaceous glands in the skin), is likely. This condition may develop or worsen during pregnancy due to hormone changes causing increased sebum production.

ACTION Try self-help treatments for acne (p.144). If these fail, you should consult your doctor. Many prescribed treatments cannot be used in pregnancy.

NO

Have you developed stretch marks? — YES

POSSIBLE CAUSE AND ACTION Stretch marks on the abdomen, thighs, and sometimes the breasts are very common in pregnancy. They are related to changes in the elastic tissue content of the skin, rather than to how much the skin stretches, and there is little you can do to prevent or minimize them. Although stretch marks are pink during pregnancy, they gradually fade to a silvery white color after the birth and are less noticeable.

NO

Does the itchy skin look normal? — YES

POSSIBLE CAUSE Itchy abdominal skin during pregnancy is usually caused by stretching as the baby grows and is not a cause for concern. If you have persistent widespread itching, consult your doctor.

ACTION Apply an emollient cream such as aqueous cream and avoid soap and perfumed bath products. Wear underwear made of natural fibers such as cotton.

NO

Do you have itching, mainly affecting the abdomen? — YES

Are you more than 28 weeks pregnant, and do you have itchy blisters on your lower abdomen? — YES

POSSIBLE CAUSE You may have a harmless condition known as pruritic urticarial papules and plaques of pregnancy, which occurs in the last 3 months of pregnancy. Consult your doctor.

ACTION Your doctor may prescribe a *corticosteroid* cream. The condition usually only lasts for around 6 weeks and often less.

NO

NO

CONSULT YOUR DOCTOR IF YOU ARE UNABLE TO MAKE A DIAGNOSIS FROM THIS CHART.

CONSULT YOUR DOCTOR IF YOU ARE UNABLE TO MAKE A DIAGNOSIS FROM THIS CHART.

146 Swollen ankles during pregnancy

Swollen ankles are very common in pregnancy, particularly during hot weather or in the later stages of pregnancy, when excess fluid tends to accumulate. Mild swelling of the ankles is usually not a cause for concern. Elevating your ankles, preferably to the same level as your hips whenever possible and wearing support panty hose may ease the swelling. Your ankles may be checked, along with your blood pressure and urine, at each prenatal visit (see ROUTINE PRENATAL CARE, below). However, swelling confined to only one ankle should always be brought to your doctor's attention immediately.

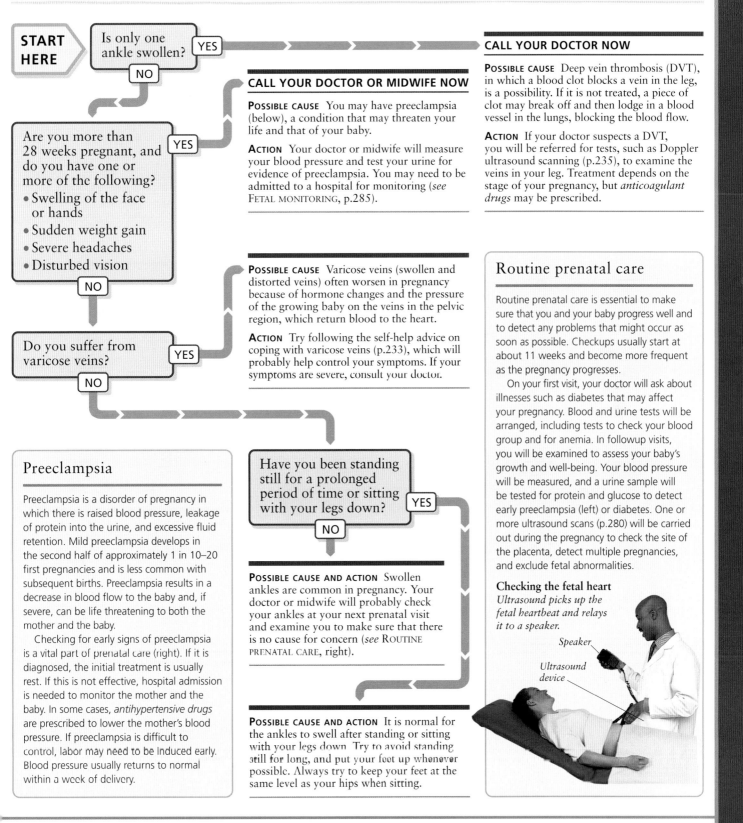

START HERE

Is only one ankle swollen? — YES →

NO

Are you more than 28 weeks pregnant, and do you have one or more of the following?
- Swelling of the face or hands
- Sudden weight gain
- Severe headaches
- Disturbed vision

YES →

NO

Do you suffer from varicose veins? — YES →

NO

Have you been standing still for a prolonged period of time or sitting with your legs down? — YES →

NO

CALL YOUR DOCTOR OR MIDWIFE NOW

POSSIBLE CAUSE You may have preeclampsia (below), a condition that may threaten your life and that of your baby.

ACTION Your doctor or midwife will measure your blood pressure and test your urine for evidence of preeclampsia. You may need to be admitted to a hospital for monitoring (*see* FETAL MONITORING, p.285).

POSSIBLE CAUSE Varicose veins (swollen and distorted veins) often worsen in pregnancy because of hormone changes and the pressure of the growing baby on the veins in the pelvic region, which return blood to the heart.

ACTION Try following the self-help advice on coping with varicose veins (p.233), which will probably help control your symptoms. If your symptoms are severe, consult your doctor.

POSSIBLE CAUSE AND ACTION Swollen ankles are common in pregnancy. Your doctor or midwife will probably check your ankles at your next prenatal visit and examine you to make sure that there is no cause for concern (*see* ROUTINE PRENATAL CARE, right).

POSSIBLE CAUSE AND ACTION It is normal for the ankles to swell after standing or sitting with your legs down. Try to avoid standing still for long, and put your feet up whenever possible. Always try to keep your feet at the same level as your hips when sitting.

CALL YOUR DOCTOR NOW

POSSIBLE CAUSE Deep vein thrombosis (DVT), in which a blood clot blocks a vein in the leg, is a possibility. If it is not treated, a piece of clot may break off and then lodge in a blood vessel in the lungs, blocking the blood flow.

ACTION If your doctor suspects a DVT, you will be referred for tests, such as Doppler ultrasound scanning (p.235), to examine the veins in your leg. Treatment depends on the stage of your pregnancy, but *anticoagulant drugs* may be prescribed.

Preeclampsia

Preeclampsia is a disorder of pregnancy in which there is raised blood pressure, leakage of protein into the urine, and excessive fluid retention. Mild preeclampsia develops in the second half of approximately 1 in 10–20 first pregnancies and is less common with subsequent births. Preeclampsia results in a decrease in blood flow to the baby and, if severe, can be life threatening to both the mother and the baby.

Checking for early signs of preeclampsia is a vital part of prenatal care (right). If it is diagnosed, the initial treatment is usually rest. If this is not effective, hospital admission is needed to monitor the mother and the baby. In some cases, *antihypertensive drugs* are prescribed to lower the mother's blood pressure. If preeclampsia is difficult to control, labor may need to be induced early. Blood pressure usually returns to normal within a week of delivery.

Routine prenatal care

Routine prenatal care is essential to make sure that you and your baby progress well and to detect any problems that might occur as soon as possible. Checkups usually start at about 11 weeks and become more frequent as the pregnancy progresses.

On your first visit, your doctor will ask about illnesses such as diabetes that may affect your pregnancy. Blood and urine tests will be arranged, including tests to check your blood group and for anemia. In followup visits, you will be examined to assess your baby's growth and well-being. Your blood pressure will be measured, and a urine sample will be tested for protein and glucose to detect early preeclampsia (left) or diabetes. One or more ultrasound scans (p.280) will be carried out during the pregnancy to check the site of the placenta, detect multiple pregnancies, and exclude fetal abnormalities.

Checking the fetal heart
Ultrasound picks up the fetal heartbeat and relays it to a speaker.

Speaker

Ultrasound device

147 Back pain during pregnancy

Consult this chart only after first consulting chart 117,
BACK PAIN *(p.238).*
Pain and aching in the middle and lower back are common
during pregnancy. They are usually caused by the effects of
hormones that soften the ligaments supporting the spine
and by difficulty maintaining good posture as a result of the

weight of the growing fetus. Backache tends to get worse as
pregnancy progresses and may make it difficult to get up from
a sitting or lying position. Although backache in pregnancy
is not usually a cause for concern, if it develops suddenly you
should contact your doctor, since it may indicate a miscarriage
in early pregnancy or the onset of labor in late pregnancy.

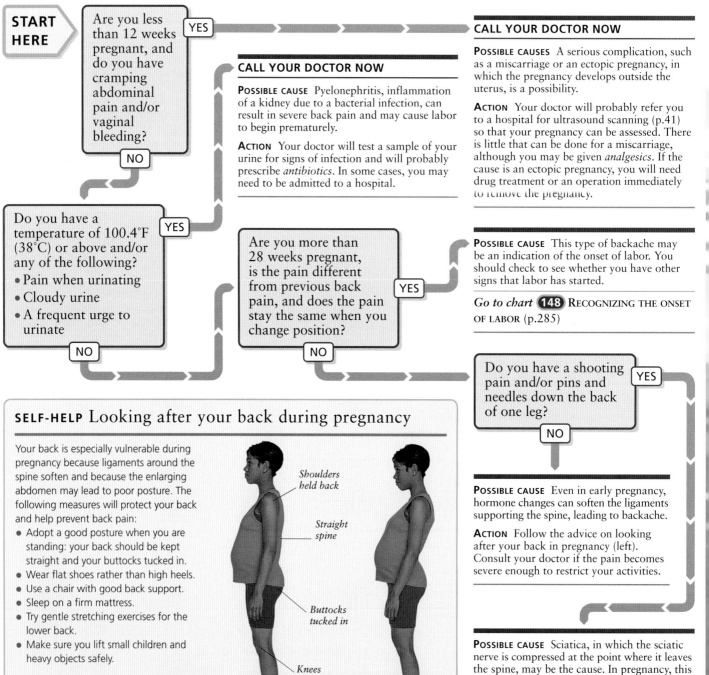

START HERE

Are you less than 12 weeks pregnant, and do you have cramping abdominal pain and/or vaginal bleeding?
— NO
— YES →

Do you have a temperature of 100.4°F (38°C) or above and/or any of the following?
• Pain when urinating
• Cloudy urine
• A frequent urge to urinate
— NO
— YES →

CALL YOUR DOCTOR NOW

POSSIBLE CAUSE Pyelonephritis, inflammation of a kidney due to a bacterial infection, can result in severe back pain and may cause labor to begin prematurely.

ACTION Your doctor will test a sample of your urine for signs of infection and will probably prescribe *antibiotics*. In some cases, you may need to be admitted to a hospital.

Are you more than 28 weeks pregnant, is the pain different from previous back pain, and does the pain stay the same when you change position?
— NO
— YES →

CALL YOUR DOCTOR NOW

POSSIBLE CAUSES A serious complication, such as a miscarriage or an ectopic pregnancy, in which the pregnancy develops outside the uterus, is a possibility.

ACTION Your doctor will probably refer you to a hospital for ultrasound scanning (p.41) so that your pregnancy can be assessed. There is little that can be done for a miscarriage, although you may be given *analgesics*. If the cause is an ectopic pregnancy, you will need drug treatment or an operation immediately to remove the pregnancy.

POSSIBLE CAUSE This type of backache may be an indication of the onset of labor. You should check to see whether you have other signs that labor has started.

Go to chart 148 RECOGNIZING THE ONSET OF LABOR *(p.285)*

Do you have a shooting pain and/or pins and needles down the back of one leg?
— NO
— YES →

POSSIBLE CAUSE Even in early pregnancy, hormone changes can soften the ligaments supporting the spine, leading to backache.

ACTION Follow the advice on looking after your back in pregnancy (left). Consult your doctor if the pain becomes severe enough to restrict your activities.

POSSIBLE CAUSE Sciatica, in which the sciatic nerve is compressed at the point where it leaves the spine, may be the cause. In pregnancy, this condition is due to hormone changes softening the ligaments supporting the spine.

ACTION Follow the self-help advice for looking after your back during pregnancy (left). Consult your doctor if the pain becomes severe enough to restrict your daily activities.

SELF-HELP Looking after your back during pregnancy

Your back is especially vulnerable during pregnancy because ligaments around the spine soften and because the enlarging abdomen may lead to poor posture. The following measures will protect your back and help prevent back pain:

• Adopt a good posture when you are standing: your back should be kept straight and your buttocks tucked in.
• Wear flat shoes rather than high heels.
• Use a chair with good back support.
• Sleep on a firm mattress.
• Try gentle stretching exercises for the lower back.
• Make sure you lift small children and heavy objects safely.

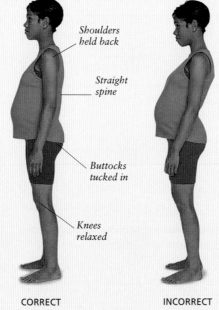

Shoulders held back

Straight spine

Buttocks tucked in

Knees relaxed

CORRECT   INCORRECT

Standing correctly
Stand with your back straight and your shoulders back. Tuck in your buttocks and relax your knees.

148 Recognizing the onset of labor

On average, pregnancy lasts for 40 weeks. However, it is quite normal for a baby to be born as early as 37 weeks or as late as 42 weeks. During labor – the series of events leading to the delivery of your baby – you experience regular contractions that dilate your cervix. Whether or not your cervix is dilating can be determined only by an internal examination. The onset of labor may be heralded by a number of different signs, including the passage of a plug of thick, perhaps bloody mucus (a "show"), abdominal or lower back pains, and water breaking (rupture of the membranes). These signs of labor vary from woman to woman. This chart is designed to help you determine whether labor may have started and how urgently you should contact your doctor or midwife for further advice.

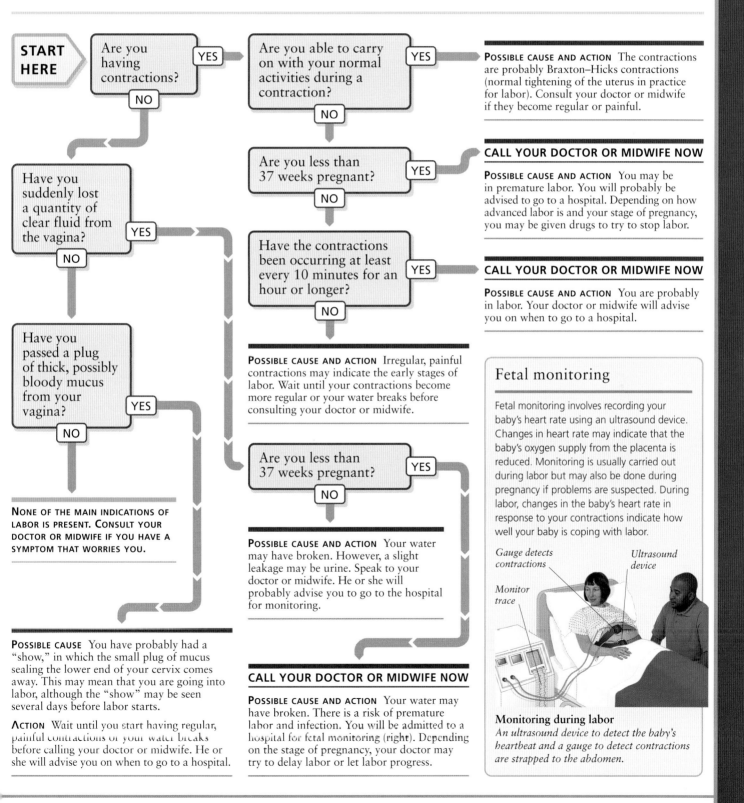

START HERE

Are you having contractions? — YES →

Are you able to carry on with your normal activities during a contraction? — YES →

POSSIBLE CAUSE AND ACTION The contractions are probably Braxton–Hicks contractions (normal tightening of the uterus in practice for labor). Consult your doctor or midwife if they become regular or painful.

Are you having contractions? — NO →

Are you able to carry on with your normal activities during a contraction? — NO ↓

Are you less than 37 weeks pregnant? — YES →

CALL YOUR DOCTOR OR MIDWIFE NOW

POSSIBLE CAUSE AND ACTION You may be in premature labor. You will probably be advised to go to a hospital. Depending on how advanced labor is and your stage of pregnancy, you may be given drugs to try to stop labor.

Are you less than 37 weeks pregnant? — NO ↓

Have the contractions been occurring at least every 10 minutes for an hour or longer? — YES →

CALL YOUR DOCTOR OR MIDWIFE NOW

POSSIBLE CAUSE AND ACTION You are probably in labor. Your doctor or midwife will advise you on when to go to a hospital.

Have the contractions been occurring at least every 10 minutes for an hour or longer? — NO ↓

POSSIBLE CAUSE AND ACTION Irregular, painful contractions may indicate the early stages of labor. Wait until your contractions become more regular or your water breaks before consulting your doctor or midwife.

Have you suddenly lost a quantity of clear fluid from the vagina? — YES →

Have you suddenly lost a quantity of clear fluid from the vagina? — NO ↓

Are you less than 37 weeks pregnant? — YES →

Are you less than 37 weeks pregnant? — NO ↓

POSSIBLE CAUSE AND ACTION Your water may have broken. However, a slight leakage may be urine. Speak to your doctor or midwife. He or she will probably advise you to go to the hospital for monitoring.

Have you passed a plug of thick, possibly bloody mucus from your vagina? — YES →

Have you passed a plug of thick, possibly bloody mucus from your vagina? — NO ↓

NONE OF THE MAIN INDICATIONS OF LABOR IS PRESENT. CONSULT YOUR DOCTOR OR MIDWIFE IF YOU HAVE A SYMPTOM THAT WORRIES YOU.

POSSIBLE CAUSE You have probably had a "show," in which the small plug of mucus sealing the lower end of your cervix comes away. This may mean that you are going into labor, although the "show" may be seen several days before labor starts.

ACTION Wait until you start having regular, painful contractions or your water breaks before calling your doctor or midwife. He or she will advise you on when to go to a hospital.

CALL YOUR DOCTOR OR MIDWIFE NOW

POSSIBLE CAUSE AND ACTION Your water may have broken. There is a risk of premature labor and infection. You will be admitted to a hospital for fetal monitoring (right). Depending on the stage of pregnancy, your doctor may try to delay labor or let labor progress.

Fetal monitoring

Fetal monitoring involves recording your baby's heart rate using an ultrasound device. Changes in heart rate may indicate that the baby's oxygen supply from the placenta is reduced. Monitoring is usually carried out during labor but may also be done during pregnancy if problems are suspected. During labor, changes in the baby's heart rate in response to your contractions indicate how well your baby is coping with labor.

Gauge detects contractions

Ultrasound device

Monitor trace

Monitoring during labor
An ultrasound device to detect the baby's heartbeat and a gauge to detect contractions are strapped to the abdomen.

149 Breast problems and pregnancy

Breast problems are common during and immediately after pregnancy but are usually easy to treat. During pregnancy, hormones cause changes in the breasts: the milk-producing glands become larger and increase in number, and the breasts may become tender. After the baby is born, the breasts can produce about 2 pints (1 liter) of milk per day. Problems soon after childbirth are often associated with establishing breastfeeding. However, these problems are usually short-lived. In most cases, breastfeeding is still possible and is the best option for the baby (*see* FEEDING YOUR BABY, below).

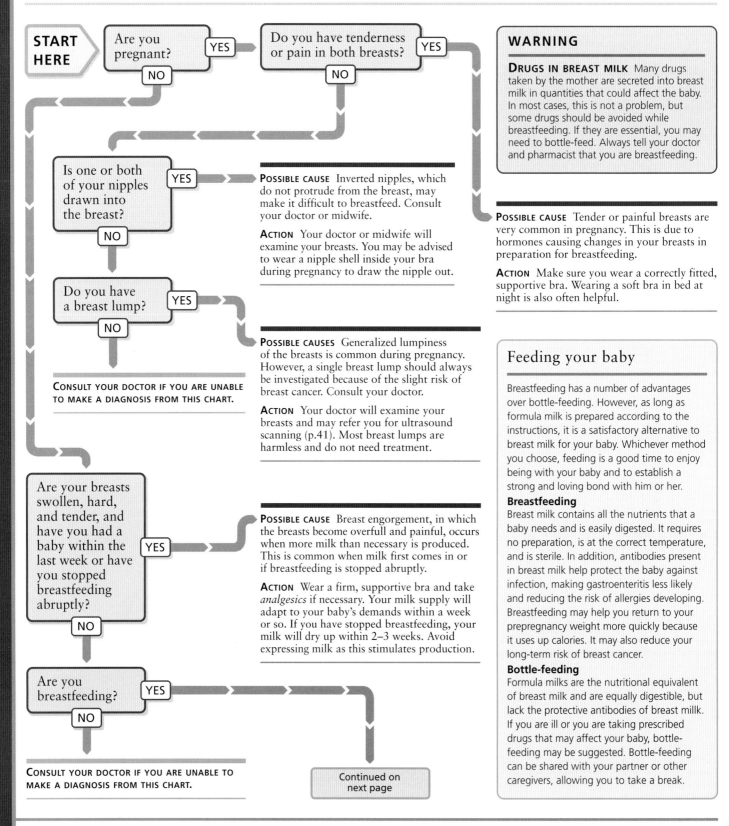

START HERE

Are you pregnant? — YES → **Do you have tenderness or pain in both breasts?** — YES →
NO

Is one or both of your nipples drawn into the breast? — YES →
NO

POSSIBLE CAUSE Inverted nipples, which do not protrude from the breast, may make it difficult to breastfeed. Consult your doctor or midwife.

ACTION Your doctor or midwife will examine your breasts. You may be advised to wear a nipple shell inside your bra during pregnancy to draw the nipple out.

Do you have a breast lump? — YES →
NO

CONSULT YOUR DOCTOR IF YOU ARE UNABLE TO MAKE A DIAGNOSIS FROM THIS CHART.

POSSIBLE CAUSES Generalized lumpiness of the breasts is common during pregnancy. However, a single breast lump should always be investigated because of the slight risk of breast cancer. Consult your doctor.

ACTION Your doctor will examine your breasts and may refer you for ultrasound scanning (p.41). Most breast lumps are harmless and do not need treatment.

Are your breasts swollen, hard, and tender, and have you had a baby within the last week or have you stopped breastfeeding abruptly? — YES →
NO

POSSIBLE CAUSE Breast engorgement, in which the breasts become overfull and painful, occurs when more milk than necessary is produced. This is common when milk first comes in or if breastfeeding is stopped abruptly.

ACTION Wear a firm, supportive bra and take *analgesics* if necessary. Your milk supply will adapt to your baby's demands within a week or so. If you have stopped breastfeeding, your milk will dry up within 2–3 weeks. Avoid expressing milk as this stimulates production.

Are you breastfeeding? — YES →
NO

Continued on next page

CONSULT YOUR DOCTOR IF YOU ARE UNABLE TO MAKE A DIAGNOSIS FROM THIS CHART.

POSSIBLE CAUSE Tender or painful breasts are very common in pregnancy. This is due to hormones causing changes in your breasts in preparation for breastfeeding.

ACTION Make sure you wear a correctly fitted, supportive bra. Wearing a soft bra in bed at night is also often helpful.

WARNING

DRUGS IN BREAST MILK Many drugs taken by the mother are secreted into breast milk in quantities that could affect the baby. In most cases, this is not a problem, but some drugs should be avoided while breastfeeding. If they are essential, you may need to bottle-feed. Always tell your doctor and pharmacist that you are breastfeeding.

Feeding your baby

Breastfeeding has a number of advantages over bottle-feeding. However, as long as formula milk is prepared according to the instructions, it is a satisfactory alternative to breast milk for your baby. Whichever method you choose, feeding is a good time to enjoy being with your baby and to establish a strong and loving bond with him or her.

Breastfeeding
Breast milk contains all the nutrients that a baby needs and is easily digested. It requires no preparation, is at the correct temperature, and is sterile. In addition, antibodies present in breast milk help protect the baby against infection, making gastroenteritis less likely and reducing the risk of allergies developing. Breastfeeding may help you return to your prepregnancy weight more quickly because it uses up calories. It may also reduce your long-term risk of breast cancer.

Bottle-feeding
Formula milks are the nutritional equivalent of breast milk and are equally digestible, but lack the protective antibodies of breast millk. If you are ill or you are taking prescribed drugs that may affect your baby, bottle-feeding may be suggested. Bottle-feeding can be shared with your partner or other caregivers, allowing you to take a break.

Continued from previous page

Are one or both nipples painful? YES / NO

SELF-HELP Avoiding cracked nipples

Cracked nipples are common at the start of breastfeeding. They are usually caused by damage to the nipple as a result of the baby not latching on properly. Make sure that your baby takes the entire nipple and most of the areola (the darker area around the nipple) into his or her mouth. Dry your nipples thoroughly after each feeding, and use absorbent breast pads and change them often. Your doctor or midwife may advise you on over-the-counter nipple creams and sprays, which may help prevent or soothe cracked nipples. If you do develop cracked nipples, they should heal by the time your breastfeeding routine is fully established.

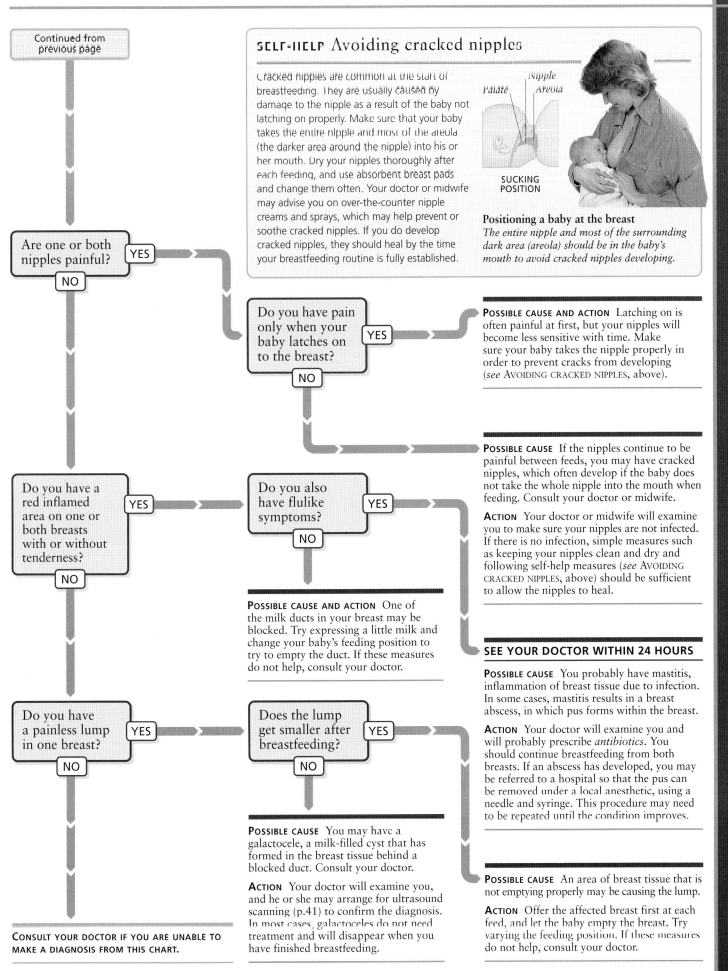

Palate — Nipple — Areola

SUCKING POSITION

Positioning a baby at the breast
The entire nipple and most of the surrounding dark area (areola) should be in the baby's mouth to avoid cracked nipples developing.

Do you have pain only when your baby latches on to the breast? YES / NO

POSSIBLE CAUSE AND ACTION Latching on is often painful at first, but your nipples will become less sensitive with time. Make sure your baby takes the nipple properly in order to prevent cracks from developing (*see* AVOIDING CRACKED NIPPLES, above).

POSSIBLE CAUSE If the nipples continue to be painful between feeds, you may have cracked nipples, which often develop if the baby does not take the whole nipple into the mouth when feeding. Consult your doctor or midwife.

ACTION Your doctor or midwife will examine you to make sure your nipples are not infected. If there is no infection, simple measures such as keeping your nipples clean and dry and following self-help measures (*see* AVOIDING CRACKED NIPPLES, above) should be sufficient to allow the nipples to heal.

Do you have a red inflamed area on one or both breasts with or without tenderness? YES / NO

Do you also have flulike symptoms? YES / NO

POSSIBLE CAUSE AND ACTION One of the milk ducts in your breast may be blocked. Try expressing a little milk and change your baby's feeding position to try to empty the duct. If these measures do not help, consult your doctor.

SEE YOUR DOCTOR WITHIN 24 HOURS

POSSIBLE CAUSE You probably have mastitis, inflammation of breast tissue due to infection. In some cases, mastitis results in a breast abscess, in which pus forms within the breast.

ACTION Your doctor will examine you and will probably prescribe *antibiotics*. You should continue breastfeeding from both breasts. If an abscess has developed, you may be referred to a hospital so that the pus can be removed under a local anesthetic, using a needle and syringe. This procedure may need to be repeated until the condition improves.

Do you have a painless lump in one breast? YES / NO

Does the lump get smaller after breastfeeding? YES / NO

POSSIBLE CAUSE You may have a galactocele, a milk-filled cyst that has formed in the breast tissue behind a blocked duct. Consult your doctor.

ACTION Your doctor will examine you, and he or she may arrange for ultrasound scanning (p.41) to confirm the diagnosis. In most cases, galactoceles do not need treatment and will disappear when you have finished breastfeeding.

POSSIBLE CAUSE An area of breast tissue that is not emptying properly may be causing the lump.

ACTION Offer the affected breast first at each feed, and let the baby empty the breast. Try varying the feeding position. If these measures do not help, consult your doctor.

CONSULT YOUR DOCTOR IF YOU ARE UNABLE TO MAKE A DIAGNOSIS FROM THIS CHART.

150 Depression after childbirth

Childbirth is followed by a dramatic alteration in the body's hormones as you begin to adjust to no longer being pregnant. Your emotions are also likely to be in turmoil. A new baby brings huge changes to your lifestyle, and you may not find it easy to come to terms with the reality of motherhood and the demands that your baby makes on you. Friends and family may be willing to help but will tend to direct all their attention toward the new baby rather than you, a huge switch from the time when you were pregnant. About 8 out of every 10 women suffer from "baby blues" soon after giving birth. Some 1 in 10 women develop a much more severe, longer-term postpartum depression.

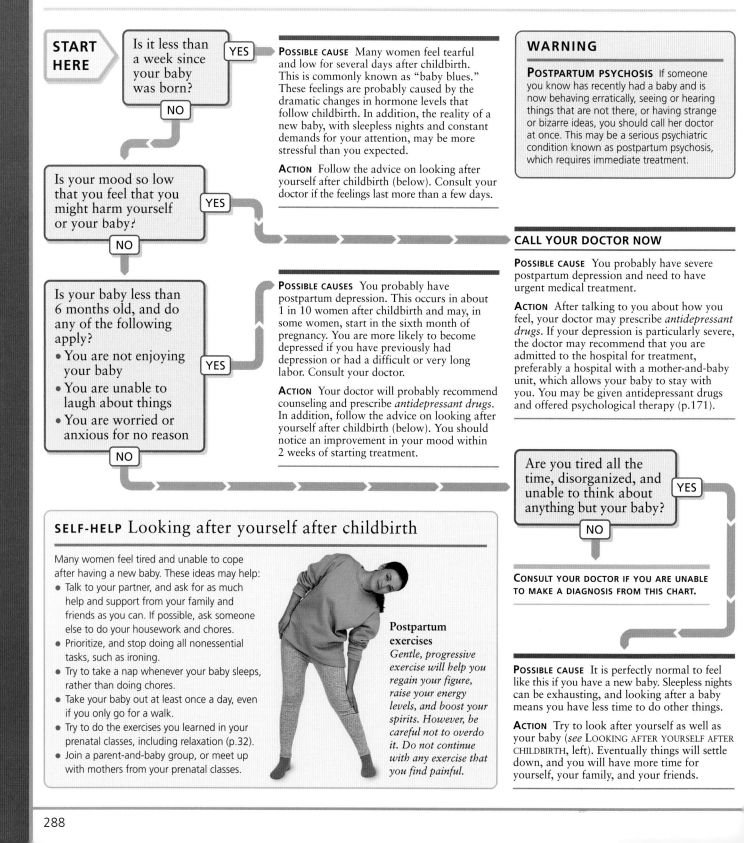

START HERE → **Is it less than a week since your baby was born?** — **YES** →

POSSIBLE CAUSE Many women feel tearful and low for several days after childbirth. This is commonly known as "baby blues." These feelings are probably caused by the dramatic changes in hormone levels that follow childbirth. In addition, the reality of a new baby, with sleepless nights and constant demands for your attention, may be more stressful than you expected.

ACTION Follow the advice on looking after yourself after childbirth (below). Consult your doctor if the feelings last more than a few days.

NO ↓

Is your mood so low that you feel that you might harm yourself or your baby? — **YES** →

NO ↓

Is your baby less than 6 months old, and do any of the following apply?
- You are not enjoying your baby
- You are unable to laugh about things
- You are worried or anxious for no reason

— **YES** →

POSSIBLE CAUSES You probably have postpartum depression. This occurs in about 1 in 10 women after childbirth and may, in some women, start in the sixth month of pregnancy. You are more likely to become depressed if you have previously had depression or had a difficult or very long labor. Consult your doctor.

ACTION Your doctor will probably recommend counseling and prescribe *antidepressant drugs*. In addition, follow the advice on looking after yourself after childbirth (below). You should notice an improvement in your mood within 2 weeks of starting treatment.

NO ↓

WARNING

POSTPARTUM PSYCHOSIS If someone you know has recently had a baby and is now behaving erratically, seeing or hearing things that are not there, or having strange or bizarre ideas, you should call her doctor at once. This may be a serious psychiatric condition known as postpartum psychosis, which requires immediate treatment.

CALL YOUR DOCTOR NOW

POSSIBLE CAUSE You probably have severe postpartum depression and need to have urgent medical treatment.

ACTION After talking to you about how you feel, your doctor may prescribe *antidepressant drugs*. If your depression is particularly severe, the doctor may recommend that you are admitted to the hospital for treatment, preferably a hospital with a mother-and-baby unit, which allows your baby to stay with you. You may be given antidepressant drugs and offered psychological therapy (p.171).

Are you tired all the time, disorganized, and unable to think about anything but your baby? — **YES** →

NO ↓

CONSULT YOUR DOCTOR IF YOU ARE UNABLE TO MAKE A DIAGNOSIS FROM THIS CHART.

POSSIBLE CAUSE It is perfectly normal to feel like this if you have a new baby. Sleepless nights can be exhausting, and looking after a baby means you have less time to do other things.

ACTION Try to look after yourself as well as your baby (*see* LOOKING AFTER YOURSELF AFTER CHILDBIRTH, left). Eventually things will settle down, and you will have more time for yourself, your family, and your friends.

SELF-HELP Looking after yourself after childbirth

Many women feel tired and unable to cope after having a new baby. These ideas may help:
- Talk to your partner, and ask for as much help and support from your family and friends as you can. If possible, ask someone else to do your housework and chores.
- Prioritize, and stop doing all nonessential tasks, such as ironing.
- Try to take a nap whenever your baby sleeps, rather than doing chores.
- Take your baby out at least once a day, even if you only go for a walk.
- Try to do the exercises you learned in your prenatal classes, including relaxation (p.32).
- Join a parent-and-baby group, or meet up with mothers from your prenatal classes.

Postpartum exercises
Gentle, progressive exercise will help you regain your figure, raise your energy levels, and boost your spirits. However, be careful not to overdo it. Do not continue with any exercise that you find painful.

FIRST AID

In some cases, immediate action can save a life. This section contains illustrated step-by-step instructions for the most common emergency situations you are likely to come across. First-aid techniques are covered for adults, as well as techniques used specifically for children and babies. In addition to familiarizing yourself with the articles here, you should obtain practical training from a recognized first-aid organization such as the American Red Cross so that you will be prepared for any emergency.

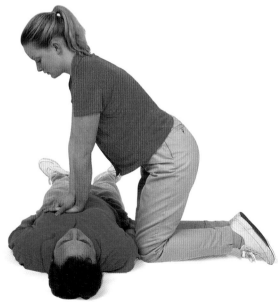

FIRST AID

First aid is the immediate care given to a sick or injured person before health-care professionals arrive. Its aims are to preserve life, prevent a condition from worsening, and promote as fast a recovery as possible. Your top priority in emergency situations, before starting first aid, is to dial 911 or call the Emergency Medical Services (EMS) for medical assistance. If possible, ask a bystander to make the call. The next priority is to check the scene for possible dangers to you, the victim, or bystanders, such as fire or dangerous fumes. You will not be able to help if you become a victim yourself; therefore, always put your own safety first. If you cannot approach the victim safely, phone for help immediately. If it is safe to approach, assess the victim's condition and give first aid.

The instructions in this section are designed to help you handle common emergency situations. There is no substitute for professional training, however, and the best form of training is a practical course in first aid. Courses are taught under the auspices of local chapters of the American Red Cross and the National Safety Council. On successful completion of a first-aid course, you are certified for 3 years. Certification in some skills, such as cardiopulmonary resuscitation, is valid for only 1 year.

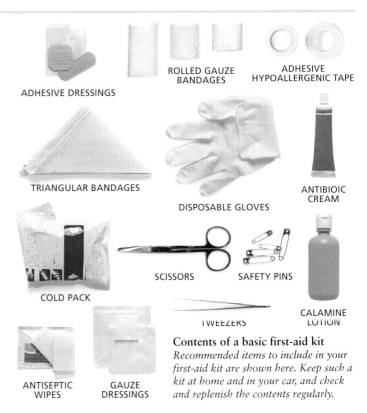

ADHESIVE DRESSINGS

ROLLED GAUZE BANDAGES

ADHESIVE HYPOALLERGENIC TAPE

TRIANGULAR BANDAGES

DISPOSABLE GLOVES

ANTIBIOIC CREAM

COLD PACK

SCISSORS

SAFETY PINS

TWEEZERS

CALAMINE LOTION

ANTISEPTIC WIPES

GAUZE DRESSINGS

Contents of a basic first-aid kit
Recommended items to include in your first-aid kit are shown here. Keep such a kit at home and in your car, and check and replenish the contents regularly.

ABC of resuscitation

Oxygen is vital for life. Normally, it is taken in by breathing and circulated around the body in the bloodstream. If either breathing or circulation fail, a procedure called resuscitation must be performed to supply the body with oxygen. The procedure is based on three checks known as the ABC of resuscitation: "ABC" stands for Airway, Breathing, and Circulation. If a person is unconscious, always follow the ABC sequence before giving any other treatment. You need to open the airway; establish if the victim is breathing; and assess whether the blood is circulating by checking for signs such as normal breathing, coughing, and movement. If the victim is not breathing, you must give artificial respiration to breathe oxygen into the body. If there are no signs of circulation, you must start cardiopulmonary resuscitation (CPR).

Adults and children

A: Airway
To open the airway, place one hand on the victim's forehead, and place two fingers of your other hand under the chin. Gently tilt the head back by pressing down on the forehead while you lift the chin.

B: Breathing
To check breathing, watch the chest for movement, listen for breath, and feel for breath on your cheek for up to 5 seconds. If there is no breathing, begin artificial respiration (p.293).

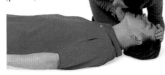

C: Circulation
Look, listen, and feel for signs of circulation, such as normal breathing, coughing or movement, for up to 10 seconds. If there is no sign of circulation, start CPR (pp.296–297).

Infants

A: Airway
To open the airway of an infant, use only one finger to lift the chin.

B: Breathing
To check breathing, watch the chest for movement, listen for breath, and feel for breath on your cheek for up to 5 seconds. If there is no breathing, begin artificial respiration (p.293).

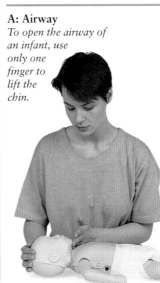

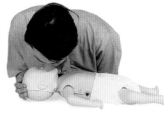

C: Circulation
Look, listen, and feel for signs of circulation, such as normal breathing, coughing or movement, for up to 10 seconds. If there is no sign of circulation, start CPR (pp.296–297).

Action in an emergency

When faced with an emergency, you should always follow a clear plan, staying calm and controlled so that you can act effectively. If necessary, take several deep, slow breaths to help yourself calm down. If possible, send someone to summon medical help while you deal with the situation. Before trying to help the victim you must be certain that you are not putting yourself in any possible danger. Remember

that you will not be able to help anyone else if you become a victim yourself. Very simple measures, such as turning off an electric switch, may be enough to eliminate danger. After you have made sure that the scene is safe, the next step is to check the victim's condition and carry out the appropriate first-aid treatment. Treat multiple injuries in order of priority, dealing with life-threatening conditions first.

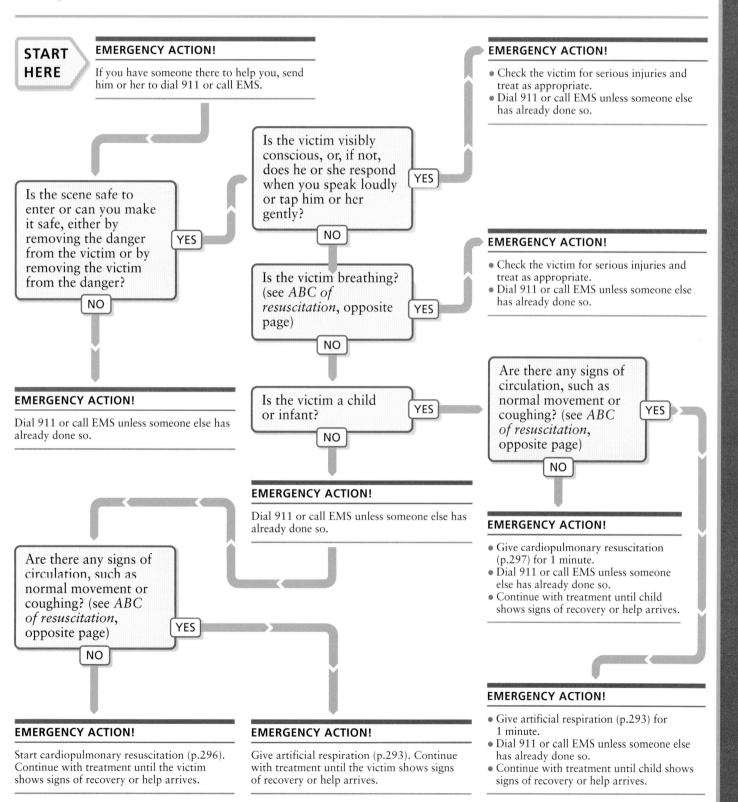

START HERE

EMERGENCY ACTION!
If you have someone there to help you, send him or her to dial 911 or call EMS.

Is the scene safe to enter or can you make it safe, either by removing the danger from the victim or by removing the victim from the danger? — YES

NO

EMERGENCY ACTION!
Dial 911 or call EMS unless someone else has already done so.

Is the victim visibly conscious, or, if not, does he or she respond when you speak loudly or tap him or her gently? — YES

NO

Is the victim breathing? (see *ABC of resuscitation*, opposite page) — YES

NO

Is the victim a child or infant? — YES

NO

EMERGENCY ACTION!
Dial 911 or call EMS unless someone else has already done so.

EMERGENCY ACTION!
- Check the victim for serious injuries and treat as appropriate.
- Dial 911 or call EMS unless someone else has already done so.

EMERGENCY ACTION!
- Check the victim for serious injuries and treat as appropriate.
- Dial 911 or call EMS unless someone else has already done so.

Are there any signs of circulation, such as normal movement or coughing? (see *ABC of resuscitation*, opposite page) — YES

NO

EMERGENCY ACTION!
- Give cardiopulmonary resuscitation (p.297) for 1 minute.
- Dial 911 or call EMS unless someone else has already done so.
- Continue with treatment until child shows signs of recovery or help arrives.

Are there any signs of circulation, such as normal movement or coughing? (see *ABC of resuscitation*, opposite page) — YES

NO

EMERGENCY ACTION!
Start cardiopulmonary resuscitation (p.296). Continue with treatment until the victim shows signs of recovery or help arrives.

EMERGENCY ACTION!
Give artificial respiration (p.293). Continue with treatment until the victim shows signs of recovery or help arrives.

EMERGENCY ACTION!
- Give artificial respiration (p.293) for 1 minute.
- Dial 911 or call EMS unless someone else has already done so.
- Continue with treatment until child shows signs of recovery or help arrives.

Choking

Choking is due to obstruction of the airway. In adults, a common cause of choking is food stuck in the throat. Infants and children often put small objects in their mouths and can easily choke. An adult or older child who is choking may cough and gasp and point to or grasp at the throat. A young child who is choking will have difficulty speaking and breathing and the face and neck will become flushed. A choking infant may squeak, turn blue, and seem to cry silently. If coughing does not clear the blockage, you need to give first aid to avoid suffocation. The techniques on these pages show how to treat conscious victims who are choking as well as those who have lost consciousness while being treated for choking or were found unconscious and known to have choked. You must reopen a blocked airway before giving any other first-aid treatment.

Conscious adults

> ### WARNING
>
> If the victim is pregnant or obese, you should give chest thrusts. Position the thumb side of your fist on the middle of the breastbone, place your other hand over your fist, and pull sharply inward.

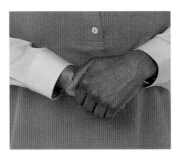

1 Encourage the victim to cough. If this does not dislodge the object, you will need to give abdominal thrusts. Stand behind the victim and reach around the body. Make a fist with one hand. Position the thumb side of your fist in the middle of the abdomen, just below the breastbone.

2 Place your other hand over your fist, and pull sharply inward and upward. Continue to give abdominal thrusts until the obstruction is cleared. If the victim continues to choke or loses consciousness (see Unconscious adults, below), dial 911 or call EMS for help.

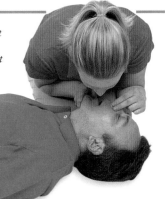

Hand is clasped over fist

Unconscious adults

> ### WARNING
>
> Only try to remove an object from a victim's throat if the object is clearly visible.

1 If you have a helper, send him or her to dial 911 or call EMS. Lay the victim on a firm surface and open the airway by pressing the forehead with one hand and lifting the chin with two fingers of the other. If you suspect spinal injury, use the modified chin lift (p.295). Remove any obvious obstruction from the mouth.

2 If the victim is not breathing, attempt 2 slow rescue breaths (p.295). If the chest does not move (a sign that air is not reaching the lungs), retilt the head and attempt to ventilate again. If the chest does not rise, assume that the airway is blocked. Check the mouth again. If unsuccessful, proceed to step 3.

Shoulders directly above chest and elbows locked

4 Kneel upright with your shoulders directly above the victim and your elbows straight. Do chest compressions as for CPR (pp.296–297). Compress the chest 15 times at a rate of about 15 compressions in 10 seconds, maintaining an even rhythm. Then attempt to give 2 rescue breaths. If air does not go in, check the mouth and then continue compressions.

Fingers interlocked and raised off chest

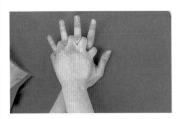

3 Place the heel of one hand on the middle of the breastbone, on an imaginary line connecting the nipples. Place the other hand on top, and interlock your fingers so that they are raised up off the victim's chest.

5 If the victim starts breathing again, place him in the recovery position (p.294) and monitor the breathing and circulation regularly (see ABC of resuscitation, p.290) until medical help arrives.

Conscious children

1 If the child is still able to breathe, encourage him or her to cough if possible because this may help to dislodge the obstruction.

2 If the child stops coughing or cannot breathe, kneel behind the child. Place a fist on the lower breastbone and put your other hand over the fist. Pull sharply inward and upward, up to 5 times. Check the mouth.

Hands positioned on chest, against lower part of breastbone

3 If chest thrusts do not dislodge the object, give up to 5 abdominal thrusts, with your fist against the child's upper abdomen. If the child is still choking or loses consciousness (see Unconscious children, right), dial 911 or call EMS, and repeat Steps 2–3 until help arrives.

Hands positioned against central upper abdomen

Unconscious children

> **WARNING**
>
> Only try to remove an object from a victim's throat if the object is clearly visible; do not feel blindly in the throat.

Feel for breath on your cheek

Tilt head back

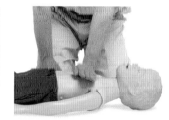

2 Place the heel of one hand on the middle of the child's breastbone as for CPR (p.296) and give up to 5 compressions. Check the mouth again to see if the obstruction has been dislodged.

Look for chest movements

1 If you have a helper, ask him or her to dial 911 or call EMS. Open the child's airway and check if he or she is breathing (see ABC of resuscitation, p.290). Remove any obvious obstruction from the child's mouth. If breathing has stopped, give up to 5 slow rescue breaths (p.295). If the child is still not breathing, go to step 2.

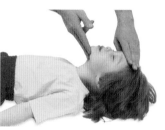

3 Attempt another rescue breath. If the child does not start to breathe, repeat the cycle of chest compressions, opening the airway, looking for an object, and breaths until medical help arrives. If the child begins to breathe again at any time, place him or her in the recovery position (p.294).

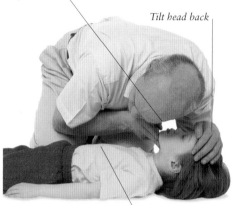

Infants

> **WARNING**
>
> • Never shake a choking infant.
> • Do not use your fingers to feel blindly down an infant's throat. Only try to remove the obstruction if you can see it clearly.

1 If the infant has a strong cough, let him or her continue. If the object is not dislodged or the victim becomes too weak or tired to cough or stops breathing, go to Step 2. If you have a helper, ask him or her to dial 911 or call EMS.

Give up to 5 back slaps

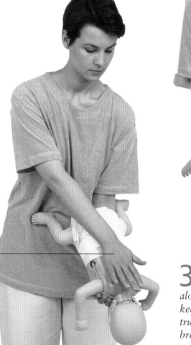

2 Lay the infant face downward on your forearm or lap, with the head lower than the trunk. Support the chin and shoulders with your hand. Give up to 5 back slaps between the infant's shoulders, then check the mouth.

3 If back slaps are not effective, lay the infant face upward along your forearm or on your lap, keeping the head lower than the trunk. Place 2 fingers on the breastbone between the nipples and give 5 chest thrusts, 1 every 3 seconds, as for CPR (p.296).

4 Dial 911 or call EMS if a helper has not already done so. Continue with cycles of 5 back slaps followed by 5 chest thrusts.

5 If at any time the infant loses consciousness, open his or her mouth, and place your finger on the tongue to allow you a clear view of the back of the mouth. Remove any obvious obstruction.

6 Tilt the head back to open the airway and give 2 rescue breaths (p.295). If the air does not reach the lungs, reposition the head and try again.

7 If the breaths still do not reach the lungs, repeat Steps 2–6 until medical help arrives or the infant starts breathing unaided again. If the infant does start breathing, hold him or her in the recovery position (p.294) and monitor breathing and circulation (see ABC of resuscitation, p.290) until medical help arrives.

Recovery position

The recovery position is a secure position in which to place a person who is unconscious but breathing. If an unconscious victim is left lying on his or her back, the tongue may block the throat and prevent air from reaching the airways to the lungs. This situation is life-threatening because the breathing and heartbeat may stop. The recovery position keeps the head, neck, and back aligned, keeps the airway open, and allows fluid to drain out of the mouth if the victim vomits. You may not need to follow all of the steps shown below if the person is found lying on his or her front or side.

Adults and children

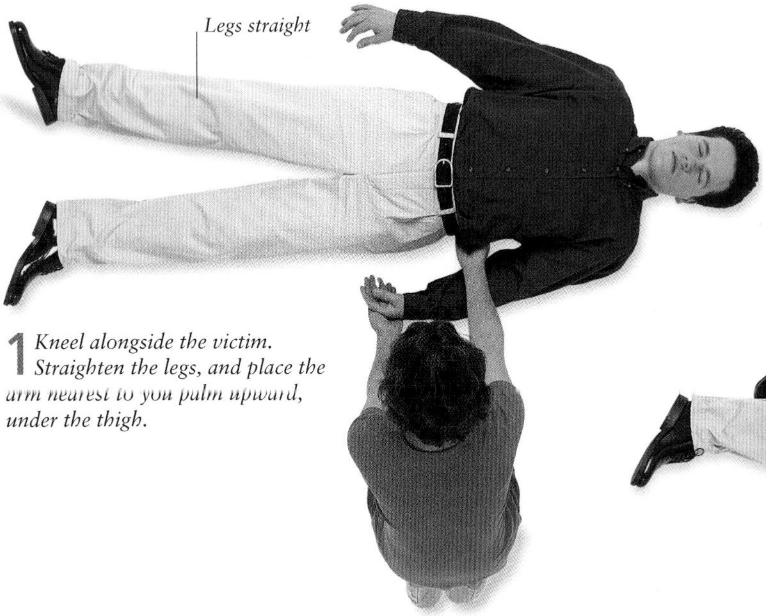

Legs straight

1 *Kneel alongside the victim. Straighten the legs, and place the arm nearest to you palm upward, under the thigh.*

2 *Bring the arm that is farthest from you across the victim's chest. Place the back of the victim's hand under the near cheek. With your other hand, pull the far leg into a bent position; keeping the foot on the floor at first, then pulling the knee toward you.*

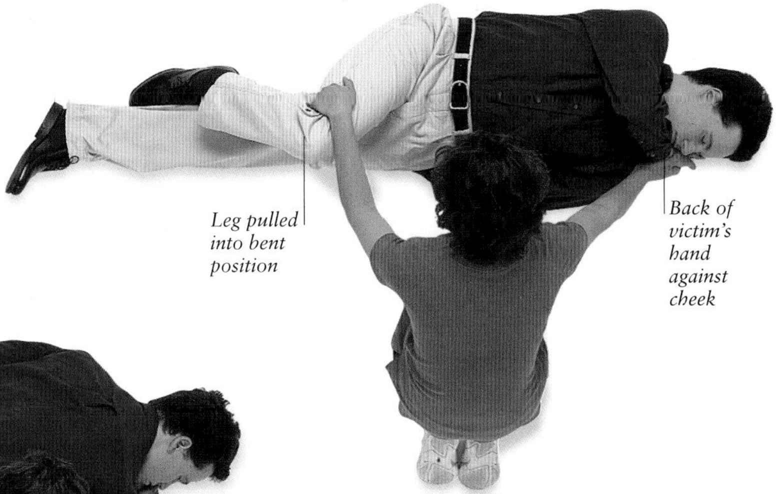

> **WARNING**
>
> If you suspect a spinal injury (p.301), do not move the victim unless breathing is impeded or the person is in danger.

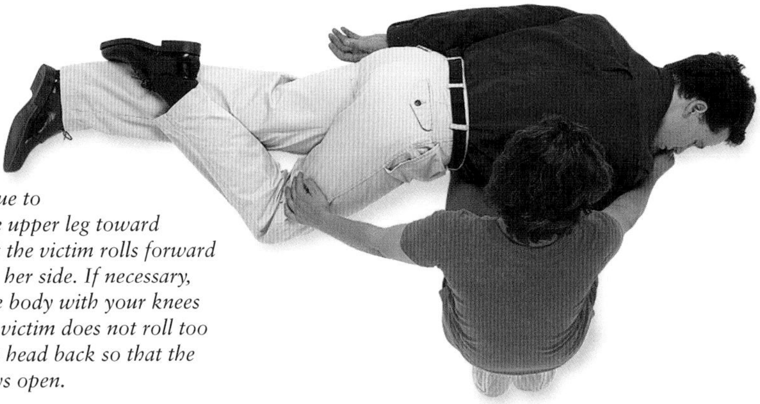

Leg pulled into bent position

Back of victim's hand against cheek

3 *Continue to pull the upper leg toward you so that the victim rolls forward onto his or her side. If necessary, support the body with your knees so that the victim does not roll too far. Tilt the head back so that the airway stays open.*

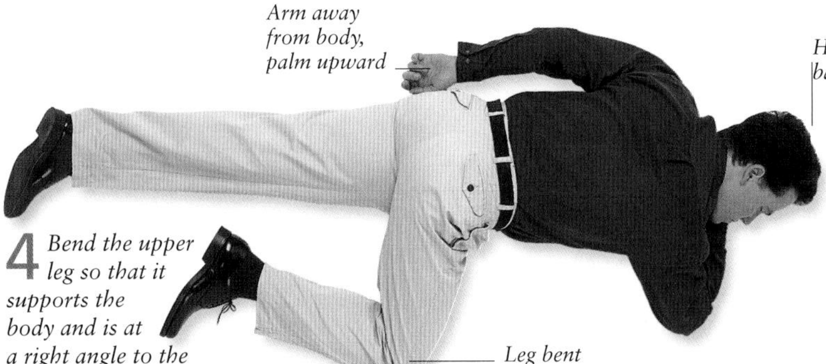

Infants

Body tilted downward

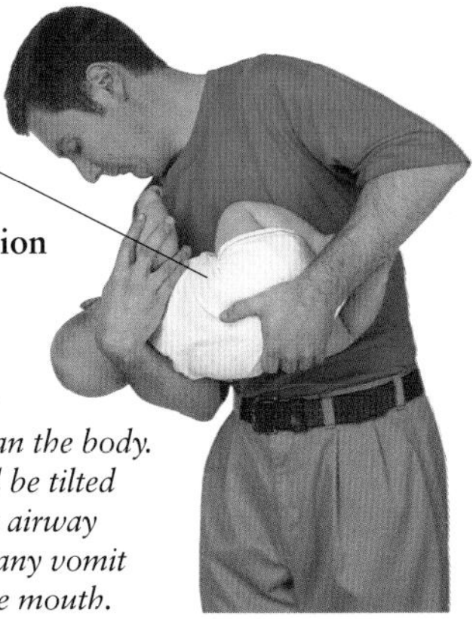

Recovery position for an infant
Hold the infant securely in your arms so that the head is lower than the body. The head should be tilted back to keep the airway open and allow any vomit to drain from the mouth.

Arm away from body, palm upward

Head tilted back slightly

4 *Bend the upper leg so that it supports the body and is at a right angle to the hip, if possible. Move the arm farthest from you so that it is away from the body. Turn the palm so that it faces upward. Check for signs of loss of circulation to the lower arm. If the skin is pale or cool to the touch, turn victim onto the opposite side after 30 minutes.*

Leg bent

5 *Dial 911 or call EMS. Regularly check the victim's breathing and signs of circulation (see ABC of resuscitation, p.290).*

> **WARNING**
>
> If you suspect a spinal injury (p.301), do not move the infant unless the breathing is impeded or the victim is in danger.

Artificial respiration

Artificial respiration is a way to force your exhaled air into the lungs of a person who is not breathing. If breathing has stopped, the victim will be unconscious, the chest will not rise or fall, and you will not be able to feel or hear breath. The face may be grayish blue. In this situation, you must give artificial respiration immediately; your exhaled air still contains enough oxygen to sustain the victim's vital organs

until help arrives. If the pulse is absent, indicating that the heart has stopped, you need to carry out cardiopulmonary resuscitation (pp.296–297) – artificial respiration combined with chest compressions. When giving artificial respiration to an infant, be careful not to blow too hard or air will go into the stomach. Use a face shield or mask, if available. However, even if you do not have one, do not hesitate to help a victim.

Adults and children

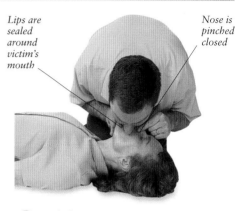

Lips are sealed around victim's mouth

Nose is pinched closed

WARNING

If you suspect spinal injury, try to open the victim's airway without tilting the head back, or tilt it only very slightly. This technique, called the modified chin lift, will minimize movement to the head and neck.

1 *If you have a helper, ask him or her to dial 911 or call EMS. If you are alone and the victim is an adult, dial 911 before proceeding to Step 2. If the victim is a child, go to Step 2 immediately.*

2 *Lay the victim on his or her back. Remove anything that is obviously loose, such as dentures, from the mouth. Open the airway by pressing down on the forehead with one hand and lifting the chin with two fingers of your other hand.*

3 *Pinch the victim's nose closed with your thumb and index finger. Take a deep breath, then place your open mouth tightly around the victim's mouth to make a good seal. Blow air into the victim's mouth for about 1½ seconds.*

Rescuer watches victim's chest

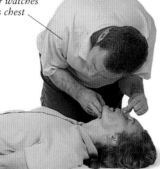

4 *Look at the victim's chest; you should see the chest fall as air leaves the lungs. Check the head position and give another breath, ensuring that you make a good seal around the mouth. If the chest does not move, assume that the airway is blocked and treat as for choking (pp.292–293). If the chest does rise and fall, go to Step 5.*

5 *Check for signs of circulation (see ABC of resuscitation, p.290). If absent, start CPR (pp.296–297). If signs of circulation are present, continue artificial respiration; give 1 breath every 5 seconds. Dial 911 or call EMS after 1 minute if it has not already been done. Check for a pulse after every minute. If the victim starts breathing, place him or her in the recovery position (p.294).*

ALTERNATIVE

If the victim has injuries to the mouth or jaw that make it difficult to use mouth-to-mouth breaths, you can blow air into the lungs through the victim's nose. Close the victim's mouth with your hand while blowing to prevent air from escaping.

Infants

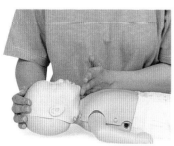

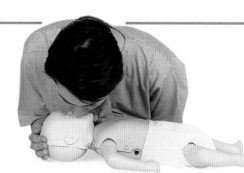

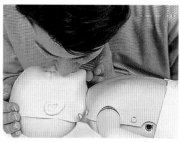

1 *Send a helper, if you have one, to dial 911 or call EMS. Place the infant on his or her back on a firm surface. Put one hand on the infant's head and tilt the head back while you lift the chin slightly with one finger of your other hand.*

2 *Carefully remove any obvious obstructions from the mouth. Seal your lips around the mouth and nose. Give 2 slow breaths of about 1½ seconds each. If the chest does not move, treat as for choking (p.293); otherwise, go to Step 3.*

3 *Check circulation by looking for signs of recovery, such as coughing, swallowing, and return of normal skin color. Dial 911 or call EMS unless this has already been done.*

4 *If there are no signs of circulation, start CPR (pp.296–297). If there are signs of circulation, keep giving breaths at a rate of 1 breath every 3 seconds. Check for signs of circulation and recovery after each minute, continuing until help arrives.*

Cardiopulmonary resuscitation (CPR)

CPR is a life-saving technique in which rescue breathing (p.295) is combined with chest compressions. It is performed on an unconscious victim who is not breathing and has no pulse to keep the blood circulating and ensure that oxygen is supplied to the tissues. Chest compressions force blood out of the heart and around the body, ensuring that the oxygen supplied by rescue breathing reaches the brain and other vital organs. Do not stop giving CPR until the victim's heart starts beating or medical help arrives. If you are too tired to continue, try to find another trained person to take over from you until medical help arrives. When you are giving chest compressions to children use slightly less pressure in order to avoid injury, and give them at a slightly different rate. Rescue breaths are also given at a different rate in infants and children, and it is important not to blow too hard, especially when treating an infant.

Adults

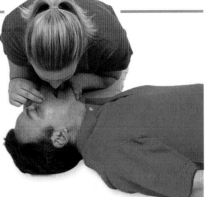

1 *Dial 911 or call EMS. Lay the victim face upward on a hard surface. Open the airway by placing one hand on the forehead to tilt the head back and lifting the chin with two fingers of the other. Look at the chest for signs of breathing and feel for breath on your cheek.*

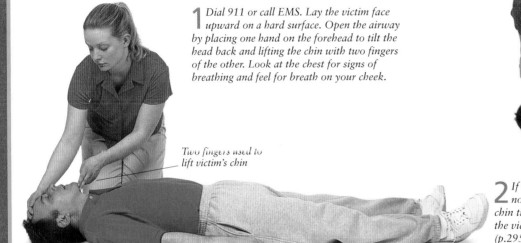

Two fingers used to lift victim's chin

2 *If the victim is not breathing, pinch the nostrils shut with one hand, and keep the chin tilted with the other. Seal your mouth over the victim's mouth, and give 2 rescue breaths (p.295). Pause to take a breath yourself between giving breaths.*

Middle finger on end of the breastbone

3 *Look for signs of circulation, such as movement, breathing, and coughing, for up to 10 seconds. If circulation is present, continue rescue breathing. If there are no signs of circulation, begin CPR (see Step 4).*

4 *Kneel to one side of the victim. Using the hand farthest from the victim's head, slide your fingers along the lowest rib to where it meets the breastbone. Place your middle finger on this point and your index finger just above it.*

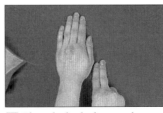

5 *Place the heel of your other hand on the breastbone, just above your index finger. This is the area of the chest where you must apply the compressions.*

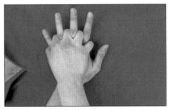

6 *Lift the fingers of the first hand away and lay the hand on top of your other hand. Interlock the fingers, so that the fingers of the bottom hand are lifted off the chest.*

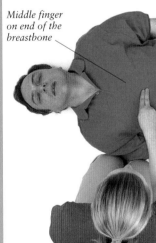

7 *Kneel upright with your shoulders directly above the victim and your elbows locked straight. Press downward, depressing the breastbone 1½–2 in (4–5 cm), then release the pressure without moving your hands. Compress the chest in this way 15 times at a rate of about 15 compressions in 10 seconds, maintaining an even rhythm. Then give 2 rescue breaths.*

Shoulders above center of victim's chest

Elbows locked

8 *Continue giving cycles of 15 chest compressions with 2 breaths of rescue breathing. After 4 cycles of compressions and breaths check breathing and circulation, and check them again every few minutes thereafter. If they are absent, continue CPR. If breathing and circulation return, stop CPR but continue to monitor until help arrives.*

Children

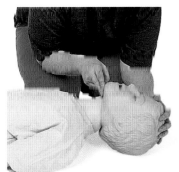

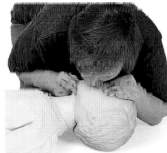

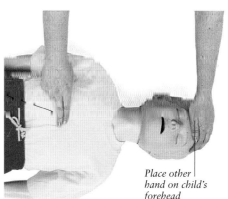

Middle finger
at end of the
breastbone

Place other
hand on child's
forehead

1 Ask a helper to dial 911 or call EMS. Lay the child face up on a firm surface. Open the airway by tilting the head back slightly. Do this by pressing down gently on the forehead with one hand and lifting the chin with 2 fingers of the other hand.

2 If there are no signs of breathing, such as chest movement or the feel of breath on your cheek, pinch the child's nose shut and seal your lips over the mouth. Give 2 rescue breaths (p.295), pausing to take a breath yourself between each one.

3 Look for signs of circulation, such as movement, breathing, and coughing, for up to 10 seconds. If circulation is present, continue rescue breathing. If there are no signs of circulation, begin CPR (see Step 4).

4 Kneel beside the victim and place one hand on the child's forehead. Locate one of the lowermost ribs with the fingers of the other hand. Slide your fingers along the rib to where it meets the breastbone. Position your middle finger at this point with the index finger just above it.

5 Place the heel of your other hand on the breastbone next to your fingers. With the heel of your hand, press down sharply on the chest, to a depth of 1–1½ in (2.5–4 cm), 5 times in 3 seconds. Count from 1 to 5 to maintain an even rhythm.

Press down sharply with the heel of one hand

6 Give 1 rescue breath. Then repeat the chest compressions and breaths for 1 minute. Dial 911 or call EMS if this has not yet been done. Repeat the cycle until the child recovers or help arrives. Recheck breathing and circulation every few minutes.

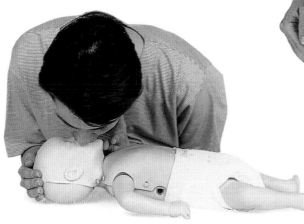

Infants

1 Dial 911 or call EMS, or ask a helper to do so. Place the infant face up on a hard surface. Tilt the head back slightly with one hand and lift the chin with one finger of the other hand. Look, listen, and feel for evidence of breathing. If the baby is not breathing, seal your lips over the mouth and nose. Give 2 slow, gentle rescue breaths (p.295), pausing to breathe yourself between the breaths.

Press down sharply on breastbone with 2 fingers of other hand

Place one hand on infant's head

3 With one hand placed on the top of the baby's head, position the tips of 2 fingers of your other hand on the breastbone, a finger's width below the nipples. Press down sharply on the breastbone, to a depth of ½–1 in (1–2.5 cm), 5 times in 3 seconds.

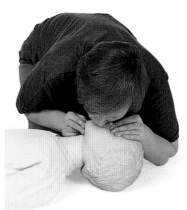

2 Look for signs of circulation, such as normal breathing, coughing, or movement. If there is circulation but no breathing, continue giving rescue breaths. If there is no breathing or circulation, start CPR (see Step 3).

4 Seal your lips over the infant's mouth and nose and give 1 breath. Check for breathing. Repeat the cycle of 5 chest compressions and 1 breath for 1 minute. If a helper has not already done so, dial 911 or call EMS. If the infant recovers at any time, stop CPR but monitor breathing and circulation until medical help arrives.

Shock

Shock can occur as a result of any severe injury or illness that dramatically reduces the flow of blood around the body, such as a heart attack or severe bleeding. It can also be due to loss of body fluids from burns or severe diarrhea and vomiting. If shock is not treated rapidly, vital organs such as the brain and heart may fail. Signs of shock may include a rapid pulse; gray-blue skin, especially on the lips; sweating; and cold, clammy skin. Later, excessive thirst and nausea and vomiting may occur. The victim may feel weak or dizzy and develop rapid, shallow breathing and a faint pulse. He or she may be restless, gasp for air, and eventually lose consciousness. It is essential to call for medical help at the first signs of shock, and to keep the victim warm and comfortable.

> **WARNING**
> - Do not leave the victim alone, except to dial 911 or call EMS. If possible, ask a helper to summon medical help.
> - Do not let the victim eat or drink unless he or she has diabetes and is hypoglycemic.

Raise legs above level of heart

1 *If you have a helper, send him or her to dial 911 or call EMS. Treat any obvious cause of shock, such as severe bleeding (opposite page).*

2 *If the person is breathing normally, lay him or her down. If you suspect a fracture (p.301), keep the person flat. Otherwise, raise the legs above the level of the heart. If the person is having difficulty breathing, help him or her sit in a comfortable position.*

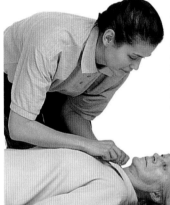

3 *Loosen any restrictions around the neck, chest, and waist, and remove the victim's shoes. Dial 911 or call EMS if a helper has not already done so.*

4 *Keep the victim from becoming cold by covering him or her with a blanket. Check the victim's level of consciousness by asking simple, direct questions. Monitor breathing and pulse and be prepared to resuscitate if necessary (see ABC of resuscitation, p.290).*

Check pulse at regular intervals

Cover the victim with a coat or blanket

Anaphylactic shock

Anaphylactic shock is a life-threatening allergic reaction to a specific food, drug, or insect sting. It can develop within seconds or a few minutes. The victim may be anxious and may have puffy eyes, a swollen face, lips, and tongue, and an itchy, red skin rash. He or she may develop wheezing and severe breathing difficulties and may lose consciousness. An injection of epinephrine and oxygen must be given as quickly as possible. If the person is aware of having an allergy and carries a supply of epinephrine, you can help him or her use this supply. Otherwise, first aid is limited to keeping the person comfortable and, if necessary, helping him or her breathe until medical help arrives.

> **WARNING**
> Do not leave the victim alone, except to dial 911 or call EMS. If possible, ask a helper to summon medical help.

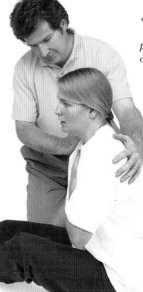

1 *Dial 911 or call EMS, or send a helper to do so immediately. If possible, provide the emergency services with details of the cause of the allergic reaction.*

2 *If the victim is conscious, help him or her sit up in the position that makes breathing easiest.*

3 *Check if the victim is carrying a syringe of epinephrine. Help him or her use it, or administer it yourself if you have been trained.*

4 *If the person loses consciousness, open the airway, check breathing and pulse, and be prepared to carry out resuscitation if necessary (see ABC of resuscitation, p.290). Monitor the person's pulse and breathing until medical help arrives.*

Severe bleeding

Severe bleeding is dramatic and distressing and can be life-threatening. Although you must try to stop the bleeding as quickly as possible, you must also be alert to the general condition of the victim. A person who is bleeding heavily may lose consciousness (see *Unconsciousness*, p.300) and is also likely to develop shock (opposite page). Severe bleeding from an injury to the face or neck can cause choking (pp.294–295). Any of these conditions may require immediate treatment. Before and after treating bleeding, wash your hands well. Wear disposable gloves if they are available and follow the procedure below to stop the bleeding.

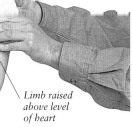

1 *Place a sterile dressing, pad, or clean cloth over the wound and press firmly in place for at least 10 minutes, or longer if necessary, until the bleeding stops. If no clean dressing is available, ask the victim to apply pressure with the palm or fingers of his or her own hands.*

2 *If the bleeding does not stop, raise the injured part above the level of the heart, if possible, and continue to apply pressure. However, if you suspect a fracture (p.301), do not move the injured part.*

Limb raised above level of heart

3 *Leaving any original pad in place, apply a pressure bandage. If blood seeps through the dressing, place another bandage on top.*

4 *Dial 911 or call EMS. Watch for signs of shock (opposite page), and treat if necessary. Continue to check the dressing for seepage of blood.*

WARNING

- Do not apply a touniquet. This can make the bleeding worse and may result in tissue damage.
- Do not try to remove a foreign body that has become embedded in a wound.

Severe burns

A severe burn may involve all layers of the skin. If it is very severe, it may also destroy the tissues underlying the skin. The affected area may appear red and may have blisters that weep clear fluid. In some cases, the area may be brown or charred. If the burn extends to very deep tissues, the skin may be white. If the nerve endings are damaged, there may be loss of feeling in the injured area. The immediate response for a serious burn is to cool the area rapidly, which minimizes damage and may help prevent loss of body fluids and the onset of shock (opposite page). It is essential to protect the wound from infection. The larger and deeper the burn, the greater the risk of shock or infection. A victim who has been burned in a fire will probably have suffered damage to the airway as a result of inhaling smoke or hot air. You should monitor his or her breathing regularly. If consciousness is lost, be prepared to resuscitate (see *ABC of resuscitation*, p.290).

WARNING

- Do not touch the burn.
- Do not apply anything to the burn other than cool liquid, preferably cool water or otherwise a cold drink.
- Do not apply ice or ice water directly to the burned area.
- Do not burst blisters.

1 *If possible, remove the victim from the source of the burn and put out any flames on the person's clothing. If you have a helper, send him or her to dial 911 or call EMS.*

2 *If the site of the burn allows you to do so, lay the victim down, protecting the burn from contact with the ground. If possible, raise the burned area above the level of the heart. Do not touch the burn or attempt to remove anything that is sticking to the burn. Dial 911 or call EMS unless a helper has done so already.*

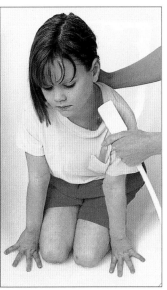

3 *Douse the burn with plenty of cool water, immerse it in water, or cover it with cold, wet towels for at least 10 minutes or until the burn has cooled down. If no tap water is available, use any other suitable source, including a garden hose, shower, or a cold soda.*

4 *Once the burn has cooled, gently remove or cut away clothing (unless sticking to the burn), shoes, belts, or jewelry before the area starts to swell or blister. Do not touch blisters. If pain persists, cool the area again. Cover the burn with a sterile dressing or any clean, non-fluffy material. Do not apply adhesive dressings to the affected skin.*

5 *Record details of the injuries and the circumstances in which they occurred. Reassure the victim while you wait for medical help to arrive. Monitor breathing and pulse (see ABC of resuscitation. p. 290), watch for signs of shock (opposite page), such as rapid pulse and cool, moist skin, and be prepared to treat appropriately.*

Wound covered with non-fluffly material

Unconsciousness

Unconsciousness results from an interruption to the normal activity of the brain. It is a potentially life-threatening condition that requires immediate medical help. A victim is likely to be unconscious if he or she does not respond to loud noises or gentle tapping or shaking. The person will make no sound or movement and his or her eyes will remain closed. If an unconscious victim is lying on his or her back, the tongue may fall back and block the airway. First-aid priorities are to maintain an open airway and to check for and treat obvious injuries.

1 *If you have a helper, send him or her to dial 911 or call EMS. If you need to leave the victim alone to call for help, place the person in the recovery position (p.292). However, if you suspect spinal injury, do not move the person unless the airway is blocked.*

WARNING

- Do not move the victim unnecessarily in case there is spinal injury.
- Do not leave the victim alone except to dial 911 or call EMS. If possible, ask a helper to summon medical help.
- Do not try to give an unconscious victim anything to eat or drink.

2 *Check the victim's breathing by looking for chest movement, listening for breaths, or feeling for breath on your face. Check the pulse and be prepared to resuscitate if necessary (see ABC of resuscitation, p.290).*

3 *Control any external bleeding (see Severe bleeding, p.299) and check for and support suspected fractures (opposite page). Look for clues to the cause of the victim's condition, such as needle marks, warning bracelets, or cards. Ask bystanders for any information to give to the medical services.*

4 *Stay with the victim until medical help arrives. Monitor the victim's breathing and pulse at regular intervals. In addition, you should periodically check whether the victim is regaining consciousness by asking simple, direct questions or tapping or shaking the person gently.*

Major seizures

A major seizure (convulsion) is a result of an electrical disturbance in the brain and consists of muscular spasms and loss of body control. Seizures that are recurrent usually indicate the brain disorder epilepsy. During a major seizure, a person falls unconscious, often letting out a cry. The body becomes rigid, the back arches, the jaw is clenched, the eyes roll upward, and the tongue may be bitten. The breathing becomes noisy and, in some cases, temporarily ceases. Convulsive shaking movements of the body may then follow, and may last for 1–3 minutes. The victim recovers consciousness within a few minutes but is left dazed and sleepy. Anyone who is giving first aid should protect the victim from injuring him- or herself during a major seizure and should remain present until recovery is complete.

1 *Attempt to support the victim if you see him or her falling. If bystanders are present, ask them to move away and remove any objects from around the victim.*

2 *Lay the victim down. Loosen clothing around his or her neck, and try to protect the head with something soft, such as a piece of folded clothing.*

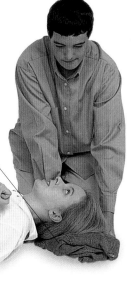

Protect victim's head

One leg kept straight

Hand under head for support

WARNING

- Do not use force in an attempt to restrain the victim.
- Do not put anything in the victim's mouth.

3 *When the convulsions have finished, place the victim in the recovery position (p.292). Check the victim's breathing and pulse at regular intervals and be prepared to resuscitate if necessary (see ABC of resuscitation, p.290).*

Other leg bent to prop up body

4 *If the victim has a severe seizure, in which he or she remains unconscious for more than 10 minutes or convulses for more than 5 minutes, or if the person has repeated seizures, dial 911 or call EMS. Stay with the victim and monitor breathing and pulse until medical help arrives.*

5 *If the victim has not had a severe seizure or repeated seizures, and you know that he or she has epilepsy, stay with the person until he or she has recovered. If you are not certain that the person has epilepsy, dial 911 or call EMS, and stay with the victim until medical help arrives.*

Spinal injury

The main risk when dealing with someone who has spinal injury is that any movement may damage the spinal cord. The most dangerous injuries are those to the neck, but any spinal injury is potentially serious. When calling the emergency services, try to tell them how the injury to the spine occurred. If you suspect an injury to the spinal cord, it is vital to keep the victim still until a doctor arrives. Signs of possible damage to the spinal cord include a burning sensation or tingling in a limb or loss of feeling in a limb. The victim may also have breathing difficulties.

WARNING

Do not move the victim from the position in which he or she was found unless he or she is in danger or loses consciousness and needs to be resuscitated.

1 Dial 911 or call EMS. Reassure the victim and keep him or her as still as possible. If the victim was found face down and must be moved, place your hands over his or her ears to hold the head aligned while helpers straighten the victim's limbs and roll him or her gently over. If the victim was found on his or her back, go to Step 2.

Rescuer's hands hold head aligned with spine

2 The safest position for a victim with a suspected spinal injury is the neutral position in which the head, neck, and spine are aligned. To check alignment, make sure that the victim's nose is in line with his or her navel.

3 If you need to realign the victim, kneel by the victim's head, place your hands firmly over his or her ears, and move the head slowly into position. Stay supporting the head in this position until the ambulance arrives.

4 If you have a helper, extra stability can be provided by getting him or her to place rolled-up clothes, towels, or blankets on either side of the victim's head and shoulders to minimize movement.

Fractures

You should suspect a fracture if the person cannot move the injured part or it is misshapen or very painful. There is likely to be swelling and bruising and possibly bleeding and a visible wound. A person with an upper limb fracture is usually able to walk and can be taken to a hospital, keeping the injured part as still as possible. Fracture of a lower limb bone is a serious injury, requiring immediate hospital treatment. Fractures of the thighbone often involve severe internal bleeding and there is a danger of shock (p.298). No weight should be placed on an injured leg.

WARNING

- Do not give anything to eat or drink, in case the victim needs general anesthesia.
- Do not move a victim with a lower limb injury unless he or she is in danger.

Upper limb fractures

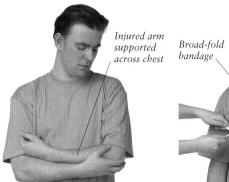

Injured arm supported across chest

Broad-fold bandage

1 Sit the victim down. If necessary, treat any bleeding (see Severe bleeding, p.299).

2 Ask the victim to hold the injured arm across his or her chest in the position that is most comfortable. Tell the victim to support the arm or wrist, if possible. Alternatively, support the part yourself.

3 Place the arm on the injured side in a sling and insert soft padding between the arm and the chest. If the arm has to be kept still, tie a broad-fold bandage around the chest and over the sling.

4 Take or send the victim to the hospital, keeping him or her seated if possible.

Lower limb fractures

1 Help the victim lie down, and treat any bleeding (see Severe bleeding, p.299).

2 Put plenty of padding, such as rolled-up blankets or towels or folded newspapers, on both sides of the injured leg. If you have a helper, send him or her to dial 911 or call EMS.

3 If you need to remove the victim from danger or leave to call for medical help, immobilize the injured limb by bandaging it to the uninjured limb. Otherwise, steady and support the injured limb with your hands until medical help arrives.

4 Try to minimize the risk of shock (p.298) developing by keeping the person warm and comfortable. Regularly check the person's breathing and pulse and be prepared to resuscitate (see ABC of resuscitation, p.290).

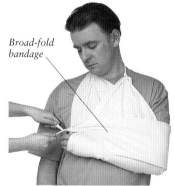

Swallowed poisons

Poisoning can be caused by swallowing toxic chemicals or poisonous plants or by overdosage of recreational or medicinal drugs. Common symptoms include pain in the abdomen or chest, nausea, vomiting, diarrhea, and breathing difficulties. There may be signs of burning around the mouth and lips. The victim may appear sluggish and confused, and may lose consciousness. Rarely, certain poisons can result in anaphylactic shock (p.298), a life-threatening allergic reaction. Signs of this condition include swelling of the face, lips, and tongue, breathing difficulties, and a rash. Call the Poison Control Center (1-800-222-1222) if you suspect poisoning, and give as much information as possible.

WARNING

Do not try to induce the victim to vomit unless you are advised to do so by a medical professional.

1 *If the victim is conscious, ask questions to obtain as much information as possible about the poisoning. If the victim is unconscious, go to step 3.*

2 *Call your doctor or Poison Control Center for instructions and give them as much information as possible. Stay with the victim and monitor his or her condition. If he or she develops signs of shock or breathing difficulties, dial 911 or call EMS.*

3 *If the victim is unconscious or loses consciousness, check his or her breathing and pulse and be prepared to resuscitate if necessary (see ABC of resuscitation, p.290).*

4 *Place the victim in the recovery position (p.292) unless you suspect that he or she has a spinal injury. Dial 911 or call EMS, then return to the victim. If alcohol poisoning is a possibility, keep the victim warm with a blanket.*

Bites and stings

In many parts of the world, certain animals, such as scorpions and snakes, have a venomous bite or sting. Rattlesnakes, coppermouths, and coral snakes are all native to the US; other snakes are kept as pets. A venomous bite or sting can cause severe pain, swelling, and discoloration at the site of the wound. Scorpion stings and snake bites can also cause vomiting, breathing problems, and an irregular heartbeat. With prompt hospital treatment, most victims recover rapidly. If possible, you should note the appearance of the snake so that the appropriate antivenom can be given. Bee and wasp stings are not usually life-threatening. However, in a few cases, a single sting can lead to anaphylactic shock (p.298), a life-threatening allergic reaction.

Insect stings

WARNING

Get medical help immediately if the victim is allergic to insect stings.

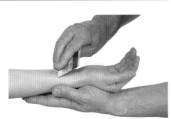

1 *If there are signs of anaphylactic shock or the sting is in the mouth or throat, dial 911 or call EMS. Give a victim stung in the mouth a piece of ice to suck or some cold water to sip. If there is no indication of shock and the sting is still in the skin, proceed to Step 2.*

2 *If the sting is still in the wound, gently scrape it out with a credit card, needle, or fingernail. Do not use tweezers or grasp the venom sac with your fingers because this may inject more venom into the victim.*

3 *Wash the injured area with soap and water, then pat dry. Cover the wound with a piece of clean cloth or gauze, and secure the material in place with a bandage.*

4 *Apply a cold compress on top of the cloth or gauze to reduce pain and swelling. Advise the victim to seek medical help if symptoms persist.*

Poisonous bites and stings

1 *Dial 911 or call EMS, and reassure the victim. If the victim has been bitten by a snake, lay him or her down, keeping the area of the bite below the level of the heart. Tell the victim not to move.*

2 *Wash the wound carefully, and pat it dry with clean swabs or other nonfluffy material. Do not rub the wound. If the wound is from a spider bite or a scorpion sting, apply a cold pack and wait for medical help. If you suspect that the bite is from a venomous snake, proceed to Step 3.*

3 *Minimize the victim's movement to stop the venom from spreading farther around the body. Immobilize the injured leg by binding it to the uninjured leg and immobilize an injured arm with a sling.*

4 *Keep the victim calm while waiting for medical help. Regularly monitor the victim's breathing and pulse and be ready to resuscitate if necessary (see ABC of resuscitation, p.290.*

WARNING

● Do not attempt to identify a venomous snake or spider by handling it.
● Do not apply a tourniquet to the affected limb or attempt to suck the venom from the bite.

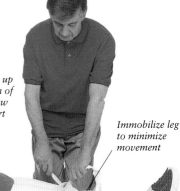

Prop victim up to keep area of wound below level of heart

Immobilize leg to minimize movement

DRUG GUIDE
& USEFUL
ADDRESSES

The Drug Guide will help you understand
prescribed and over-the-counter drugs and
how to use them safely. It explains the general
principles of drug treatment and contains
information on specific drug groups. Useful
Addresses provides sources for additional
health information and tells you how to
contact self-help and support groups.

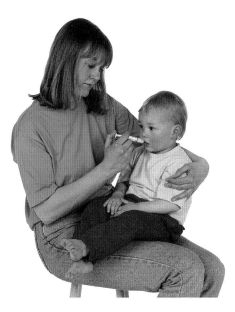

DRUG GUIDE

A vast range of drugs is available for treating disorders. Drugs are used not only to cure many conditions but, in some cases, to control symptoms in disorders such as epilepsy and rheumatoid arthritis, as well as to relieve common, minor symptoms such as wheezing or itching. Some drugs can be bought over the counter (OTC) at pharmacies. Other types can be obtained only with a prescription from your doctor. Drugs may be given in a variety of different forms, depending on considerations such as the part of the body needing treatment and the age of the user. Most drug treatments act systemically: they are introduced into the body and circulate in the bloodstream, which carries the drugs to the tissues where they are needed. Drugs may also be given as topical preparations, which are applied to a particular area of the body and act only on that area.

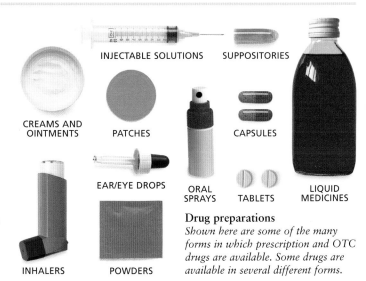

INJECTABLE SOLUTIONS · SUPPOSITORIES
CREAMS AND OINTMENTS · PATCHES · CAPSULES
EAR/EYE DROPS · ORAL SPRAYS · TABLETS · LIQUID MEDICINES
INHALERS · POWDERS

Drug preparations
Shown here are some of the many forms in which prescription and OTC drugs are available. Some drugs are available in several different forms.

How drugs affect you

A drug may have several effects on your body in addition to the intended action. These include side effects, tolerance, and dependence. Side effects are unwanted effects resulting from a normal dose. Tolerance occurs as the body adapts to a drug's actions. As a result of tolerance, side effects may disappear, but the effectiveness of a drug may be reduced and you may need larger doses to get the same benefit. Dependence is a psychological or physical need for a drug. A drug's effects can vary from one individual to another, depending on a number of factors such as age and body size.

Side effects

Almost all systemic drugs – drugs that can affect the whole body – can cause side effects. These effects occur because drugs act on cells throughout the body and not just on the area to be treated. Certain side effects are predictable; for example, the action of some analgesics (p.309) on the body can also result in constipation. Most side effects are not serious and may disappear as your body becomes more tolerant. However, some may be serious or even potentially fatal. For example, high doses of certain anticancer drugs (p.305) can lead to heart failure. Drugs can also produce unpredictable side effects. One such effect is an allergic reaction, which may be caused by any type of drug; the symptoms can vary from a mild rash to severe breathing problems (anaphylaxis).

People at special risk

Some people are at a higher risk than others of having an adverse reaction to a drug. This variation occurs because people's bodies absorb and excrete drugs at different rates, so that the same dose of a drug may reach different concentrations in the blood. How the body processes a drug may be partly genetically determined and also depends on factors such as body size and kidney function. Groups at higher risk of adverse effects include fetuses (drugs taken by the mother can cross the placenta), babies and children (especially breast-fed babies whose mothers are taking drugs that pass into breast milk), people who have liver or kidney disease (drugs may not be broken down and eliminated from the body), and elderly people (kidney and liver function may have declined with age).

Using drugs safely

Before taking medication, read the instructions carefully and talk to your doctor or pharmacist if you have any questions. Find out if the drug may affect everyday tasks such as driving, if you should take it on an empty stomach, and what to do if you miss a dose. Inform the doctor or pharmacist about any drugs that you have taken recently or that have affected you adversely; in addition, say if you are pregnant or planning a pregnancy, because some drugs can be harmful to a fetus.

Taking drugs correctly

When taking tablets or capsules, swallow them with plenty of water so that they do not become stuck in your esophagus. If you are taking liquid medicine, shake the bottle well before use to mix the ingredients thoroughly, and measure the dose carefully. Devise a routine to help you remember when to take your drugs, especially if you are taking more than one medication. Make sure that you complete the full course of any treatment, even if your symptoms seem to have disappeared. Never take someone else's prescribed drug or give yours to anyone else. Do not use OTC remedies for more than a few days unless you know the cause of your symptoms and are sure that the condition is improving.

Giving medicine with a syringe
Drugs for small children often come in liquid form. Use a syringe to measure doses accurately and administer them without spillage.

Storing drugs safely

To prevent drugs from deteriorating, follow the directions given for storage. Keep the drugs in their original containers. Some drugs need to be stored in a cool, dry place and others in the refrigerator or away from light. Always keep drugs out of reach of children; if possible, put them in a locked cabinet. Since medicines that have passed their expiration dates may become ineffective or even harmful, dispose of them carefully. It is best to return old medicines to a pharmacist.

A–Z of drugs

This section is an alphabetical guide to the major drug groups. The entries give the uses and possible side effects of the drugs. They also tell you if the drugs are available over the counter or a prescription is needed. When appropriate, warning boxes draw attention to important information about the effects of certain drugs.

Drug group names appearing in *italic typeface* cross-refer to other drug groups within the A–Z of drugs.

ACE inhibitors

A group of drugs that, because of their ability to widen blood vessels, are used to treat hypertension (high blood pressure) and heart failure (a reduction in the pumping efficiency of the heart). ACE (angiotensin-converting enzyme) inhibitors may also be used to treat diabetic kidney disease, in which the small blood vessels in the filtering units of the kidneys are damaged. These drugs are often prescribed with others, such as *diuretics* or *calcium channel blockers*. ACE inhibitors may harm a fetus and should not be used during pregnancy. Always tell your doctor if you are planning a pregnancy or are pregnant.

POSSIBLE SIDE EFFECTS
These include light-headedness, persistent dry cough, muscle cramps, diarrhea, and hives. Because the first dose may reduce the blood pressure dramatically, causing light-headedness, people are often advised to take the first dose at bedtime. Kidney damage is a rare but serious side effect.

> **WARNING**
>
> If you are taking an ACE inhibitor drug, do not take a *nonsteroidal anti-inflammatory drug* without first consulting your doctor because the combination may increase the risk of kidney damage.

Analgesics

Drugs that relieve pain. The two main types are opioid (also called narcotic) and non-opioid (also called non-narcotic) analgesics. A number of commonly used analgesics are combinations of more than one drug. Opioid analgesics are mainly used to relieve severe pain. Nonopioid analgesics, most of which are *nonsteroidal anti-inflammatory drugs* (NSAIDs), may be used to ease mild or moderate pain such as headaches. Combinations of two or more analgesics and, in some cases another drug such as caffeine, may provide greater pain relief than a single analgesic.

Opioid drugs are the strongest analgesics available. They may be given for pain during a heart attack or following surgery or serious injury and are widely used in the relief of pain caused by cancer. Opioids may be given orally or, if the pain is severe or accompanied by vomiting, by injection. Some opioids are available in combination with nonopioids.

Nonopioid analgesics are less potent than opioids, and a number are available over the counter, including acetaminophen, aspirin, and NSAIDs such as ibuprofen. Nonopioids are used mainly for pain such as headache, toothache, or menstrual pain. They are also effective in treating fever, and NSAIDs reduce the inflammation that occurs in conditions such as arthritis. One group of NSAIDs, the COX2 antagonists such as celecoxib and rofecoxib, may have a less damaging effect on the stomach than other NSAIDs.

POSSIBLE SIDE EFFECTS
Side effects of opioid analgesics include nausea, vomiting, drowsiness, constipation, and difficulties with breathing. Nonopioid analgesics rarely cause side effects if they are used occasionally and are taken only at the doses recommended. Aspirin and other NSAIDS, when they are taken repeatedly, may damage the lining of the stomach or intestines, leading to bleeding or ulceration. However, taking NSAIDs with food may reduce these side effects. Acetaminophen is dangerous if it is taken in doses higher than the recommended maximum daily intake. An overdose of acetaminophen can cause severe liver and, rarely, kidney damage.

> **WARNING**
>
> Do not give aspirin to children under 12 years because it increases the risk of Reye syndrome, a rare brain and liver disorder.

Antacids

Drugs taken to relieve indigestion, heartburn, gastritis (inflammation of the stomach lining), and gastroesophageal reflux (the regurgitation of stomach acid into the esophagus). Antacid drugs also help relieve ulcers that have developed in the wall of the stomach or duodenum.

Antacid drugs neutralize stomach acids, which helps prevent or relieve inflammation and pain in the upper digestive tract. Antacids also give the stomach or duodenal lining time to heal after damage by an ulcer and is therefore sensitive to normal amounts of stomach acid. Antacids can be bought over the counter.

POSSIBLE SIDE EFFECTS
Most antacids have few serious side effects. However, some may cause fluid retention or belching and/or constipation.

Antianginal drugs

Drugs used to treat angina (chest pain due to impaired blood supply to heart muscle). Antianginal drugs include *beta blockers*, *nitrates*, and *calcium channel blockers*.

For people who have only occasional attacks of angina, a fast-acting antianginal drug is needed at the first sign of an attack. A nitrate drug such as sublingual nitroglycerine is usually prescribed for this purpose. If the attacks become more frequent or severe, preventive treatment may be necessary. If they are taken regularly, beta blockers, calcium channel blockers, or long acting nitrate patches can control the angina, but none of these drugs cure the underlying disorder.

POSSIBLE SIDE EFFECTS
Antianginal drugs can produce a variety of minor side effects, including dizziness and, sometimes, fainting due to lowered blood pressure. Other effects include throbbing headaches at the start of treatment and flushing.

Antianxiety drugs

Drugs used to relieve the symptoms of severe anxiety. Benzodiazepines are the main type of antianxiety drug. Some *antidepressants* and buspirone may also be used to treat anxiety.

Antianxiety drugs provide temporary relief from anxiety when it limits a person's ability to cope with everyday life. In most cases, the underlying disorder is best treated by counseling, psychotherapy, or other therapy.

Benzodiazepines reduce feelings of restlessness and agitation, slow mental activity, and often produce drowsiness. You should not drink alcohol while taking benzodiazepines because it increases their sedative effect.

Beta blockers are sometimes used to calm a person before surgical treatment or anxiety that occurs before a public performance, known as situational anxiety. Beta blockers reduce the physical symptoms of anxiety, such as shaking and palpitations.

POSSIBLE SIDE EFFECTS
Benzodiazepines often cause drowsiness and can also cause confusion, dizziness, poor coordination, and lethargy. There is a risk of dependence if they are taken for longer than 1–2 weeks. If you are taking beta blockers, your sleep may be disturbed and your hands and feet may feel cold.

> **WARNING**
>
> Benzodiazepines often cause drowsiness and may affect your ability to drive vehicles or operate machinery.

Antiarrhythmic drugs

Drugs used to treat abnormal heart rates and rhythms (arrhythmias). Commonly used antiarrhythmics include *beta blockers*, *calcium channel blockers*, and the digitalis drug digoxin. However, there are many other oral antiarrhythmics used, depending upon the specific arrhythmia, including amiodarone, quinidine, procainamide, disopyramide, flecainide, tocainide, and propafenone. Many of these must be started in the hospital. Once an antiarrhythmic drug is required, you may have to take it indefinitely. In many cases, your doctor may arrange for you to have regular blood tests to check levels of the drug.

POSSIBLE SIDE EFFECTS
Some types of antiarrhythmics reduce blood pressure, and this may cause light-headedness when you stand up. Others may cause other

types of arrhythmias, requiring an adjustment or a change in therapy. Other side effects are specific to particular drugs.

Antibiotics

A group of drugs used to treat infections caused by bacteria. They are also used to prevent infection if a person's immune system is impaired or if there is a risk of endocarditis (inflammation of the lining of the heart).

Some antibiotic drugs are effective against only certain types of bacteria. Others, known as broad-spectrum antibiotics, are effective against a wide range of bacteria. The choice of antibiotic drug depends on the type of bacterium as well as the site of the infection. This choice is most effectively made by growing a culture of the bacterium and checking its sensitivity to various types of antibiotics. More than one antibiotic drug may be prescribed in order to increase the efficiency of treatment and to reduce the risk of antibiotic resistance.

POSSIBLE SIDE EFFECTS

Most antibiotics can cause nausea, diarrhea, or a rash, as well as adverse effects typical of particular types. Antibiotics may disturb the normal balance between certain types of bacteria and fungi in the body, leading to proliferation of the fungus that causes thrush. Some people occasionally experience a severe allergic reaction to antibiotics. Many antibiotics affect the action of other medications.

Anticancer drugs

Drugs used to treat cancer. Most anticancer drugs are cytotoxic (kill or damage rapidly dividing cells). Others alter the body's hormone balance and play an important part in controlling the spread (metastasis) of cancers.

Several different anticancer drugs may be prescribed together to maximize their effects. The choice of drugs depends on the type of cancer, its stage of development, and the general health of the patient. Anticancer drugs may be given with the aim of curing the cancer, prolonging life, or relieving symptoms. In some cases, drugs are given in combination with surgery and/or radiation therapy.

Anticancer drugs are especially useful in the treatment of lymphomas, leukemias, and cancer of the ovary or testis. They are also used to treat cancers of the breast, prostate, and endometrium. Since many anticancer drugs are potentially harmful to a developing fetus, always consult your doctor about contraception before starting treatment.

POSSIBLE SIDE EFFECTS

In the early stages of treatment, nausea, vomiting, and diarrhea may occur, which in some cases may be sufficiently serious to make hospitalization necessary. Anticancer drugs may also cause hair loss, anemia, increased susceptibility to infection, and/or abnormal bleeding. To minimize adverse effects, anticancer drugs are usually given in short courses with time between each course.

Anticoagulant and antiplatelet drugs

Drugs used to prevent unwanted blood clots from forming in the blood vessels. They are also used to stabilize clots that have already formed, preventing an embolism, in which a piece of existing clot breaks off, travels, and blocks a blood vessel supplying a vital organ. Anticoagulant drugs cannot dissolve blood clots, however, and *thrombolytic drugs* are used for this purpose.

In general, antiplatelet drugs are used to prevent unwanted clots from forming in arteries; anticoagulants are prescribed to prevent clots from developing or enlarging in veins. The drugs are usually taken orally, but anticoagulants may be given by injection or infusion if clotting must be controlled quickly, such as during or after surgery.

Warfarin, the most frequently used oral anticoagulant, is used long-term to prevent deep vein thrombosis, in which an unwanted clot forms in a vein, or pulmonary embolism, in which a clot lodges in the lungs. The drug is also prescribed to people at risk of a stroke. Because oral anticoagulants interact with many other drugs, patients are given a warning card that lists prohibited drugs.

If you have angina or you have had a heart attack or a stroke, you may be advised to take an antiplatelet drug for life. Aspirin is the most commonly used antiplatelet drug. It should not be taken with any anticoagulants except on the direction of a doctor.

Oral anticoagulants can be harmful to a fetus. You should tell your doctor if you are planning to become pregnant or are pregnant.

POSSIBLE SIDE EFFECTS

Easy bruising is a side effect of warfarin and, more rarely, rashes, hair loss, and diarrhea may occur. People taking oral anticoagulants are given regular blood tests because too high a dose can cause more serious bleeding.

> ## WARNING
>
> Contact your doctor immediately if you are taking an oral anticoagulant and you have nosebleeds or excessive bruising, or notice blood in your urine.

Anticonvulsants

Drugs used in the treatment of epilepsy and other types of seizures. Anticonvulsant drugs are taken regularly to reduce the frequency and severity of seizures and as an emergency treatment to stop a prolonged seizure.

Anticonvulsant drugs are also administered to prevent seizures following a serious head injury or some types of brain surgery. They may be given to a child with a high fever who has a history of febrile convulsions (seizures brought on by a high temperature).

The choice of drug is largely determined by the type of seizure to be treated. Long-term treatment may require the use of more than one type of anticonvulsant drug. You should

always consult your doctor before planning a pregnancy because some anticonvulsants affect the development of the fetus.

POSSIBLE SIDE EFFECTS

Anticonvulsant drugs can produce various adverse effects, including reduced concentration, impaired memory, poor coordination, and fatigue. Your doctor will try to establish a dose that prevents seizures while minimizing adverse effects. Regular monitoring of blood levels of the drug may be necessary in order to achieve this.

Antidepressants

Drugs that help relieve many of the symptoms of depression, such as loss of interest in everyday activities, poor appetite, lethargy, insomnia, despair, and thoughts of suicide.

There are many types of antidepressants, including selective serotonin reuptake inhibitors (SSRIs), tricyclics, monoamine oxidase inhibitors (MAOIs), and others. The antidepressant effect of these drugs begins after 10–14 days, but the full effect may not be felt for up to 8 weeks. People with moderate to severe depression are most commonly prescribed SSRIs or tricyclics because there are fewer side effects than with MAOIs. MAOIs react adversely with certain foods, such as cheese, and with many other drugs. Therefore, they are usually prescribed only when other types of antidepressants have not been effective. People taking MAOIs are given a card listing foods and drugs they must avoid.

POSSIBLE SIDE EFFECTS

SSRIs can cause headaches, diarrhea, nausea, and reduced sex drive. Restlessness and anxiety may also occur. A dry mouth, difficulty urinating, constipation, and blurred vision are common with tricyclics, but these effects tend to diminish as treatment continues. Side effects of MAOIs include dry mouth, drowsiness, light-headedness, and digestive disturbances.

Antidiarrheal drugs

Drugs used to relieve diarrhea, either as a short-term measure to control an acute attack of diarrhea, or long-term for intestinal disorders such as irritable bowel syndrome.

Diarrhea usually clears up in about 48 hours, and drug treatment is not required. Drinking plenty of fluids is usually all that is needed. Do not give antidiarrheal drugs to children.

The main types of antidiarrheal drugs are opioids, bulk-forming agents, and adsorbents. Some are available over the counter. Opioids are the most effective antidiarrheal. They are used when the diarrhea is severe and debilitating. Opioids also help relieve abdominal pain associated with diarrhea. Bulk-forming agents and adsorbents have a milder effect and are often used to regulate bowel action over a prolonged period in people with irritable bowel syndrome. Do not take a bulk-forming agent when taking opioids; the combination could cause feces to compact and block the intestine.

POSSIBLE SIDE EFFECTS

All types of antidiarrheals can cause constipation and therefore need to be taken with plenty of water. There is a risk of dependence with prolonged use of opioids.

Antiemetics

A group of drugs used to treat nausea and vomiting caused by motion sickness, vertigo, inner ear disorders such as Ménière's disease, certain drugs (especially *anticancer drugs*), and occasionally severe vomiting during pregnancy. Some antiemetic drugs are available over the counter. If you need to take an antiemetic for any reason other than to prevent or relieve motion sickness, you should consult your doctor so that he or she can determine the cause of the vomiting and the correct treatment. Do not take antiemetics during pregnancy except when you are advised to do so by a doctor. Antiemetics are normally taken orally, but they may be given by injection or as a suppository if vomiting is severe.

POSSIBLE SIDE EFFECTS

Many antiemetics can cause drowsiness. Therefore, you should not drive or operate machinery until you know how the drugs affect you. Some may result in dry mouth, difficulty urinating, and dizziness.

Antifungal drugs

A group of drugs prescribed to treat infections caused by fungi. Antifungal drugs are commonly used to treat athlete's foot and ringworm. They are also used to treat oral or vaginal thrush and rare fungal infections that affect internal organs.

Antifungal preparations are available as tablets, lozenges, liquids, creams, injections, and vaginal suppositories. Some of these can be bought over the counter.

POSSIBLE SIDE EFFECTS

Preparations applied to the skin, scalp, mouth, or vagina may occasionally increase irritation. Antifungal drugs given by mouth or injection can cause more serious side effects, including liver or kidney damage.

Antihistamines

Drugs that block the effects of histamine, a natural chemical that is released during allergic reactions. Antihistamines are used in the treatment of rashes such as urticaria (hives) to relieve itching, swelling, and redness. They are also used in the treatment of allergic rhinitis to relieve sneezing and a runny nose.

Antihistamines are sometimes included in *cough remedies* and *cold and flu remedies* and are also used as *antiemetics*. Because many of these drugs have a sedative effect, they are sometimes used to induce sleep, especially when itching prevents sleep at night. Some of the most recently introduced antihistamines have very little sedative effect.

Usually, antihistamine drugs are taken orally but some types are available as nasal sprays, eyedrops, or skin lotions. Some of these preparations are available over the counter. Antihistamines may be given by injection in an emergency for anaphylactic shock (severe allergic reaction).

POSSIBLE SIDE EFFECTS

Many antihistamines cause drowsiness and dizziness, but the new generation of antihistamines have virtually no soporific effect. Other possible side effects include loss of appetite, nausea, dry mouth, blurred vision, and difficulty urinating.

Antihypertensive drugs

Several groups of drugs used in the treatment of high blood pressure (hypertension) to prevent the development of complications such as stroke, heart failure (reduced pumping efficiency), heart attack (myocardial infarction), and kidney damage.

There are several types of antihypertensive drugs. *Diuretics*, *beta blockers*, *calcium channel blockers*, and *ACE inhibitors* are commonly used, but there are others that are also used for this purpose. A combination of several antihypertensive drugs is usually used to control severe hypertension.

POSSIBLE SIDE EFFECTS

Apart from the side effects typical of specific groups, all antihypertensive drugs may cause dizziness and fainting as a result of lowering the blood pressure too much.

Antispasmodic drugs

A group of drugs that relax spasm of the smooth (involuntary) muscle in the wall of the intestine or bladder. Antispasmodic drugs are used mainly in the treatment of irritable bowel syndrome and diverticular disease.

There are two main types of antispasmodic drugs: direct smooth muscle relaxants, which have a direct effect on the smooth muscle in the intestinal wall, and anticholinergics, which work by reducing the transmission of nerve signals to the intestinal walls.

POSSIBLE SIDE EFFECTS

Possible adverse effects of antispasmodic drugs include dry mouth, blurred vision, and difficulty urinating.

Antiviral drugs

Drugs used in the treatment of infection by viruses. To date, no drugs have been developed that can reliably eradicate viruses and cure the illnesses that they cause. However, some antiviral drugs have already been proven useful in treating a few viral infections, particularly herpes. The antiviral drugs reduce the severity of these infections but may not eliminate them completely, and attacks may therefore recur.

Substantial advances have been made in the treatment of HIV infection and CMV (cytomegalovirus) infections that occur in patients with AIDS and others whose immune systems are suppressed. Research into HIV infection has shown that drug treatment should be started before the immune system has been damaged irreparably. The risk of drug resistance can be reduced by using a combination of antiviral drugs.

Treatment with antiviral drugs is also recommended in some circumstances for people, such as nurses and doctors, who have been exposed to HIV infection in their occupation.

POSSIBLE SIDE EFFECTS

Antiviral drugs used in the treatment of AIDS carry a high risk of causing anemia due to bone marrow damage. Most other antiviral drugs rarely cause side effects. Antiviral creams, which are available over the counter, may irritate the skin. Antiviral drugs given by mouth or injection can cause nausea and dizziness, and, rarely, kidney damage if the treatment is long-term.

Beta blockers

A group of drugs widely prescribed to treat disorders of the heart and circulation, as well as some other conditions.

Beta blocker drugs, which are also known as beta-adrenergic blocking agents, are used in the treatment of angina (chest pain due to insufficient oxygen reaching the heart muscle), high blood pressure, and irregular heartbeat. Beta blockers are sometimes given after a heart attack (myocardial infarction) to reduce the likelihood of further damage to the heart muscle. Beta blockers may also be given to prevent attacks of migraine and to reduce the physical symptoms of anxiety (such as palpitations, tremor, and excessive sweating). They may be given to control the symptoms of thyrotoxicosis, in which the thyroid gland is overactive. A beta blocker may be given in the form of eyedrops to treat glaucoma (raised fluid pressure in the eyeball).

POSSIBLE SIDE EFFECTS

Beta blockers can exacerbate some respiratory disorders, and they are not normally given to people who have chronic bronchitis, emphysema, or asthma. If you are taking a beta blocker, your sleeping pattern may be disrupted, and your hands and feet may feel cold because the blood circulation in the extremities is reduced. Men may experience erectile dysfunction, but normal sexual function usually returns when the drug is stopped. Rarely, beta blockers cause rashes and dry eyes. All of these side effects tend to be more common and more severe in elderly people.

> **WARNING**
>
> Do not suddenly stop taking a beta blocker drug without first consulting your doctor. Abrupt withdrawal of the drug can cause a rise in blood pressure, worsening of angina, or an increased risk of a heart attack (myocardial infarction).

Bronchodilators

A group of drugs that widen the airways in the lungs and are used to ease breathing difficulties due to asthma or chronic bronchitis. Bronchodilators can be given by inhaler, in pill form, or, in severe cases, by nebulizer (a device that delivers high doses in aerosol form through a mask or mouthpiece) or injection.

Three main groups of drugs are used as bronchodilators: sympathomimetics, anticholinergics, and xanthines. When inhaled, some sympathomimetics take effect within 10 minutes and are often used for the rapid relief of shortness of breath. Anticholinergics and xanthines are slower-acting and are often used in the long-term prevention of breathing difficulties. Two or more types of bronchodilators may be used simultaneously.

POSSIBLE SIDE EFFECTS
Sympathomimetics can cause palpitations and trembling. Anticholinergics can cause a dry mouth, blurred vision, and difficulty urinating. Xanthines can cause headaches and palpitations.

Inhaled bronchodilator drugs are not absorbed by the body in large amounts, and serious side effects are therefore uncommon. However, they can cause palpitations, anxiety, and abdominal pain.

Calcium channel blockers

A group of drugs used in the treatment of angina (chest pain due to an inadequate blood supply to heart muscle) and high blood pressure. Some calcium channel blockers may be taken regularly to reduce the frequency of migraine attacks. Nifedipine, is used to treat Raynaud's phenomenon, in which fingers and toes become painful and pale due to constriction of small arteries in the hands or feet. Verapamil is used to treat some abnormal heart rhythms (arrhythmias).

Calcium channel blockers may be used alone or in combination with other drugs used for the treatment of high blood pressure, angina, or arrhythmias. Usually, the drugs are initially prescribed at a low dose and gradually increased to an effective level. The ideal dose for you will be one that is high enough to allow the drug to be effective without causing troublesome side effects.

POSSIBLE SIDE EFFECTS
The most common side effects of calcium channel blockers are constipation, headaches, facial flushing, dizziness (usually on standing up), and edema in the lower extremeties. However, these effects generally disappear with continued treatment. Nausea, fatigue, and palpitations are less common side effects.

WARNING

Do not suddenly stop taking a calcium channel blocker drug without consulting your doctor. Abrupt withdrawal can cause worsening of angina.

Cold and flu remedies

Preparations for the relief of symptoms of the common cold and flu. Many different preparations are available over the counter. The main ingredient is usually a mild *analgesic*, such as acetaminophen or aspirin, which helps relieve aches and pains. Other common ingredients include *antihistamines* and decongestants, which help reduce nasal congestion, and caffeine, which acts as a mild stimulant. Those remedies containing antihistamines can cause drowsiness. Vitamin C is frequently included in cold relief products, but there is no evidence that it speeds recovery. Zinc tablets are claimed to shorten the duration of colds, but this effect is as yet unproven, and indigestion is one of their side effects.

Corticosteroids

Drugs similar to the corticosteroid hormones produced by the adrenal glands. Corticosteroid drugs have a wide variety of uses. They are available as topical creams, ointments, lotions, and nasal sprays. They can also be taken orally or given by inhaler or injection. Corticosteroids are prescribed to people with Addison's disease, in which the level of the natural hormone cortisol is inadequate due to destruction of the adrenal glands by disease. Corticosteroids are also prescribed following surgical removal of the adrenal glands or when the pituitary gland has been destroyed by disease, surgery, or irradiation.

Corticosteroids are used in the treatment of inflammatory intestinal disorders, such as ulcerative colitis and Crohn's disease. Urgent corticosteroid treatment is required to reduce inflammation in temporal arteritis, a condition in which inflammation of the artery supplying the retina can lead to blindness.

Corticosteroids are also used in the treatment of autoimmune diseases (in which the body attacks its own tissues), such as rheumatoid arthritis, and in asthma, eczema, iritis (inflammation of the iris), and allergic rhinitis. The injection of corticosteroids around an inflamed tendon or joint may relieve pain in disorders such as tennis elbow and arthritis. Corticosteroid drugs are also used to suppress the immune system in order to prevent the rejection of a transplanted organ and in the treatment of certain types of cancers, such as those of the lymphatic system (lymphomas) and of the blood (leukemias).

POSSIBLE SIDE EFFECTS
Short-term use of corticosteroids rarely produces side effects. Prolonged use of strong topical corticosteroids can cause local damage to the skin. Long-term treatment with oral corticosteroids may cause easy bruising, acne, a moon-shaped face, and weight gain. It can also cause raised blood pressure, osteoporosis, slow growth in children, and increased risk of infection.

Abrupt withdrawal from long-term, high-dose corticosteroids can lead to a rapid fall in blood pressure and, in some cases, shock, which can be fatal. If your doctor prescribes corticosteroid drugs for you for more than several weeks, you should inform any health professional treating you that you have received this dosage of medication.

Cough remedies

Preparations containing various drugs used to treat coughing. Coughing is a natural reflex action that helps clear the lungs of sputum. The effectiveness of cough medicines is doubtful, which is why doctors rarely prescribe them for minor respiratory disorders. However, a wide variety of cough remedies is available over the counter. Most consist of a syrupy base to which various drugs and flavorings have been added.

The main groups of drugs used to treat coughs are expectorants, mucolytics, and suppressants. Expectorants are supposed to encourage productive coughs (that produce sputum). The benefit of these is not proven, however. Mucolytics make sputum less sticky and easier to cough up. Cough suppressants, which often contain drugs such as codeine, are usually effective in relieving a troublesome cough but are not available over the counter. Cough suppressants may have a sedative effect and cause drowsiness.

Diuretics

A group of drugs that help remove excess water and salt from the body by increasing the amounts that are lost as urine. Diuretic drugs are commonly used in the treatment of high blood pressure and heart failure (a reduction in the heart's pumping efficiency). Diuretics are also used to treat other conditions in which excess fluid accumulates in the body, such as liver or kidney disorders and glaucoma. Some diuretics may be used to prevent altitude sickness and to treat the inner ear disorder Menière's disease.

The most frequently prescribed diuretic drugs are thiazides, potassium-sparing diuretics, and loop diuretics. Thiazide drugs are the most commonly prescribed diuretic for the treatment of hypertension. Loop diuretics are more powerful than thiazides and are used to treat accumulation of fluid caused by heart failure and some kidney and liver disorders. They may also be given by injection for the emergency treatment of heart failure. Both thiazide and loop diuretics can cause excessive loss of potassium from the body, which can result in confusion and weakness. If your potassium levels become low you may be given a potassium-sparing diuretic, either alone or in combination with a thiazide or loop diuretic. Alternatively, you might be given oral or intravenous potassium supplements.

POSSIBLE SIDE EFFECTS
All diuretics increase the frequency with which you need to urinate, an effect that is most noticeable at the start of treatment.

Some diuretics may raise the level of uric acid in the blood, and thereby increase the risk of gout. They can also raise blood sugar levels, which can cause or aggravate diabetes mellitus. Potassium-sparing diuretics can cause a dry mouth, digestive disturbances, and rash.

Immunosuppressants

Drugs that reduce the activity of the immune system (the body's natural defenses). They are prescribed following transplant surgery to prevent foreign tissues from being rejected. Immunosuppressants are also given to halt the progress of autoimmune disorders (in which the body's immune system attacks its own tissues) such as rheumatoid arthritis. Recently, immunosuppressant drugs have been given in the early stages of these disorders with the aim of preventing tissue damage. They are unable, however, to restore tissue that has already been damaged.

There are two main types of immunosuppressants: *corticosteroids* and cytotoxic immunosuppressants. The drugs cyclosporin and tacrolimus are also used. Corticosteroids are usually used initially for autoimmune disorders. If they are not effective, cytotoxic drugs may used in addition; cyclosporin is also an option. To prevent rejection of transplants, the most commonly used drugs are cyclosporin, tacrolimus, and azathioprine.

Some immunosuppressants can harm a fetus. You should tell your doctor if you are planning a pregnancy or are pregnant.

POSSIBLE SIDE EFFECTS
All immunosuppressants have potentially serious adverse effects. By reducing the activity of the immune system, they increase the risk of infection. These drugs also increase the risk of certain cancers and can make the body's blood clotting mechanism less effective.

> **WARNING**
>
> When taking immunosuppressant drugs, it is important that you immediately report any signs of infection, such as a sore throat or fever, or any unusual bruising or bleeding to your doctor.

Laxatives

Drugs that make feces pass more easily through the intestines. Laxatives are most commonly used to treat constipation, in which the bowels are not opened as frequently as usual and the feces are hard. They may also be given to clear the intestines before surgery or investigational procedures.

Laxatives can be bought over the counter. If you are taking them for constipation, use them only until your bowel movements have returned to normal. See your doctor if constipation continues for more than a few days.

Laxatives are classified into different types, depending on how they work. Bulk-forming agents, osmotic laxatives, and fecal softeners

all make feces softer and easier to pass. Stimulant laxatives make the intestinal muscles move feces more rapidly. Bulk-forming laxatives are the safest type for long-term use and are therefore the most commonly used for long-term disorders, such as irritable bowel syndrome. You must drink plenty of water when taking this type of laxative because the bulky feces could block the intestines.

POSSIBLE SIDE EFFECTS
Stimulant laxatives and the osmotic laxative lactulose can cause abdominal cramps and flatulence. Bulk-forming laxatives can cause abdominal discomfort and flatulence. Some fecal softeners may interfere with the absorption of fat-soluble vitamins.

Lipid-lowering drugs

Drugs that are used to reduce excessive levels of lipids (fatty substances), especially cholesterol and triglycerides, in the bloodstream. Lipid-lowering drugs reduce the risk of severe atherosclerosis (narrowing of the arteries) and especially coronary artery disease in people with a family history of high blood lipid levels for whom dietary measures have not worked. The drugs may also be given to people with angina (chest pain due to insufficient oxygen reaching the heart muscle) to reduce the risk of having a heart attack (myocardial infarction), and after a heart attack in order to minimize the risk of further attacks.

The main types of lipid-lowering drugs include statins, fibrates, anion-exchange resins, and nicotinic acid and its derivatives. These drugs work in different ways to lower the levels of lipids in the blood. Your doctor's choice of drug treatment will depend largely on which type of lipid is causing your condition. In some instances, your doctor may prescribe a combination of several different drugs. Lipid-lowering drugs are taken orally on a daily basis, and most need to be taken long-term. Since statins and fibrates can harm a fetus or baby, you should notify your doctor if you are planning a pregnancy, are pregnant, or are breast-feeding.

You may be advised to incorporate natural products such as fish oil into your diet. Fish oil helps reduce triglyceride blood levels. It occurs naturally in oily fish, such as mackerel, and is available as a dietary supplement.

POSSIBLE SIDE EFFECTS
Side effects that may occur while taking lipid-lowering drugs include nausea, diarrhea or constipation, headaches, and muscle pain. Statins can affect the liver, requiring periodic blood tests.

Nitrates

A group of drugs that widen blood vessels used in the treatment of angina (chest pain due to impaired blood supply to the heart muscle) and severe heart failure (a reduction in the heart's pumping efficiency).

Possible adverse effects of nitrate drugs include headache, flushing, and dizziness.

Tolerance (the need for greater amounts of a drug for it to have the same effect) may develop when the drug is taken regularly.

Nonsteroidal anti-inflammatory drugs

Nonsteroidal anti-inflammatory drugs, or NSAIDs, are nonopioid *analgesics* that are used to relieve the discomfort and inflammation caused by a variety of musculoskeletal disorders. These drugs are also commonly used to treat other types of pain such as headaches and menstrual pain.

Commonly used NSAIDs include ibuprofen, diclofenac, naproxen, and indomethacin. Although aspirin is technically an NSAID, it is not normally classed with other NSAIDs since it has only a limited anti-inflammatory effect at normal doses. NSAIDs are used to treat acute conditions, such as ligament damage and muscle sprains and tears, and they usually relieve symptoms within a few hours. In addition, NSAIDs are used to treat long-term musculoskeletal disorders such as osteoarthritis and rheumatoid arthritis. They can relieve pain rapidly but may take as long as 2 weeks to reduce levels of inflammation. Although NSAIDs are effective in alleviating the symptoms of musculoskeletal disorders, they do not cure the underlying condition.

NSAIDs are most commonly taken orally, although occasionally they may be applied as a gel or given by injection. For many conditions, NSAIDs are used with other treatments such as physical therapy. Ibuprofen and naproxen can be bought over the counter.

POSSIBLE SIDE EFFECTS
NSAIDs can cause a wide range of side effects, the most important of which are nausea, indigestion, and sometimes ulceration of or bleeding from the stomach. Some NSAIDs irritate the stomach more than others. People with a past history of indigestion may be advised against taking NSAIDs, or an NSAID with fewer gastrointestinal side effects may be recommended. People with the respiratory disorder asthma are advised not to take NSAIDs because these drugs can exacerbate the condition.

Oral rehydration solutions

Over-the-counter preparations used to treat dehydration resulting from diarrhea and vomiting. Oral rehydration solutions are made up of water, essential minerals such as sodium and potassium, and the sugar glucose. Usually, drinking plenty of fluids to replace the water that the body loses in diarrhea or vomiting is the only treatment needed for adults. However, it may be necessary to give oral rehydration solutions to treat fluid loss that occurs in infants and young children. These groups are at a much greater risk of dehydration than adults because any water lost accounts for a higher proportion of the total water content in their bodies.

Rehydration solutions can be bought over the counter as ready-to-drink liquids or in frozen form to be eaten as a popsicle. When used according to the instructions, oral rehydration solutions do not cause side effects.

Sex hormone preparations

Preparations that contain synthetic versions of the naturally occurring sex hormones. Synthetic versions of the female sex hormones estrogen and progesterone, known respectively as estrogens and progestins, are most commonly used as oral contraceptives. They are also used in the treatment of some cancers and in hormone replacement therapy (HRT) to relieve menopausal symptoms and prevent osteoporosis. Higher doses of female hormones are used to treat menstrual disorders such as heavy menstrual periods. Progestins should not be used during pregnancy.

The male hormone testosterone is used to treat delayed puberty and decreased libido.

POSSIBLE SIDE EFFECTS

Side effects of female sex hormones include fluid retention, headaches, and depression. Premenopausal women may experience some bleeding between menstrual periods. Taking HRT for more than 5 years slightly increases the risk of breast cancer. In some women, estrogens increase the risk of deep vein thrombosis, the formation of an unwanted clot in a vein. Side effects of testosterone are rare, but include adverse effects on the liver, prostate, and cholesterol levels.

Skin preparations

Various preparations applied to the skin that usually consist of a base such as an ointment, cream, or lotion, to which active ingredients may be added. The main types are emollients, antipruritics, topical *corticosteroids*, anti-infective preparations, and retinoids.

Emollients moisturize the skin and are used to treat dry, scaly skin in disorders such as eczema and psoriasis. Antipruritics are used to control itching. Some antipruritics are simple emollients or cooling lotions, such as calamine, and are available over the counter. Others may include drugs, usually corticosteroids, *antihistamines*, or anesthetics. Topical corticosteroids reduce inflammation due to eczema, psoriasis, or dermatitis. Topical anti-infective preparations may contain *antibiotics* for bacterial infections, *antiviral* or *antifungal drugs* for viral or fungal infections, respectively, or antiparasitic drugs for skin infestations with parasites.

Topical retinoids, used for conditions such as acne, psoriasis, and the roughness and fine wrinkles of sun-damaged skin, are chemically related to vitamin A. Since retinoid drugs can harm a fetus, you should discuss contraception with your doctor before starting treatment.

POSSIBLE SIDE EFFECTS

Some preparations may irritate the skin. Long-term use of strong topical corticosteroids may eventually result in thinning of the skin in the affected area. Topical retinoids may cause the skin to peel and to become red and inflamed.

Sleeping drugs

Drugs that are used in the treatment of insomnia. Sleeping drugs may be prescribed to reestablish sleep patterns after a period of insomnia or when insomnia is the result of a stressful event, such as a death in the family. They may also be used if your sleep pattern needs adjusting to suit your work. Sleeping drugs do not treat the cause of the insomnia, which may be anxiety or depression. Do not drink alcohol while taking sleeping drugs because the sedative effect is enhanced.

Many sleeping drugs cause dependence and are therefore usually prescribed only for a week or two when other measures (such as a warm bath before bed or relaxation exercises) have failed.

Benzodiazepines, which are also used to treat anxiety disorders, may be used to treat insomnia. Over-the-counter remedies containing *antihistamines* are also available. Other drugs that may be prescribed are zaleplon and zolpidem. If the insomnia is caused by depression, your doctor may prescribe *antidepressants*. Sleeping drugs should not be used during pregnancy.

POSSIBLE SIDE EFFECTS

Benzodiazepines can cause confusion, dizziness, and poor coordination, even between doses. Elderly people need to take extra care because of the increased risk of falling. Preparations that contain antihistamines have few side effects, but you should not take these drugs for longer than a few days without consulting your doctor. In some cases, they sometimes cause a dry mouth and blurred vision. Side effects of zaleplon and zolpidem include nausea, vomiting, headache, dizziness, and confusion.

> **WARNING**
> Sleeping drugs can affect your ability to drive or to operate machinery; these effects may persist the following day.

Thrombolytic drugs

Drugs that rapidly dissolve unwanted clots in blood vessels. Thrombolytics are most commonly used as emergency treatment for heart attacks (which are due to blockage in an artery supplying the heart muscle) or for certain types of stroke, which are usually caused by a blood clot blocking the blood supply to part of the brain. Given in the early stages of a heart attack or stroke, thrombolytics can significantly increase the chance of survival. The drugs are administered by injection, and treatment is carefully monitored because of the risk of abnormal bleeding. An allergic reaction to thrombolytic drugs, causing breathing difficulties, may also occur.

Thyroid drugs

Drugs that are used to treat under- and over-activity of the thyroid gland (known as hypothyroidism and hyperthyroidism, respectively). Synthetic thyroid hormones are given to treat hypothyroidism, and antithyroid drugs are used for hyperthyroidism.

Synthetic thyroid hormones are usually taken orally every day. Drugs are started at a low dose, and the dose is increased gradually until an effective level is reached without causing side effects.

Antithyroid drugs are used as preparation for thyroid surgery or for long-term treatment of hyperthyroidism. The drugs are taken daily, and levels of thyroid hormone are usually reduced to normal over a period of 2–3 months. Treatment usually continues for 12–18 months. The most commonly used antithyroid drug is methimazole.

POSSIBLE SIDE EFFECTS

Given at the correct dose, synthetic thyroid hormones cause no side effects. Regular blood tests are carried out to ensure that the correct dose is maintained.

Side effects of antithyroid drugs are usually minor and include nausea, headache, rashes, itching, and joint pains. However, the drugs also have the potentially serious effect of reducing the body's ability to fight infection.

> **WARNING**
> If you are taking methimazole and have symptoms of an infection, or a severe sore throat, contact your doctor at once. Do not take any more pills until your doctor tells you that it is safe to do so.

Ulcer-healing drugs

Drugs prescribed to treat peptic ulcers, which occur when excess production of stomach acid or damage to the mucous lining of the esophagus, stomach, or duodenum exposes and erodes the underlying tissue.

The symptoms of an ulcer can be relieved by *antacids*, but healing is slow and an ulcer-healing drug is often required. There are several types. The most commonly used are H_2 blockers and proton pump inhibitors, which work by reducing the amount of stomach acid released. They may be prescribed in combination with *antibiotics* to eradicate *Helicobacter pylori*, a bacterium that is commonly present in the stomach and causes ulcers. Some H_2 blockers can be bought over the counter. Other ulcer-healing drugs work by protecting the stomach lining from acid. Pain is reduced within a few hours of starting treatment, and the ulcer heals in 4–8 weeks.

POSSIBLE SIDE EFFECTS

Proton pump inhibitors do not usually cause serious side effects but can cause headache, rash, and diarrhea. Side effects with H_2 blockers are rare but can include dizziness, fatigue, rash, headache, and diarrhea.

USEFUL ADDRESSES

Throughout the US, hundreds of organizations, from government agencies such as the National Institutes of Health to nonprofit organizations such as the Red Cross, are dedicated to helping people deal with most conditions.

This list is a limited sample of such organizations, but further information is available from local libraries, hospitals, and health clinics. Most organizations provide information about resources for specific medical or emotional conditions, and many have support groups or can provide information about groups in your area.

The American College of Physicians–American Society of Internal Medicine (ACP–ASIM) cannot accept responsibility for information provided by the onsites or organizations listed here. Inclusion in this list does not indicate endorsement by the ACP–ASIM, and you should always to consult your doctor on personal health matters.

GENERAL INFORMATION

American College of Physicians-American Society of Internal Medicine
190 N. Independence Mall
West Sixth Street and Race
Philadelphia, PA 19106-1572
Tel: (800) 523-1546
Tel: (215) 351-2400
Online: www.acponline.org

American Medical Association
515 North State Street
Chicago, IL 60611-3211
Tel: (312) 202-5000
Online: www.ama-assn.org

The Centers for Disease Control and Prevention
1600 Clifton Road NE
Atlanta, GA 30333
Tel: (888) 232-3228
Tel: (800) 311-3435
Online: www.cdc.gov

Medic Alert Foundation International
323 Colorado Avenue
Turlock, CA 95382
Tel: (800) 825-3785
Online: www.medicalert.org

Medline
Online: www.nlm.nih.gov

National Institutes of Health
9000 Rockville Pike
Bethesda, MD 20892
Tel: (301) 496-4000
Online: www.nih.gov

Office of Rare Diseases
31 Center Drive
Bethesda, MD 20892
Tel: (301) 402-4336
Online:
www.rarediseases.info.nih.gov/ord

US Food and Drug Administration (FDA)
5600 Fishers Lane
Rockville, MD 20857
Tel: (800) INFO-FDA
Online: www.fda.gov

AGING

American Association of Retired People
601 E Street NW
Washington, DC 20049
Tel: (800) 424-3410
Tel: (877) 434-7598 (TTY)
Online: www.aarp.org

ALZHEIMER'S DISEASE

Alzheimer's Association
919 North Michigan Avenue
Chicago, IL 60611-1676
Tel: (800) 272-3900
Tel: (312) 335-8700
Online: www.alz.org

ALCOHOL-RELATED PROBLEMS

Alcoholics Anonymous
PO Box 459
Grand Central Station
New York, NY 10163
Tel: (212) 870-3400
Online:
www.alcoholicsanonymous.org

ALLERGY AND ASTHMA

Asthma and Allergy Foundation of America
1233 20th Street NW
Washington, DC 20036
Tel: (800) 7-7ASTHMA
Tel: (202) 466-7643
Online: www.aafa.org

ARTHRITIS

American College of Rheumatology
1800 Century Place
Atlanta, GA 30345
Tel: (404) 633-3777
Online: www.rheumatology.org

Arthritis Foundation and American Juvenile Arthritis Organization
1330 West Peachtree Street
Atlanta, GA 30309
Tel: (800) 283-7800
Online: www.arthritis.org

BRAIN TUMORS

American Brain Tumor Association
2720 River Road
Des Plains, IL 60018-4110
Tel: (800) 886-2282
Tel: (847) 827-9910
Online: www.abta.org

BREAST-FEEDING

La Leche League International
PO Box 1209
Franklin Park, IL 60131
Tel: (800) LA-LECHE
Online: www.lalecheleague.org

CANCER

American Cancer Society
1599 Clifton Road, NE
Atlanta, GA 30329-4251
Tel: (800) ACS-2345
Tel: (404) 320-3333
Online: www.cancer.org

Cancer Care
275 Seventh Avenue
New York, NY 10001
Tel: (800) 813-4673
Tel: (212) 302-2400
Online: www.cancercare.org

Leukemia & Lymphoma Society
1311 Mamaroneck Avenue
White Plains, NY 10605
Tel: (800) 955-4572
Tel: (914) 949-5213
Online: www.leukemia-lymphoma.org

National Alliance of Breast Cancer Organizations
9 East 37th Street
New York, NY 10016
Tel: (212) 889-0606
Online: www.nabco.org

National Cancer Institute
9000 Rockville Pike
Bethesda, MD 20892
Tel: (800) 422-6237
Online: www.nci.nih.gov

COMPLEMENTARY THERAPIES

National Center for Complementary and Alternative Medicine
NICCAM Clearinghouse
PO Box 7923
Gaithersburg, MD 20898-7923
Tel: (888) 644-6226
Tel: (888) 644-6226 (TTY)
Online: www.nccam.nih.gov

COUNSELING AND PSYCHOLOGICAL THERAPIES

American Counseling Association
5999 Stevenson Avenue
Alexandria, VA 22304-3300
Tel: (800) 347-6647
Tel: (703) 823-9800
Tel: (703) 823-6862 (TTY)
Online: www.counseling.org

CRISIS SUPPORT

The Samaritans of USA
9 Wild Harbour Road North
Falmouth, MA 02556
Tel: (800) 893-9900
Online: www.befrienders.org

DEATH AND BEREAVEMENT

Choice in Dying
1620 I Street NW
Washington, DC 20006
Tel: (800) 989-WILL
Tel: (202) 338-9790
Online:
www.partnershipforcaring.org

Hospice Foundation of America
2001 S Street NW
Washington, DC 20009
Tel: (800) 854-3402
Online:
www.hospicefoundation.org

DENTISTRY

American Dental Association
211 E. Chicago Avenue
Chicago, IL 60611
Tel: (312) 440-2500
Online: www.ada.org

DIABETES

American Diabetes Association
1701 North Beauregard Street
Alexandria, VA 22311
Tel: (800) 342-2383
Online: www.diabetes.org

Juvenile Diabetes Foundation
120 Wall Street
New York, NY 10005-4001
Tel: (800) JDF CURE
Tel: (212) 875-9500
Online: www.jdrf.org

DIGESTIVE DISORDERS

Crohn's and Colitis Foundation of America
386 Park Avenue South
New York, NY 10016-8804
Tel: (800) 932-2423
Tel: (212) 685-3440
Online: www.ccfa.org

International Foundation for Functional Gastrointestinal Disorders
PO box 170864
Milwaukee, WI 53217

Tel: (414) 964-1799
Online: www.iffgd.org

DISABILITY

National Organization on Disability
910 16th Street NW
Washington, DC 20006
Tel: (202) 293-5960
E-mail: ability@nod.org
Online: www.nod.org

DRUG-RELATED PROBLEMS

Narcotics Anonymous
PO Box 9999
Van Nuys, CA 91409
Tel: (818) 773-9999
Online: www.na.org

Partnership for Drug Free America
405 Lexington Avenue
New York, NY 10174
Tel: (212) 922-1560
Online: www.drugfreeamerica.org

EATING DISORDERS

The National Eating Disorders Association
165 West 46th Street
New York, NY 10036
Tel: (212) 575-6200
E-mail: members.aol.com
Online: www.edap.org

EPILEPSY

American Epilepsy Society
342 North Main Street
West Hartford, CT 06117
Tel: (860) 586-7505
Online: www.aesnet.org

EYE AND VISION PROBLEMS

American Academy of Ophthalmology
PO Box 7424
San Francisco, CA 94120-7424
Tel: (415) 561-8500
Online: www.eyenet.org

American Council of the Blind
1155 15th Street NW
Washington, DC 20005
Tel: (800) 424-8666
Tel: (202) 467-5081
E-mail: info@acb.org
Online: www.acb.org

Glaucoma Research Foundation
200 Pine Street
San Francisco, CA 94104
Tel: (800) 826-6693
Tel: (415) 986-3162
Online: www.glaucoma.org

FAMILY PLANNING

Planned Parenthood Federation of America
26 Bleecker Street
New York, NY 10012
Tel: (800) 230-PLAN
Tel: (212) 965-7000
Online:
www.plannedparenthood.org

FIRST AID

American Red Cross
430 17th Street NW
Washington, DC 20006
Tel: (800) HELP-NOW
Online: www.redcross.org

GENETIC DISORDERS

National Cystic Fibrosis Foundation
New York Chapter
60 East 42nd Street
New York, NY 10165
Tel: (212) 986-8783
Online: www.cff.org

HEAD INJURY

Brain Injury Association
105 North Alfred Street
Alexandria, VA 22314
Tel: (703) 236-6000
Online: www.biausa.org

HEADACHE

National Headache Foundation
428 West St. James Place
Chicago, IL 60614-2750
Tel: (800) 843-2256
Online: www.headaches.org

HEARING DISORDERS

American Speech-Language-Hearing Association
10801 Rockville Pike
Rockville, MD 20852
Tel: (800) 498-2071
Tel: (301) 897-5700
Tel: (301) 897-0157 (TTY)
Online: www.asha.org

American Tinnitus Association
PO Box 5
Portland, OR 97207
Tel: (503) 248-9985
Online: www.ata.org

HEART AND CIRCULATION DISORDERS

American Heart Association National Center
7272 Greenville Avenue
Dallas, TX 75231
Tel: (800) 242-8721
Online: www.americanheart.org

HIV INFECTION AND AIDS

AIDS Action Council
1875 Connecticut Avenue NW
Washington, DC 20009
Tel: (202) 986-1300
Online: www.aidsaction.org

CDC National HIV/AIDS Hotline
Tel: (800) 342-2437
Online: www.cdc.gov

HOME CARE

Family Caregiver Alliance
90 Market Street
San Francisco, CA 94108
Tel: (415) 434-3388
Online: www.caregiver.org

INCONTINENCE

American Foundation for Urologic Disease
1126 North Charles Street
Baltimore, MD 21201
Tel: (800) 242-2383
Tel: (410) 468-1800
Online: www.afud.org

INFECTIOUS DISEASES

Infectious Disease Society of America
99 Canal Center Plaza
Alexandria, VA 22314
Tel: (703) 299-0200
Online: www.idsociety.org

Lyme Disease Foundation
One Financial Plaza
Hartford, CT 06103
Tel: (860) 525-TICK
Online: www.lymefind@aol.com

CFIDS Association of America (chronic fatigue syndrome)
PO Box 223098
Charlotte, NC 28222-0398

Tel: (800) 442-3437
Online: www.cfids.org

INFERTILITY

Resolve, Inc.
1310 Broadway
Somerville, MA 02144-1779
Tel: (617) 623 1156
Tel: (617) 623 0744 (helpline)
Online: www.resolve.org

LEARNING DISABILITIES

Learning Disabilities Association
4156 Library Road
Pittsburg, PA 15234-1349
Tel: (412) 341-1515
Online: www.ldaamerica.org

LIVER DISEASE

American Liver Foundation
1425 Pompton Avenue
Cedar Grove, NJ 07009
Tel: (800) 223-0179
Online: www.liverfoundation.org

LUNG DISEASE

American Lung Association
1740 Broadway
New York, NY 10019
Tel: (800) 586-4872
Online: www.lungusa.org

MENTAL HEALTH PROBLEMS

National Alliance for the Mentally Ill
Colonial Place 3
2107 Wilson Boulevard
Arlington, VA 22201-3042
Tel: (800) 950-6264 (helpline)
Tel: (703) 524-7600
Tel: (703) 516-7991 (TTY)
Online: www.nami.org

National Depressive and Manic-Depressive Association
730 North Franklin Street
Chicago, IL 60610-3526
Tel: (800) 826-3632
Online: www.ndmda.org

NEUROLOGICAL DISORDERS

National Multiple Sclerosis Society
30 West 26th Street
New York, NY 10010
Tel: (800) 344-4867
Online: www.msnyc.org

Myasthenia Gravis Foundation
5841 Cedar Lake Road
Minneapolis, MN 55416
Tel: (800) 541-5454
Online: www.myasthenia.org

OSTEOPOROSIS

National Osteoporosis Foundation
1232 22nd Street NW
Washington, DC 20037
Tel: (800) 223 9994
Tel: (202) 223-2226
Online: www.nof.org

PAIN RELIEF

American Chronic Pain Association
PO Box 850
Rocklin, CA 95677
Tel: (916) 632-0922
Online: www.theacpa.org

PARKINSON'S DISEASE

American Parkinson's Disease Association, Inc.
1250 Hylan Boulevard
Staten Island, NY 10305
Tel: (800) 223-2732
Tel: (718) 981-8001
Online: www.apdaparkinson.org

National Parkinson Foundation
1501 NW 9th Avenue
Bob Hope Road
Miami, FL 33136-1494
Tel: (800) 327-4545
Online: www.parkinson.org

PROSTATE DISORDERS

American Foundation for Urologic Disease
1128 North Charles Street
Baltimore, MD 21201
Tel: (800) 242-2383
Online: www.afud.org

PREGNANCY AND CHILDBIRTH

American College of Obstetricians and Gynecologists
409 12th Street SW
Washington, DC 20090-6920
Tel: (202) 638-5577
Online: www.acog.org

America's Crisis Pregnancy Helpline
1423 Greenway Drive
Irving, TX 75038
Tel: (800) 67-BABY-6
Online: www.thehelpline.org

Healthy Mothers, Healthy Babies Coalition
121 North Washington Street
Alexandria, VA 22314
Tel: (703) 836-6110
Online: www.hmhb.org

SAFETY AND HEALTH

Occupational Safety and Health Administration
US Department of Labor Public Affairs Office
200 Constitution Avenue
Washington, DC 20210
Tel: (800) 321-OSHA
Tel: (202) 693-1999
Online: www.osha.gov

SKIN DISORDERS

American Academy of Dermatology
930 N. Meacham Road
Schaumburg, IL 60173-4965
Tel: (888) 462-3376
Tel: (847) 330-0230
Online: www.aad.org

SEXUAL PROBLEMS

Sexuality Information and Education Council of the United States
130 West 42nd Street
New York, NY 10036
Tel: (212) 819-9770
Online: www.siecus.org

SMOKING

Smoking, Tobacco and Health Information Line
Centers for Disease Control and Prevention
Tel: (800) 232-1311
Online: www.cdc.gov

SLEEP DISORDERS

The American Academy of Sleep Medicine
6301 Bandel Road
Rochester, MN 55901
Tel: (507) 287-6006
Online: www.aasmnet.org

SPEECH AND LANGUAGE DISORDERS

American Speech-Language-Hearing Association
10801 Rockville Pike
Rockville, MD 20852
Tel: (800) 498-2071
Tel: (301) 897 5700
Tel: (301) 897-0157 (TTY)
Online: www.asha.org

STROKE

American Stroke Association
7272 Greenville Avenue
Dallas, TX 75231
Tel: (800) 787-6537
Tel: (303) 649-9299
Online: www.strokeassociation.org

TRAVEL HEALTH

CDC Travel Information Hotline
Tel: (404) 332-4559
Online: www.cdc.gov/travel

URINARY SYSTEM DISORDERS

American Foundation for Urologic Disease
1128 North Charles Street
Baltimore, MD 21201
Tel: (401) 468-1800
Online: www.afud.org

Interstitial Cystitis Association
51 Monroe Street
Rockville, MD 20850
Tel: (301) 610-5300
Online: www.ichelp.org

WOMEN'S HEALTH

American College of Obstetricians and Gynecologists
409 12th Street SW
Washington, DC 20090-6920
Online: www.acog.org

National Women's Health Resource Center
5255 Loughboro Road NW
Washington, DC 20016
Tel: (202) 537-4015
Online: www.healthywomen.org

INDEX

This index gives entries for the major symptoms covered in the book as well entries for many of the diseases and disorders that may be the cause of symptoms. There are also entries for drug groups, parts of human anatomy, and issues covered in the first part of the book. However, as with any index, it cannot be comprehensive. Page numbers that appear in **bold** indicate a reference to an entire symptom chart. Page numbers that appear in *italics* indicate a reference to an illustration. For detailed advice on how to use the 150 charts, see pp.44–45. In addition to this index, the chartfinders on pp.46–48 (the system-by-system chartfinder and the symptom-by-symptom chartfinder) can also be used to help find the particular charts you need.

ACKNOWLEDGMENTS

DK Publishing would like to thank the following for their assistance :

ADDITIONAL EDITORIAL ASSISTANCE
Ann Baggaley, Alyson Lacewing, Nick Mulcahy, Jane Perlmutter, and, for their help on the first aid section of the US edition, Jemima Dunne and Janet Mohun

ADDITIONAL DESIGN AND DTP ASSISTANCE
Chloe Burnett, Kirsten Cashman, Terence Clarke/Housewren, Megan Clayton, Andrew Nash, Schermuly Design Company

PHOTOGRAPHERS
Steve Bartholomew, Andy Crawford, Jo Foord, Steve Gorton, Dave King, Ranald Mckechnie, Tracy Morgan, Gary Ombler, Susanna Price, Tim Ridley, Jules Selmes, Steve Shott, Debi Treloar

ILLUSTRATORS
Evi Antoniou, Joanna Cameron, Gary Cross, John Egan, Mick Gillah, Debbie Maizels, Patrick Mulrey, Peter Ruane, Richard Tibbits, Halli Verrinder, Philip Wilson, Deborah Woodward

PROJECT ADMINISTRATION
Joanna Benwell, Delyth Hughes

INDEXER
Julie Rimington

The growth charts on pp.26–27 were derived from data collected by the National Center for Health Statistics in collaboration with the National Center for Chronic Disease Prevention and Health Promotion (2000) (www.cdc.gov/growthcharts).

Childhood immunization schedule information on p.37 according to the recommended childhood immunization schedule, United States, 2002 (American Academy of Pediatrics).

PICTURE CREDITS
Abbreviations: t = top; c = center; b = bottom; l = left; r = right
Biofotos: 11tr; **Robert Harding Picture Library:** Front jacket bc, 12tr; © **Mothercare:** 33bl; **National Meningitis Trust:** 79br; **Philips PR Dept:** 41tr; **Dr. Janet Page:** 13tr, 13cr, 39c, 40tl; **Science Photo Library:** Front jacket bl, 15cl, 42br; CNRI 40cr, 41cr; **Dr. Robert Friedland:** 42tl; **Gca - CNRI:** 40br; **James King-Holmes:** 253tr, 253tr2; **Petit Format/CSI:** 21tr; **Professor P. Motta/Dept. of Anatomy/University "La Sapienza" Rome:** 21bl; **Secchi, Lecaque, Roussel, UCLAF, CNRI:** 19br; **St. John's Institute of Dermatology:** 183br.

PREVIOUS EDITIONS
MEDICAL EDITORS Dr. Tony Smith, Dr. Charles Clayman; MEDICAL CONSULTANTS Dr. S.M.M. Kinder, Dr. T.J.L. Richards, Dr. H.B. Valman EDITORIAL DIRECTOR Amy Carroll; ART DIRECTOR Chez Picthall; PROJECT EDITORS Cathy Meeus, Christine Murdoch; EDITORS Jillian Agar, Candace Burch, Jane Farrell, Terence Monaighan; EDITORIAL ADVISER Donald Berwick; ART EDITOR Dinah Lone; DESIGN ASSISTANTS Peter Cross, Simone End, Sarah Ponder, Sally Powell, Jane Tetzlaff, Ellen Woodward

Every effort has been made to acknowledge those individuals, organizations, and corporations that have helped with this book and to trace copyright holders. DK Publishing apologizes in advance if any omission has occurred. If an omission does come to light, the company will be pleased to insert the appropriate acknowledgment in any subsequent editions of this book.